Geriatric Audiology

Second Edition

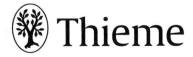

Geriatric Audiology

Second Edition

Barbara E. Weinstein, PhD
Professor and Executive Officer
Doctor of Audiology Program
Graduate Center, City University of New York
New York, New York

Thieme
New York • Stuttgart

Thieme Medical Publishers, Inc.
333 Seventh Ave.
New York, NY 10001

Acquisitions Editor: Emily Ekle
Editorial Assistant: Christopher Malone
Senior Vice President, Editorial and Electronic Product Development: Cornelia Schulze
Production Editor: Barbara A. Chernow
International Production Director: Andreas Schabert
Vice President, Finance and Accounts: Sarah Vanderbilt
President: Brian D. Scanlan
Compositor: Carol Pierson, Chernow Editorial Services, Inc.
Cover image: Courtesy of Starkey Hearing Technologies
Printer: Sheridan Books, Inc.

Library of Congress Cataloging-in-Publication Data

Weinstein, Barbara E.
 Geriatric audiology / Barbara Weinstein. — 2nd ed.
  p. ; cm
 Includes bibliographical references and index.
 ISBN 978-1-60406-174-1 — ISBN 978-1-60406-775-0 (eISBN)
 I. Title
 [DNLM: 1. Hearing Disorders. 2. Aged. 3. Aging—physiology. 4. Health Services for the Aged. 5. Hearing—physiology. WV 270]
 618.97′78—dc23   2012033254

Important note: Medical knowledge is ever-changing. As new research and clinical experience broaden our knowledge, changes in treatment and drug therapy may be required. The authors and editors of the material herein have consulted sources believed to be reliable in their efforts to provide information that is complete and in accord with the standards accepted at the time of publication. However, in view of the possibility of human error by the authors, editors, or publisher of the work herein or changes in medical knowledge, neither the authors, editors, nor publisher, nor any other party who has been involved in the preparation of this work, warrants that the information contained herein is in every respect accurate or complete, and they are not responsible for any errors or omissions or for the results obtained from use of such information. Readers are encouraged to confirm the information contained herein with other sources. For example, readers are advised to check the product information sheet included in the package of each drug they plan to administer to be certain that the information contained in this publication is accurate and that changes have not been made in the recommended dose or in the contraindications for administration. This recommendation is of particular importance in connection with new or infrequently used drugs.

Some of the product names, patents, and registered designs referred to in this book are in fact registered trademarks or proprietary names even though specific reference to this fact is not always made in the text. Therefore, the appearance of a name without designation as proprietary is not to be construed as a representation by the publisher that it is in the public domain.

Printed in the United States

5 4 3 2 1

ISBN 978-1-60406-174-1
eISBN 978-1-60406-775-0

This second edition of *Geriatric Audiology* is dedicated to my husband,
Louis Bernstein, and to our adult children, Michael, Benjamin, and Rachel Bernstein.
Thank you for helping to ensure that my life is rich, balanced, and fulfilling.

This edition is written in loving memory of my twin sister and best friend, Robin; our older brother, Ira;
and our parents, who barely reached their golden years yet instilled in each of us the importance
of pursuing our passions and never compromising our moral compass and standards.

Contents

Preface

In the first edition of *Geriatric Audiology*, Dr. Mark Ross bemoaned the fact that we as a profession are "losing the balance, that too much stress has been placed upon the diagnostic and medical aspects of the profession." He reflected that Doctor of Audiology (AuD) students at the time the first edition was published did not have an adequate background in understanding and managing the psychosocial implications of hearing loss. Since the publication of the first edition, the core component of quality health care, which is the concept of patient-centered care, whereby the provider partners with care recipients and family members, has gained momentum. When patients are active participants in their health care, they become the recipient of services and technologies that focus on their needs and preferences (Agency for Healthcare Research and Quality [AHRQ], 2012).

Evaluating the patient experience is critical to the implementation of a patient-centered approach. In short, identifying and understanding the varied needs of persons with hearing impairment and their communication partners will help to usher in a patient-centered approach to care. Increasingly, receptivity to patient needs and preferences are the drivers of patient-centered health care (Davis, Schoenbaum, & Audet, 2005). Davis and colleagues (2005) describe seven attributes of patient-centered care, two of which are patient engagement in care and routine feedback to the health care provider, both of which should inform diagnosis and management. The variety of tools available to help audiologists gauge the acceptability of outcomes achieved with a given intervention should be embraced, as the information can help patients make more sound decisions relative to their hearing health care and can help to make audiologists more accountable.

Armed with the knowledge that the more patients and family members are involved with their own health care, the greater the improvement in the health outcomes and satisfaction levels, I decided to distribute a ten-item survey to hearing aid users to gain insight into the perceived effects of their hearing loss, their experience purchasing hearing health care services, and the advice they would offer dispensing audiologists. I felt that beginning the text by discussing responses from 25 experienced hearing aid users, with a mean age of 84 years, would help set the stage for practicing patient-centered care.

Respondents to the survey reported using hearing aids for an average of 10 years. The majority of respondents have been using hearing aids for at least 3 years, and some reported using hearing aids for more than 20 years. All respondents live independently in urban settings. Although the majority of respondents purchased their hearing aids from an audiologist in private practice, several purchased them from a hospital-based audiologist, and some purchased their hearing aids from an audiologist at Costco.

The responses were exceedingly informative. Regarding price, most felt the cost was excessive. Those purchasing hearing aids from Costco did so because the purchase price was significantly less and relatively reasonable. Informa-

tive, poignant, and inspiring, responses indicated that most felt that their hearing loss is alienating and socially limiting; creates significant participation restrictions; is embarrassing, a nuisance, and frustrating; and compromises and diminishes their ability to communicate on a day-to-day basis. One person with hearing impairment suggested that any sensory loss, especially hearing loss, affects one's quality of life. Another respondent indicated that she was afraid to participate in conversation out of fear that others will view her as "off the wall" because of the inability to respond correctly to what is being said.

Experiences with hearing aids were very mixed, as was the purchase experience. The majority of respondents said they would recommend hearing aids to friends and would recommend their dispenser. One piece of advice many wished to offer audiologists is the importance of maintaining contact with their patients. Respondents felt that they heard better with the hearing aids than without and that hearing aids do enrich their lives. One wise respondent said that hearing aids contribute positively to one's self-image, whereas not using them actually detracts from one's personal image. Several respondents who were pleased with their hearing aids remain frustrated by the difficulty of hearing in noisy places. One astute respondent advised persons with hearing impairment not to fear new technology and suggested that a strategy for dealing with their hearing loss is to "lead the conversation," as this allows the person with hearing loss to control the topic of conversation!

Those respondents with a negative experience likened their audiologist to a used-car dealer; they were frustrated because they were not given a choice regarding the hearing aid manufacturer or offered the inclusion of a "t-coil" for use with a hearing loop, and because the audiologist did not take the time to explain why he or she recommended a specific hearing aid and seemed to be more interested in the sale than in the person with hearing loss. One respondent advised audiologists not to promise what they could not deliver with hearing aids, and cautioned that it is important to listen to the patient. One of my favorite comments came from an 83-year-old with 4 years of hearing aid experience, who said that with the hearing aids she did not feel any loss, and that she was very satisfied with the bright red Miracle-Ear hearing aids she wears daily as they are preferable to the dull beige option!

Although I am primarily an academic who preaches more than I practice, collaborating with and learning from persons with hearing loss and their communication partners informs my teaching, writing, and clinical work. It is my fervent hope that the material covered in this text, be it the anatomical or psychological changes associated with aging or the in-depth discussion of audiologic rehabilitation, will lend itself to a change in orientation from the medical model to a person-centered focus. Mark Ross's vision for our profession and training programs continues to resonate both in this text and, it is hoped, through the voice of individuals with hearing loss whom we treat.

References

AHRQ. (2012). http://www.ahrq.gov/qual/ptcareria.htm

Davis, K., Schoenbaum, S., & Audet, A. (2005). A 2020 vision of patient-centered primary care. The Commonwealth Fund. www.commonwealthfund.org/Publication

Acknowledgments

My deepest thanks to Christopher Malone and Emily Ekle, who oversaw the rewrite of the bulk of the text through its many iterations.

I

Aging: Normal and Abnormal Aspects

Chapter 1

The Demography and Epidemiology of Aging

A gray head is a crown of glory. It is found in the righteous.
—*Proverbs 16.31*

◆ Learning Objectives

After reading this chapter, you should be able to

- ◆ outline the demographic revolution, which is taking place in the 21st century;
- ◆ explain how the aging of the population will influence caseloads and the practice of audiology; and
- ◆ understand health disparities in the elderly.

◆ Global Demographic Changes: A Cross-National Perspective

Improvements in public health coupled with technological advances have led to a global demographic revolution. In light of changing demographics and the movement of the world's population into cities, the World Health Organization (WHO) has coined the term *active aging* as a way to approach and treat this large demographic (WHO, 2007). In this paradigm shift, the concept of active aging entails enhancing the quality of life by considering economic and social factors, the physical environment, health and social services, and behavioral and personal determinants. It is in this context that this chapter on demographics is written.

We are living in historic times. Worldwide, the older population is growing at a dramatic rate. The world's 65-and-older population is projected to triple by midcentury, from 516 million in 2009 to 1.55 billion in 2050 (U.S. Bureau of the Census, 2007). According to projections, by 2050 the number of older people in the world will exceed the population of children. Specifically, 13% of the total population, or one billion persons, will be 65 years of age or older by 2030 (U.S. Department of State, 2007). The most rapid growth in the older populations is occurring in less developed countries, such that between 2006 and 2030 the percentage increase in persons aged 65 years or over will increase by 140% in less developed countries as compared with 51% in more developed countries (U.S. Department of State, 2007). For the first time in history, the percentage of

persons aged 65 or over will outnumber the percentage of children under 5 years of age (U.S. Department of State, 2007).

Between 1975 and 2025, the percentage of persons over 60 years old is projected to increase by 224%, compared with only 102% for the general population. In 2006, the United States had the second largest elderly population (38,690,169) after China, which reported a 65+ population of 106,125,141. In that same year, the U.S. reported the second largest oldest-old population, also behind the more populous China. Despite its very large older population, the U.S. is considered one of the younger of the developed countries, whereas Sweden has the highest proportion (17.9%) of older adults as compared with the U.S., Canada, and other industrialized countries. It is projected that by the year 2025, Japan, Italy, and Germany will have the largest proportion of older adults of the eight countries with the largest older adult population. Although the relative number of older persons is higher in developed countries, the number of those in less developed countries is growing rapidly, such that by the year 2025 more than two thirds of the world's older citizens will be living in poorer geographic regions. With 60 percent of the world's population, Asia has one of the largest concentrations of aging persons. **Figure 1.1** depicts the global trends that will be taking place over the next several decades.

Pearl

The worldwide older population is growing at a much faster rate than the overall population. It is projected that by 2050 the number of people 65 or older worldwide will grow to 1.55 billion (U.S. Bureau of the Census Public Information Office, 2012).

◆ Size and Growth of the Older Population in the United States

The rate of growth of the population aged 65 or over has exceeded that of the general U.S. population (U.S. Bureau of the Census, 2008b). Between 1900 and 2000, the total U.S. population increased threefold, whereas the population of people aged 65 years or over increased by a factor of close to 11. During the

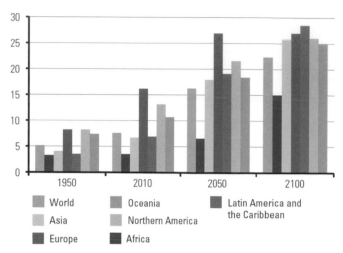

Fig. 1.1   Global growth in percentage of population over 65 years of age. [From United Nations Department of Economic and Social Affairs Population Division. (2011). *World population prospects: The 2010 revision graphs and maps from the world population 2010 wall chart. The 2011 revision.* New York: United Nations. (Reprinted by permission) http://esa.un.org/unpd/wpp/Documentation/pdf/WPP2010 _Wallchart_Plots.pdf.]

next several decades, the growth rate for the population of persons 65 years of age or over is expected to outpace that for the total population rather dramatically, such that by 2040 one in five persons, or 75 million persons in the U.S., will have reached 65 years of age, representing 20% of the total U.S. population (Beers, 2005; Centers for Disease Control and Prevention [CDC], 2006). Interestingly, it is projected that by 2050, 1% of the U.S. population will be 100 years of age or over (i.e., 4.1 million) (Manton, Gu, & Lamb, 2006). **Table 1.1** depicts the changes over time quite dramatically. In 1940 the population aged 65 or over represented 6.8% of the total U.S. population and in 2000 it constituted 12.4% of the population; by 2020 this age group will represent 16.3% and, by 2040, 20.4% of the U.S. population. Thus, in the year 2000 more than 35 million Americans were 65+, approximately half the number of persons projected by the year 2040 to be 65+ years of age. The most rapid increase in the 65+ population is expected between the years 2010 and 2030, when the baby boom generation reaches age 65. In summary, by 2030, the number of older Americans

is projected to more than double to approximately 71 million. Close to 20% of persons in the U.S. aged 65+ are members of a minority group. The fact that baby boomers began to reach age 65 by 2011 accounts in large part for the aforementioned trend.

Pearl

Of the total U.S. population (301,237,703), 37,980,136 citizens of the United States are 65 years of age or older.

Special Consideration

The 65 and older population is projected to increase to between 80 and 90 million by 2050, and the 85 and older population is projected to increase to close to 21 million (U.S. Bureau of the Census, 2004).

The older population itself is getting older, with the most dramatic growth among the "oldest old," namely those 85 years of age or over (Beers, 2005). Although the 85+ population accounted for 12% of the elderly population in the year 2000, it is projected to account for nearly 20% of the elderly population in the year 2050. In absolute terms, 5.5 million people, or 2% of the U.S. population, was 85 or older as of July 1, 2007, and by 2020 it is projected that the 85+ population will reach 6.6 million, representing a 15% increase from the previous decade (U.S. Bureau of the Census, 2007). More than half of the world's oldest old live in six countries: China, the U.S., India, Japan, Germany, and Russia. In many countries, the oldest old are now the fastest growing portion of the total population. On a global level, the 85-and-over population is projected to increase 151% between 2005 and 2030, compared with a 104% increase for the population aged 65 and over and a 21% increase for the population under age 65. The percentage of oldest old varies considerably from country to country. The most striking increase will occur in Japan, which is one of a few countries considered to be aging rapidly. By 2030, nearly 24% of all older Japanese are expected to be at least 85 years old (Hayutin, 2007).

Special Consideration

Within the older population, the fastest growing segment is the oldest old, a group with greater needs in all areas of health care. The oldest old will number 19 million in 2050. The growth of the 85+ population, a major outgrowth of improved disease prevention/ health promotion activities and health care, will have a marked impact on the health care system and, accordingly, implications for hearing health care.

The shift in the proportion of persons 65+ and persons under 18 years is also noteworthy. In 1900 persons under the age of 18 years constituted 40% and persons 65+ constituted 4% of the total U.S. population. In contrast, by the year 2030, the proportion of the population under 18 will be comparable to

Table 1.1   Actual and Projected Growth of Persons 65+ (in Thousands) and 85+ (in Thousands): 1940 to 2040

Year	Total Population (All Ages)	≥65 Years of Age: Number (%) of Total Population	≥85 Years of Age: Number (%) of Total Population
1940	132,122	9031 (6.8)	370 (4.1)
1960	179,323	16,560 (9.2)	929 (5.6)
1980	226,546	25,550 (11.3)	2240 (8.8)
2000	281,422	34.992 (12.4)	4240 (12.1)
2020	335,805	54,632 (16.3)	7269 (13.3)
2040	391,946	80,049 (20.4)	15,409 (19.2)

Source: Adapted from U.S. Bureau of the Census. (2004). *U.S. interim projects by age, sex, race, and Hispanic origin.* http://www.census.gov/ipc/www/ usinterimproj/.

that of 65+. That is, by the year 2030, 21% of the U.S. population will be under 18 years and 22% will be 65+ years. One of the fastest growing segments of the U.S. population is centenarians (those age 100 or older); in 2010, there were 80,000 centenarians, and their numbers are rising dramatically, such that by 2045 the number of centenarians in the U.S. is projected to reach 757,000. Supercentenarians, people who are 110+ years old, occur at a rate of 1 per 7 million, and in 2010 there were 60 to 70 supercentenarians in the U.S. With the increase in the number of centenarians and supercentenarians, interventions to promote an increased quality of life become increasingly important, especially regarding hearing health care and its potential for helping to forestall cognitive aging (New England Centenarian Study, 2011). The increase in the number of centenarians is a global phenomenon; in Canada there were 4635 centenarians in 2006, or 1.5 centenarians per 10,000 population, and Japan reported the highest prevalence of centenarians in 2006, with 2.3 per 10,000 population (Perls, 2010).

Minority Aging

The racial and ethnic composition of the elderly population will be changing profoundly in the next 50 years owing to immigration patterns, fertility, and mortality rates. In 2000, 16% or 5.7 million older adults in the U.S. were classified as minorities, and it is projected that by 2010, 8.1 million or 20% of individuals 65+ will be minorities. By 2020, 23.6% of the elderly will be members of the minority population (Administration on Aging, 2007). Population projections suggest that between 2004 and 2030 the older white population will grow by 74%, the older African American population will grow by 147%, and the older Hispanic population will grow by 254%. It is noteworthy that the older population of American Indians, Aleuts, and Eskimos will grow by 143% and of Asians and Pacific Islanders by 208% (Administration on Aging, 2007). The proportion of elderly within the Hispanic population is projected to increase from 6% in 1995 to close to 14% in 2050. The proportion of blacks and the "other races" category within the elderly population is also expected to increase in this time period, such that in 2050, 33% of the elderly population will be black, Hispanic, or "other races." Conversely, the proportion of whites in the elderly population will decrease dramatically during that time frame (Administration on Aging, 2007).

These trends have implications for health care and health literacy. Rather than narrowing, the disparities in major health indicators between whites and nonwhites are widening. For example, on most health indices including health behavior and practices, African Americans, American Indians, and Hispanic ethnic and racial groups are disadvantaged relative to whites. In contrast, on most indicators, Asian Americans appear to be as healthy as, if not healthier than, white Americans. Further, socioeconomic status and educational level interact in complex ways with race and gender to further contribute to differences in health status between white Americans and non-white groups. Interestingly, disparities in health risk behavior prevalence among adults with and without hearing loss are most apparent among those 65 years of age or older (Schoenborn & Heyman, 2008). Audiologists must make every attempt to ensure that members of all ethnic groups have access to audiology services, and that literacy levels are considered when developing educational materials.

Life Expectancy

The length of a healthier old age is increasing at a rather remarkable rate. Average life expectancy has increased substantially since 1900, such that for both sexes a person born in 2005 could expect to live to 77.8 years (National Center for Health Statistics, 2007). This represents an increase of 2.4 years since 1990. Gender and race have an impact on life expectancy such that at birth females have a higher life expectancy than males. Overall, African-American females born in 2005 have a life expectancy at birth of 76.5 as compared with African-American males, whose life expectancy is 70 years, the first time this barrier has been broken (CDC, 2006). In contrast, white females born in 2005 have a life expectancy of 80.8 years as compared with white males, whose life expectancy is 75.7 years. It is important to note that between 1900 and 2005 the gap in life expectancy between the white population and the black population narrowed. Although average life expectancy declines with advancing age, after age 65 years the interaction between age and gender is rather interesting. On average, 25% of women aged 75 years will be expected to live an additional 17+ years, 25% will live 7 years or less, and 50% will live an additional 12 years or longer (Durso, 2006). Finally, according to CDC data gathered through 2007, the average 65-year-old can expect to live until 84 years of age, thanks in large part to decline in the death rate.

Life expectancy differs by country of origin as well. Life expectancy in Japan is considered to be the world's highest, at 82 years (Hayutin, 2007). Girls born in China between 2000 and 2005 have a life expectancy of 73 years, those born in Hong Kong have a life expectancy of 85 years, and those born in South Africa have a life expectancy of 51 years. Boys born in China between 2000 and 2005 have a life expectancy of 70 years, those born in Hong Kong have a life expectancy of 79 years, and those born in South Africa have a life expectancy of 47 years. Life expectancy is also influenced by the multiplicity of geriatric conditions from which older adults suffer. For example, the fact that older adults with diabetes are at increased risk for such conditions as depression, falls, polypharmacy, and cognitive impairment has an impact on life expectancy, making it increasingly variable among older adults (Durso, 2006).

Pearl

An individual who has reached age 65, as of this writing, is expected to have a life expectancy of an additional 20 years. Increased longevity is accompanied by an increase in prevalence of multiple chronic conditions, associated disability, and activity limitations.

Living Arrangements

Overall, about one third (30%) of noninstitutionalized elderly persons live alone, with the very old and women being the most likely to do so. In 2006, 10.7 million older adults lived alone—2.9 million older men and 7.8 million older women

(Administration on Aging, 2007). According to a 2007 report, 71% of men aged 65+ lived with their spouse or other family members as compared with 42% of women in this age group (Administration on Aging, 2007).

Approximately half of the women 75 years or older lived alone. Interestingly, more than 670,000 grandparents aged 65 years or over lived in households in which only their grandchildren were present, and over 800,000 resided in homes with the adult children and grandchildren (Administration on Aging, 2007). It is of interest that there are considerable disparities by race and gender among older adults. In 2006, 52% of older African-American men lived with their spouse, 18% with other relatives, and 26% lived alone. Among older African-American women, 23% lived with their spouse, 34% with other relatives, and 41% lived alone (Administration on Aging, 2007). In 2007, 84% of older Asian men lived with their spouse and 8% lived alone, whereas 47% of older Asian woman lived with their spouse and 20% lived alone. In 2006, 69% of older Hispanic men lived with their spouse and 17% lived alone, whereas 40% of Hispanic older women lived with their spouse and 25% lived alone. Trends in living arrangements are of relevance to audiologists when attempting to gauge the impact of hearing loss on the individual and family members and when deciding about candidacy for hearing aids or hearing assistance technologies. Further, with the advent of home health care as an alternative to institutionalization, health literacy of caregivers and family members as it relates to hearing impairment and communication will assume greater importance.

Pearl

It is critical that audiologists appreciate that living alone brings with it a series of concerns for the hearing-impaired elderly. It may be a threat to personal safety, as individuals who suffer from hearing loss may not be able to hear warning signals. Hence, a discussion about hearing assistance technology is always indicated for the hearing impaired who live alone.

◆ Geographic Considerations: A Domestic Perspective

In the U.S. more than half of persons aged 65+ lived in one of nine states in 2008, and in 2007 persons aged 65+ made up nearly 15% of the total population in ten states including Connecticut, Massachusetts, Arkansas, and North Dakota (Administration on Aging, 2007). As would be expected, the most populous states are also the ones with the largest numbers of elderly: California (4 million elderly), Florida (3.1 million), New York (2.6 million), Texas (2.4 million), and Pennsylvania (1.9 million). Although the most populous state, California, has the largest number of persons aged 65+, Florida has a higher proportion of persons aged 65+; in 2007 it was 17%, as compared with Virginia, 15.5%, and in Pennsylvania, 15.2% (U.S. Bureau of the Census, 2007). In contrast, Alaska has the lowest absolute number and lowest proportion of individuals aged 65+ (7.9%). Interestingly, the majority of older adults reside in metropolitan areas, with only 19.5% living in nonmetropolitan areas (Administration on Aging, 2007).

Pearl

The states with the greatest proportion of older adults are different from those with the greatest number. In 2006, most persons 65+ resided in metropolitan areas and this trend is projected to continue.

Also notable in the U.S. has been the proportional increase in the elderly population in selected regions, and the projected increase in the proportion of older adults residing in selected states between 1989 and 2010. The states projected to have the largest percent increase in the 65+ population during the latter time frame are Hawaii, Alaska, Arizona, and Georgia, whereas those with the smallest increase are North Dakota, Iowa, and Montana. By the year 2010 California's elderly population increased by 52% to more than 4.7 million, maintaining its rank as the state with the largest number of older adults. Florida will continue to have the largest percentage of older adults, rising to nearly 20% of its population. It is projected that by the year 2020, 32 states will have more than 16% of their population 65 years of age or over. These demographic changes have implications for the demand for hearing health care services. In short, retirement areas will need hearing health care services as their population ages.

Economic Status

The economic resources and status of older adults must be considered in terms of both cash and noncash resources. In general, the elderly have substantially lower average cash incomes than do the nonelderly. However, when lifetime accumulations of wealth, government in-kind transfers, real estate, and other assets are taken into account, some of the differences in economic status are erased. Specifically, as reported by older adults in a 2005 survey, Social Security accounted for 35% of aggregate income, pensions accounted for 19%, earnings accounted for 28%, and asset income accounted for 13%. Hence, income from Social Security is the major source of income for the elderly, accounting for 90% or more of income for some 34% of beneficiaries (Administration on Aging, 2007).

Assessing economic status based on income, older Americans emerge as having a lower economic status than do younger adults. In 2007, the median income of families whose head of the household was 65+ was approximately $41,851 versus close to $50,000 for the general population. The median income was $24,323 for older men and $14,021 for older women (Administration on Aging, 2007). Median incomes for households headed by Asians aged 65+ was $47,135, for non-Hispanic whites $43,654, for African Americans $30,025, and for Hispanics $31,544. Interestingly, in 2007, 8% of family households with a person 65+ had incomes less than $15,000 and 53% had incomes of more than $35,000. Within the 65+ population, the oldest old have the lowest family incomes.

In 2007, 3.6 million (9.7%) persons aged 65+ had incomes below the poverty level (Administration on Aging, 2007). This poverty rate represents an increase of 10% from 2006. A smaller number (2.4 million) of the elderly are considered near poor, meaning their income is between the poverty level and 125% of the poverty level. Poverty levels are affected by gender, race, and geography. The oldest elderly are the most likely to have incomes below the poverty level. But it is reassuring that the proportion of all people 65 or older living in poverty has dropped from 35% in 1959 to the present rate of 9.4%. Similarly, in 1965, 63% of blacks 65 or older lived below the poverty level versus 22.7% today. In sum, as of a 2009 report, poverty rates for people 65 or older in 2007 were statistically unchanged from 2006. There were 3.6 million seniors in poverty in 2007, up from 3.4 million in 2006 (U.S. Bureau of the Census, 2008a). Change in income status as one ages is an additional incentive for audiologists to promote hearing interventions early, as shifts in priorities take place and expenditures for hearing aids may be unrealistic for many.

Educational Attainment

It is projected that, in 2015, 76% of older adults will have completed high school and 20% will hold a bachelor's degree. Educational attainment influences life expectancy and economic status such that the better educated live longer and are less likely to be at the poverty level. Projected improvements in educational attainment vary by race such that improvements continue to lag for nonwhites including blacks and Hispanics. Differences in education level have a profound impact on health status and disparities. Educational attainment is an important indicator, as it influences health literacy, physical vulnerability, and health outcomes. Interestingly, people with limited education have limited material resources and are also more vulnerable physically (Clark, Stump, Miller, & Long, 2007). Further, although education is a stronger predictor than income of whether an individual develops functional limitations or chronic conditions, income level has a stronger effect on whether the condition worsens (Herd, Goesling, & House, 2007). The more rapid increase in the minority older adult population and the disparity in educational level have implications for delivery of health care services in general and hearing health care services in particular.

Pearl

Adults with hearing loss have higher rates of health risk behaviors, including smoking and alcohol use, than do those with good hearing (Schoenborn & Heyman, 2008).

◆ Health Care Expenditures and Utilization of Health Care Services

Over 80% of persons 65 years of age or over have chronic conditions that account for 46% of the global burden of disease. The economic impact of longevity, with its attendant increase in chronic illness and comorbidities, is profound. National health care expenditures in the U.S. totaled $2.1 trillion in 2006 representing, a 6.7% increase from 2005. This amounts to 15% of the gross domestic product. In 2005 older adults averaged $4331 in out-of-pocket health care expenditures, which is an increase of 57% over 1995 expenditures (Administration on Aging, 2007). In contrast, during the same time frame, the general population averaged $2776 in out-of-pocket costs. The major health care expenditures for the elderly in that year were on health insurance, medication, medical services, and medical supplies. Hospital spending, which accounted for 31% of national health expenditures, increased by 7% in 2006. Interestingly, spending for prescription drugs accounted for 10% of national health expenditures in 2006, with 60% of people aged 65+ reporting that they had three or more drugs prescribed during the month prior to completing the health survey (U.S. Department of Health and Human Services [USDHHS], 2009). Given the high prevalence of chronic conditions, the elderly use more prescription drugs, dental care services, vision aids, hearing aids, and medical equipment than do younger adults. Older adults use health care services more frequently than do younger adults, and their health care costs are correspondingly higher. Health care utilization is highest among the oldest old. One important indicator of health service utilization is use of physician services. Physician contacts for persons 45 to 64 years were 3.9 in 2005, versus a mean of 10 contacts per year for persons 65 to 74 years and 15 per year among persons 85+ (Pompei & Murphy, 2006).

Consumption patterns of the elderly are most revealing as are expenditures for care of chronic conditions experienced by the elderly. As 88% of the population aged 65 years or over have at least one chronic condition, it is not surprising that 75% of U.S. health care expenditures go to treating chronic conditions (Wolff, Starfield, & Anderson, 2002). According to Anderson and Horvath (2002), health care costs for persons with at least three chronic conditions accounted for 89% of the annual Medicare budget. People aged 65+ spend a good proportion of their economic resources on essentials, including health care and transportation. In light of their health care expenditures, and the state of the economy, older adults are likely to spend money on hearing health care only if they can see that the benefit justifies the expense. That is to say, increasingly the health care consumer is asking whether the cost and health care effects of a hearing aid, for example, can be seen as providing value given the financial outlay. Disease-specific health-related quality of life outcome measures are gaining acceptance as the gold standard against which to justify the cost of hearing aids.

Perceptions of Health Status

Gains in life expectancy bring with it changes in patterns of illness, a decrease in mobility, an increase in dependency, and an increase in the utilization of health services. Yet Crimmins (2004) reported that the health status of older adults has improved dramatically over the past several decades, with greater longevity and technological advances. Chronic rather than acute conditions predominate with increased longevity. Approximately 82% of older adults have at least one chronic disease, with hypertension, chronic joint symptoms, and heart disease being the three most prevalent according to the 2006 Health Interview Survey (Pleis & Lethbridge-Cejku, 2007). According to a recent report by the Institute of Medicine (2008), 20% of persons 55 years of age or older reported mental health conditions including anxiety disorders, cognitive impairment, and mood disorders. Further, 31% of persons with disabilities and 45% of severely disabled community-dwelling older adults reported symptoms of depression, with nearly half of nursing home residents in a 2005 report presenting with dementia and 20% with other psychological diagnoses (Institute of Medicine, 2008).

Nearly 39% of older Americans report their health status to be very good or excellent with only 27.5% of adults aged 75 years or older self-assessing their health status to be fair or poor (Administration on Aging, 2007; Pleis & Lethbridge-Cejku, 2007). Although both health status and the subjective component of health, referred to as self-rated health, are dramatically influenced by age, the perception of one's health status declines less rapidly than does one's actual health status (Henchoz, Cavalli, & Girardin, 2008). The divergence between objective and perceived health status with advancing age, or the observation that older adults tend to view their health status favorably relative to actual health status, is due to several interesting variables. Henchoz et al (2008) contend that cognitive factors, adaptive strategies, expectations regarding the normal changes with age, temperament, and a sense of acceptance tend to explain why self-ratings of one's health is at odds with actual health status. Of interest as well is that, as people age, the gap between number of acute or chronic conditions and perception of health becomes wider. An interesting trend reported by Henchoz et al is that robust octogenarians differ from frail octogenarians in terms of the congruence between perceived and actual health status. For example, 46% of frail older adults in their sample tended to rate their health status as satisfactory as compared with 23% of robust older adults. Stated differently, those in their sample who were frail or dependent, and therefore in poor health, self-rated their health more positively than would be warranted by reality. This finding has implications for acceptance of hearing loss and management of its consequences.

Perceptions of health status vary with race as well, such that 24% of older African Americans and 29% of older Hispanics were less likely than were older whites (40%) and Asians (30%) to rate their health as excellent or good. The latter results from improvements in medical care, changes in lifestyle patterns (e.g., more exercise, decline in smoking rates, better control of blood pressure), and living conditions. Health literacy, or the degree to which individuals have the capacity to obtain, process, and understand information about health and health care services, influences perceptions of health status (Institute of Medicine, 2004). In short, health illiteracy compromises the ability to use health information from any source, and influences health-related decision making and, accordingly, how one judges one's health status (Bennett, Chen, Soroui, & White, 2009).

Individuals aged 65 years or older represent the largest single group in the U.S. with limited general and health literacy skills (White, 2008). In addition to age, health literacy varies with race and income level. These variations influence the rate of chronic conditions, self-reported physical functional status, and mental health status as measured by responses to subscales of the Medical Outcomes Study (MOS) Short-Form Health Survey (SF-36) (Wolf, Gazmararian, & Baker, 2005). Specifically, inadequate health literacy (e.g., measured by reading fluency) is a significant predictor of poor physical health status, when controlling for chronic conditions (Wolf et al, 2005). Further, inadequate health literacy is associated with more activity limitations, limitations in activity because of physical health status, mortality, and limitations in instrumental activities of daily living, even after controlling for sociodemographic factors, including income level, and chronic conditions (Baker et al, 2007; Wolf et al, 2005). Persons with low health literacy tend to be less likely to use preventive health care services, which quite possibly may explain the causal relationship between inadequate health literacy and self-reported physical and mental functioning. The extent to which health literacy impacts hearing health care service delivery remains unexplored.

◆ Chronic Conditions

It is noteworthy that as people age, acute conditions become less frequent and there is an increased likelihood of experiencing one or more chronic conditions or long-term illnesses that are rarely cured. Chronic disease, which affects older adults most dramatically, is associated with diminished quality of life and increased costs for health care. As of this writing, 80% of older adults have at least one chronic condition, with 50% having at least two. The increase in prevalence of chronic conditions, and disability with the increase in age is associated with increased comorbidity of chronic illnesses. In 2005, the prevalence of multiple co-occurring chronic conditions was large; 21% of Americans had more than one chronic condition or multiple longstanding illnesses (Vogeli et al, 2007). Among Americans aged 65 years or over, 62% had multiple chronic conditions (MCC) in 2005; this number was expected to have increased dramatically by 2020. Interestingly, a seminal report issued by the Institute of Medicine revealed that 23% of Medicare beneficiaries have five or more chronic conditions (Institute of Medicine, 2001). The fact that persons with more chronic conditions become more functionally impaired sooner than persons with fewer chronic conditions is an important consideration when trying to convince older adults of the value of hearing aids to reduce the functional impact of a multiplicity of chronic conditions (Vogeli et al, 2007).

In addition to advancing age, gender, economic status, race, and ethnicity influence the prevalence of chronic disease. For example, diabetes, heart disease, and any cancer are more prevalent in men, whereas arthritis is more prevalent in women. In 2005 and 2006, 70% of non-Hispanic blacks reported a diagnosis of hypertension versus 51% for non-Hispanic whites. Similarly, 29% of non-Hispanic blacks suffered from diabetes versus 16% of non-Hispanic whites. Hispanics reported higher levels of diabetes (25%) than non-Hispanic whites (16%), lower levels of arthritis, and comparable levels of hypertension. The prevalence of comorbidity of disease increases with age, and among the oldest old comorbidity occurs in most people.

Hearing Loss and Related Chronic Conditions

Chronic conditions, which include stroke, heart disease, cancer, and diabetes, are among the most common and the most costly to treat, and have the most significant impact on quality of life. The most prevalent conditions among the 65+ population, according to data from the Medicare Current Beneficiary Survey (MCBS), are arthritis (57%), hypertension (55%), pulmonary disease (38%), and diabetes (17%) (Vogeli et al, 2007). Interestingly, the majority of people with these illnesses are prone to age-related hearing impairment, which has the potential to exacerbate functional declines in the elderly.

Hearing difficulties, vision limitations, and absence of teeth are prevalent conditions among persons aged 65 and over. In fact, 31.9% of persons aged 65 to 74 years and 50% of persons aged 75 or older reported trouble hearing, whereas 13.6% of persons aged 65 to 74 years reported vision limitations with glasses or contacts and 21.7% of persons aged 75 or older reported vision limitations with glasses or contacts (Pleis & Lethbridge-Cejku, 2007). By 2020, the number of Americans aged 40 or older who will be blind is expected to rise by 70% to 1.6 million, and the number with low vision is expected to exceed 5.5 million. It is noteworthy that the prevalence of hearing impairment among persons aged 65 or over is demonstrably higher than that of visual impairment, and the prevalence of each condition increases dramatically among those aged 75 years or over. Overall, 17% of the total U.S. population, more than 36 million, experience chronic hearing impairment (Bainbridge, Hoffman, & Cowie, 2008). According to the National Institute on Deafness and Other Communication Disorders (NIDCD), more people are losing their hearing earlier in life due to the combination of noise exposure and environmental factors, such that nearly 10 million people between 45 and 64 years of age experience chronic hearing impairment (Rosenbloom, 2007). According to the NIDCD, almost 12% of men between the ages of 65 and 74 years report tinnitus, with tinnitus identified more frequently in white individuals.

The prevalence of selected chronic conditions tends to vary somewhat with race, with the prevalence of hearing impairment being higher among whites than blacks (Lim, Thorpe, Gordon-Salant, & Ferrucci, 2011). In contrast, the prevalence of hypertension is higher among blacks than whites. Lam, Lee, Gómez-Marín, Zheng, and Caban (2006) analyzed data on self-reported visual and hearing impairment from the National Health Interview Survey (NHIS) to determine the rate of concurrent visual and hearing impairment (self-report) and the influence of race on prevalence rates. Confirming the data from the 1989 NHIS, African-American participants reported less hearing impairment as compared with white respondents, men were more likely to report hearing impairment, and 1.3% of respondents claimed a concurrent visual and hearing impairment. These findings are predictable from the literature on health literacy.

The natural clustering of chronic conditions has been studied in depth, but the extent to which hearing impairment and vestibular dysfunction co-occur with conditions such as heart disease, diabetes, pulmonary conditions, and arthritis has not been fully explored. According to the National Health and Nutrition Examination Survey (NHANES) for 2001 to 2004, 35% of Americans (69 million) 40 years of age or older present with vestibular dysfunction and hypertension, and diabetes is associated with higher rates of vestibular dysfunction (Agrawal, Carey, Della Santina, Schubert, & Minor, 2009). Further, data from the NHANES for 1999 to 2004 revealed that the prevalence of hearing impairment is higher among men and women with self-reported diabetes between the ages of 20 and 59 years (Bainbridge et al, 2008). Interestingly, care of older adults with more than one chronic condition accounts for 95% of all Medicare spending and for 66% of Medicare spending for those with five or more chronic conditions (Vogeli et al, 2007). When depression is one of the comorbidities, individuals with chronic conditions have an increased likelihood of using emergency department services, and when hearing impairment is present, as is very probable, quality of care can be further compromised. Finally, comorbidity is associated with multiple medication use, an increased risk for adverse reactions, an increased likelihood of ototoxic effects, and an increased likelihood of hospitalizations (Boyd et al, 2005).

Audiologists should emphasize to hospital workers, especially emergency room workers, how to best communicate with patients, as this might help ensure the patients' understanding of instructions and their ultimate compliance or adherence with treatment regimens. Emergency room workers should not start walking away when they are speaking to patients, should face the listener at all times when speaking, and should not look down at the computer when taking a history or preparing patients for discharge. Strategies for educating health care workers about communication are discussed at length in subsequent chapters.

Special Consideration

Eighty-eight percent of persons aged 65+ experience at least one chronic condition (Wolff et al, 2002). The average 75-year-old suffers from three chronic conditions and takes five prescription medications. The two most prevalent chronic diseases are hypertension and chronic joint symptoms (arthritis), and hearing impairment is among the most prevalent of disabilities or limitations (Pleis & Lethbridge-Cejku, 2007).

Activity Limitations

In 2005 and 2006, the percentage of older adults with limitation of activity ranged from 25% of 65- to 74-year-olds to 60% of adults 85 years old and over (National Center for Health Statistics [NCHS], 2009). According to the most recent NCHS survey (2009), arthritis and other musculoskeletal conditions were the most frequently mentioned chronic conditions causing limitation of activity, with heart and circulatory conditions emerging as the second leading cause. Interestingly, among adults aged 85 years or over living at home, senility or dementia, vision conditions, and hearing problems were frequently mentioned causes of activity limitation. Age was a major determinant of activity limitations, such that among those aged 65 to 74 years, 10 out of every 1000 reported hearing loss as a major cause of activity limitations, versus 78 out of every 1000 Americans 85 years of age and older. Hearing loss was matched with senility as a major cause of activity limitations among older adults 85 years and over (NCHS, 2009).

Special Consideration

In light of the high number of physician visits among older adults, it is incumbent on audiologists to educate physicians about hearing loss in older adults, its consequences, and the devices available to help overcome the handicap resulting from hearing impairment. Physicians should be taught to routinely screen for possible handicapping hearing impairments using referral criteria that have good specificity, sensitivity, and predictive accuracy.

◆ Workforce and Retirement Trends

The increase in longevity in this century brings with it an increase in the amount of time spent in all major activities, including work and retirement. Interestingly, a recent report by the U.S. Bureau of Labor Statistics (2008) revealed that the number of workers aged 65 or over increased 101% between 1977 and 2007, with the increase being greatest for woman over 65 years of age (for men the increase was 75%, and for women the increase was 147%). According to the Bureau of Labor Statistics (BLS), by 2014 the number of workers aged 55 or over will grow to 20% of the labor force, up from the 15% it is today. Although the number of people aged 75 or over who are employed is relatively small (0.8% of the employed in 2007), this age group had the most dramatic gain in employment, increasing by close to 170% from 1977 to 2007. Increasingly, job growth for older workers is most dramatic in the service sector. Examples of jobs in this sector include grocery clerks, waitresses, and substitute teachers, all positions previously held by young people (Amadeo, 2007). According to the BLS, over half of older workers are continuing to work rather than retiring. Those who cannot afford to retire are taking bridge jobs (a stopgap or "bridge" between a full-time career and full retirement), whereas those who can are exploring career options that are of more interest to them as they mature. In the wake of the financial crisis of 2008 to 2009, one in five workers responding to a survey conducted in September 2009 by Bankrate indicated that they plan to leave the office between 1 and 5 years later than they first planned. Interesting, 18% of respondents indicated that they would never be able to retire (Bankrate, 2009). Another interesting trend for the next decade is the opportunity for part-time work among persons aged 65+ and an emphasis on volunteerism among those living longer and remaining healthy.

Special Consideration

These educational and workforce trends suggest that hearing health care interventions will take on increasing importance, as the ability to hear and understand is typically viewed as essential to job performance.

◆ Nursing Home Care

With current trends toward a rapidly aging U.S. population with increasing longevity, the health care system and long-term-care services will face many challenges. According to current projections, 35% of Americans of age 65 will receive some nursing home care in their lifetime, with 18% potentially living in a nursing home for at least 1 year, and 5% for at least 5 years. There are 1.8 million residents living in 17,000 nursing homes in the U.S. (National Nursing Home Survey [NNHS], 2004). Most of today's nursing homes are free standing, but increasingly retirement communities or continuing care retirement communities are including a nursing home as an option, given the increasing numbers of people who wish to age in place. Although the percentage of older adults living in nurs-

ing homes has declined from 8.1% of those 75 or older in 2000 to 7.4% in 2006, it is projected that by 2020 the nursing home population will increase to 2.6 million. Almost 50% of nursing home residents are 85 years of age or older, with the average age of residents being 79 years. The majority of nursing home residents require assistance with their regular activities of daily living, which includes transferring, bathing, dressing, eating, and toileting (NNHS, 2004).

Mental disorders were the second leading cause of nursing home admission in 2004. Of particular relevance to audiologists is the fact that nearly 50% of residents suffer from some level of dementia, and more than 30% from depression; 33.9% of all nursing home residents reportedly had at least one fall in the 180 days prior to the interview, and 8.9% of residents had fallen in the 30 days prior to the interview. Specifically, residents aged 65 years or older (35.3%) were more likely than those under age 65 (22.4%) to have fallen in the 180 days prior to the survey (NNHS, 2004; Samos, Aguilar, & Ouslander, 2010). The minimum data set (MDS), a structured tool designed to assess residents from a clinical and functional point of view, triggers the use of resident assessment protocols that address 18 conditions common to residents in nursing homes. The conditions, which include cognitive loss, communication difficulties, problems with psychosocial well-being, falls, and behavioral problems, all could be exacerbated by an untreated hearing loss and could be addressed in part via auditory interventions (Samos et al, 2010). It is incumbent on audiologists working in nursing homes to make sure those working directly with residents know how to recognize individuals with hearing impairment and individuals prone to falls, how to communicate with the hearing impaired, and how to operate hearing aids or assistive technologies. It is also important that included in the front of the medical record is a statement regarding the resident's hearing status, and some sort of symbol should be placed outside the resident's room so that in case an emergency bell goes off the hearing impaired are notified, as often warning sounds are not audible.

Pearl

In light of the fact that the majority of nursing home residents are 75 years of age or over, the prevalence of significant hearing loss is rather high, necessitating the need for hearing aids or, more appropriately, hearing assistance technologies. Institutional long-term care takes place either in nursing homes or in assisted living facilities that offer a housing alternative for older adults who are relatively independent.

◆ Home Health Care

Home health care encompasses services for persons of any age who are disabled, chronically ill, or recovering from an acute illness (National Association for HomeCare and Hospice, 2008). The trend toward caring for someone medically in the home reduces the need for long-term hospitalization. In light of economic considerations, approximately eight million Americans require some type of medical care in the home, with over 20,000 home health care providers delivering service. To qualify for home care, recipients must be homebound, and a physician must state that the patient needs skilled care at home and needs at least one of the following services: part-time or intermittent skilled nursing care or physical therapy, or speech-language services (National Association for HomeCare and Hospice, 2008).

Traditionally, recipients of home care have chronic conditions requiring attention or are terminally ill. Conditions requiring home health care most frequently include diabetes, heart failure, chronic ulcer of the skin, osteoarthritis, and hypertension, and often most of these individuals will have a hearing impairment that is likely to interfere with care (Scharpf et al, 2006). Medical and social home health care services available in the home include physician care; nursing care; physical, occupational, and speech therapy; and care from home health aides. More than 66% of recipients of home health care services are elderly. Considered a cost savings to Medicare, the home care portion of Medicare's total budget has increased dramatically (Corazzini, 2003). In 2007, annual expenditures for home health care were $57.6 million (National Association for HomeCare and Hospice, 2008). Medicare is the largest single payer of home health care services. In 2006, Medicare spending accounted for 37% of home health expenditures, including hospice and home health care. Medicare home health spending grew to 13.7% in 2007, with a 10.2% projected growth rate per year from 2008 to 2017. In 2007, the home health benefit accounted for 3.6% of total Medicare spending; 35% was spent for hospital care, 14% for physician services, and 2% for hospice care (National Association for HomeCare and Hospice, 2008). Home health care is expanding not only in the U.S. but also in other countries. In Spain, 57% of homes have at least one person who requires care, and in 66% of those cases the family is the sole caregiver.

◆ Palliative Care and Hospice Care

The terms *palliative care* and *hospice care* are often used interchangeably, but there are subtle differences. Palliative care may be defined as interdisciplinary care of patients and families focused on the relief of suffering and improving quality of life in individuals whose disease is no longer responsive to curative treatment (von Gunten, 2002). Palliative care may be provided at any time during a person's illness, from the time of diagnosis, or it may be given at the same time as curative treatment. In contrast, hospice care, a model of quality care, always provides palliative care and is focused on the terminally ill patient who no longer seeks curative treatments and is expected to live for only 6 months or less. In individuals receiving palliative care, communication and psychological, social, and spiritual support are of paramount importance. Benefiting both patients and their families, palliative care communication and support for the family are the main goals along with symptomatic care. The team helps patients and families make medical decisions and choose treatments that are in line with their goals (National Association for HomeCare and Hospice, 2008).

Hospice care agencies provide supportive and palliative care to people at the end of their life. Hospice agencies focus on comfort and quality of life rather than curative treatments (National Association for HomeCare and Hospice, 2008). Nursing care, medical social work services, physician services, counseling, inpatient care, home care and homemaker services, medical appliances and supplies, physical and occupational therapies, speech-language pathology services, and bereavement services are available for families and patients as necessary for palliative treatment for terminal illnesses.

Clinical palliative care is made available at three distinct levels: primary, secondary, and tertiary. Primary palliative care refers to the basic skills and competencies required of all physicians and other health care professionals. Secondary palliative care refers to the specialist clinicians and organizations that provide consultation and specialty care. Tertiary palliative care refers to the academic medical centers where specialist knowledge for the most complex cases is practiced, researched, and taught (von Gunten, 2002). Audiologists have an important role to play in the delivery of palliative care. For example, in the early stages when the patient is involved in decision making, it is critical to ensure that the patient is able to understand health professionals with whom he or she is interacting. The physician consults with the patient to set short- and long-term goals. Further, throughout the process interpersonal relationships are paramount, such as communicating with loved ones. Interestingly, exploration is currently underway to determine the utility of videophone technology to provide psychological support and symptom monitoring in selected cases (Dang, Golden, Cheung, & Roos, 2010).

Pearl

The goal of palliative care is to improve the quality of life and to provide support at the end of life. The emphasis on hospice care is caring and not curing.

◆ Telemedicine, Telehealth, and Health Informatics

The role of telemedicine, telehealth, and health informatics in the effective delivery of health care to the elderly is increasing. As these fields are newly emerging, a definition of the jargon being used in health care follows. The development of information and communication technology (ICT)-based methods for medicine, health care, and prevention is one aspect of the emerging field of health informatics (Koch & Hägglund, 2009). As a substitute for face-to-face contact between patient and provider, telemedicine employs telecommunication and computer technologies to provide and support health care when distance separates the participants (Institute of Medicine, 1996; Norris, 2002). Telecommunications technology, which could include voice, video, and other electronic information processing technologies, is used to gather and transmit data relevant to diagnosis (e.g., monitor blood pressure, heart rate, and other vital information), treatment, and therapeutic interventions where distance or time separates the patient and health care service provider (Koch, 2006). The terms *telehealth* and *telecare* are often used interchangeably by health care professionals, but in my view telehealth is distinctive in that it focuses on education and on the use of telecommunications as a means of protecting and promoting health (Charness, 2006). Potential preventive and educational applications of telemedicine include remote monitoring, patient education, and data collection (Dang et al, 2010). Advances in information and communication technology coupled with participation of federal and private health insurers have made home telemedicine both feasible and financially affordable (Hersh et al, 2006).

In general, the ultimate aim of telemedicine and ICT is to improve the quality of patient-based health care in a cost-effective way (Koch & Hägglund, 2009). Electronic communication between the elderly patient and the health care provider is beneficial because it can be used in the public health arena for health promotion activities, to address common issues such as difficulty with transportation, especially for those in remote areas, and to address concerns about home safety and isolation. At present, home-based telemedicine is most commonly used for management of chronic diseases or specific conditions, such as heart disease or diabetes mellitus. It is also used for monitoring falls and by psychiatrists and neurologists when verbal communication is a key component of the diagnostic assessment (Hersh et al, 2006). Further, monitoring patients via electronic communication technologies can help reduce the burden on the family member as caregiver. I have participated in a form of telemedicine in which I have worked with the homebound elderly to help resolve questions about their hearing aids, to troubleshoot hearing aids, and to promote communication with family members. It was an invaluable experience. Finally, e-health, an emerging field, refers to delivery of information and health services via the Internet or related technologies (Dang et al, 2010). Increasingly, older adults are "mining" the Internet for health information and services. The Internet also offers online support groups. Its promise can be fulfilled as long as Web sites are simple, user friendly, reliable (Dang et al, 2010).

◆ Implications of the Demographic Changes for Hearing Health Care Professionals

The composition of the older adult population has been changing dramatically over the past few decades, with the aging of the baby boomers, the increase in average life expectancy, the increase in racial and ethnic minority populations, and the increase in racial and ethnic health disparities emerging in the 21st century (Centers for Disease Control and Prevention and the Merck Company Foundation, 2007). The projected demographic shifts will pose great challenges for society in general, and health care professionals in particular, in helping individuals grow old with dignity, independence, and an adequate quality of life. As we enter this new era, with older adults living longer than ever before, we must respond to the increase in the multiplicity of chronic conditions, including hearing loss with which older adults will live as they continue to work longer and live decades in retirement. According to a recent survey by the Pew Research Center, 28% of older adults volunteered that what they valued most about the chance to grow old is the opportunity to spend more time with family, with 25% of respondents indicating that, above all, they valued the time spent with their grandchildren (Pew Research Center,

2009). Respondents indicated that they have more time to spend doing volunteer work and more time traveling. On the down side, 20% of those aged 65 to 84 years responding to the survey said they felt sad or depressed. Hence, adequate hearing and communication can by association enhance the value of the experience of growing older.

Special Consideration

Audiologists must be cognizant of the demographic changes and the characteristics of this large subsample of the U.S. population that will impact on the demand for hearing health care services.

These demographic imperatives are as follows:

◆ The older population will continue to grow in the future, with the most rapid increase taking place between the years 2010 and 2030.
◆ By 2030 there will be 70 million older persons, representing 20% of the population.
◆ Minority populations are projected to represent 25% of the elderly population in 2030, with the growth rate being greatest for Hispanics.
◆ The number of older adults will exceed the number of children 0 to 17 years by the year 2030.
◆ The 85+ population is expected to triple in size between 1980 and 2030.
◆ The prevalence of hearing loss will rise dramatically with the increase in the absolute numbers and relative proportion of older adults.
◆ The elderly spend more in dollars than do the nonelderly on health care, including services and products.
◆ The proportion of life spent in retirement has increased dramatically, and is projected to increase further as we move into the 21st century.
◆ Some 5.8 million people aged 65 or older were in the labor force in 2007; projections indicate that by 2016 the number will reach 10.1 million (Statistical Abstract of the United States, 2009).
◆ The use of physician services is more widespread among older adults than younger persons.
◆ The National Healthy People Objectives for 2010 includes goals to reduce the prevalence of hearing loss and to eliminate health disparities among persons with functional hearing impairment (USDHHS, 2000).
◆ Health disparities and low health literacy are contributors to functional decline and are likely mediated in part by untreated hearing impairments.

The increase in the number and proportion of older adults who are 65+ coupled with the high prevalence of hearing loss in this age group is likely to expand the ranks of persons requiring hearing health care services. Shifting demographics will impact on the proportion of persons aged 65+ in the audiologist's caseload. At present, persons between ages 65 and 84 years constitute 26%, and persons aged 85+ years constitute 6.78% of the audiologist's caseload. In contrast, children from birth to 2 years of age constitute 11%, children from 3 to 5 years constitute 14.57%, and children and teenagers from 6 to

17 years constitute 17% of the audiologist's caseload. Many of the elderly individuals will be healthier and will be spending a good deal of time retired. Many will be better educated, and gainfully employed through their ninth decade. Their sense of hearing and the ability to communicate on all levels with all media will become even more critical. Tomorrow's old people will probably expect more in terms of service and will want control over what happens to them (Kane, 1994).

In delivering hearing health care services to older adults, the professional must be cognizant of the impact of their social, physical, and psychological characteristics on the nature of our services. Older adults will look toward hearing health care professionals to restore a lost sense that is interfering with their ability to function on a variety of levels in a very dynamic world. They will demand that the services provide tangible benefits to them and their family members, enhancing or allowing them to maintain an adequate quality of life. Living well—not merely living longer—and making productive use of the years that have been added to their lives will be the goal for healthy older adults surviving into the 21st century (Friedan, 1993). Audiologists should be the professional of choice to ensure adequate hearing health care for the aging adult.

References

Administration on Aging. (2007). *Aging into the 21st century.* http://www.aoa.gov/AoARoot/Aging_Statistics/future_growth/aging21/demography.aspx

Agrawal, Y., Carey, J. P., Della Santina, C. C., Schubert, M. C., & Minor, L. B. (2009, May). Disorders of balance and vestibular function in US adults: Data from the National Health and Nutrition Examination Survey, 2001–2004. *Archives of Internal Medicine, 169,* 938–944

Amadeo, K. (2007). *The impact of an aging labor force on the U.S. economy.* In *About.com: U.S. Economy.* http://useconomy.about.com/od/supply/p/Aging_Workers.htm

Anderson, G., & Horvath, J. (2002). *Chronic conditions: Making the case for ongoing care.* Princeton, NJ: Robert Wood Johnson Foundation's Partnership for Solutions

Bainbridge, K. E., Hoffman, H. J., & Cowie, C. C. (2008, Jul). Diabetes and hearing impairment in the United States: audiometric evidence from the National Health and Nutrition Examination Survey, 1999 to 2004. *Annals of Internal Medicine, 149,* 1–10

Baker, D. W., Wolf, M. S., Feinglass, J., Thompson, J. A., Gazmararian, J. A., & Huang, J. (2007, Jul). Health literacy and mortality among elderly persons. *Archives of Internal Medicine, 167,* 1503–1509

Bankrate. (2009). *Retirement income planning.* http://www.bankrate.com/finance/financial-literacy/retirement-income-planning.aspx

Beers, M. (2005). *The Merck Manual of Geriatrics,* 3rd ed. http://www.merck.com/mrkshared/mmg/home.jsp (online update). Rahway, NJ: Merck

Bennett, I. M., Chen, J., Soroui, J. S., & White, S. (2009, May–Jun). The contribution of health literacy to disparities in self-rated health status and preventive health behaviors in older adults. *Annals of Family Medicine, 7,* 204–211

Boyd, C. M., Darer, J., Boult, C., Fried, L. P., Boult, L., & Wu, A. W. (2005). Clinical practice guidelines and quality of care for older patients with multiple comorbid diseases: Implications for pay for performance. *Journal of the American Medical Association, 294,* 741–743

Centers for Disease Control and Prevention (CDC). (2006). *Trends in health and aging.* National Center for Health Statistics Data Warehouse. http://www.cdc.gov/nchs/agingact.htm

Centers for Disease Control and Prevention and the Merck Company Foundation. (2007). *The state of aging and health in America 2007 report* Division of Population Health, National Center for Chronic Disease Prevention and Health Promotion (www.cdc.gov/aging/data/stateofaging.htm)

Charness, N. (2006). *Telehealth/telemedicine: Value for blind and visually impaired persons?* Presentation at the Josephine L. Taylor Leadership Institute, Public Health and Aging Session, Atlanta, GA

Clark, D. O., Stump, T. E., Miller, D. K., & Long, J. S. (2007, May). Educational disparities in the prevalence and consequence of physical vulnerability. *Journal of Gerontology, 62,* S193–S197

Corazzini, K. (2003, Oct). How state-funded home care programs respond to changes in Medicare home health care: resource allocation decisions on the front line. *Health Services Research, 38,* 1263–1281

Crimmins, E. M. (2004). Trends in the health of the elderly. *Annual Review of Public Health, 25,* 79–98

Dang, S., Golden, A., Cheung, H., & Roos, B. (2010). Telemedicine applications in geriatrics. In H. Fillit, K. Rockwood, & K. Woodhouse (Eds.), *Brockelhurst's textbook of geriatric medicine and gerontology* (7th ed.). Philadelphia: Saunders Elsevier

Durso, S. C. (2006, Apr). Using clinical guidelines designed for older adults with diabetes mellitus and complex health status. *Journal of the American Medical Association, 295,* 1935–1940

Friedan, B. (1993). *The fountain of age.* New York: Simon & Schuster

Hayutin, A. (2007). *How population aging differs across countries: A briefing on global demographics.* Stanford Center on Longevity. http://longevity.stanford.edu/files/BriefingGlobalDemographics_0.pdf

Henchoz, K., Cavalli, S., & Girardin, M. (2008). Health perception and health status in advanced old age: A paradox of association. *Journal of Aging Studies, 22,* 282–290

Herd, P., Goesling, B., & House, J. S. (2007, Sep). Socioeconomic position and health: the differential effects of education versus income on the onset versus progression of health problems. *Journal of Health and Social Behavior, 48,* 223–238

Hersh, W., Hickham, D., Severance, S., Dana, T., Krages, K., & Helfand, M. (2006). Diagnosis, access and outcomes: update of a systematic review of telemedicine services. *Journal of Telemedicine and Telecare, 12,* 3–31

Institute of Medicine. (1996). *Telemedicine: A guide to assessing telecommunications in health care.* Washington, DC: National Academy Press

Institute of Medicine. (2001). *Crossing the quality chasm: A new health system for the 21st century.* Committee on Quality of HealthCare in America. Washington, DC: National Academies Press

Institute of Medicine. (2004). *Health literacy: A prescription to end confusion.* Washington, DC: National Academies Press

Institute of Medicine. (2008). *Retooling for an aging America: Building the health care workforce.* Washington, DC: National Academies Press

Kane, R. L. (1994, Apr). Looking toward the next millennium. *ASHA, 36,* 34–35

Koch, S. (2006, Aug). Home telehealth—current state and future trends. *International Journal of Medical Informatics, 75,* 565–576

Koch, S., & Hägglund, M. (2009, Jul). Health informatics and the delivery of care to older people. *Maturitas, 63,* 195–199

Lam, B. L., Lee, D. J., Gómez-Marín, O., Zheng, D. D., & Caban, A. J. (2006, Jan). Concurrent visual and hearing impairment and risk of mortality: The National Health Interview Survey. *Archives of Ophthalmology, 124,* 95–101

Lim, F., Thorpe, R., Gordon-Salant, S., & Ferrucci, L. (2011). Hearing loss prevalence and risk factors among older adults in the United States. *J Gerontol A Biol Sci Med Sci* http://biomedgerontology.oxfordjournals.org/content/early/2011/02/27/gerona.glr002.full.pdf+html

Manton, K., Gu, X., & Lamb, V. (2006). Long-term trends in life expectancy and active life expectancy in the United States. *Population and Development Review, 32,* 81–106

National Association for HomeCare and Hospice. (2008). *Basic statistics about homecare.* http://www.nahc.org/facts/08HC_Stats.pdf

National Center for Health Statistics (NCHS). (2009). *United States, 2008 with Chartbook.* Hyattsville, MD: NCHS

National Center for Health Statistics (NCHS). (2007). *With Chartbook: On trends in the health of Americans.* Library of Congress Catalog Number 76–641496. Hyattsville, MD: U.S. Government Printing Office. *Medical Care, 10,* 28

National Nursing Home Survey (NNHS). (2004). *National Center for Health Statistics.* DHHS Publication No. (PHS) 2009–1738. Hyattsville, MD: U.S. Department of Health and Human Services Centers for Disease Control and Prevention

New England Centenarian Study. (2011). *Why study centenarians? An overview.* http://www.bumc.bu.edu/centenarian/overview/

Norris, A. (2002). *Definitions of telemedicine, telehealth and telecare. Essentials of telemedicine and telecare.* New York: Wiley

Perls, T. (2010). Successful aging: the centenarians. In H. Fillit, K. Rockwood, & K. Woodhouse (Eds.), *Brockelhurst's textbook of geriatric medicine and gerontology* (7th ed.). Philadelphia: Saunders Elsevier

Pew Research Center. (2009). *Growing old in America: Expectations vs. reality.* http://pewresearch.org/pubs/1269/aging-survey-expectations-versus-reality

Pleis, J., & Lethbridge-Cejku, M. (2007). *Summary health statistics for U.S. adults: National health interview survey, 2006.* Hyattsville, MD: National Center for Health Statistics

Pompei, P., & Murphy, J. B. (2006). *Geriatrics review syllabus: A core curriculum in geriatric medicine* (6th ed.). New York: American Geriatrics Society

Rosenbloom, S. (2007). The day the music died. *New York Times*, July 12

Samos, L., Aguilar, E., & Ouslander, J. (2010). Institutional long term care in the United States. In H. Fillit, K. Rockwood, & K. Woodhouse (Eds.), *Brockelhurst's textbook of geriatric medicine and gerontology* (7th ed.). Philadelphia: Saunders Elsevier

Scharpf, T. P., Colabianchi, N., Madigan, E. A., Neuhauser, D., Peng, T., Feldman, P. H., et al. (2006). Functional status decline as a measure of adverse events in home health care: an observational study. *BMC Health Services Research, 6*, 162

Schoenborn, C., & Heyman, K. (2008). *Health disparities among adults with hearing loss: United States, 2000–2006.* National Center for Health Statistics (NCHS) Health E Stats

Statistical Abstract of the United States. (2009). Table 568. http://www.census.gov/compendia/statab

United Nations Department of Economic and Social Affairs Population Division. (2011). *World population prospects: The 2010 revision graphs and maps from the world population 2010 wall chart. The 2011 revision.* New York: United Nations. http://esa.un.org/unpd/wpp/Documentation/pdf/WPP2010_Wallchart_Plots.pdf

U.S. Bureau of the Census. (2004). *U.S. interim projects by age, sex, race, and Hispanic origin.* http://www.census.gov/ipc/www/usinterimproj/

U.S. Bureau of the Census. (2007). *News.* http://www.census.gov/Press-Release/www/releases/archives/population/011910.html

U.S. Bureau of the Census. (2008a, August 26). News: Household income rises, poverty rate unchanged, number of uninsured down. U.S. Department of Commerce. http://www.census.gov/Press-Release/www/releases/archives/income_wealth/012528.html

U.S. Bureau of the Census. (2008b). *Population profile of the United States.* http://www.census.gov/population/www/pop-profile/elderpop.html

U.S. Bureau of the Census Public Information Office. (2012). http://www.census.gov/newsroom/releases/archives/facts_for_features_special_editions/cb11-ff08.html

U.S. Bureau of Labor Statistics. (2008). *Spotlight on older workers.* http://www.agingworkforcenews.com/2008/07/us-bureau-of-labor-statistics-spotlight.html

U.S. Department of Health and Human Services. (2000, Nov). *Healthy people 2010* (2nd ed.). *With understanding and improving health* (2 vols.). Washington, DC: U.S. Government Printing Office

U.S. Department of Health and Human Services. (2009). *Health, United States, 2008.* Centers for Disease Control and Prevention. National Center for Health Statistics. http://www.cdc.gov/nchs/data/hus/hus08.pdf#highlights

U.S. Department of State. (2007). *Why population aging matters: A global perspective.* Department of State and the Department of Health and Human Services National Institute on Aging, National Institutes of Health

Vogeli, C., Shields, A. E., Lee, T. A., Gibson, T. B., Marder, W. D., Weiss, K. B., et al. (2007, Dec). Multiple chronic conditions: prevalence, health consequences, and implications for quality, care management, and costs. *Journal of General Internal Medicine, 22*(Suppl 3), 391–395

von Gunten, C. F. (2002, Feb). Secondary and tertiary palliative care in US hospitals. *Journal of the American Medical Association, 287*, 875–881

White, S. (2008). *Assessing the nation's health literacy: Key concepts and findings of the National Assessment of Adult Literacy (NAAL).* Chicago: American Medical Association Foundation

Wolf, M. S., Gazmararian, J. A., & Baker, D. W. (2005, Sep). Health literacy and functional health status among older adults. *Archives of Internal Medicine, 165*, 1946–1952

Wolff, J. L., Starfield, B., & Anderson, G. (2002, Nov). Prevalence, expenditures, and complications of multiple chronic conditions in the elderly. *Archives of Internal Medicine, 162*, 2269–2276

World Health Organization (WHO). (2007). *Global age-friendly cities: A guide.* Geneva: WHO

Chapter 2

The Biology of Aging

Age is a question of mind over matter. If you don't mind, it doesn't matter.

—*Satchel Paige*

◆ Learning Objectives

After reading this chapter, you should be able to

- become familiar with the theories of aging and the distinction between normal aging and disease;
- apply your knowledge of the physical changes in the organ systems to your audiology practice; and
- understand the implications of these changes for audiology interventions.

◆ What Is Aging?

The terms *aging* and *disease* are often used interchangeably when referring to the condition of being old, yet aging is *not* a disease (Miller, 2009). A determinant of disease that produces many changes, aging is associated with increased risk of physical and cognitive decline. For the purposes of this text, *aging* is a global, complex, synchronized biological process that occurs across all species at a rate that varies considerably (Galasko, 2009; Miller, 2009). Characterized by a decline in the ability to respond to stress and by an increase in homeostatic imbalance, which tends to affect numerous cells, tissues, organs, and systems, the term *aging* refers to all time-associated events that take place in the life span of an organism (Masoro, 2010; Miller, 2009). It is well established that while aging is a unitary, coordinated, and continuous process that takes place gradually over time, the rate at which aging progresses can be decelerated, thereby extending the life span (Kirkwood, 2009a; Miller, 2009). The rate at which and the degree to which aging impacts an individual depends on the interaction among intrinsic living processes (nature), such as aerobic metabolism; extrinsic factors (nurture) associated with environmental effects; and damage from age-associated diseases (Tremblay & Ross, 2007). Caloric restriction, which involves restricting food intake by close to half of what is typically eaten, is an example of an extrinsic environmental factor that increases longevity

in certain species by retarding the aging of physiological processes (Masoro, 2010).

Although most experts agree that genetic endowment is a "limiting factor" on the biological and behavioral aspects of aging (Schulz & Albert, 2009, p. 97), two forms of aging—intrinsic and extrinsic—seem to interact to help us understand the mechanisms of this universal process. Intrinsic aging refers to characteristics and processes that occur universally with aging in all members of the same gender within a given species (Peterson, 1994). Understanding intrinsic aging assists in clarifying the relation between aging and disease, and in specifying how biologists may better identify why and how the body becomes more vulnerable to disease and disability as we age (Kirkwood, 2009a). According to the literature on the biology of intrinsic aging, this process appears to be driven by a variety of random molecular events that begin early in life and tend to build up in cells and tissues. Busse (1969) used the term *primary aging* synonymously with *intrinsic aging*, which he defined as a time-related biological process not contingent on stress, trauma, or disease. In contrast, *extrinsic aging* refers to outside factors, such as lifestyle, caloric intake, or environmental factors that influence the varying degree and rate at which people age. Normal aging can be conceived of as the sum of intrinsic and extrinsic aging plus idiosyncratic or genetic variables unique to each individual (Peterson, 1994). Straus and Tinetti (2009) emphasize that cultural and societal factors influence extrinsic aging and must guide diagnostic and therapeutic decision making.

In summary, the normal biological aging process has several features that distinguish it. First, the aging process is ubiquitous, universal, and developmental, occurring to some extent in everyone after maturation (Evans, 1994; Miller, 2009). It is an individualized and variable process such that organ systems within individuals age at different rates, and thus as people get older less alike they become (Kirkwood, 2009a; Lewis, 1990; Peterson, 1994; Williams, 1994). Yet aging is characterized by a predictable, inevitable evolution and maturation until death (Williams, 1994). It is progressive, so that the probability of developing age-related conditions increases with time. Further, normal biological aging processes cause irreversible changes in cells or organs and permanently increase the probability that a given individual will suffer from harmful consequences (Peterson, 1994). Similarly, there is an increased vulnerability to disease with increasing age and a reduced ability to adapt to environmental change (Cristofalo, 1990) According to Cristofalo (1990, p. 6), "aging is a process which is quite distinct from disease; the fundamental changes of aging can be thought of as providing the substratum in which the age-associated diseases can flourish."

> **Pearl**
>
> Aging is a "process that turns young adults into old ones" (Miller, 2009, p. 4). Aging is not a disease. Age changes occur in all members of a species and takes place in virtually all species (Hayflick, 2000). Although the underlying mechanisms of aging follow a certain course, there is considerable variability in how aging affects individuals (Kirkwood, 2009a).

◆ Theories of Aging

The scientific study of aging began about 75 years ago, and since that time multiple perspectives on the aging process have emerged. The latest theories on aging have a more interdisciplinary focus, with emphasis placed on how and why specific changes take place as part of the aging process, and why there is so much variability across individuals in how they age (Bengtson, Gans, Putney, & Silverstein, 2009). In general, the theories of aging can be classified as biological, psychological, and sociological. This chapter addresses primarily the biological and the psychological; the latter relates to changes within the brain with age. Environmental factors, evolution, technological advances, and public health considerations also have an impact on the aging process and hence the theories of aging.

Biological Theories of Aging

Biological aging can very simply be defined as the gradual and progressive changes in physical function that occur in all species and that begin in adulthood and end at death (Austad, 2009). The biological mechanisms responsible for the aging process include both a stochastic process and a nonstochastic or programmed senescence process (Bengtson et al, 2009). Stochastic (chance) theories posit that aging events occur randomly as genetic mutations and accumulate with time, whereas the programmed senescence theories hold that aging is predetermined and is a function of structured genetic expression.

Evolutionary senescence theory, the immunological theory, the free radical theory, and the programmed longevity theory have garnered the most research over the years and will be discussed below. **Table 2.1** categorizes the various theories.

Evolutionary Senescence Theory

In his review of existing biological theories of aging, Austad (2009) concludes that the evolutionary senescence theory has considerable empirical evidence to support it. Evolutionary theorists argue that aging results from a decline in the force of natural selection, and that longevity will be selected if it is beneficial to one's fitness to survive (Weinert & Timiras, 2003). The evolutionary senescence theory appears to explain why animals of different species age at all; it explains the different patterns in aging rate across species, and exceptions to the various patterns. The theory posits that antagonistic pleiotropy is the form of gene action that determines the rate at which species age (i.e., genes early in life may have good effects but may have deleterious effects later in life). Further, antagonistic pleiotropy theory suggests that late-acting deleterious genes may be favored by natural selection and be actively accumulated in populations if they have any beneficial effects early in life (Gavrilov & Gavrilova, 2002). An interesting tenet of this theory is that aging evolves only in species that have an age structure (e.g., there is a distinction between reproductive and somatic cells), and in species that have evolved in low levels of environmental hazards. It is worth noting that various classes of gene action mediate the evolutionary biology theory (e.g., germ-line mutations that one is born with). Further, according to the evolutionary theory, it seems that for each species, the environment and genetics interact such that determining which genes are robust and can withstand negative forces depends in part on the challenges presented by the environment (Bengtson et al, 2009). According to evolutionary biologists, favorable gene actions may take place late in life, thereby escaping the forces of natural selection that will not be passed on to future generations (Martin, 2009). Similarly, some evolutionary biologists suggest that benign mutations with which some people are born may not manifest until late in life, thereby escaping the forces of natural selection yet having a negative impact on health and, by extension, the life span (Effros, 2009). One final tenet of the evolutionary biology theories is that the later a mutation expresses itself, the smaller the probability that it will be removed by the forces of natural selection (Gonidakis & Longo, 2009). In summary, the evolu-

Table 2.1 Biological Theories of Aging

Theory	Tenet
Immune system theory (organ system based)	As individuals age, the immune system becomes less functional, thereby leading to breakdown.
Free radical theory (stochastic or cellular based)	Age-related changes take place due to an accumulation of free radicals.
Evolutionary senescence theory	Natural selection of a gene is advantageous at one point in life but detrimental at later points in life.
Programmed longevity/aging by design theory	The length of one's life and timing of one's death are preprogrammed and influenced by gene switch.

Source: Modified from Pankow, L., & Solotoroff, J. (2007). Biological aspects and theories of aging. In J. Blackburn & C. Dulmus (Eds.), *Handbook of gerontology: Evidence-based approaches to theory, practice, and policy.* Hoboken, NJ: John Wiley.

tionary theory of aging posits that aging is a balance between wear and tear and prevention and repair, which is genetically controlled (Shringarpure & Davies, 2009).

The Immunological Theory

The immunological theory of aging posits that the adaptive immune system plays an important role in aging. To understand this theory, the reader must accept that the role of the immune system is to combat harmful agents that arise early in life and that the success of this process early on will influence one's life span (Effros, 2009). However, as will become clear from the examination of the many aging theories, what is beneficial at an early stage in life may prove to be detrimental or less beneficial as one ages. The immune system theory of aging first proposed by Walford (1969) holds that aging is due in large part to faulty immunological processes (Effros, 2009). It has its basis in biologists' understanding of the characteristics of the normal immune system. The immune system provides a crucial mechanism for the individual's interaction with the environment. Considered to have an innate component and an adaptive component, the immune system is the body's line of defense against parasites, viruses, and bacteria that may enter the body; it also produces antibodies to foreign proteins or chemicals introduced from outside the body (Effros, 2009; Hayflick, 1994). The immune system comprises several cell types, which form a network of interacting elements (Abrams, Beers, & Berkow, 1995). These interacting elements work together to generate cell-mediated immunity (T lymphocytes or T cells), humoral immunity (B lymphocytes or B cells), and nonspecific immunity (monocytes and polymorphonuclear neutrophil leukocytes) (Abrams et al, 1995). Each T and B lymphocyte cell derives from hematopoietic stem cells that have on their surface a unique set of receptors that enable it to recognize a foreign substance, referred to as an antigen (Effros, 2009). The immune system of humans has evolved to a point where it is capable of responding to an infinite variety of foreign antigens that we encounter throughout life.

The B and T cells evolved so that they perfectly complement each other in terms of their functional activities (Effros, 2009). The B cells secrete antibodies that inactivate pathogens in the bloodstream, whereas the T cells serve as effector cells, recognizing and responding to infected cells or pathogens in the bloodstream. In light of the small number of cells that can recognize and respond to a single antigen, the cytotoxic T cells that recognize a particular virus must undergo clonal expansion as a way of proliferating (cell division). Hence, clonal expansion is critical to T-cell responses. It is noteworthy that as people age, the level of telomerase, an enzyme that makes or synthesizes telomeres (e.g., small units of DNA that seal the tips of chromosomes, the structures at the end of chromosomes) decreases, and in turn this is associated with the shortening of the telomeres (ends of the chromosomes). Interestingly, telomeres can be considered a kind of a clock that keeps track of the number of divisions a cell has undergone such that when a critical length is reached, the cell enters a stage of "irreversible growth arrest" (Effros, 2009, p. 166). It seems that T cells undergo dramatic changes with age (e.g., shortened telomere length), often referred to as replicative senescence of T cells, which explains in part why the immune system tends

to work less effectively with age. In short, with age, the body becomes less able to resist the effects of the infinite number of foreign antigens invading it. Finally, the concept of antagonistic pleiotropy is integral to the immunological theory. In short, the human body develops many systemic responses to protect itself from foreign antigens, yet this fine-tuned system breaks down in aging, thereby interfering with the ability to resist or fight off these foreign bodies (Bengtson et al, 2009). Hence, this "dysregulated immune system" may account for the development of cardiovascular disease, Alzheimer's disease, and other diseases that have an increased incidence with aging.

In summary, T-cell functional capacity or the ability of the immune system to produce the appropriate antibodies in adequate numbers declines with age, and this decline in functional capacity contributes to a deficiency in cell-mediated immunity as these cells are integral to the body's ability to fight disease (Hayflick, 1994). The immune system influences critical defense reactions against foreign pathogens and is implicated in disease progression (e.g., age-associated loss in bone mass is due in part to immunological factors) (Adler & Nagel, 1994; Effros, 2009). Three examples of the interplay among aging, immunology, and disease are the development of Alzheimer's disease, diabetes, and cardiovascular disease. It is of interest that changes in T-cell telomere length correlates with the severity of Alzheimer's disease as determined by scores on the Mini-Mental Status Exam (Effros, 2009). Further, people with shorter telomeres in their blood cells have an increased rate of diabetes, cardiovascular disease, and Alzheimer's disease, and individuals with longer telomeres have an increased life expectancy beyond 60 years of age (DePinho, 2010).

Pearl

It has been speculated, and shown in mice that reactivating telomerase can halt or reverse the shortening of telomeres, thereby essentially turning back the clock on aging (DePinho, 2010). This is referred to as the telomere rejuvenation strategy. There is a positive correlation between telomere length and healthy aging (Warner, Sierra, & Thompson, 2010).

The Free Radical Theory

First proposed in 1957, the free radical theory of aging remains one of the oldest and most popular mechanistic theories of aging, which posits that wear and tear are the root causes of aging (Bengtson et al, 2009; Warner et al, 2010). A free radical is any molecule with an unpaired electron in its outer ring, and it seems that oxygen-based molecules are predominant in the free radical species (Mattson, 2009). Free radicals are produced during aerobic respiration. Harman (2006) suggests that certain types of mitochondria that generate a disproportionately large amount of reactive oxygen species (ROS) in cells and are induced by oxidative stress play an important role in aging as well. There is evidence to suggest that aging is associated with an increase in the production and accumulation of oxyradicals in all bodily tissues (Mattson, 2009). The free radical theory of aging posits that aging is due to the deleterious effects of oxidative damage, and that free radical reactivity inherent in biology results in cumulative damage and senescence (Warner et al, 2010; Weinert & Timiras, 2003). Regarding the term *oxidative*, it is important to keep in mind that the processes essential to life, including respiration and metabolism, are oxidative, so it is noteworthy that according to this theory the accumulation of "oxidative stress leads to disease" (Bengtson et al, 2009). Having originated in radiation biology, the seed for the free radical theory was first planted by Gerschman, Gilbert, Nye, Dwyer, and Fenn (1954); Denham Harman is a chief proponent of this theory of aging (Hayflick, 1994). Harman (2006) speculates that one's life span is determined, in large part, by the rate of oxidative damage to mitochondrial DNA.

There has been a flurry of research over the past two decades documenting the impact of oxidants on reactive oxygen species in aging (Beckman & Ames, 1998). Free radicals, which are unstable molecular fragments formed by complex chemical reactions, are produced during aerobic respiration and other physiological processes including mitochondrial electron transport (Cristofalo, 1990; Hayflick, 1994; Martin, 1992). Free radicals are highly reactive elements that lead to cumulative oxidative damage, ultimately resulting in aging and death in humans (Shringarpure & Davies, 2009). As free radicals contain an unpaired electron or are missing an electron from the outer shell, they are capable of and eager to react or pair with available molecules from any part of the cell, including in the DNA, protein, and lipids (Martin, 1992). Free radical damage to lipids has been noted in the aging heart, liver, and kidney. Free radicals can quickly be destroyed by protective enzyme systems, yet according to the free radical theory, some escape destruction and cause damage in important biological structures (Cristofalo, 1990). Upon uniting with neighboring molecules, free radicals can cause considerable destruction because the molecules to which they attach are prevented from performing their designated function in the cell (Martin, 1992). This accumulation of damage, which ultimately interferes with function, can cause death.

> **Pearl**
>
> Mitochondria are the main sites for the generation of reactive oxygen species, and the rate of mitochondrial damage may determine one's life span. It is widely accepted that mitochondrial DNA damage tends to increase with age (Shringarpure & Davies, 2009).

Examples of the damage created by free radicals include the accumulation of lipofuscin, an "age pigment" that accumulates in aging cells, such as those in the inner ear, and the formation of the neuritic plaques characteristic of dementia of the Alzheimer's type (Hayflick, 1994). Skeletal muscle is vulnerable to oxidative stress, and it has been hypothesized that deterioration of muscle function is associated with oxidative damage of muscle proteins (Warner et al, 2010). Evidence in support of the free radical theory of aging is the observation that chemicals, known as antioxidants, can inhibit the formation of free radicals by preventing unpaired oxygen electrons from attaching to susceptible molecules (Hayflick, 1994). Most organisms

are equipped with lines of defense against oxidative stress, thereby minimizing the release or formation of free radicals. Several small molecules produced by the human body acts as antioxidants or "scavengers of free radicals," including vitamin E, ascorbic acid (i.e., vitamin C), and glutathione (GSH) (Shringarpure & Davies, 2009); the latter can also be raised by taking vitamins orally. It is important to note that while most organisms are equipped with antioxidant defenses, damage to cellular macromolecules cannot be avoided, increasing with age.

Although the free radical theory enjoys considerable popularity as a theory of cellular aging, a causal relationship between oxidative stress and aging has not been proven categorically as a major theory of human aging and longevity (Bengtson et al, 2009; Hayflick, 1994). It is safe to say, however, that oxidative damage is related to aging and age-related disease.

> **Pearl**
>
> The aging process is associated with a gradual accumulation of damage to cells and tissues that begins early and is due to multiple processes, including genetic and nongenetic factors (Kirkwood, 2009a).

Programmed Longevity

Programmed longevity is considered by some authorities to be an evolutionary theory. I consider it to be a hybrid theory providing a link between the evolutionary and mechanistic theories of aging. It holds that the healthy portion of an individual's life is programmed to optimize fitness (Gonidakis & Longo, 2009). Further, proponents agree that aging produces tangible effects on an individual or members of a given species without producing an ailment per se. Stated differently, as organisms age, systems break down; there are age-associated markers for cell damage and death, and the organisms become less likely to survive. These theorists hold that aging is intrinsically programmed, and the genome in large part determines life expectancy (Shringarpure & Davies, 2009). For example, with time age changes take place in the DNA, and the DNA has reduced repair capabilities. Further, proponents of the concept that aging is genetically programmed suggest that the expression of genes is specifically programmed to either extend life or to trigger senescence. Although it is enticing to think that DNA is encoded for a lifetime, this type of thinking conflicts with evolutionary theorists (Pankow & Solotoroff, 2007). Kirkwood (2005) is not of the opinion that there are specific genes for aging, and he argues that this theory is flawed. He does acknowledge that underlying the aging process is a lifelong, bottom-up accumulation of molecular damage and cellular defects that are both intrinsic and occur at random, and that genetic mechanisms contribute to maintenance and repair of the organism throughout life. According to Kirkwood (2009b), support for the theory that there are genes that actively underlie aging and are specifically programmed to "end life" is weak.

Discussion of the Various Biological Theories of Aging

Biological aging, which is associated with major losses, is a progressive process, associated with gradual impairment of function and susceptibility to environmental stressors, which ultimately is associated with disease and death (Kirkwood, 2005). My review of the major biological theories of aging, including the rate of living (wear and tear), programmed aging, and evolutionary senescence, suggests that empirical evidence may not support any of the theories as acting independently to explain the phenomenon of aging, nor does it support the idea that any of the theories exist in a vacuum (Austad, 2009). The evidence is compelling that genes that have deleterious effects later in life accumulate because of evolutionary processes whereby they escaped natural selection (Austad, 2009; Bengtson et al, 2009). However, it also seems clear that aging may in fact be "a balance between wear and tear and genetically controlled mechanisms of prevention and repair" (Shringarpure & Davies, 2009, p. 229). The sentiment of Harman (2006) that aging is the accumulation of changes that one can attribute to development, genetic defects, the environment, disease, and an inborn aging process is probably the most sound.

Based on my review of aging theories, it appears safe to conclude the following: (1) Aging is a series of biological changes associated with the passage of time, which occurs in biological as well as nonbiological systems. (2) There is no single theory that explains why or how we age. (3) Aging is unavoidable, universal, and has many causes. (4) Aging is an extremely variable phenomenon across biological, cognitive, personality, and social characteristics. (5) There is no specific gene for aging, and in fact it seems clear that multiple genes contribute to the aging phenotype. (6) Natural selection and environment play an important role in aging. (7) The aging process is progressive and deleterious (Blass, Cherniack, & Weiss, 1992; Kirkwood, 2009a).

Kirkwood (2009a,b) proposed a model for the mechanism of aging that I support. Kirkwood (2009b) suggests that aging is driven by a lifelong accumulation of random molecular damage that increases the number of cells that carry defects. This accumulation of cellular defects leads to age-associated frailty, disability, and disease, which can be delayed by environmental factors such as good diet, exercise, and other lifestyle factors, but can be accelerated by stress, poor diet, and adverse environmental conditions. It seems also from evolutionary biology that genetic factors are influenced by the mechanisms (e.g., environmental accumulation) listed in **Fig. 2.1,** which attempts to capture Kirkwood's conception of the mechanisms of aging. It is important to add that chance figures into the individuality of the aging process (Kirkwood, 2009b).

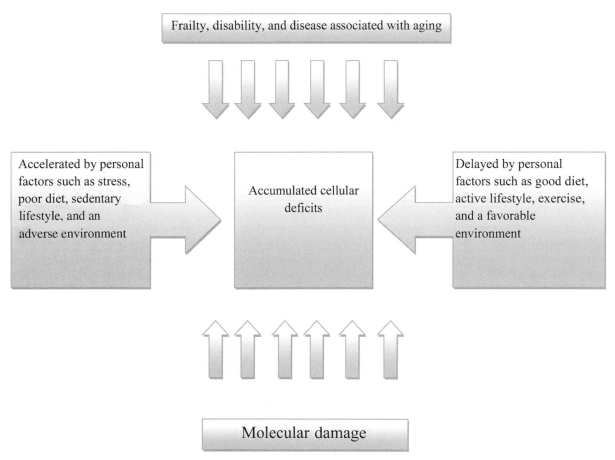

Fig. 2.1 Mechanism of aging. [Modified from Kirkwood, T. (2009b). Genetics of age-dependent human disease. In J. Halter, J. Ouslander, M. Tinetti, S. Studenski, K. High, & S. Asthana (Eds.), *Hazzard's geriatric medicine and gerontology* (6th ed.). New York: McGraw-Hill.]

Consistent with Kirkwood's perspective on aging, the convoy model of social relations provides a life span perspective on how personal, situational, and environmental factors may shape and impact the health and well-being of individuals (Antonucci, Birditt, & Akiyama, 2009). The word *convoy* refers here to the close social relationships that surround individuals, providing them with the base for personal development and exploration. According to this model, social networks and social relations are central to development, with the quality and quantity of social relations influenced by personal and situational variables. Interestingly, a personal assessment of one's satisfaction or dissatisfaction with one's social networks contributes to the understanding of how social relations impact psychological and physiological health and well-being. Hence, negative social interactions, which may ensue from impaired hearing, according to the convoy model, may have negative outcomes for the individual. Similarly, stress mediates the impact of personal and social factors on relationships and ultimate well-being. Hence, for example, social relations can buffer the effect of stress on well-being. In my view, untreated hearing impairment and associated deficits in speech under-

standing could be stressors that interfere with interpersonal relations, resulting in negative outcomes for the individual. Interestingly, as shown in **Fig. 2.2**, self-efficacy, or the belief that one can master a situation, appears to mediate the support–health relationship (Antonucci et al, 2009). Specifically, **Fig. 2.2** illustrates how personal characteristics, situational characteristics, and self-efficacy interact to impact mental and physical well-being.

◆ Structural and Functional Changes Associated with Aging

Several changes in organ systems occur gradually as people age. Many of the changes can be explained on the basis of the theories of aging previously discussed. Although several thousands of age changes have been identified, this discussion focuses on morphological changes in the organ systems and on those functional implications that may have a potential impact on hearing status and on the delivery of comprehensive audiology services to older adults.

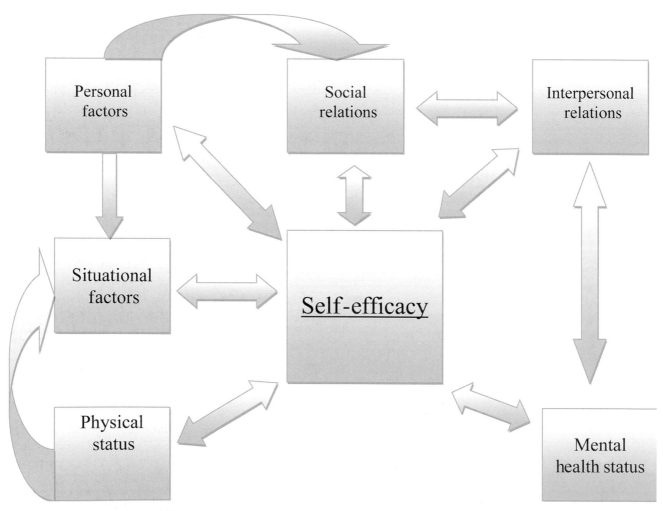

Fig. 2.2 Interplay among personal factors influencing biological aging. [Modified from Antonucci, T., Birditt, K., & Akiyama, H. (2009). In V. Bengtson, M. Silverstein, N. Putney., & D. Gans (Eds.), *Handbook of theories of aging* (2nd ed.). New York: Springer.]

Body Configuration and Composition

As humans age, there are several changes taking place that contribute to overall declines in body systems. Most notable is the loss of body water or decline in the proportion of body weight attributable to water. Water makes up two thirds of the body weight, and is found in extracellular and intracellular compartments and in the form of plasma, lymph fluid, and spinal fluid. Accordingly, changes in water metabolism contribute to several changes within organ systems (Morley, 1990). Further, as will become evident, aging is associated with reductions in lean body mass, in protein synthesis and protein degradation rates, and in the amount of potassium in the human body (Morley, 1990). On average, by age 75, the number of cells in the human body may have declined by as much as 30%, exacting a toll on major systems. Bone mineral density (BMD), which accounts for close to 70% of bone strength, declines as we advance from middle age to old age (Masoro, 2010). These changes in body composition, structure, and function contribute to many of the changes within the human body that are described below.

Changes in Appearance and in Body Temperature

Overall, there is a gradual decrease in height in both genders as we age, along with a decrease in weight after age 55. Reductions in height are attributable to changes in the skeleton, including calcification of tendons and ligaments; thinning of vertebral disks associated with osteoporosis; and weakening and shrinkage of muscle groups (Tideiksaar & Silverton, 1989). Characteristically, as people age they assume a more stooped posture with the head and neck bent slightly forward and the hips and knees flexed. It is likely that normal aging changes in height contribute to instability and an increased prevalence of falls among older adults.

Declines in weight are due to a decline in lean tissue mass, a decrease in total body water, a decline in muscle mass, and bone loss (Kane, Ouslander, & Abrass, 1994). Whereas slight weight loss is common with increasing age, significant weight loss may be symptomatic of an active disease process. For example, it is well recognized that weight loss is common in individuals who are undernourished or malnourished, have Alzheimer's disease, suffer from depression, undergo drug-nutrient interactions, or have cancer. The changes in body composition can have a significant effect on level of function.

Overall, aging is associated with a decline in bone mass, skeletal muscle mass, strength, and work capacity. Loss of skeletal muscle mass has been known to occur with advancing age in both men and women (Andreoli, Scalzo, Masala, Tarantino, & Guglielmi, 2009). Yet studies have shown that elderly men lose more skeletal leg muscle than do women, and such skeletal mass muscle loss is often masked by weight stability due to an increase in total body fat mass through middle age and a decrease after 70 years of age. Significant decreases in lean body mass are also known to occur in both men and women with increasing age. Such changes to body composition may occur as early as 40 years of age (Andreoli et al, 2009). Weight stability is also important for maintaining health with advancing age, as weight loss or gain could be indicative of illness and an increase in the inability to perform activities of daily living (ADL), and could increase mortality (Newman et al, 2001). Elderly individuals with stable weight tend to maintain an optimal health status and lower disability status as compared with those who are prone to lose or gain weight. Aging is also associated with a progressive decline in the ability to sense absolute temperature (e.g., hot and cold), and in the ability of the body to generate heat and to dissipate heat (Masoro, 2010). The deficits in regulation of body temperature render older adults very vulnerable to the effects of high and low temperatures.

The Skin

Human skin has several major roles. It serves as a protective barrier against homeostatic regulation and against mechanical, thermal, or chemical injuries and from loss of fluid; as an interface with the external environment; as a thermoregulator; and as a window through which the body reveals its internal pathology (Kaminer & Gilchrest, 1994; Veysey & Finlay, 2010). Specialized mechanoreceptors in the skin register pressure, touch, and vibration; hence, it is critical for sensory perception (Frick, Leonhardt, & Starck, 1991; Veysey & Finlay, 2010). The skin also participates in immunobiological defense reactions. In general, the skin shows dramatic changes with age. In fact, some of the changes in the skin lining the external ear canal are of particular relevance to audiologists during selected procedures (e.g., cerumen management, earmold/hearing-aid impressions, and diagnostic tests including immittance testing and otoacoustic emissions). A brief overview of skin anatomy will facilitate the discussion.

The skin is composed of several interrelated functional layers that tend to undergo changes with age. The layers include the epidermis, the dermis, the subcutaneous fat, and the cutaneous appendages (Balin, 1990). The layers are shown in **Fig. 2.3**. The epidermis is the outer or most superficial layer of the skin. The epidermis serves as the cutaneous surface of the skin. It comprises several layers, and it functions primarily to protect the deeper tissues from drying, invasion by organisms, and trauma. The epidermis is composed primarily of keratinocytes, with smaller populations of Langerhans' cells and melanocytes (Veysey & Finlay, 2010). Keratinocytes are constantly being reproduced after being pushed to the surface, replacing other keratinocyte cells that have died and are subsequently shed (Kaminer & Gilchrest, 1994). It takes about 28 days for the turnover of keratinocyte cells to take place; however, the

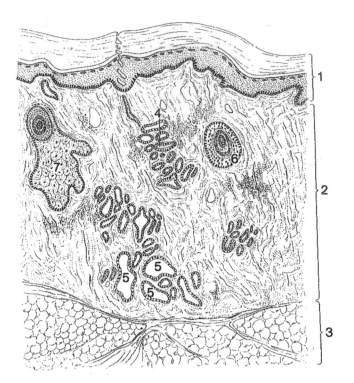

Fig. 2.3 Functional layers of the skin: 1, epidermis; 2, dermis; 3, subcutaneous connective tissue; 4, sweat gland; 5, apocrine sweat gland; 6, hair root sheath; 7, sebaceous gland with hair root sheath. [Data from Frick, H., Leonhardt, H., & Starck, D. (1991). *Human anatomy 1. General anatomy, special anatomy: limbs, trunk wall, head and neck* (1st ed.). New York: Thieme Medical Publishers. Reprinted by permission.]

turnover time of these epidermal cells is reduced dramatically as people age (Kaminer & Gilchrest, 1994). As a result of the decrease in epidermal cell turnover with age, there is a decrease in the rate at which wounds heal (Veysey & Finlay, 2010). In addition to keratinocytes, the epidermis contains melanocytes and Langerhans' cells. The melanocytes contain melanin, which is responsible for defining skin color and serves as the body's protection against solar radiation (Kaminer & Gilchrest, 1994). There is a steady decrease in melanocytes with each decade, which occurs in both sun-protected and sun-exposed skin. The loss of melanin in the skin that occurs with age means that as people age they have less protection against the negative effects of ultraviolet (UV) radiation. Graying of hair, for example, is a manifestation of loss of function of the melanocytes (Balin, 1990). The Langerhans' cells, which derive from the bone marrow, are important for antigen recognition. With age, there is a dramatic decrease in the number of Langerhans' cells. This decrease is greatest in photo-aged skin.

The dermis or inner layer of skin lies beneath the epidermis. It consists predominantly of connective tissue and contains blood vessels, lymphatics, sweat glands, and sebaceous glands. It serves to provide a tough layer that supports the epidermis and binds to the subcutaneous layer (Veysey & Finlay, 2010). The dermis also contains specialized cellular components that are produced by fibroblasts and include collagen (a protein) and elastin. Collagen gives skin its strength and support, whereas

elastin provides it with its elasticity and resilience (Veysey & Finlay, 2010). With few exceptions, throughout the body the dermis contains hair follicles and the major sensory fibers that help humans distinguish among pain, touch, heat, and cold. Sebaceous glands, such as those located in the outer third of the ear canal, have primary responsibility for protecting the skin against dryness through the production of an oily substance known as sebum. In contrast, sweat glands produce perspiration, allowing for the elimination of water and electrolytes (Falvo, 1991). The dermis has an extensive microvasculature network that contributes to thermoregulation and the inflammatory response of the skin (Kaminer & Gilchrest, 1994).

During aging, the epidermis becomes structurally thinner; there is a flattening of the dermo-epidermal junction, and the corneocytes adhere less to one another, causing a reduction in their water-binding capacity, which leads to skin dryness. With age there is a depletion of certain types of melanocytes; hair graying is also a consequence of aging of the epidermal layer of the skin. Similarly, decreased blood flow slows healing and provides pathogens the opportunity to enter broken skin. Overall, the skin becomes dry and itchy, and its integrity decreases over time (Scheinfeld, 2005).

The dermis undergoes significant anatomical and physiological change with age as well. Many of these changes may impact considerably on audiological practice. Overall, there is an approximate 20% loss in dermal thickness with age that can account for the paper-thin appearance of the skin of some older adults (Kaminer & Gilchrest, 1994). There are changes in the collagen and elastin fibers, which degenerate, resulting in less bulk and structure to the dermis (Giangreco, Qin, Pintar, & Watt, 2008). Further, the number of mast cells, which serve a protective function, and fibroblasts, which help to heal wounds, decreases, resulting in a diminished ability for healing (Lawton, 2007). The most pertinent anatomical and physiological changes are displayed in **Table 2.2**. There is a reduced vascular response of old skin to chemical irritants and microbial invasion. Apocrine gland activity is diminished, and the sebaceous glands in the dermis become larger, hyperplastic, and less active (Veysey & Finlay, 2010). Changes in the dermis with age account in large part for the tendency for people to be prone to wrinkle formation as they age. In sun-exposed sites there tends to be more abnormalities in the collagen and elastin fibers in the dermis. With age (>70 years), most elastin fibers in the dermis appear abnormal, and thus the skin loses the elasticity and resilience provided by these fibers (Veysey & Finlay, 2010). The latter age-related changes have implications for hearing-aid fittings and for pure-tone hearing sensitivity. With age the density of Langerhans' cells in the skin decreases, and there is a decline in their number. In light of their role in immune function, age-related changes in the Langerhans' cells are associated with delayed hypersensitivity reactions. Further, older adults have a diminished capacity to manifest characteristic reactions when exposed to known allergens, and they are more susceptible to skin infections. Finally, age-related changes in the skin and its vasculature contribute to a decrease in sensory perception and an increase in the pain threshold, which places older adults at risk for burns and infections. Further, the diminished tensile strength of the dermis, which is produced by the decrease in collagen, and the reduction in microvascu-

Table 2.2 Age-Related Anatomic and Physiological Change Within the Dermis

Decrease in number of cells
Decrease in elasticity
Decrease in thickness
Reduction in microvasculature
Decrease in number of fibroblasts and amount of collagen and elastin
Loss of efficiency of nerve cells
Decreased sensitivity to sensory perception (e.g., pain) and pressure
Increase in the size of sebaceous glands and decrease in sebum output
Skin more easily damaged
Altered thermal regulation
Decreased sweating
Decreased wound healing
Muted inflammatory reactions

Sources: From Veysey, E., & Finlay, A. (2010). Aging and the skin. In H. Fillit, K. Rockwood, & K. Woodhouse (Eds.), *Brockelhurst's textbook of geriatric medicine and gerontology* (7th ed.). Philadelphia: Saunders Elsevier; and Balin, A. (1990). Aging of human skin. In W. Hazzard, R. Andres, E. Bierman, & J. Blass (Eds.), *Principles of geriatric medicine and gerontology* (2nd ed.). New York: McGraw-Hill.

lature account in part for the diminished wound healing in older adults (Kaminer & Gilchrest, 1994). Another consequence of changes in the dermis is that the cutaneous end organs responsible for pressure, vibration, and light-touch sensation decrease to about one third of their density with advancing age, leading to an increase in pain threshold and resulting susceptibility to skin injury.

Skin aging involves increased susceptibility to injury and infection, reduced wound healing, loss of dermal elasticity or poor dermal elasticity, poor epidermal barrier maintenance, and increased cancer risk, and therefore skin complaints are a major reason for ambulatory care visits among older adults (McCullough & Kelly, 2006; Patel, Ragi, Lambert, & Schwartz, 2010; Veysey & Finlay, 2010). Skin infections in the elderly are more common than in younger individuals, as they are complicated by the multiple medications used to control diseases that accompany normal aging. Diabetes and neoplasms particularly undermine the function of the immune system, and diseases such as hyperlipidemia and hypertension decrease blood flow to the skin, decreasing the ability of the elderly body to fight off infection. The skin lining the ear canal is particularly susceptible to skin lesions, especially for hearing-aid users.

In summary, with aging the epidermis undergoes an overall thinning and a decrease in the size and proliferation rate of keratinocytes. Similarly, the thickness, density, and cellularity of the dermis decrease, leading to a thin feeling to the skin. Further, collagen fibers become thicker and correspondingly less flexible, resulting in increased susceptibility to tear. There is a loss of vascularity of the skin especially in the superficial dermis, which disturbs thermoregulation (Veysey & Finlay, 2010). Of relevance to audiologists fitting hearing aids, the function of sweat glands decreases and moisture content of the skin declines as well (Scheinfeld, 2005). Finally, the above changes in older skin often affect the skin that lines structures of the ear, making it more sensitive to trauma, disorders, and

compromised wound healing relative to younger adults. Cutaneous disorders with a predilection for the ear include pruritus, or itching; seborrheic dermatitis, a chronic superficial inflammatory disorder of the skin; seborrheic keratoses, a benign lesion of the skin; and basal or squamous cell carcinoma. Dermatological pathology warrants referral to the dermatologist.

> **Special Consideration**
>
> Audiologists who engage in cerumen management and hearing-aid dispensing must keep in mind the aforementioned dermatological concerns and should be ever vigilant about cutaneous pathology and the importance of infection control.

The Nervous System

The human body is endowed with a nervous system that is quite complex given the diversity of functions it subserves. The nervous system serves as the command center, or as a relayer of information, for a variety of body functions. It coordinates and controls behavioral activities throughout the body in response to the internal and external environment by sending, receiving, and sorting electrical impulses (Falvo, 1991). Hence, it is concerned with enteroception, the perception of processes taking place inside of the body, and with exteroception, the perception of processes taking place outside of the body (Schuenke, Schulte, & Schumacher, 2007). Morphologically, the nervous system can be divided into the central (CNS) and peripheral nervous systems (PNS). **Figure 2.4** displays the left lateral view of the CNS, consisting of the brain and spinal cord.

The nerves that extend from the brain (cranial nerves) and spinal cord (spinal nerves) comprise the peripheral nervous system (Schuenke et al, 2007). When the brain is sectioned, macroscopically it is clear that the CNS consists of gray brown regions known as gray matter, which can be distinguished from glistening white areas known as white matter. The surface of the brain appears gray because of the presence of nerve cell bodies, whereas the surface of the spinal cord appears white because of the lipid content of a myelin sheath surrounding the axons. That is to say the white matter of the CNS contains axons of neurons that conduct nerve messages, whereas the gray matter of the brain, made up of cell bodies, is responsible for receiving, sorting, and processing nerve messages (Falvo, 1991). The meninges are connective tissue membranes that cover and protect the brain and spinal cord, which in turn are encased in bone. The meninges consist of three membranes known as the pia mater, the dura mater, and the arachnoid.

The brain consists of three main parts, namely the forebrain, midbrain, and hindbrain. The cerebrum (telencephalon), thalamus, and hypothalamus comprise the forebrain; the tectum and tegmentum constitute the midbrain (mesencephalon); and the cerebellum, pons, and medulla comprise the hindbrain. Collectively, the midbrain, pons, and medulla are referred to as the brainstem, a midline structure flanked by the cerebrum and cerebellum. **Figure 2.5** depicts a midsagittal section of the three main parts of the brain, and **Fig. 2.6** shows a midsagittal section of the brainstem, with the cerebellum apparent.

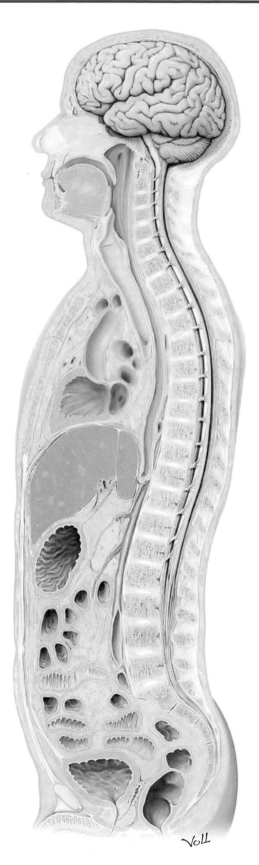

Fig. 2.4   A left lateral view of central nervous system. (From *THIEME Atlas of Anatomy, Head and Neuroanatomy,* © Thieme 2007, Illustration by Markus Voll.)

Anatomy of the Head and Neuroanatomy

The cerebrum (cortex), the largest part of the human brain, is divided into two hemispheres—right and left—and four lobes—frontal, parietal, occipital, and temporal. The corpus callosum, a bundle of axons, connects the right and left hemispheres. **Figure 2.7** shows a left lateral view of the left hemisphere and the four lobes. The cerebrum, which contains convolutions known as gyri and depressions known as sulci, is responsible for higher brain function such as thought and action. Interestingly, in conditions associated with brain atrophy, such as Alzheimer's disease, the sulci are actually enlarged (Schuenke et al, 2007).

The major functional unit of the nervous system is the neuron, or nerve cell, that transmits neural impulses. The component parts of the neuron, namely the soma or cell body, the dendrites or receptor segments, and the axons or nerve fibers, are shown in **Fig. 2.8**. Collectively, the dendrites and axons are referred to as processes. Dendritic spines are specialized membrane compartments that extend from the dendritic shaft of neurons (Dickstein et al, 2007). Unlike axons, dendrites are not insulated by a myelin sheath. The myelin serves to insulate the axons electrically, significantly boosting nerve conduction velocity (Schuenke et al, 2007). It is noteworthy that almost all axons in the CNS are myelinated, whereas the axons in the PNS are selectively myelinated according to the need for rapid information transfer along the axon (e.g., fast conduction velocity). The PNS and CNS also differ in terms of their myelinating cells, such that Schwann cells myelinate the axons in the PNS (e.g., auditory nerve). Oligodendrocytes are responsible for the formation of myelin in the brain (Wong, 2002). Neurological conditions have a differential impact on the myelin sheaths such that peripheral myelin sheaths may stay intact in conditions in which the central myelin sheath degenerates.

Each neuron has only one axon, which relays messages to other neurons or cells, whereas one neuron may have multiple dendrites, which conduct impulses to the cell body (Schuenke et al, 2007). Dendrites, which are profusely branched and variable, have primary responsibility for neuronal information processing (Dickstein et al, 2007). Dendrites account for nearly 90% of the total surface area of the receptive surface area of neurons (Wong, 2002). The brain contains approximately 100 billion neurons and trillions of neuroglial cells, which surround the neurons and provide functional and structural support. Accounting for about 2% of our body weight, the adult human brain weighs approximately 1400 g, surpassed only by the weight of the brain of the bottle-nosed dolphin (1500–1600 g)!

The nerves within the PNS that bring information toward the CNS from other parts of the body constitute the afferent division of the PNS. Those nerves that carry impulses from the CNS to other parts of the body make up the efferent division of the PNS. **Figure 2.9** shows the 12 cranial nerves, which enter and exit the brainstem, along with the organs to which they connect.

The neurons in the brain are postmitotic differentiated cells that do not duplicate or replicate themselves following cell death. The cells of the auditory sense organ and neural pathways are nonmitotics. That is, after specialized function

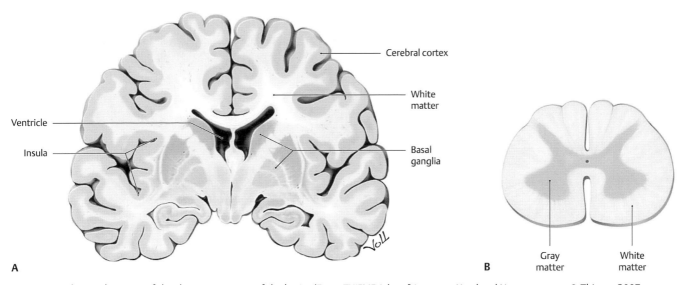

Fig. 2.5 Midsagittal section of the three main parts of the brain. (From *THIEME Atlas of Anatomy, Head and Neuroanatomy*, © Thieme 2007, Illustration by Markus Voll.)

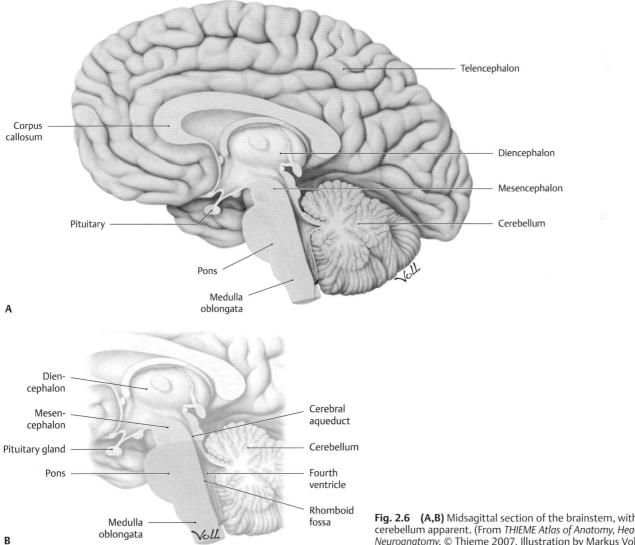

Fig. 2.6 (A,B) Midsagittal section of the brainstem, with the cerebellum apparent. (From *THIEME Atlas of Anatomy, Head and Neuroanatomy*, © Thieme 2007, Illustration by Markus Voll.)

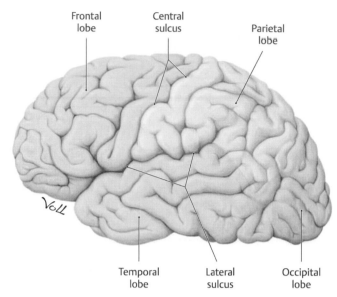

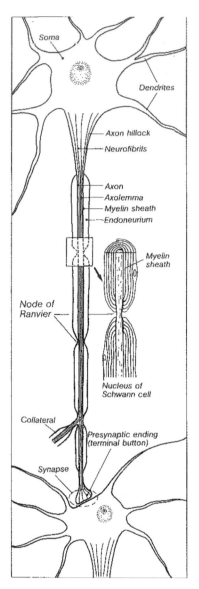

Fig. 2.7 A left lateral view of the left hemisphere and the four lobes. (From *THIEME Atlas of Anatomy, Head and Neuroanatomy,* © Thieme 2007, Illustration by Markus Voll.)

has been established, they too pursue the course of aging and dying.

Special Consideration

The brain is plastic, so it can adapt and strengthen connections or form new connections between neurons and circuits (Galasko, 2009). In short, remaining neurons tend to sprout new connections and "repair or compensate for the short or broken circuits that occur when a neighboring neuron dies" (Hayflick, 1994, p. 163).

Neurotransmitters, or chemicals released by the axons, enable nerve impulses to be transmitted between neurons. Examples of neurotransmitters within the brain include dopamine, norepinephrine, epinephrine, serotonin, and acetylcholine. Serotonin and norepinephrine are considered monamine neurotransmitters in the brain. Acetylcholine is a neurotransmitter in selected populations of neurons in the brain, most notably in the hippocampus, the region that is central to learning and memory. Enzymes such as acetyltransferase or acetylcholinesterase work with the neurotransmitters to enable neurons to communicate with each other. Calcium regulates neurotransmitter release from presynaptic terminals and postsynaptic changes, which, in adults, are associated with learning and memory (Mattson, 2009). Dopaminergic receptors are present in the frontal regions of the brain and have a critical role to play in cognitive function, especially working memory. Cells in the nervous system produce a variety of proteins that serve to both protect the neurons against injury and death and promote neuronal survival and growth (Mattson, 2009).

Fig. 2.8 Component parts of the neuron. [From Despopoulos, A., & Silbernagl, S. (1991). *Color atlas of physiology* (4th ed.). New York: Thieme Medical Publishers. Reprinted by permission.]

Pearl

Lipofuscin, which consists of protein and lipids, is the most common age-related marker seen in tissues throughout the body, evident in considerable amounts in the inferior olive, the dentate nucleus of the cerebellum, and large areas in the cerebral cortex.

Age-related declines in brain structure and neurobiology are well documented in the literature. It is well established that the human brain loses significant volume over time, which is associated with shrinkage as we age. The human brain undergoes a progressive decrement in weight such that by age 85 it reaches its lowest weight, having decreased by 11% as

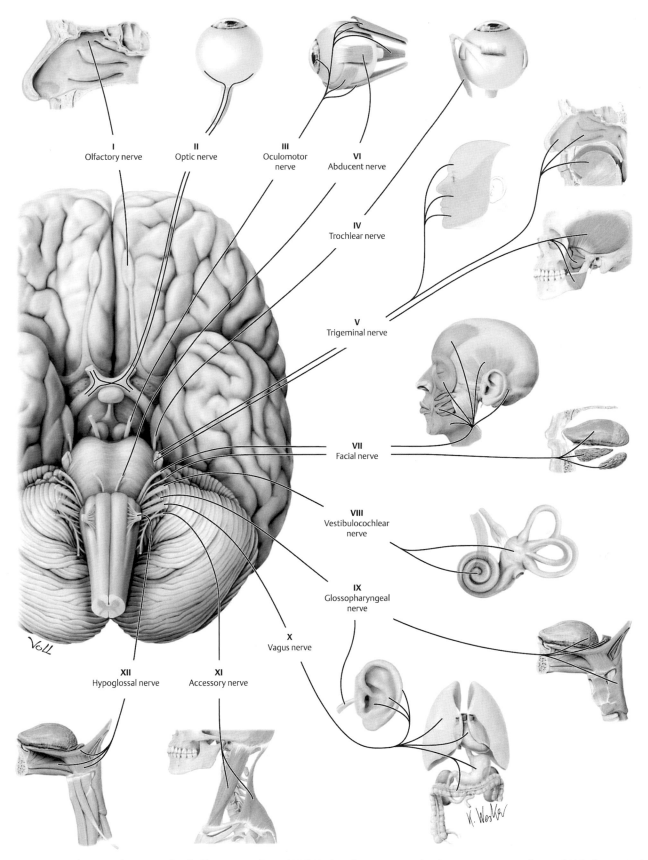

Fig. 2.9 Twelve cranial nerves at level of brainstem. (From *THIEME Atlas of Anatomy, Head and Neuroanatomy,* © Thieme 2007, Illustration by Markus Voll and Karl Wesker.)

compared with maximum (Galasko, 2009). Interestingly, it can shrink up to 15%, but such extreme shrinkage is associated with pathology such as dementia and poor memory. In light of the weight loss, the brain also undergoes a change in shape, especially on its surface, with a narrowing of the gyri/convolutions and a widening of the sulci/grooves between the gyri. All of the major cell types in the brain undergo structural changes with age. Some of the cell changes include nerve cell death, shrinkage of brain tissue, neuronal cell loss in selective brain regions, loss of myelinated fibers, synapse loss, dendritic expansion and retraction, reductions in brain volume, and reductions in cortical thickness and in white matter integrity (Galasko, 2009; Goh & Park, 2009; Mattson, 2009).

Normal aging is also associated with shrinkage in soma size, loss or regression of dendrites and dendritic spines, alterations in neurotransmitter receptors, and decline in the white matter fibers that connect gray-matter regions (Goh & Park, 2009). Further, older adults typically have fewer motor neurons, less branching per neuron, a reduction in the number of myelinated nerve fibers, and diminished nerve fiber diameters and impairment of neurotransmitters (Carmeli, Patish, & Coleman, 2003).

Pearl

Normal age-related changes are due to progressive and irreversible changes associated with aging of tissue and the inability of the nervous system to repair and regenerate (Galvin, 2009). However, exercise and mental training is associated with increases in brain volume and functional responses in selected regions including the frontal cortex (Dickstein et al, 2007; Goh & Park, 2009).

The frontal and temporal lobes undergo age-related changes that directly affect speech recognition ability and cognitive function. Similarly, age-related atrophy in cortical volume takes place in the prefrontal regions, with less atrophy in the parietal and temporal regions. These changes may in part explain the age-related decline in executive control, fluid intelligence, and some memory processes (Willis, Schaie, & Martin, 2009). Age-related shrinkage is site specific, such that the extrapyramidal and orbital cortex show substantial shrinkage, whereas no shrinkage is exhibited in the parietal and occipital cortex (Wong, 2002). The decrease in weight is associated in part with loss of white matter, neuron atrophy, and the loss of chemical constituents of the brain, including selected proteins and lipids, which occurs with aging (Poirier & Finch, 1994). During aging there is reportedly a change in the neurotransmitter system, including a decrease in the amount of chemical associated with neurotransmitter activity and corresponding loss in the synthetic ability of certain catecholaminergic and serotoninergic neurons. According to Mattson (2009), norepinephrine levels appear to increase in selected brain regions with age, yet levels of serotonin tend to decrease in the hippocampal region and the cerebral cortex. Researchers have speculated that neuronal alterations (e.g., dendritic changes with age) impact parameters of the cholinergic, serotonergic, and dopaminergic systems, and also impact the distribution of neurofilament proteins (Dickstein et al, 2007). In turn, changes

in these systems leave the neurons vulnerable to impaired transmission. Interestingly, age-related increases in neurofilament proteins render neurons more prone to neurofibrillary tangles (NFTs), leading eventually to neurodegenerative diseases and dementia (Dickstein et al, 2007). Age-related loss of synapses and modifications of synaptic structure have been reported based on studies using electron microscopy (Wong, 2002). Neurochemical changes associated with aging account in part for the slowing of cognitive processing with increasing age. Further, age-related decrease in levels of serotonin has been implicated as contributing to the increased prevalence of affective disorders (e.g., depression) in older adults (Mattson, 2009).

Pearl

The histological changes that are universal in the aging brain include accumulation of lipofuscin and the appearance of neurofibrillary tangles in mesial temporal structures (Mrak, Griffin, & Graham, 1997).

The number of nerve cells decreases and neurons become smaller with normal aging as well. Age-related changes in the dendrites include shortening, a reduction in the number of dendritic branches, and loss of dendritic spines (Wong, 2002). Neuronal loss within the brain is quite variable between regions of the brain and among individuals. Nerve cell loss is minimal in the brainstem nuclei, yet neuron death is considerable in the cerebral cortex. In general, neuronal loss ranges from 10 to 60%. With respect to the auditory system, it has been reported that the superior temporal gyrus may lose as much as 55% of its neuronal content, whereas the tip of the temporal lobe may show only a 10 to 35% loss (Poirier & Finch, 1994). Neurons that remain tend to accumulate lipofuscin, or aging pigment, which is most pronounced in the cell body. In certain individuals the accumulation of lipofuscin and the aggregation of microtubule-associated protein tau contribute to the development of NFTs upon which metals such as aluminum may deposit (Galasko, 2009). There is evidence to suggest that after age 50, NFTs occasionally appear in the medial temporal gyrus (Dickstein et al, 2007). In the extreme case, the appearance of NFTs in areas in the temporal neocortex is associated with senile dementia of the Alzheimer's type. Although plaques and tangles are a hallmark of Alzheimer's disease, they also appear, albeit in lesser numbers, in the brains of older persons without clinical evidence of the disease (Abrams et al, 1995). Amyloid B peptide accumulates as a part of the normal aging process and forms plaque in the parenchyma and vasculature of the brain (Galasko, 2009). The plaque tends to accumulate most heavily in the hippocampus, a region of the brain important for memory and learning. Aging is also associated with an increase in production and accumulation of oxygen-based molecules (a dominant free radical species) in tissues of the brain (Mattson, 2009). Whereas Alzheimer's disease selectively damages specific brain regions and is associated with amyloid-β plaques, NFTs, and significant neuron and synapse loss, neuronal death and accumulation of NFTs is minimal in normal aging (Dickstein et al, 2007).

Aging is accompanied by a decrease in neuronal inhibition and an increase in the threshold for induction of the action potential in cranial nerves. Further, the amount of sheath surrounding the axons of peripheral nerves decreases with age, perhaps contributing to a reduction in neural conduction time. Populations of dopaminergic neurons also show changes with age. These changes in the nerve fibers explain in part the decrease in the speed with which action potentials travel with age in both the afferent and the efferent systems. Aging is also associated with deficits in choline transport, acetylcholine synthesis, and acetylcholine release (Mattson, 2009). In addition, dopamine levels and dopamine transport levels decrease with age, and these changes have been implicated as contributing to age-related deficits in motor control. In general, aging is accompanied by a microscopic loss in the number and integrity of peripheral receptors, most notably in the lower extremities, and a lower concentration of touch corpuscles in the skin. Further, as was noted earlier, nerve conduction velocity slows with age, and the latency period for sensory and motor nerves increases. As a result of these alterations, aging is associated with a decrease in response to tactile stimuli; an increase in the threshold for vibration sense; and a decline in sensitivity to light touch, to deep pain perception, to position sense, and to pinprick sensation. These changes can impact on hearing-aid fittings with older adults. Decline in evoked cortical activity with age has been documented in older adults as well and is associated with decline in working memory (Wong, 2002). Declines in working memory are most apparent when older adults are exposed to information that is presented at a rapid rate or in the presence of competing stimuli, challenging the ability to store and process information. Age-related hippocampal atrophy is associated with a reduction in recollection but not familiarity. It is also possible that frontal lobe changes could influence recollection across the life span (Yonelinas et al, 2007). Finally, vessels that supply blood to the brain are vulnerable to age-related changes that render them susceptible to rupture or stroke (Mattson, 2009). Similarly, there tends to be age-related reduction in brain perfusion, decrease in cerebral blood flow, and decline in cerebral metabolic rate for oxygen and glucose use. Although age-related reduction in glucose use is not dramatic, changes in the cerebral blood vessels may result in a reduction in the amount of energy available to neurons.

The behavioral implications of the changes in the nervous system include a slowing of central processing, which may manifest as slowed psychomotor responses, decreased motor reaction time, increased motor response time, and decreased performance on selected intellectual tasks, including a slowing in the ability to learn new information, and noncritical forgetfulness (Tarawneh & Galvin, 2010). Intellectual performance peaks during the 30s, plateaus throughout the 50s and 60s, and variably declines during the late 70s (Beers, 2005). It is important to note that as the brain has a surplus of brain cells, it is not the number of cells lost that accounts for behavioral changes, but rather the location of the brain cell loss and the ability of cells in that region to make new connections with remaining neurons. Further, certain properties of the brain including its redundancy, the availability of compensatory mechanisms, and plasticity at the level of the nerve cell may mitigate some of the adverse effects of age-related changes in the brain (Abrams et al, 1995). For example, studies have shown that the gradual deterioration and dying off of nerve cells may be accompanied by compensatory lengthening and an increasing number of dendrites in the remaining nerve cells. Thus, possible new connections within the dendritic tree may make up for fewer cells. In light of neuroplasticity, the brain continues to change and adapt to aging and to increase the breadth and of its function (Goh & Park, 2009). The fact that the mature brain does retain the capacity for neural plasticity or to adapt to new sensations (e.g., auditory) after varying periods of deprivation has implications for audiologists (Polley et al, 2008).

Cognitive Aging Theories Associated with Age-Related Changes in the Brain

Prior to discussing the connection between age-related changes in the brain and cognitive aging theories, a few terms need to be defined. These terms include cognitive processes, cognitive resources, working memory, executive function, and inhibitory function, among others. The term *cognitive processes* refers to how people acquire, store, manipulate, and use information, and *cognitive processing speed* refers to the speed with which new information can be acquired and manipulated (Wingfield, Tun, McCoy, Steward, & Cox, 2006). The term *cognitive resources* is often used in the context of memory and loosely refers to the degree of deliberate processing required to perform a task. The cognitive resources one has depends in part on perceptual speed, attentional capacity, working memory, and inhibitory function. *Working memory* is the ability to hold and to manipulate information in immediate memory. Critical for carrying out complex tasks such as learning and comprehension, working memory is typically assessed using tests that quantify word or digit span. Working memory is often taxed during recognition tasks that require recall of sentences. The term *inhibitory function* refers to one's ability to focus on information relevant to the task and to suppress irrelevant information that may be activated during a particular task. Older adults are at the greatest disadvantage, inhibiting irrelevant information when performing memory tasks (Lemke, 2009).

Cognitive Reserve Theory

The term *cognitive reserve* refers to the ability of individuals to continue to function adequately despite the presence of neural deficits or pathology (Willis et al, 2009). There is a distinction between passive and active cognitive reserve, and this model is relevant to an understanding of the cognitive reserve (CR) theory. *Passive cognitive reserve* is defined in terms of the amount of neuropathology that can be sustained before clinical or functional deficits become apparent. In contrast, *active cognitive reserve* is based on the premise that the brain compensates for deficits by enlisting alternative processes or compensatory strategies. Hence, it can be theorized that individuals with higher cognitive reserve can be more successful in coping with the same amount of age-related changes, and in fact the individual variability may explain in part the differences among older adults in speech understanding in complex situations. It is noteworthy that two types of neural mechanisms underlie cognitive reserve (Willis et al, 2009). A normal process used by healthy and brain damaged individuals to cope with demanding tasks, *neural reserve* entails using more efficient and flexible brain networks or cognitive paradigms. In contrast, *neural compensation* implies the need to adopt new compensatory brain networks because pathology or age-related changes have negatively impacted those networks that were previously used.

The CR theory posits that greater levels of reserve can protect against cognitive impairment in the face of compromised integrity of the brain. As neurons become damaged due to various factors along the life course, the physiological integrity of the brain deteriorates, resulting in reduced cognitive efficiency and expression of cognitive impairment or dementia at a certain threshold of damage. The threshold at which age-related changes in the brain is associated with functional impairments depends on the level of cognitive reserve. Greater cognitive reserve may reflect some combination of greater overall cognitive efficiency, greater proliferation of neurons in the brain, more connections between neurons, or greater ability to compensate for declines in cognition through the use of alternative problem-solving strategies (Vance & Crowe, 2006). It is notable that according to the interpretation of Willis et al (2009), the cognitive reserve hypothesis posits that high-functioning individuals may process tasks in a more efficient manner, rather than because there is an anatomical difference between those with high and low levels of cognitive reserve. Hence, cognitive reserve is a malleable entity that some suggest is under the control of the individual as active agents in developing reserve and compensatory strategies to forestall the effects of age-related changes in the brain (Willis et al, 2009).

Cognitive Plasticity

Recently neuroscientists have focused on the issue of plasticity in adult cognition. To this end, various terms have been used to discuss the concept of plasticity, including neural plasticity, neural reserve, and cognitive reserve (Willis et al, 2009). A life-span perspective of cognitive plasticity has emerged, impacting my perspective on how this relates to audiology in general and audiologists in particular. Two terms are of relevance to this discussion: neural plasticity and cognitive plasticity. The term *neural plasticity* refers to the potential for morphological changes in the brain to occur as an organism is exposed to stimuli that promote learning or challenge to existing cognitive structures, and the resulting adaptation that best describes the potential role of neural plasticity for increasing cognitive reserve. If neural plasticity shrinks, then the potential for morphological change decreases (Vance & Crowe, 2006). Various health and activity factors influence the amount of neural plasticity in older adults.

The term *cognitive plasticity* has been defined with reference to an individual's latent cognitive potential under specific conditions, or it can be defined in terms of one's capacity to acquire cognitive skills (Willis et al, 2009). There are three different levels at which cognitive plasticity occurs: at the level of the brain (brain plasticity), at the behavioral level, and at the sociocultural level. Neural plasticity at the level of the brain refers to the capacity of neural circuits to change in response to changes in neural activity and is associated with such physiological changes as increased myelinization of axons, changes in the size and shape of neurons, and changes in synaptic connections between neurons (Willis et al, 2009). The relationship between age and neural plasticity has been studied using positron emission tomography (PET) and functional magnetic resonance imaging (fMRI), and the data are interesting. It appears that older adults show reduced activation in selected brain regions and on a wide array of tasks (Kramer, Bherer, Colcombs, Dong, & Greenough, 2004). It is unclear as to why reduced activation takes place, but one theory is possibly that aging is associated with the loss of neural resources, whereas an alternate theory holds that neural resources are available but are not enlisted (Willis et al, 2009). Another age-related finding is that as compared with younger adults, older adults show recruitment of different brain regions and also nonselective recruitment of brain regions (Kramer et al, 2004).

Cognitive plasticity at the behavioral level has been studied at multiple levels, with the focus being on those cognitive processes known to decline with age, including processing speed and inhibition, inductive reasoning and episodic memory, and fluid intelligence and executive functioning (Willis et al, 2009). Specifically, the effect of cognitive training on behavioral cognitive plasticity has been studied in older adults, and available data suggest the following: (1) performance improves in such areas as working memory and speed of processing; (2) training effects in selected functions, including primary mental abilities such as memory, reasoning performance, and speed of processing, can be sustained for 5 years; (3) training effects can transfer to a reduction in functional decline (Willis et al, 2006); (4) booster sessions that supplement training are helpful in terms of maintenance; and (5) transferability of training effects on cognitive function and in slowing down decline in selected cognitive functions. Finally, with regard to behavioral and cognitive plasticity, experiences at the behavioral level seem to shape the capacity of the brain to reconfigure its networks and to acquire new cognitive skills as individuals age (Willis et al, 2009). Similarly, cognitive stimulation at the behavioral level and resultant neural configuration can occur in old age. Data on behavioral and cognitive plasticity have tremendous implications for benefit from hearing aids and assistive technologies in older adults.

Pearl

Regarding plasticity, the literature is replete with data showing the neural plasticity of the central auditory system, which physiologically is seen by the reorganization of sensory maps associated with the lack of stimulation from peripheral receptors, and behaviorally is shown by improved auditory skills.

Several variables have been identified that may influence plasticity (Vance & Crowe, 2006). Greater physical activity is associated with better overall health and probably better cerebrovascular fitness, which would benefit cognition. Education is the single most important predictor of cognitive viability in later life. Many studies have shown that adults with higher levels of educational attainment have better performance on cognitive testing and are at a lower risk of age-related cognitive loss and dementia. Obtaining a formal education appears to be an important environmental experience that may promote the formation of neural connections or may represent a propensity to engage in mentally stimulating activities throughout life. There is evidence that having an extensive social network or socially integrated lifestyle is associated with intact cognitive function in older adulthood. Researchers have also posited that reducing the experience of stress and depression through antidepressant use may facilitate synaptic plasticity and in turn augment maintenance of cognitive function. People engaged in more stimulating cognitive activities are less likely to undergo age-related cognitive decline or the onset may be delayed.

A diet rich in vitamin E may also be beneficial in maintaining cognitive abilities despite the aging process, and oxidative stress negatively affects neuroplasticity in the aging CNS (Casoli, Stefano, Delfino, Fattoretti, & Bertoni-Freddari, 2004). Cognitive training represents a formalized method of training for maintaining or increasing cognitive function in the face of physiological and functional changes.

Pearl

The changes in response time have implications for pure-tone testing. The slowing in the ability to learn new information impacts on aspects of audiological rehabilitation. The fact that overall intellectual performance is maintained well into the 80s underlines the importance of treating the older adult as an intelligent human being deserving of respect and support.

In summary, cognitive changes associated with normal age-related structural and physiological changes within the brain include decrease in processing speed, cognitive flexibility, sustained attention, slowing of psychomotor and cognitive speed, visuospatial perception, and working memory (Craft, Cholerton, & Reger, 2009; Tarawneh & Galvin, 2010). In light of the cognitive and sensorimotor changes with age, the following approach to testing is recommended:

- Respect the patient.
- Do not be condescending.
- Do not infantilize.
- Allow extra time in the testing schedule.
- Provide extra pacing between stimulus presentations and patient responses.
- Repeat the instructional set.
- Verify that the patient understands the response task required.
- Use facilitatory strategies to make sure that the patient learns new tasks.
- Repeat or review material from the previous lesson of the lesson plan before moving on to the next lesson.
- Write down important information at end of each lesson.
- Use all modalities to ensure or promote recall of new information.
- Determine the best response strategy for pure-tone testing based on manual dexterity and wrist and arm mobility.
- Encourage sensory stimulation, be it hearing-aid use, hearing-assistive technologies, cochlear implant, or a bone-anchored hearing aid.

The Musculoskeletal System

The skeletal system is made of 206 bones, which support the framework of the body. It is classified into two types of bone: cortical (i.e., compact), which is primarily found in the shafts of long bones and the extremities, and trabecular (cancellous), which is typically located in the vertebrae, pelvis, and the ends of long bones (Duque & Troen, 2009; Francis, 2009). Further, bone is composed of both inorganic and organic compounds, is metabolically active, and its structural integrity relies on the metabolic processes of its bony tissue (Abrams et al, 1995; Duque & Troen, 2009). Bones store calcium and other mineral salts and, along with ligaments, tendons, and cartilage, are connective tissue, which support and connect other tissue and tissue parts.

In addition to bone, the musculoskeletal system includes several tissues including joints, tendons, ligaments, intervertebral disks, cartilage, and muscle. The musculoskeletal system subserves three functions: limb movement, support, and protection of soft tissue and calcium homeostasis (Gregson, 2010; Loeser & Delbono, 2009). The skeletal system supports the surrounding tissues and assists in movement, providing leverage and attachment of muscles. Tendons, made of cells and macromolecules (e.g., collagen), are bands of connective tissue that connect muscle to bone, enabling muscle movement. They convey the forces of muscle contraction directly to bone (Loeser & Delbono, 2009). Collagen makes up most of the weight of tendons. Collagen fibers form the main supportive protein in skin, tendon, bone, cartilage, and connective tissue, and provide the necessary rigidity and strength. Ligaments are tough bands of tissue that connect bone to bone at the joint site and provide stability to joints during movement. Bones are bound together at joints, of which there are several different varieties. Thus, a joint is the place where two or more bones come together. *Articulation* is the term that defines the coming together of two bones at a joint. Joints are classified according to different criteria depending for the most part on the number of skeletal elements articulating at a joint cavity (Frick, Leonhardt, & Starck, 1991). Some joints are synovial or freely movable; others are ball and socket and allow for circular movements. Some joints are fibrous or fixed, and still others are cartilaginous, allowing for slight movements.

In general, the skeleton undergoes dramatic change with age, becoming considerably weaker. Overall, normal aging produces a loss of bone tissue beginning between the ages of 30 and 50, proceeding at a more rapid rate for women than for men, with women losing more of their bone mass (i.e., total amount of calcium in the skeleton) with age (Francis, 2009; Hayflick, 1994). Menopause in women accelerates bone loss (Francis, 2009; Gregson, 2010). Further, tensile strength of tendons and ligament–bone connections declines with age, and there are age-related changes in the intervertebral disks. Interestingly, the age-related decline in bone density appears to be associated with falling testosterone levels in men and estrogen levels in women (Gregson, 2010). There is a decrease in skeletal muscle mass, muscle efficiency, and muscle strength with aging (Loeser & Delbono, 2009; Morley, Baumgartner, Roubenoff, Mayer, & Nair, 2001). The decrease in muscle efficiency is responsible for the decline in muscle power that occurs with aging. The decrease in muscle mass, strength, and power with aging is caused by atrophy in protein synthesis (Morley et al, 2001). Muscle weakness in the lower limbs is a risk factor for falls. Aging is also associated with decline in range of motion of joints and changes in tendons and ligaments. Similarly, the strength of ligaments and tendons and where they insert into bone tends to be reduced with age (Loeser & Delbono, 2009).

Collagen becomes irregular in shape, bound more tightly together, and more rigid with age. Articular cartilage thins and changes color with age, and there is a decrease in tensile stiffness. Further, the fibers are less likely to be in a uniform parallel formation. As noted earlier in this chapter, less collagen is degraded and less is synthesized with age. The changes in collagen tissue are in part responsible for decreased mobility in the body's tissue with advancing age (Lewis & Bottomley, 1990). When collagen in the fibers surrounding joints undergoes age-related changes, joints become stiff and their range of motion limited. In addition, cartilage becomes less pliable with age. The tissue water content of normal-aged cartilage decreases with age. However, osteoarthritis, a disorder of hyaline cartilage and subchondral bone, which is a leading cause of physical disability in persons over 65, is associated with an increase in tissue water content (Fife, 1994).

Additionally, as people age, muscle fiber is replaced by fatty tissue, which leads to a decrease in muscle mass. Aging is also associated with a decrease in the size and number of available muscle fibers, and a decline in the number of muscle motor units. The speed of muscle contraction, muscular strength, endurance, and muscle mass tend to decrease with age (Lewis & Bottomley, 1990; Tideiksaar & Silverton, 1989). As a consequence, grip strength tends to decline with age as do exercise tolerance and performance. Although the numerous age-related changes in the tissues that make up the musculoskeletal system take place gradually over time, the changes do contribute in large part to the stiffness, back pain, many chronic conditions, and physical disability experienced as people grow old.

Special Consideration

Changes within the musculoskeletal system and musculoskeletal disease have major rehabilitative implications for audiologists working with the hearing impaired. For example, pharmacological therapy can have ototoxic effects, and loss of range of motion can interfere with independent use of hearing aids and assistive listening devices.

In summary, the musculoskeletal system undergoes several changes as individuals' age, and the implications for the auditory system relate mostly to gait and middle ear function.

The Visual System

The visual system is quite complex. The aging process has several effects on the eye, some of which have variable effects on vision. Further, there are several ocular diseases that are quite prevalent in the elderly. A brief overview of the anatomy and physiology of the eye follows.

The visual organ consists of a globe and its adnexa (Schuenke et al, 2007). The important anatomical landmarks of the eye are shown in **Fig. 2.10**. The globe has three coats and is embedded in the adnexa. The coats of the globe include the outer fibrous layer, namely the cornea and sclera; the middle layer or tunica vasculosa, which includes the uvea, and consists of the iris, ciliary body, and choroid; and the inner layer, consisting of the retina and pigment epithelium (Schuenke et al, 2007). Note that the sclera is merely a whitish layer of connective tissue, and at the front of the eye it becomes the transparent cornea. The adnexa are the upper and lower lids, including the eyelashes, the eyebrows, the muscles that open and close the lids, the lacrimal glands, and the lacrimal drainage system.

The retina, the innermost of the three ocular coats, is a thin, semitransparent, netlike membrane. The retina, which comprises 10 layers of tissue, is continuous with the optic nerve. The retina contains two kinds of photoreceptors, namely the rods and the cones, which are the antennae of the visual system. The color-sensitive cones are concerned with visual acuity and color discrimination, whereas the rods are concerned with peripheral vision, especially when a room is dim (Tabbara, 1989). The rods are sensitive to differences in degree of

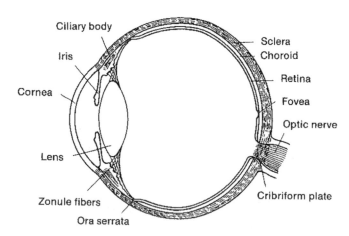

Fig. 2.10 Section through the globe.

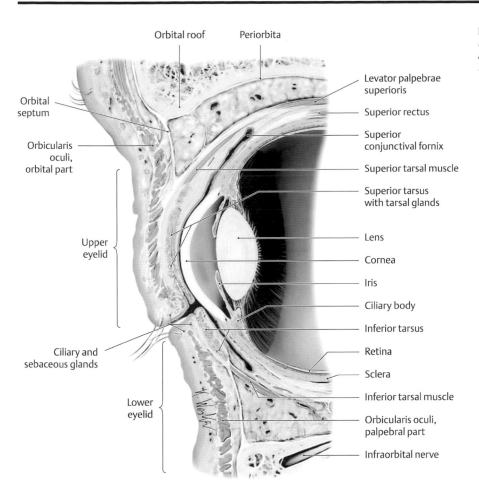

Orbital roof   Periorbita

Orbital septum

Orbicularis oculi, orbital part

Upper eyelid

Ciliary and sebaceous glands

Lower eyelid

Levator palpebrae superioris

Superior rectus

Superior conjunctival fornix

Superior tarsal muscle

Superior tarsus with tarsal glands

Lens

Cornea

Iris

Ciliary body

Inferior tarsus

Retina

Sclera

Inferior tarsal muscle

Orbicularis oculi, palpebral part

Infraorbital nerve

Fig. 2.11 Sagittal section through the anterior orbital cavity. (From *THIEME Atlas of Anatomy, Head and Neuroanatomy,* © Thieme 2007, Illustration by Karl Wesker.)

illumination and function with reduced illumination responsible for dark adaptation (Schuenke et al, 2007). The macula, an oval, yellowish spot in the center of the retina, is the key focusing area of the retina, and is responsible for central vision. The macula is the area of sharpest vision. The major functions of the retina are to receive visual images, to partly analyze the visual image, and to send the latter information to the brain.

The outer coat of the visual organ consists of the cornea and the sclera, which together provide a tough resistant coat and capsule for the globe, a highly mobile structure that moves in all directions (Schuenke et al, 2007). The cornea is a transparent avascular tissue that inserts into the sclera. It has a high water content. It functions as a protective membrane and a window through which light rays pass on their way to the retina. In contrast, as noted above, the sclera is the dense, white, opaque, outer coat of the eye that is continuous with the cornea. It prevents scattered light from entering the eye so that the optical pathway through the pupil is not disturbed (**Fig. 2.11**).

The middle ocular coat contains several important structures. The uvea is spongy and blood-filled and divided into three parts: the choroid lining of the sclera, the iris, and the ciliary body. The iris, which gives the eyes their color, is a colored circular membrane that is suspended behind the cornea and immediately in front of the lens. The round aperture in the center of the iris is the pupil, which controls the amount of

light entering the eye. The iris contains fibers that constrict to control the pupil, regulating pupillary size and reaction to light. The ciliary body in conjunction with the ciliary muscle and ciliary processes alters the tension of the lens, helping it to focus on near and distant objects. Two chambers make up the bulk of the eye: the vitreous humor and the aqueous humor. The central portion of the eye is filled with vitreous humor. The vitreous, which is the large chamber behind the lens, is a clear, avascular gelatinous body constituting two thirds of the volume and weight of the eye. It helps maintain the shape and transparency of the eye (Tabbara, 1989). The aqueous humor is the small chamber in front of the lens, which is much thinner and helps to maintain the shape of the eyeball. The aqueous humor circulates throughout its chamber. The lens, whose sole purpose is to focus light and images on the retina, is an avascular, colorless, transparent structure that is suspended behind the iris. The conjunctiva is a thin mucous membrane that helps keep the outside of the eye moist.

The eye undergoes several morphological and functional changes as an individual ages, and hence visual impairment disproportionately affects older adults. In fact, population estimates indicate that in the United States more than 26 million people over the age of 40 years have some type of visual disorder, with more than 4 million people aged 55 years or older experiencing severe vision impairment (Watson, 2009). A recent study by Cigolle, Langa, Kabeto, Tian, and Blaum (2007) reviewed data from the Health and Retirement Study and found that prevalence of visual impairment increases dramatically with age, with the absolute prevalence of visual impairment rising from 5% in those between 65 and 69 years of age to 12% among those between 80 and 84 years of age. As the prevalence of hearing impairment in the former cohort was 19% and in the latter cohort 33%, the authors reported that the co-occurrence of these two chronic conditions is rather high in persons over 65 years of age.

It is noteworthy that visual impairment can be defined in two different ways, and the definition helps determine estimates regarding functional impacts. Normal visual acuity is defined as 20/20 vision, which means that at a distance of 20 feet each eye can read the line of letters in the eye chart designated for 20 feet. Although in the United States *visual impairment* is defined as visual acuity worse than 20/40 but better than 20/200 (legal blindness) in the better eye, even with corrective lenses, the World Health Organization defines *visual impairment* as visual acuity worse than 20/70 but better than 20/400 (legal blindness) in the better eye, even with corrective lenses (Servat, Risco, Nakasato, & Bernardino, 2011). Visual acuity can be further divided into static and dynamic. Static acuity refers to the ability to resolve stationary details, and dynamic acuity refers to the ability to resolve the details of moving objects. Both static and dynamic acuity decline with increasing age. It is noteworthy that the ability to detect movement is influenced in part by the amount of light present, which explains why, for speech reading, the speaker's face must be well lit and without glare. Specifically, older people require more light to achieve equal improvement in visibility of a target under different levels of illumination. Finally, accommodation, or the process by which the eye changes optical power to focus on an object as its distance changes, also decreases with age. This change explains why we recommend an optimal distance of 3 to 6 feet between the speaker and the listener.

The age-related physiological changes within the eye and their functional correlates are listed in **Table 2.3**. Consistent with changes in the dermis, the eyelid experiences a loss of tone and elasticity (Servat et al, 2011). Older adults are prone

to dry eye because of two age-related changes in the eye. First, the lacrimal glands are less active and tear production tends to decrease with aging, and second because there is a decline in production of conjunctival mucin by the goblet cells and stabilizing surface oil by the meibomian glands with age, as well. The lens of the eye undergoes a host of changes. It tends to thicken, becoming rigid and inelastic, hence limited in its ability to change shape. The latter changes may be due in part to age-related changes in the structural proteins of the lens. These changes interfere with visual accommodation or the ability to shift focus from distant to near objects. As a result, the majority of individuals become farsighted as they age, as exhibited by the tendency to hold things at arm's length for greater clarity. Presbyopia, or the diminished ability to focus clearly on objects at a normal distance, is the most apparent of the visual changes associated with aging and is a major common cause of refractive errors and visual impairment in older adults. The lens tends to yellow and become more opaque with age, causing the cooler colors to be filtered out, whereas the warm colors (e.g., red, yellow, orange) remain more easily seen. Therefore, it becomes difficult to distinguish between blues and greens. The aging lens develops pinpoint opacities, which produces dazzle from sources of bright light. In addition, the vitreous gel tends to liquefy as individuals age.

The iris becomes more rigid and there is a corresponding decrease in the size of the pupil with age. Further, aging is associated with an impaired ability to increase pupillary diameter. That is, pupillary diameter decreases and direct and consensual reaction to light tends to be reduced. Further, the vasculature of the retina ages along with the vasculature in other parts of the body. As a result, far less light reaches the retina in older adults than in young adults. In fact, the retina of a 60-year-old receives only one third of the light received by a 20-year-old. This explains, in part, why older adults require more illumination for reading and to get around safely indoors. The ability to adjust to abrupt changes in illumination is decreased as a result of changes in the pupil. That is, both light and dark adaptation require greater time with age. This difficulty in adjusting when moving from a light to a dark area has implications for speech-reading ability. Older adults may com-

Table 2.3   Normal Age-Related Changes in the Eye and Functional Implications

Physiological Changes	Functional Implications
Lens	
Increased stiffness and loss of flexibility	Reduced ability to focus on nearby objects
Ciliary muscles lose tone	
Reduction in light transmission through lens	Decreased depth perception
	Decline in color discrimination
	Reduced visual acuity
Yellowing	Decreased color sensitivity
Pupil	
Narrowing of the pupil's dilation; decrease in size and diameter	Slowed dark and light adaptation
	Decrease in color discrimination
Visual Field	
Reduced visual field over which one can process visual information presented rapidly	Loss of peripheral vision
Retina	
Decreased function of the rods and cones	Decreased visual acuity
Eyelid	
	Loss of elasticity and tone

Table 2.4 Solutions to Age-Related Visual Changes that May Impact on Assessment, Audiological Rehabilitation, and Communication Ability

Visual Change	Functional Effects and Management Implications
Decrease in visual activity	Increase illumination without increasing glare; increase contrast during interactions with patient, use large-print materials and large images on written instructions and when performing paper-and-pencil evaluations; establish eye contact and position yourself in the person's line of vision.
Presbyopia	Increase illumination, advise use of corrective lenses to focus the light, especially during audiological rehabilitation.
Decrease in contrast sensitivity	Use magnifiers, good illumination, bright colors (e.g. red and yellow); add a contrast between colors (e.g. dark image on a light surface); use contrasting colors, such as yellow and blue, for identifying and locating information. This is especially important when highlighting hearing-aid controls.
Decrease in dark adaptation	Advise the patient to take a moment to dark/light adapt; use sunglasses to facilitate speech-reading ability; avoid abrupt changes in lighting when moving from light to dim environments.
Delayed recovery from glare; increased sensitivity to glare in the environment	Advise the patient to use less fluorescent lighting; use of hats and visors can both promote better speechreading ability; light should be even and from multiple source to ensure adequate light levels without glare; curtains or blinds should be adjusted to diffuse sunlight and to prevent direct illumination; shiny surfaces, reflective fixtures, or waxed floors add to the problems created by glare.
Loss of accommodation	Patient has difficulty focusing on close targets.
Decline in color discrimination	Patient has increased difficulty detecting differences between dark colors (e.g. blue and black) and difficulty with pastels.
Decrease in visual reading ability	Patient's reading rate and efficiency decrease.

plain that objects are not bright because a small pupil allows less light to enter the eye.

Table 2.4 lists the normal visual changes with age that result from the above structural changes along with suggestions for minimizing their functional effects. By far the most common age-related cause of visual impairment in older adults are macular degeneration, diabetic retinopathy, glaucoma, and cataract (Watson, 2009). The normal functional visual changes that arise from the age-related changes in vision include decreased contrast sensitivity, decreases in dark/light adaptation, and delayed glare recovery (Carter, 1994; Watson, 2009). These functional changes impact on speech-reading ability, legibility of hearing-aid informational brochures, battery manipulation, mobility, and functional independence, heightening the import of audition in those with compromised vision. Contrast sensitivity, which refers to the ability to discern the difference between an object and its background, decreases with age due to a decrease in retinal sensitivity, retinal luminance, and CNS changes with age. The major complaint of individuals with decreased contrast sensitivity is that they do not see well under conditions of poor lighting or contrast. A partial solution is to increase illumination, as most older adults require two to three times more light than do younger persons for a comparable task, to wear amber-tinted lenses indoors, and to use a handheld magnifier to enhance functioning. Dark/light adaptation decreases because the retinal rod photosensitive disks are not replaced efficiently with age, resulting in an inability of the eye to respond to changes in light intensity. The best solution is to use illumination controls such as sunglasses or a visor on sunny days, and to allow time for adaptation when entering or exiting a dark room (Carter, 1994). Older adults often suffer from delayed glare recovery, which interferes with optimal visual function. Glare arises when scatter from bright lights does not form part of the retinal image. Additionally, older

adults often have a restriction of visual fields, decreased visual localization, age-related deficits in spatial ability, and age-related changes in visual pursuit, and they have difficulty finding a target from among distracters (Cross et al, 2009). The latter age-related changes in detection and visual pursuit may explain why speech reading when multiple speakers are talking is problematic. A major challenge when working with older adults with age-related vision impairment is to provide enough light without creating disabling glare. Environmental lighting is effective in increasing the light level without glare. The information contained in **Table 2.4** should be reviewed with older adults with hearing impairment who are instructed to use visual cues to supplement audition. Some of the suggestions can enhance the amount of information derived from vision especially when combined with compromised audition.

Pearl

When communicating with older adults, audiologists should attempt to avoid poor sources of light such as fluorescent lights, a major source of light scatter. Use of incandescent bulbs decreases disturbing glare, as does use of antireflective coatings on the surface of eyeglasses (Carter, 1994).

Several ocular diseases, prevalent among older adults, cause abnormal visual changes. In particular four eye diseases, namely cataracts, glaucoma, macular degeneration, and diabetic retinopathy, as well as refractive errors are the leading cause of visual impairment in older adults; **Table 2.5** provides a brief description of each of these. Audiologists should be familiar with each of the above, given the high prevalence of adults 65 years of age or older who are classified as having low vision, which results from one or more of these conditions. It is note-

Table 2.5   Age-Related Causes of Vision Impairment

Condition	Etiology	Functional Consequence
Macular degeneration	Intracellular residue on the macular region between the retinal pigment epithelial cells and Bruch's membrane. The hard drusen appears as dots of yellow or white lying below retinal vessels, and loss of central visual field and central vision.	Loss of acuity and contrast sensitivity, which leads to difficulty reading print and identifying faces, difficulty with depth cues and distance, and loss of color and contrast sensitivity, leading to mobility difficulty; image distortion; blurred vision
Open-angle glaucoma	Occurs when a sustained increase in the intraocular pressure damages the retinal nerve fibers; results in gradual degeneration of the optic nerve	Decreased ability to function in dim light, decreased dark adaption, glare disability, and gradual loss of visual fields, severe visual impairment, possible blindness, difficulty reading and writing due to narrowed visual field; visual field loss
Cataracts	Opacity or clouding of the crystalline lens, which interferes with passage of light	Decreased visual acuity, contrast sensitivity, and color perception, difficulty with detail vision, loss of perception of depth and distance; blurred vision
Diabetic retinopathy	Retinopathy associated with diabetes mellitus; damage to the retina associated with complications from diabetes mellitus	Glare disability, decreased acuity, and decreased dark/light adaptation, possible blindness, loss of color and contrast sensitivity, difficulty reading recognizing faces, reading print material, difficulty with distance and depth cues, fluctuating vision; floaters
Refractive errors	A defect in the ability of the lens or cornea to focus on an image accurately	Blurred vision, difficulty reading, difficulty seeing distant objects

Sources: Adapted from Watson, G. (2009). Assessment and rehabilitation of older adults with low vision. In J. Halter, J. Ouslander, M. Tinetti, S. Studenski, K. High, & S. Asthana (Eds.), *Hazzard's geriatric medicine and gerontology* (6th ed.). New York: McGraw-Hill; and Carter, T. L. (1994, Sep). Age-related vision changes: a primary care guide. *Geriatrics, 49,* 37–42, 45, quiz 46–47.

worthy that African Americans are at increased risk for primary open-angle glaucoma. In fact, the Baltimore Eye Survey (Tielsch et al, 1991) found that blacks had a prevalence of glaucoma four to five times that of whites, whereas Friedman et al (2004) found the age-adjusted prevalence of glaucoma to be nearly three times higher in blacks than in whites. Further, the anatomical microstructure of the posterior sclera of African Americans differs significantly from that of whites, possibly contributing to earlier development and severity of ocular disease in this population (Yan, McPheeters, Johnson, Utzinger, & Vande Geest, 2011). The rates of eye diseases such as glaucoma, cataracts, macular degeneration, and diabetic retinopathy are higher among Latinos of Mexican descent living in Los Angeles as compared with non-Hispanic whites living in the United States (Varma et al, 2010).

The above conditions will affect speech-reading ability and the environment in which hearing-aid orientation and group counseling sessions should be designed to maximize auditory-visual communication. The term *low vision* refers to persons with corrected visual acuity between 20/70 and 20/200 (as noted above, acuity measurements are based on the Snellen eye chart, with optimal acuity rated at 20/20 and reduced vision indicated by a higher number in the denominator). The diagnosis of low vision is made when vision cannot be fully corrected by lenses, medical treatment, or surgery. A low vision loss can be central (reduced visual acuity) or peripheral (reduced visual field). Loss of peripheral or side vision can result from glaucoma or stroke. The major functional implication of a central loss is difficulty with detail discrimination (e.g., reading positive and negative on hearing-aid battery doors, reading volume control numbers), whereas the major func-

tional implication of a peripheral problem is difficulty in orientation and mobility. In older adults, the most frequent type of vision loss is central, as a result of macular degeneration (Fletcher, 1994).

In summary, vision impairment is a major health issue for older adults that often interferes with routine activities, including hearing-aid battery insertion and removal of wax guards on hearing aids. As with hearing loss, people with impaired vision underutilize both vision rehabilitation services and high- and low-tech adaptive devices. Audiologists should encourage persons with hearing impairment to be sure that their vision is maximized, as auditory visual speech recognition and manipulation of hearing aids and hearing-assistive technologies can be optimized with corrected vision. Specifically, audiologists must make every effort to ensure that vision acuity is maximized during counseling sessions by using, for example, handheld or stand magnifiers to demonstrate the function of various hearing-aid controls, appropriate lighting, large-print reading materials, and raised-dot markings on hearing aids to help in locating particular controls. Audiologists should refer clients with low-vision problems to the appropriate professional for evaluation and management. **Table 2.6** lists some strategies for promoting communication with older adults with hearing, as well as visual, impairments.

Pearl

Nearly every person will experience changes in vision with age. As with hearing loss, the impact of the changes will vary considerably.

Table 2.6 Strategies for Promoting Communication for People with Visual Problems

Improving Verbal Communication
  Introduce yourself by name.
  Let the patient know when you enter or leave the room.
  Speak before touching the person.
  Approach the patient on the side of his or her better eye.
  Allow the patient with visual loss to speak for him- or herself; talk directly to the person with the visual impairment.
  Let the person with visual loss do as much as possible; this builds confidence.
Making Text More Legible for Persons with Visual Impairment and Low Vision
  Text should be printed with the highest possible contrast of light against dark.
  Printed material is most readable in black and white.
  Use wide spacing between letters.
  Use extra-wide margins, especially for bound material, which makes it easier to use on a flat surface.
  Use large fonts, 16- to 18-point.
  Use ordinary typeface, upper and lower case, or boldface.
  Do not use paper with a glossy finish.
Telephone Features for Patients with Visual Impairments
  Suggest that the patient use telephones with large buttons and good contrasts.
  Suggest that the patient use telephones with paging, memory, and redial features.

The Hand, the Wrist, and the Fingers

As hand function declines with aging and the ability to manipulate hearing aids, implantable devices and hearing-assistance technologies relies on hand function, a review of the particular structural and functional changes with age is pertinent. Hand function diminishes with age because of age-related declines in multiple systems including the musculoskeletal systems, sensory systems, CNS, and PNS (Singh, 2009). Primary factors accounting for changes in hand function with age include changes that occur at the level of the bones and joints, changes in bone mass that occur with age, changes in muscle mass that are highly correlated with muscle strength and hand-grip strength and associated changes in dexterity which interfere with small movements (Singh, Pichora-Fuller, Hayes, et al., 2012). Further, musculoskeletal changes that account in part for decreases in strength with age come into play as well. Older adults demonstrate reduced tactile sensitivity in their fingers as compared with younger adults, due most likely to age-related loss of sensory mechanoreceptors (Singh, 2009). With age, there is a decrease in the vibratory sense and in proprioception due to a combination of factors including degeneration in the nerve fibers and arteriosclerotic changes in arterioles. Further, aging is associated with a decline in muscle bulk especially in the intrinsic muscles of the hands. Along with a decline in muscle bulk comes a decline in muscle strength, which will have an influence on hand grip strength. Speed of repetitive hand movements change as well, and this could impact the choice of response mode used during pure-tone testing (e.g., switch versus hand-raising).

Arthritis, osteoarthritis (OA), and rheumatoid arthritis (RA) are prevalent conditions in older adults that affect the wrist and the hand and restrict mobility. OA of the hand, defined as a bony inflammation of a joint or joints, is more prevalent than RA of the hand and typically involves the thumb (Lewis & Bottomley, 1990; Ling & Ju, 2009), which is important for manipulation of hearing technologies and implantable devices. A key feature of OA is stiffness in the morning and after periods of inactivity. Hand osteoarthritis tends to affect more women than men. RA, a systemic autoimmune inflammatory disease characterized primarily by joint swelling and pain, is associated with joint destruction and disability. Highest among woman, the prevalence of RA among persons over 60 years in the United States is approximately 2%. It is projected that by 2012 there would be more than 29 million individuals aged 70 years or older living in the United States with RA, which translates to more than half a million adults in this age demographic living with RA and requiring care (Manno & Bingham, 2011). In contrast to OA, RA typically involves the small joints of the hands and wrists, and therefore this condition, which is associated with significant disability, will interfere with manipulation of hearing aids. In summary, compromised manual dexterity associated with age changes in the hand combined with the various types of arthritis, will have a deleterious effect on handling of hearing aids and manipulation of selected controls, including wax guards, battery doors, toggle switches, and rotating wheels, so audiologists should assess dexterity when deciding on the features and the style of hearing aid to recommend.

◆ Physiological Changes in Remaining Systems

Several other systems undergo physiological changes with age. These include the metabolic system, the renal system, the respiratory system, the cardiovascular system, the immune system, and the endocrine system. The basic changes are cited below, along with the implications of the changes for audiologists.

The Metabolic System

Metabolism is the sum of all of the numerous and complex chemical events taking place in the human body (Hayflick, 1994). *Metabolic rate* is a term that refers to the rate at which the substances that run our body are utilized to provide energy for the physiological activities in which humans engage. Protein tissue is the most metabolically active body compartment. Additional energy sources within our body include fat tissue, which is metabolized as we exercise, and carbohydrates. A large amount of energy is necessary to maintain homeostasis, and this amount of energy is referred to as the basal metabolic rate (BMR) (Fried, Walston, & Ferrucci, 2009). The BMR tends to be expressed as energy expenditure per total body mass; thus, the latter is a key determinant of BMR. Age is associated with a reduction in total body protein. Further, protein, or lean body mass, and BMR tend to decline with age. The mass of fat stored within the body tends to increase. Further, as people age, less energy is required to maintain metabolically active body mass (Chernoff, 1990). Chernoff (1990) cautioned that these changes occur in all people as they age, albeit at different rates. Chronic disease states, exercise, tendency toward a sedentary lifestyle, and nutritional status may influence the rate at which they occur. The metabolic changes that occur with age may account for some of the age-related changes occurring in the inner ear.

The Renal System

The ordinary function of the renal system is to remove wastes and to adequately regulate the volume and content of extracellular fluid. A substantial reduction in renal function accompanies normal aging, for the most part due to age-related anatomical and physiological changes within the kidneys. The changes in renal function reduce the older adult's ability to respond to a variety of physiological and pathological stresses, with substantial implications for overall function (Abrams et al, 1995). The size and weight of the kidneys tend to decline with age, with weight decreasing from 250 to 270 g in young adulthood to 180 to 200 g in the eighth decade of life. Further, there is a decrease in the number and functioning of glomeruli and tubules. The role of the kidney is to maintain the internal environment of the body by eliminating many of the products of metabolism and regulating the body's water content. A well-known end product of metabolism is creatinine. Kidney function, measured by the ability to clear nitrogenous wastes from the blood, declines with age. Further, using age-adjusted standards for creatinine clearance (CrCl), the Baltimore Longitudinal Study of Aging (BLSA) confirmed a progressive decline of renal function with aging specifically, or CrCl has been shown to decrease with increasing age. However, as with other aging functions, kidney function varies dramatically across persons at all ages, and when declines are noted, they occur at substantially different rates (Vlassara, Ferrucci, Post, & Striker, 2009). The correlation with age may be due to the fact that skeletal muscle is a major source for creatinine, and with age comes changes in body composition, especially the crude and relative decline of muscle mass. The tendency for, or capacity of, the kidney to hypertrophy is lost, and blood flow is reduced with aging (Kenney, 1988). In general, the functional changes in the kidney leave the older adult more vulnerable to a variety of environmental or drug-induced stresses, but do not generally lead to disease or disability.

The kidney has primary responsibility for clearance of drugs. Renal drug clearance decreases with increasing age, and this effect is exaggerated when older adults do not receive the correct dosing of medications. In older adults, the doses of drugs excreted by the kidneys (e.g., aminoglycosides, antibiotics, digoxin preparations) require adjustment to compensate for age-related changes in renal function. If not, older adults will be vulnerable to drug overdose. It is often the case that drugs that are misprescribed and do not clear properly are toxic to the auditory or vestibular system. The latter system can have vestibulotoxic (balance problems), ototoxic (hearing problems), or combined otovestibulotoxic effects. Aminoglycoside antibiotics, furosemides, chemotherapeutic agents, and digoxin, commonly prescribed drugs for the elderly, may require dosage adjustments based on gender and age-adjusted CrCl values to prevent toxicity associated with age-related changes in renal drug clearance. Finally, audiologists should familiarize themselves with the chronic diseases prevalent among older adults and the medications used to treat these diseases, as large enough doses of some of the medications can be ototoxic. A familiar example is arthritis, for which large doses of salicylates may be prescribed, resulting in temporary hearing loss and possibly tinnitus. Monitoring of hearing status with otoacoustic emissions is recommended in older adults with compromised renal systems.

Pearl

In light of age-related changes in pharmacodynamics, professionals should be attuned to possible drug-induced causes of hearing and balance problems. Similarly, audiologists should be familiar with the names of medications commonly prescribed for the elderly and associated with oto- and vestibulotoxic effects. Monitoring of hearing status is important in individuals for whom ototoxic or vestibulotoxic medications are prescribed.

The Endocrine System

The endocrine system consists of several glands, cells, and tissues scattered throughout the body that produce hormones. Some of the glands of the endocrine system are autonomous, secreting hormones in response to chemical changes within the blood, whereas others do so through such endocrine organs as the pituitary gland and the hypothalamus. Neuroendocrine function, neurotransmitter regulation, and the hypothalamic-pituitary-adrenal axis all fall into this system. The endocrine system, which affects virtually all cells of the body, undergoes changes with age that may in fact reduce the physiological reserve of tissues and organ systems (Hayflick, 1994). The major age-related change in this system is a decrease in production and secretion of hormones that control many essential bodily functions. For example, the production, metabolism, and secretion of testosterone, insulin, aldosterone, thyroid, adrenal, and growth hormones decrease with normal aging (Belchetz & Hammond 2009). Similarly, there is decrease in adrenal androgen (synthesized by the adrenal cortex) production in old age. Further, the ability of the blood to maintain a normal level of glucose declines with age. Hayflick (1994) suggested that the latter age-related hormonal changes may erode the body's responsivity to stresses and hence interfere with such variables as healing, recovery from trauma, and adaptation to heat and cold. In addition to the above changes, the thyroid gland undergoes morphological changes including change in its appearance, a decrease in follicle size, and a reduction in the amount of colloid produced (Miller, 2009). Typically, thyroid hormone action is diminished as part of the normal aging process, and because oxygen consumption appears to decrease with age, the basal metabolic rate tends to decline as well (Belchetz & Hammond, 2009).

The Immune System

The role of the immune system is protective and defensive. It defends the body against infections and disease and is responsible for internal homeostasis (Gameiro, Romão, & Castelo-Branco, 2010). It includes anatomical, physiological, phagocytic, and inflammatory barriers. Natural killer (NK) cells of the innate immunity system represent an important line of protection against tumor and infected cells. They consist of a group of mechanisms that detect, inactivate, and remove foreign materials and pathogens from the body. The thymus gland, which contains lymphocytes, is integral to the performance of the immune system (Hayflick, 1994). T cells are thymus-derived lymphocytes that circulate in the peripheral blood and in the lymph channel (Adler & Nagel, 1994). In addition to T lymphocytes, immune reactions are coordinated by the interaction among B lymphocytes and antigen-presenting cells. The immune system performs these duties primarily through the release of a class of proteins known as antibodies, which come in different varieties and are uniquely tailored to combat particular microorganisms or foreign cells. For the most part, the immune system develops antibodies that detect and deactivate foreign protein bodies and to a lesser extent "self" proteins essential to vital life processes (Hayflick, 1994).

The immune system undergoes significant changes with age, including lymphocyte subsets, in cytokines, and in immunological tolerance (Tonet & Nóbrega, 2008). As people age, there is a decline in the mass of the thymus, and the proportion of lymphocytes within the thymus changes as well. Whereas it is generally accepted that T-cell function declines with age, there is no consensus on the effects of age on the B-cell response (Adler & Nagel, 1994; Miller, 1990). As we age, self proteins undergo some minor changes, and the antibodies produced by the immune system may attack as foreign what is really a slightly changed self protein (Hayflick, 1994). Similarly, there are changes in immune tolerance with age (Gameiro et al, 2010). The natural immune defenses of the body are also reduced in part because of the increased fragility of the skin and a decrease in the amount of antibody produced by mucous membranes. The end result of this phenomenon is the development of autoimmune diseases, which tends to increase in prevalence as people age and is more prevalent in women than in men. Examples of autoimmune diseases prevalent in older adults include some forms of arthritis and some forms of lupus.

In summary, the immune system undergoes some significant functional changes with age, including a decline in the ability to produce antibodies to foreign substances, an increase in the tendency to produce antibodies to self proteins, and a general decline in the ability to mount an immune response against pathogens. The decline in protective immune reactions with age increases the susceptibility of older adults to infection and neoplasia (Miller, 1990). It is also important to emphasize the large individual variability that characterizes the age changes within the immune system, and that behavioral or lifestyle variables also influence immunosenescence. The pharmacological management of individuals with autoimmune disease has implications for audiologists, as some of the medication is potentially ototoxic or vestibulotoxic. Further, autoimmune disease is associated with hearing impairment and auditory processing difficulties, which often fluctuate when the condition exacerbates.

The Cardiovascular System

Circulatory organs, which consist of the heart, blood vessels, and lymphatics, are responsible for transporting and distributing blood to cells in the body (Schuenke et al, 2007). The system of blood vessels includes arteries, capillaries, and veins. The shape of a pear and the size of a fist in shape, the normal heart acts as a pump, circulating blood throughout the body (Frick et al, 1991). Although in males the healthy heart weighs about 300 g, its size and weight vary with body size and degree of physical activity. The relative weight of the female heart tends to be a little less than the weight of the typical male heart. Located somewhat to the left of the center of the chest, the heart is a combined suction and pressure pump. The heart muscle, which requires oxygen and nutrients to survive, is composed of muscle that contracts continuously with only brief periods of rest between contractions. Blood carries oxygen and nutrients to all parts of the body. Arteries convey blood from the heart and distribute it throughout the body; thus, coronary arteries are vessels that carry the blood with oxygen and nutrients to the myocardial muscle. In contrast, veins return the blood to the heart. The blood flow in the vascular system, which is a closed network, is maintained by the pumping action of the heart (Schuenke et al, 2007). The contraction phase of the heart's work is called the systole, whereas the time when the heart is relaxed and the chambers are filled is called diastole. Blood pressure is the ratio between these two pressures. The amount of pressure produced varies with the force with which the heart pumps and the degree to which the blood vessels resist blood flow (Falvo, 1991).

The cardiovascular system undergoes considerable structural changes with age that can lead to some significant changes in cardiac function. Certain regions of the aging heart undergo calcification (e.g., mitral and aortic valves) with age. The muscular mass of the normal adult heart, known as the myocardium, tends to enlarge with age. Yet the total number of cardiac myocytes (muscle cells in the heart) declines with age with a gender effect as well. The decrease in myocytes is greater in males than in females (Howlett, 2010). In general, there is an increase in elastic and collagenous tissue in all parts of the conduction system of the heart. Specifically, the heart contains collagen and elastin in addition to cardiac myocytes. The amount of collagen (fibrous protein that holds heart cells together) in the heart increases with age, and the elastin undergoes structural changes, reducing the elastic recoil that characterizes healthy hearts (Howlett, 2010). The latter changes increase the stiffness of the myocardium and have implications for cardiac function.

Although the heart itself demonstrates little change in chamber size with age, heart weight tends to increase because of increased ventricular wall thickness, especially in the area of the left ventricle (Howlett, 2010). The aorta and its valves tend to undergo an increase in rigidity/stiffness and a decrease in elasticity and increased arterial stiffening with age. Arterial stiffening is due in part to a thickening of the innermost tissue constituting the arterial pipeline that leads to a narrowing of the diameter of the artery and increased rigidity. The diameter of the aorta increases with age, the mitral and aortic leaflets increase in thickness, and the circumference of the four cardiac valves increases with age (Kitzman & Taffet, 2009). With age the coronary arteries also become more dilated and more susceptible to calcification. Interestingly, due to the anatomical changes noted above, it seems that the shape of the heart changes somewhat with age. The implications of the age-related structural changes in the heart are profound for cardiac function.

Cardiovascular function results from an interaction among several different variables. Thus, in discussing the age effects, the individual factors that tend to regulate cardiovascular performance will be isolated. There is widespread agreement that due to an age-associated increase in the stiffness of central elastic arteries, aging is associated with an increase in peak systolic blood pressure, but diastolic pressure does not seem to change (Hayflick, 1994; Kitzman & Taffet, 2009). Resting heart rate does not change with age; however, there is an age-related decrease in maximum heart rate in response to exercise. In general, aging is associated with a diminished maximum heart rate in the sitting position, decreased myocardial contractility, and a decrease in stroke volume or the volume of blood pumped during each contraction (Lakatt, 1990). Although most studies suggest a decline in cardiac output with age, some suggest that resting cardiac output does not change with age in healthy active individuals. Decreased cardiac output can lead to reductions in cerebral blood flow and cardiac syncope; thus the area continues to be investigated. There is general agreement that the heart's ability to respond to stress declines with age, as does the maximum heart rate achieved during exercise (Lakatt, 1990). With regard to the latter, this age-related limit in the ability of the cardiovascular system to respond to age is present in both fit and sedentary individuals, but regular exercise does reduce the adverse effects of age on the heart (Howlett, 2010). Further, the amount of oxygen delivered to and used by muscles (i.e., maximum oxygen consumption) progressively declines with age, with the decline modifiable with certain lifestyle changes. The reduced ability of the cardiovascular system to deliver raw materials (e.g., proteins) to working muscles changes the chemical composition of muscle fibers, contributing in part to a generalized decline in muscular strength and function with age. Further, the decline in pumping ability of the aging heart under stress can lead to limited endurance, easy and early fatigability, compromised ability to maintain prolonged sustained activity, reduced exercise tolerance, and a lowered threshold for the development of clinical conditions (Kitzman & Taffet, 2009; Roth, 1991). Additionally, there is general agreement that with increasing age, there is an increase in workload on the heart, as it has the job of pumping blood against less compliant arteries. It is noteworthy that coronary artery or ischemic heart disease is the most common disease in individuals over the age of 60, and cardiovascular disease (CVD) remains the most common cause of death in the world (Haigis & Sinclair, 2011). As is discussed in Chapter 5, several cardiovascular risk factors for hearing loss have recently been identified.

The Respiratory System

The respiratory system has two major components: the pulmonary system, which consists of the lungs and the lower airways, including the bronchioles and associated tissue, and the chest wall, which consists of the rib cage and the diaphragm-abdomen, which is essentially a large dome-shaped muscle (Kent & Vorperian, 2006; Rochet, 1991). The lungs essentially occupy the thoracic cavity. In general, the lungs assume the gross shape of the chest wall, and as the dimensions of the chest wall change, so do the lungs. The left lung tends to be smaller than the right due in part to the left displacement of the apex of the heart (Frick et al, 1991; Kent & Vorperian, 2006). The right lung is also shorter and broader. The lungs provide an interface between the atmosphere with which the body exchanges gases, and the blood that transports gases to and from active cells where oxygen is used and carbon dioxide produced (Kenney, 1988). In essence, the primary task of the lungs is respiration; however, they play a role in metabolism as well (Despopoulos & Silbernagl, 1991). Millions of alveoli, or small air sacs, are housed in the walls of the terminal bronchioles.

The overall function of the respiratory system is gaseous exchange between the human organism and the environment. In short, the respiratory system transports oxygen, inspired from the air, in the blood to the tissues. In turn, the carbon dioxide, a waste product of tissue metabolism, moves in the opposite direction (Despopoulos & Silbernagl, 1991). The respiratory gases are thus alternately transported over distances. Abnormal functioning of the respiratory system adversely affects every system of the body by diminishing the oxygen supply (Falvo, 1991). The functioning of the respiratory system is closely linked to proper function of the neuromuscular and cardiovascular systems; thus, anatomical changes in the latter systems may result in functional changes in the pulmonary system. In general, lung structure and function reach their maximum level of development and efficiency early in the second decade of life, declining slowly thereafter (Saltzman, 1992). It is important to note that respiratory muscle strength and endurance are vital to respiratory function (Supiano, 2009). There are several types of respiratory muscles that are responsible for moving air into and out of the lungs, and aging has a differential effect on the proportion of each type of fiber (Kent & Vorperian, 2006).

Selected parts of the respiratory system undergo structural and functional changes with age (Davies & Bolton, 2010). Changes in elastin and collagen structures within the lung and resulting stiffening of the lung is associated with reduced chest wall compliance with age. The latter changes in compliance may account in part for the alteration in pulmonary function with aging. Examples of age-related changes in pulmonary function include a decline in vital capacity, impaired mobility of the thoracic cavity, decrease in elastic recoil due to increased lung tissue compliance, increased airflow resistance, and a potential decrease in forced expiratory volume (Enright, 2009; Saltzman, 1992).

Further, there is a loss in the alveolar surface area as both alveoli and the alveolar ducts enlarge. The shape of the chest wall changes, becoming more barrel shaped with age. The joints of the thorax become more rigid, the cartilage becomes calcified, the rib cage stiffens, and, correspondingly, chest wall compliance decreases. Further, medium and small airways, which are composed primarily of smooth muscle, tend to narrow due to a decrease in elasticity. In general, respiratory muscle strength and mass decrease with age interfering in part with exercise tolerance (Enright, 2009; Saltzman, 1992). The principal muscle of respiration, the diaphragm, tends to flatten as a consequence of the age-related changes in lung compliance and hyperinflation of the chest wall (Davies & Bolton, 2010; Dean, 1994). Diaphragm muscle strength also declines with age, and vital capacity is normally reduced when the latter muscle weakens, as occurs with age (Enright, 2009). Similarly, there is a weakening of intercostal muscle strength and of abdominal muscles with age. The latter changes contribute to decreased elasticity of the lung. Further, the tissues of the respiratory system undergo changes with age. The alveolar sacs and ducts enlarge progressively with age and join together with adjacent alveoli. The pulmonary vessels undergo an increase in internal fibrosis and thickening of the vessel walls. A notable functional change in the respiratory system associated with age is a decrease in lung function and reserve especially during stress. Maximal ventilation, which is the process of moving air from the environment to the alveoli during inspiration, and from the alveoli to the environment during expiration, tends to decline with age. Aging is associated with a breakdown of the mucosal barrier of the lung and reduced mucociliary action, with resulting alterations in respiratory defense mechanisms (Davies & Bolton, 2010). Specifically, there is a decrease in ciliary action and secretory immunoglobulin of nasal and respiratory passages, which can in some cases neutralize viral activities (Abrams et al, 1995).

In summary, changes in pulmonary structure and progressive declines in pulmonary function have been noted with aging. The extent of the functional implications depends in large part on alterations in related systems, especially the cardiovascular, immunological, and neuromuscular systems. Older adults with respiratory problems are susceptible to the development of middle ear disease, and smoking can increase the risk.

The Vocal Mechanism

Speech production involves three systems: the respiratory, laryngeal, and articulatory (oral cavity) (Kent & Vorperian, 2006). The vocal mechanism or laryngeal system consists of the larynx or voice box and an elaborate system of cartilage, muscles, and tissues. The vocal folds, which are muscular cushions or bands, run lengthwise from the front to the back of the larynx. They are the vibrating structures of the larynx, and the actions of the vocal folds is controlled by several cartilages (e.g., thyroid) and muscles. The glottis, or space between the vocal folds, is formed by the true vocal folds, which include the vocal ligament, the vocalis muscle, and the mucosal covering. The epiglottis is a cartilage that closes over the entry to the elevated larynx during swallowing so as to prevent food

from reaching into the respiratory system (Becker, Naumann, & Pfaltz, 1989; Kent & Vorperian, 2006). The joints and muscles of the larynx adjust the position and tension of the vocal chords, with efficient joint production depending on intact respiratory and vocal mechanisms. The respiratory system includes the trachea and lungs, and the articulatory cavity includes the lips, tongue, jaw, oral, and nasal and pharyngeal cavities (Kent & Vorperian, 2006). The oral and nasal cavities are separated by the hard and soft palate. The human voice, an organ of communication, can be viewed as a wind instrument. In short, air from the lungs, bronchi, and trachea (the wind space) is driven past a narrow slit (vocal chords), causing vibration, whose character is influenced by the chest and movement of structures in the oral and nasal cavities (i.e., the resonance chamber) (Anderson & Shames, 2006; Despopoulos & Silbernagl, 1991). The upper aerodigestive tract, which includes the oral cavity, larynx, pharynx, and esophagus, is involved in swallowing as well (Sonies, 2006). The structure and action of the larynx is shown in **Fig. 2.12**.

The laryngeal system undergoes several changes with age, which tends to have implications for voice production. In general, age-related changes in muscle tension, fiber density, muscle strength, and muscle contraction take place in the muscles involved in mastication, speaking, voice production, lingual movements, and swallowing (Robbins, Hind, & Barczi, 2009). Edema, atrophy of laryngeal musculature, reduction and degeneration of nerve fibers serving laryngeal cartilages, degeneration of the cricoarytenoid joint, reduction of the lamina propria, and epithelial cell thickness and density can occur with age (Awan, 2006). As the vocal mechanism is truly a system of cartilage, glands, joints, nerves, ligaments, and muscles, it is susceptible to many of the changes that take place in these systems as people age. In general, the laryngeal cartilage calcifies and ossifies. The latter occurs earlier in males than in females. The true vocal folds undergo fatty degeneration and atrophy. The laryngeal muscles atrophy and undergo degeneration as well. The laryngeal ligaments in many cases stiffen, and thinning and breakdown have been observed in some of the joints, most notably the cricoarytenoid. These changes have

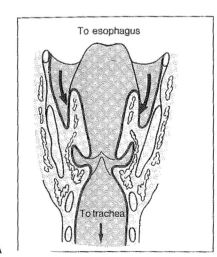
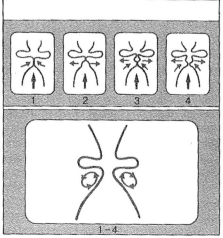

A   B

Fig. 2.12 **(A)** Structure of the larynx. **(B)** Motion of the vocal chords. [From Despopoulos, A., & Silbernagl, S. (1991). *Color atlas of physiology* (4th ed.). New York: Thieme Medical Publishers. Reprinted by permission.]

been attributed to a reduction in blood supply to the laryngeal muscles. The laryngeal nerves undergo changes with age by virtue of the thickening of the capillary walls and reduction in the diameter of the vessels. Salivary function changes with age, and diminished salivary flow is associated with dryness in the mouth (Sonies, 2006). The cells lining the nasopharynx atrophy with age, leading to decrements in the sense of smell (olfaction), and taste buds lining some of the tongue change with age, leading to a reduced sensitivity for a broad range of tastes (Sonies, 2006; Tarawneh & Galvin, 2010).

It is important to note that the swallowing mechanism undergoes considerable age-related changes in part due to changes in respiratory function, postural changes that occur with aging, changes in the tone of muscles involved in swallowing, the ossification of laryngeal cartilages, and decrease in tongue pressure, to name a few (Sonies, 2006). Similarly, as numerous muscles, afferent and efferent sensory fibers, portions of the brainstem, and cerebral and midbrain fibers are all involved in swallowing, the extent to which age-related changes take place in these structures will determine the nature and expression of age-related changes in swallowing. Finally, it is important to note that in light of the latter changes, it tends to take longer to swallow as we age.

As a result of physiological changes in the vocal mechanism, the aging voice is characterized by slight hoarseness, increased variability in pitch, declines in pitch control and pitch range, and a decrease in loudness (Kahane & Beckford, 1991). Once again, it is important to emphasize that there is large individual variability among older persons in vocal characteristics, due to the highly variable rate in the onset and progression of physiological aging in the vocal mechanism (Burzynski, 1987). The latter vocal changes can interfere with communication, especially when hearing loss is present. The rehabilitative implications of changes in the laryngeal system as they pertain to audiology primarily derive from the fact that older voices can be difficult for the hearing impaired to hear and understand. This is especially problematic in group audiological rehabilitation sessions.

Special Consideration

A voice amplifier, similar to the pocket talker, can be used with older adults whose vocal intensity is so weak as to interfere with expressive communication. Voice amplifiers are helpful with individuals who can produce voice consistently, yet at a reduced loudness level (Yorkston & Garrett, 1997). Amplifiers are especially helpful during group hearing-aid orientation or counseling sessions.

The Gastrointestinal System

The gastrointestinal (GI) system includes the stomach, liver, esophagus, mouth, colon, small intestine, and pancreas. Each of these systems undergoes structural and functional changes with age. For the most part, the great functional reserve of the digestive tract reduces the clinical impact of age-related changes. The sense of taste is subserved by selected structures within the GI system, specifically the mouth within the oral cavity. The mouth has an intricate sensory control system with receptors for pain, taste, texture, and temperature. Taste receptors are collected in the taste bud located on the tongue

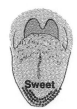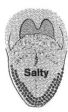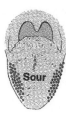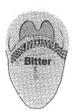

Fig. 2.13 Localization of taste qualities on the tongue. [From Despopoulos, A., & Silbernagl, S. (1991). *Color atlas of physiology* (4th ed.). New York: Thieme Medical Publishers. Reprinted by permission.]

and palate. Four basic taste qualities are recognized: salt, sour, bitter, and sweet. As is shown in **Fig. 2.13**, these receptors are unevenly distributed over the tongue. The sense of taste is mediated in part by three nerves—the chorda tympani, the greater superficial petrosal, and the glossopharyngeal—that innervate various parts of the tongue. The chorda tympani, a branch of the seventh cranial nerve, which passes across the eardrum en route to the brain, innervates a portion of the front of the tongue. The greater superficial petrosal, also a branch of the seventh cranial nerve, innervates taste buds on the palate. Age is associated with decreased sensation of taste due to a progressive loss of taste buds predominantly on the anterior tongue. Aging is primarily associated with a decrease in detection of sweet and salty taste. Further, space-occupying lesions on selected cranial nerves may also alter taste sensation. Professionals working with older adults must ask case history questions that enable them to distinguish between changes in gustation related to age and changes associated with head trauma, surgical trauma, disease, or pathology such as an acoustic tumor.

Age-related changes in the jaw and temporomandibular joint (TMJ) may also be of relevance to audiology. The TMJ is located between the maxillary glenoid fossa and the condylar process of the mandible (Abrams et al, 1995). It is essential to all articulated maxillary and mandibular functions. In general, the structures constituting the TMJ undergo degenerative changes, which are similar to changes in the joints throughout the body (Baum & Ship, 1994). TMJ disorders, which may include osteoarthritis, displacement of the TMJ disk, and myofascial pain in the masseter and temporal muscles, are often associated with otalgia and neck pain (Abrams et al, 1995). Joint noises such as a click are often present in persons with TMJ dysfunction.

Pearl

Joint noises may be mistaken for tinnitus, a common symptom experienced by older adults, and TMJ dysfunction should be ruled out as a cause of tinnitus in older adults.

◆ Future Considerations

Stem Cells and Aging

Stem cell biology is relevant to audiology to the extent that it may have therapeutic potential, which pertains to the peripheral or central auditory system. Before discussing how stem cell function changes during aging, a brief overview of the biology of aging that pertains to stem cells is relevant. Embryonic stem cells (ESCs) and adult somatic stem cells are two types of naturally occurring stem cells (Liu & Rando, 2011). ESCs are derived from the inner cell mass of blastocysts in 3- to 5-day-old embryos and give rise to the billions of specialized cells in the human body. ESCs can survive in vitro, and in this state they retain their ability to differentiate and morph into specialized cell types throughout the human body. Adult somatic stem cells exist throughout the lifetime of an individual, and have the ability to replicate; there is probably a mechanism that replenishes stem cells (Liu & Rando, 2011). Although they have the ability to divide and to differentiate and are present in bone marrow, skeletal muscle, skin, brain, and adipose tissue, they tend to remain in a quiescent state until recruited to maintain or repair tissue homeostasis. It seems that stable microenvironments house stem cells, and they tend to gather with subsets of differentiated cells that have a particular "niche," taking on the characteristics of the cells with which they reside. Hence, when stem cells are transplanted, they often take on the characteristics of the neighboring cells. Cells in the niche transmit environmental cues to neighboring stem cells, thereby helping to regulate stem cell activity.

In short, stem cell activity is determined by the needs of the cells and tissues in which they reside. As would be expected, stem cell function changes during aging. Stem cells are not protected from the changes at the molecular level that take place as a natural by-product of aging. In addition, mutations take place in mitochondrial DNA in stem cells, leading to irreversible alterations. Because stem cells are reliant on the tissues in which they reside, stem cell aging tends to be tissue cell specific, yet stem cells do help sustain the integrity of the cells that reside within their niche. Further, extrinsic factors and systemic factors can contribute to stem cell aging and loss of functionality. If a stem cell resides in a host that is aging, then the extent to which the stem cell will function optimally depends on the status of the cells in the niche. Researchers have begun to explore the aging of muscle stem cells, of intestinal epithelial stem cells, and of neural stem cells, and it is hoped that the findings from these studies will have implications for stem cells in selected tissues within the auditory system. Research must focus on the environment or the "niche" in which the stem cells are transplanted due to their interdependence.

Sirtuins, Aging, and Prevention of Disease

Sirtuins are longevity assurance genes or longevity genes that are found in the genomes of most living things including bacteria, plants, animals, and humans (Haigis & Sinclair, 2011). Researchers believe that sirtuins sense the environment and modulate the protective mechanisms of cells to maximize survival of individuals when adversity sets in, thereby helping to prevent the onset of disease especially those associated with aging. Interestingly, the work of Haigis & Sinclair (2011) suggests that certain types of sirtuin alleles influence susceptibility to disease, and in fact are able to slow the onset of disease. A growing area of research is the role of sirtuins in the regulation of energy metabolism and metabolic responses central to disease and aging. One type of sirtuin is highly expressed in endothelial cells and is responsible for suppressing the development of atherosclerosis, and may play a role in preventing cerebrovascular disease. Sirtuins also interact with regulators of immune responses and therefore may slow the development of inflammatory disease, which is so common in older adults. Sirtuins can also suppress T-cell activation. The study of sirtuin biology is relatively new, but given the role in energy metabolism, inflammatory disease, and tumor suppression, to name a few areas, the role of sirtuin enzymes in ear disease remains a promising area of study.

◆ Functional Implications of Age-Related Changes Within the Organ Systems

Older adults tend to overestimate their healthiness or underestimate the significance of a specific age-related change in the function of organ systems and associated medical condition(s). This tends to cause delay in their seeking medical assistance for potentially grave diseases and for potentially reversible conditions (Besdine, 1990). A major reason for the tendency to underreport symptoms relates to "ageism." Older adults come to expect that the aging process is associated with irremediable physiological and functional declines as well as selected chronic conditions and disease processes. Accordingly, they regard the changes they experience as conditions they must accept and live with. Also, health care professionals lack familiarity with the normal aging process. Normal old age is increasingly characterized by good health and independence, which are components of successful aging, according to Rowe and Kahn (1998). As Besdine (1990, p. 177) states:

> Although decline in some biologic functions accompanies normal human aging, these declines and their functional impact are gradual, and their impact is further softened by the decades over which they occur and by remaining, if shrinking, physiologic reserve. Major functional decline occurring abruptly in an already aged person should be assumed to be caused by disease, not aging.

Another characteristic of the aging process is the presence of multiple disease processes or chronic conditions. The prevalence of chronic conditions and the potential for co-occurring diseases is directly proportional to age. The oldest and frailest adults may have multiple diseases (Besdine, 1990). A unique characteristic of older adults is the role of functional disability rather than acute disease. In light of the poor correlation among the type and severity of functional disability, age-related changes in organ systems, and disease, a complete examination of older adults entails a comprehensive functional assessment as well as a thorough medical evaluation. The major premise underlying this recommendation is that as we age, several organ systems undergo changes that in isolation or in combination have functional implications for older adults. Often the client's perception of the functional impact of age-related changes in selected organ systems guides referral and management. That is, the functional consequences of disease often take priority over the medical consequences, assuming the change is not life threatening. Finally, one of the most interesting aspects of aging is evidence that supports the existence of cortical plasticity in old age associated with cognitive memory training as well as the positive effects of an active lifestyle on shaping the brain and body (Lemke, 2009). In short, the human brain can be shaped by external influences like learning and practicing.

Knowing about the biological changes accompanying aging is a precondition for meeting the needs and providing appropriate intervention services to the growing number of hearing impaired elderly. The clinical assessment of older adults must by virtue of the changes associated with age be multidimensional, interdisciplinary, and above all functional (Williams, 1994). A multidimensional approach entails quantifying the older adult's medical, psychosocial, and functional capabilities (Brockelhurst & Williams, 1989). An interdisciplinary approach implies collaboration between health professionals and health agencies. Members of the team might include a nurse, social worker, psychologist, audiologist, nutritionist, and physician. A functional approach implies that the physician's reality, namely the etiological and anatomical-pathophysiological diagnoses, is supplemented by the patient's reality, namely the functional diagnosis (Kane et al, 1994). The information that emerges from a comprehensive functional assessment assists in determining overall health, well-being, need for health and social services, and, ultimately, quality of life. Similarly, the audiological history of an older adult should have a functional basis. Self-report scales are used to obtain information about the functional implications of age-related changes throughout the auditory system. The ability of the physician, physician's assistant, nurses, and physical therapists to communicate with older adults with hearing impairment is integral to the quality of care; hence, it is incumbent on audiologists to educate health professionals regarding hallmarks of hearing impairment and how to communicate with older adults with hearing impairments. This is imperative as typically physicians do not have adequate training in the intricacies of hearing loss in older adults.

◆ Implications of Age-Related Changes for Audiological Assessment

In addition to impacting on the questions asked during the case history, the functional implications of changes in the organ systems influence procedures during the routine diagnostic assessment, as well as aspects of audiological rehabilitation. **Table 2.7** summarizes the functional declines and their impact on aspects of assessment and intervention. Keep the test modifications in mind, as they will increase the reliability and validity of test results.

◆ Conclusion

As of this writing, more than 600 million people in the word are 60 years of age or older, representing 10% of the world's population. It is projected that by the year 2050, 21% of the world's population will be 60 years of age or over, a dramatic

Table 2.7 Implications of Age-Related Changes in Organ Systems for Assessment and Intervention

Age-Related Change	Modification	Age-Related Change	Modification
1. Intellectual performance maintained into the 80s	Do not be condescending, do not infantilize.	6. Confusion associated with Alzheimer's disease	Do not correct incorrect responses. If patient cannot answer questions during the case history, assuming the clinician is sure that the question was heard, do not get angry or lose patience. This strategy will avoid emotional responses to failure and catastrophic reactions that can worsen performance on selected tasks.
2. Performing tasks may take longer	Allow extra time in schedule for hearing-aid fitting and post-fitting. Allow enough time between stimulus presentations and patient response.	7. Decrease in recall	During hearing-aid orientation, review material learned at previous session before moving on to new procedures. Use all modalities to ensure or promote recall of new information.
3. More difficulty in learning new tasks	Repeat instructional set. Verify that patient understands response tasks. Verify that patient understands material presented during the hearing-aid orientation and counseling sessions. Use facilitatory strategies to make sure patient learns tasks required.	8. Decreased visual acuity	Make sure test suite and management rooms have adequate illumination. Handouts from audiological rehabilitation sessions should have enlarged print, with highest possible contrast. Printed material is best in black and white.
4. More plasticity at the nerve cell level	Fitting a previously unamplified ear may result in recovery of speech understanding ability.		
5. Motor reaction time decreases	Evaluate difference in response patterns during pure-tone test (e.g., yes/no versus hand-raising or button pushing).		

increase and a call to action for audiologists. It is notable that most of the elderly live in developing countries underscoring the contribution of environment, sanitation, and public health to longevity (Sowers & Rowe, 2007). Hence, for a variety of reasons, the life span of humans is longer than ever before; however, it is notable that the environment does interact with one's genetic makeup to influence longevity (Aviv, 2011). Further, individuals are healthier than ever before well into their eighth or ninth decade of life. As we age, the human body undergoes dramatic changes, yet its resilience is remarkable, as is the ability of organ systems such as the brain to reconfigure their networks. There is great variation in the rate of decline for each organ system, and a decline in function in one organ system does not necessarily imply a similar decline in other organ systems. Similarly, the individual differences in the rate and nature of aging is humbling. It is important to emphasize that environment and lifestyle influence to a great extent the actual and perceived effects of aging on the individual, contributing to the individual variations in the rate at which organ systems age. Further, while physiological reserve diminishes with aging, it often remains adequate unless disease intervenes. There are modifiable life course factors that influence health and aging, and individuals have the ability to influence their life course, including the onset of age-associated functional changes (Sowers & Rowe, 2007).

As individuals age, the ability to communicate with family members, friends, and health care professionals assumes greater importance, and it is the responsibility of audiologists to continue to accumulate evidence for the integral role hearing plays in the quality of the prolonged lives of older adults. Audiologists must be active proponents for hearing health promotion activities, as emerging evidence suggests that our interventions can forestall cognitive aging and enhance life quality. In short, "Good hearing is a precondition for staying active, being involved, participating in social life, and preserving one's cognitive and functional level" (Lemke, 2009, p. 41).

Special Consideration

The response to age-related changes in structure and function is variable and has an impact on management decisions. Audiologists should be cognizant of normal age-related changes to the extent that they may affect the evaluation process, the formulation of an effective rehabilitative approach, and the client's response to management.

References

Abrams, W., Beers, M., & Berkow, R. (1995). *The Merck manual of geriatrics* (2nd ed.). Whitehouse Station, NJ: Merck

Adler, W., & Nagel, J. (1994). Clinical immunology and aging. In W. Hazzard, E. Bierman, J. Blass, W. Ettinger, & J. Halter (Eds.), *Principles of geriatric medicine and gerontology* (3rd ed.). New York: McGraw-Hill

Anderson, N., & Shames, G. (2006). *Human communication disorders: An introduction* (7th ed.). Boston: Allyn & Bacon

Andreoli, A., Scalzo, G., Masala, S., Tarantino, U., & Guglielmi, G. (2009, Mar). Body composition assessment by dual-energy X-ray absorptiometry (DXA). *La Radiologia Medica, 114,* 286–300

Antonucci, T., Birditt, K., & Akiyama, H. (2009). In V. Bengtson, M. Silverstein, N. Putney., & D. Gans (Eds.), *Handbook of theories of aging* (2nd ed.). New York: Springer

Austad, S. (2009). Making sense of biological theories of aging. In V. Bengtson, M. Silverstein, N. Putney., & D. Gans (Eds.). *Handbook of theories of aging* (2nd ed.). New York: Springer

Aviv, A. (2011). Leukocyte telomere dynamics, human aging, and life span. In E. Masoro & S. Austad (Eds.), *Handbook of the biology of aging* (7th ed.). New York: Elsevier

Awan, S. N. (2006, Apr-May). The aging female voice: acoustic and respiratory data. *Clinical Linguistics & Phonetics, 20,* 171–180

Balin, A. (1990). Aging of human skin. In W. Hazzard, R. Andres, E. Bierman, & J. Blass (Eds.), *Principles of geriatric medicine and gerontology.* New York: McGraw-Hill

Baum, B., & Ship, J. (1994). The oral cavity. In W. Hazzard, E. Bierman, J. Blass, W. Ettinger, & J. Halter (Eds.), *Principles of geriatric medicine and gerontology* (3rd ed.). New York: McGraw-Hill

Becker, W., Naumann, H., & Pfaltz, C. (1989). *Ear, nose and throat diseases—a pocket reference.* Stuttgart: Georg Thieme Verlag

Beckman, K. B., & Ames, B. N. (1998, Apr). The free radical theory of aging matures. *Physiological Reviews, 78,* 547–581

Beers, M. (2005). The merck manual of geriatrics. http://www.merck.com/mkgr/mmg/home.jsp

Belchetz, P., & Hammond, P. (2009). Adrenal and pituitary disorders. In H. Fillit, K. Rockwood, & K. Woodhouse (Eds.), *Brockelhurst's textbook of geriatric medicine and gerontology.* Philadelphia: Saunders Elsevier

Bengtson, V., Gans, D., Putney, N., & Silverstein, M. (2009). Theories about aging: handbook of theories of aging. In V. Bengtson, M., Silverstein, N., Putney., D., & Gans, D. (Eds.), *Handbook of theories of aging* (2nd ed.). New York: Springer

Besdine, R. (1990). Clinical evaluation of the elderly patient. In W. Hazzard, R. Andres, E. Bierman, & J. Blass (Eds.), *Principles of geriatric medicine and gerontology* (2nd ed.). New York: McGraw-Hill

Blass, J., Cherniak, P., & Weksler, M. (1992). Theories of aging. In E. Calkins, A. Ford, & P. Katz (Eds.), *Practice of geriatrics.* Philadelphia: W.B. Saunders

Brockelhurst, J., & Williams, T. (1989). Multidisciplinary health assessment of the elderly. *Danish Medical Bulletin. Gerontology, Special Supplement,* 7

Burzynski, C. (1987). The voice. In H. G. Mueller & V. Geoffrey (Eds.), *Communication disorders in aging.* Washington, DC: Gallaudet University Press

Busse, E. (1969). Theories of aging. In E. Busse & E. Pfeiffer (Eds.), *Behavior and adaptation in late life.* Boston: Little, Brown

Carmeli, E., Patish, H., & Coleman, R. (2003, Feb). The aging hand. *J Gerontol Biol Sci Med Sci, 58,* 146–152

Carter, T. L. (1994, Sep). Age-related vision changes: a primary care guide. *Geriatrics, 49,* 37–42, 45, quiz 46–47

Casoli, T., Stefano, G., Delfino, A., Fattoretti, P., & Bertoni-Freddari, C. (2004). Vitamin E deficiency and the aging effect on expression levels of GAP-43 and MAP-2 in selected areas of the brain. *Annals of the New York Academy of Sciences,* Wiley Online Library. http://onlinelibrary.wiley.com/doi/10.1196/annals.1297.008/full.

Chernoff, R. (1990). Nutritional rehabilitation and the elderly. In C. Lewis (Ed.), *Aging: The Health Care Challenge* (2nd ed.). Philadelphia: F. A. Davis

Cigolle, C. T., Langa, K. M., Kabeto, M. U., Tian, Z., & Blaum, C. S. (2007, Aug). Geriatric conditions and disability: the Health and Retirement Study. *Annals of Internal Medicine, 147,* 156–164

Craft, S., Cholerton, B., & Reger, M. (2009). Cognitive changes associated with normal and pathological aging. In J. Halter, J. Ouslander, M. Tinetti, S. Studenski, K. High, & S. Asthana (Eds.), *Hazzard's geriatric medicine and gerontology* (6th ed.). New York: McGraw-Hill

Cristofalo, V. (1990). Biological mechanisms of aging: An overview. In W. Hazzard, R. Andres, E. Bierman, & J. Blass (Eds.), *Principles of geriatric medicine and gerontology* (2nd ed.). New York: McGraw-Hill

Cross, J. M., McGwin, G., Jr., Rubin, G. S., Ball, K. K., West, S. K., Roenker, D. L., et al. (2009, Mar). Visual and medical risk factors for motor vehicle collision involvement among older drivers. *The British Journal of Ophthalmology, 93,* 400–404

Davies, G., & Bolton, C. (2010). Age related changes in the pulmonary system. In H. Fillit, K. Rockwood, & K. Woodhouse (Eds.), *Brockelhurst's textbook of geriatric medicine and gerontology* (7th ed.). Philadelphia: Saunders Elsevier

Dean, E. (1994). Cardiopulmonary development. In B. Bonder & M. Wagner (Eds.), *Functional performance in older adults.* Philadelphia: F. A. Davis

DePinho, R. (2010, Nov). Telomerase reverse aging. *Nature.* http://www.nature.com/news/2010/101128/full/news.2010.635.html

Despopoulos, A., & Silbernagl, S. (1991). *Color atlas of physiology* (4th ed.). New York: Thieme Medical Publishers

Dickstein, D. L., Kabaso, D., Rocher, A. B., Luebke, J. I., Wearne, S. L., & Hof, P. R. (2007, Jun). Changes in the structural complexity of the aged brain. *Aging Cell, 6,* 275–284

Duque, G., & Troen, B. (2009). Osteoporosis. In J. Halter, J. Ouslander, M. Tinetti, S. Studenski, K. High, & S. Asthana (Eds.), *Hazzard's geriatric medicine and gerontology* (6th ed.) New York: McGraw-Hill

Effros, R. (2009). The immunological theory of aging revisited. In V. Bengtson, M. Silverstein, N. Putney., & D. Gans (Eds.), *Handbook of theories of aging* (2nd ed.). New York: Springer

Enright, P. (2009). Aging of the respiratory system. In J. Halter, J. Ouslander, M. Tinetti, S. Studenski, K. High, & S. Asthana (Eds.), *Hazzard's geriatric medicine and gerontology* (6th ed.). New York: McGraw-Hill

Evans, J. (1994). Aging and disease. In D. Evered & J. Whalen (Eds.), *Research and the aging population.* Chichester, England: John Wiley

Falvo, D. (1991). *Medical and psychosocial aspects of chronic disease and disability.* Gaithersburg, MD: Aspen

Fife, R. (1994). Osteoarthritis. In W. Hazzard, E. Bierman, J. Blass, W. Ettinger, & J. Halter (Eds.), *Principles of geriatric medicine and gerontology* (3rd ed.). New York: McGraw-Hill

Fletcher, D. C. (1994, May). Low vision: the physician's role in rehabilitation and referral. *Geriatrics, 49,* 50–53

Francis, R. (2009). Metabolic bone disease. In H. Fillit, K. Rockwood, & K. Woodhouse (Eds.), *Brockelhurst's textbook of geriatric medicine and gerontology* (7th ed.). Philadelphia: Saunders Elsevier

Frick, H., Leonhardt, H., & Starck, D. (1991). *Human anatomy 1. General anatomy, special anatomy: limbs, trunk wall, head and neck* (1st ed.). New York: Thieme Medical Publishers

Fried, L., Walston, J., & Ferrucci, L. (2009). Frailty. In J. Halter, J. Ouslander, M. Tinetti, S. Studenski, K. High, & S. Asthana (Eds.), *Hazzard's geriatric medicine and gerontology* (6th ed.). New York: McGraw-Hill

Friedman, D. S., Wolfs, R. C., O'Colmain, B. J., Klein, B. E., Taylor, H. R., West, S., et al. Eye Diseases Prevalence Research Group (2004, Apr). Prevalence of open-angle glaucoma among adults in the United States. *Archives of Ophthalmology, 122,* 532–538

Galasko, D. (2009). The aging brain. In B. Sadock, V. Sadock, & Ruiz, P. (Eds.), *Comprehensive textbook of psychiatry* (9th ed.). Baltimore: Wolters Kluwer/ Lippincott, Williams & Wilkins

Galvin, J. (2009). Mental status and neurological examination older adults. In J. Halter, J. Ouslander, M. Tinetti, S. Studenski, K. High, & S. Asthana (Eds.), *Hazzard's geriatric medicine and gerontology* (6th ed.). New York: McGraw-Hill

Gameiro, C. M., Romão, F., & Castelo-Branco, C. (2010, Dec). Menopause and aging; changes in the immune system—a review. *Maturitas, 67,* 316–320

Gavrilov, L. A., & Gavrilova, N. S. (2002, Feb). Evolutionary theories of aging and longevity. *TheScientificWorldJournal, 2,* 339–356

Gerschman, R., Gilbert, D. L., Nye, S. W., Dwyer, P., & Fenn, W. O. (1954, May). Oxygen poisoning and x-irradiation: a mechanism in common. *Science, 119,* 623–626

Giangreco, A., Qin, M., Pintar, J. E., & Watt, F. M. (2008, Mar). Epidermal stem cells are retained in vivo throughout skin aging. *Aging Cell, 7,* 250–259

Goh, J. O., & Park, D. C. (2009). Neuroplasticity and cognitive aging: the scaffolding theory of aging and cognition. *Restorative Neurology and Neuroscience, 27,* 391–403

Gonidakis, S., & Longo, V. (2009). Programmed longevity and programmed aging theories. In E. Maroro & S. Austad (Eds.), *Handbook of the biology of aging* (7th ed.). New York: Elsevier

Gregson, C. (2010). Bone and joint aging. In H. Fillit, K. Rockwood, & K. Woodhouse (Eds.), *Brockelhurst's textbook of geriatric medicine and gerontology* (7th ed.). Philadelphia: Saunders Elsevier

Haigis, M., & Sinclair, D. (2011). Sirtuins in aging and age-related diseases. In E. Maroro & S. Austad (Eds.), *Handbook of the biology of aging* (7th ed.). New York: Elsevier

Harman, D. (2006, May). Free radical theory of aging: an update: increasing the functional life span. *Annals of the New York Academy of Sciences, 1067,* 10–21

Hayflick, L. (1994). *How and why we age.* New York: Ballantine Books

Hayflick, L. (2000). The future of aging. *Nature, 408,* 267–269

Howlett, S. (2010). Effects of aging on the cardiovascular system. In H. Fillit, K. Rockwood, & K. Woodhouse (Eds.), *Brockelhurst's textbook of geriatric medicine and gerontology* (7th ed.). Philadelphia: Saunders Elsevier

Kahane, J., & Beckford, N. (1991). The aging larynx and voice. In D. Ripich (Ed.), *Geriatric communication disorders.* Austin: Pro-Ed

Kaminer, M., & Gilchrest, B. (1994). Aging of the skin. In W. Hazzard, E. Bierman, J. Blass, W. Ettinger, J. & Halter (Eds.), *Principles of geriatric medicine and gerontology* (3rd ed.). New York: McGraw-Hill

Kane, R., Ouslander, J., & Abrass, I. (1994). *Essentials of clinical geriatrics* (3rd ed.). New York: McGraw-Hill

Kenney, R. (1988). Physiology of aging. In B. Shadden (Ed.), *Communication behavior and aging.* Baltimore: Williams & Wilkins

Kent, R., & Vorperian, H. (2006). The biology and physics of speech. In N. Anderson & G. Shames (Eds.), *Human communication disorders* (7th ed.). Boston: Pearson

Kirkwood, T. B. (2005, Feb). Understanding the odd science of aging. *Cell, 120,* 437–447

Kirkwood, T. (2009a). Evolution theory and the mechanism of aging. In H. Fillit, K. Rockwood, & K. Woodhouse (Eds.), *Brockelhurst's textbook of geriatric medicine and gerontology* (7th ed.). Philadelphia: Saunders Elsevier

Kirkwood, T. (2009b). Genetics of age-dependent human disease. In J. Halter, J. Ouslander, M. Tinetti, S. Studenski, K. High, & S. Asthana (Eds.), *Hazzard's geriatric medicine and gerontology* (6th ed.). New York: McGraw-Hill

Kitzman, D., & Taffet, G. (2009). Effects of aging on cardiovascular structure and function. In J. Halter, J. Ouslander, M. Tinetti, S. Studenski, K. High, & S. Asthana (Eds.), *Hazzard's geriatric medicine and gerontology* (6th ed., pp. 883–895). New York: McGraw-Hill

Kramer, A., Bherer, L., Colcombe, S., Dong, W., & Greenough, W. (2004). Environmental influences on cognitive and brain plasticity during aging. *Journal Of Gerontology: Medical Sciences, 59,* 940–957

Lakatt, E. (1990). Heart and circulation. In E. Schneider & J. Rowe (Eds.), *Handbook of the biology of aging* (3rd ed.). San Diego: Academic Press

Lawton, S. (2007). Addressing the skin-care needs of the older person. *British Journal of Community Nursing, 12,* 203–204, 206, 208

Lemke, U. (2009). The challenge of aging-sensory, cognitive, socio-emotional and health changes in old age. In *Hearing care for older adults.* Http://www .Phonak.Com/Us/B2b/En/Events/Proceedings/Archive/Adult_Conference _Chicago2009.Html

Lewis, C. (1990). *Aging: The health care challenge* (2nd ed.). Philadelphia: F. A. Davis

Lewis, C., & Bottomley, J. (1990). Musculoskeletal changes with age: clinical implications. In C. Lewis (Ed.), *Aging: The health care challenge* (2nd ed.). Philadelphia: F. A. Davis

Ling, S., & Ju, Y. (2009). Osteoarthritis. In J. Halter, J. Ouslander, M. Tinetti, S. Studenski, K. High, & S. Asthana (Eds.), *Hazzard's geriatric medicine and gerontology* (6th ed.). New York: McGraw-Hill

Liu, L., & Rando, T. A. (2011, Apr). Manifestations and mechanisms of stem cell aging. *Journal of Cell Biology, 193,* 257–266

Loeser, R., & Delbono, O. (2009). Aging of the muscles and joints. In J. Halter, J. Ouslander, M. Tinetti, S. Studenski, K. High, & S. Asthana (Eds.), *Hazzard's geriatric medicine and gerontology* (6th ed.). New York: McGraw-Hill

Manno, R., & Bingham, C. (2011). Rheumatoid arthritis in the older patient. *Clinical Geriatrics, 19,* 43–51

Martin, G. (1992). Biological mechanisms of aging. In J. Evans & T. F. Williams (Eds.), *Oxford textbook of aging.* Oxford: Oxford University Press

Martin, G. (2009). Modalities of gene action predicted by the classical evolutionary theory of aging. In E. Maroro & S. Austad (Eds.), *Handbook of the biology of aging* (7th ed.). New York: Elsevier

Masoro, E. (2010). Physiology of aging. In H. Fillit, K. Rockwood, & K. Woodhouse (Eds.), *Brockelhurst's textbook of geriatric medicine and gerontology* (7th ed.). Philadelphia: Saunders Elsevier

Mattson, M. (2009). Cellular and neurochemical aspects of the aging human brain. In J. Halter, J. Ouslander, M. Tinetti, S. Studenski, K. High, & S. Asthana (Eds.), *Hazzard's geriatric medicine and gerontology* (6th ed.). New York: McGraw-Hill

McCullough, J. L., & Kelly, K. M. (2006, May). Prevention and treatment of skin aging. *Annals of the New York Academy of Sciences, 1067,* 323–331

Miller, R. (1990). Aging and the immune response. In E. Schneider & J. Rowe (Eds.), *Handbook of the biology of aging* (3rd ed.). San Diego: Academic Press

Miller, R. (2009). Biology of aging and longevity. In J. Halter, J. Ouslander, M. Tinetti, S. Studenski, K. High, & S. Asthana (Eds.), *Hazzard's geriatric medicine and gerontology* (6th ed.). New York: McGraw-Hill

Morley, J. (1990). Nutrition and aging. In W. Hazzard, R. Andres, E. Bierman, & J. Blass (Eds.), *Principles of geriatric medicine and gerontology* (2nd ed.). New York: McGraw-Hill

Morley, J., Baumgartner, R., Roubenoff, R., Mayer, J., & Nair, K. (2001). Sarcopenia. http://www.sociciens.org/Morley%20et%20al%202001.pdf

Mrak, R., Griffin, S. T., & Graham, D. I. (1997, Dec). Aging-associated changes in human brain. *Journal of Neuropathology and Experimental Neurology, 56,* 1269–1275

Newman, A. B., Yanez, D., Harris, T., Duxbury, A., Enright, P. L., & Fried, L. P.; Cardiovascular Study Research Group (2001, Oct). Weight change in old age and its association with mortality. *Journal of the American Geriatrics Society, 49,* 1309–1318

Pankow, L., & Solotoroff, J. (2007). Biological aspects and theories of aging. In J. Blackburn & C. Dulmus (Eds.), Handbook of gerontology: Evidence-based approaches to theory, practice, and policy. Hoboken, NJ: John Wiley

Patel, G., Ragi, G., Lambert, W., & Schwartz, R. (2010). Skin diseases and old age. In H. Fillit, K. Rockwood, & K. Woodhouse (Eds.), *Brockelhurst's textbook of geriatric medicine and gerontology* (7th ed.). Philadelphia: Saunders Elsevier

Peterson, M. (1994, Feb). Physical aspects of aging: is there such a thing as "normal"? *Geriatrics, 49,* 45–49, quiz 50–51

Poirier, J., & Finch, C. (1994). Neurochemistry of the aging human brain. In W. Hazzard, E. Bierman, J. Blass, W. Ettinger, & J. Halter (Eds.), *Principles of geriatric medicine and gerontology* (3rd ed.). New York: McGraw-Hill

Polley, D. B., Hillock, A. R., Spankovich, C., Popescu, M. V., Royal, D. W., & Wallace, M. T. (2008, Nov-Dec). Development and plasticity of intra- and intersensory information processing. *Journal of the American Academy of Audiology, 19*, 780–798

Robbins, J., Hind, J., & Barczi, S. (2009). Disorders of swallowing. In J. Halter, J. Ouslander, M. Tinetti, S. Studenski, K. High, & S. Asthana (Eds.), *Hazzard's geriatric medicine and gerontology* (6th ed.). New York: McGraw-Hill

Rochet, A. (1991). Aging and the respiratory system. In D. Ripich (Ed.), *Geriatric communication disorders.* Austin: Pro-Ed.

Roth, E. (1991). The aging process. In R. Hartke (Ed.), *Psychological aspects of geriatric rehabilitation.* Gaithersburg, MD: Aspen

Rowe, J., & Kahn, R. (1998). *Successful aging.* New York: Random House

Saltzman, A. (1992). Pulmonary disorders. In E. Clakins, A. Ford, & R. Katz (Eds.), *Practice of geriatrics* (2nd ed.). Philadelphia: W. B. Saunders

Scheinfeld, N. (2005). Infections in the elderly. *Dermatology Online Journal, 11*, 8. http:/dermatology.cdlib.org/113/reviews/elderly/scheinfeld.html

Schuenke, M., Schulte, E., & Schumacher, U. (2007). *Atlas of anatomy—head and neuroanatomy.* New York: Thieme Medical Publishers

Schulz, R., & Albert, S. (2009). Psychosocial aspects of aging. In J. Halter, J. Ouslander, M. Tinetti, S. Studenski, K. High, & S. Asthana (Eds.), *Hazzard's geriatric medicine and gerontology* (6th ed.). New York: McGraw-Hill

Servat, J. J., Risco, M., Nakasato, Y. R., & Bernardino, C. R. (2011). Visual impairment in the elderly: impact on functional ability and quality of life. *Clinical Geriatrics, 19*, 49–56

Shringarpure, R., & Davies, K. (2009). Free radicals and oxidative stress in aging. In V. Bengtson, M. Silverstein, N. Putney, & D. Gans (Eds.), *Handbook of theories of aging* (2nd ed.). New York: Springer

Singh, G., Pichora-Fuller, K., Hayes, D., Schroeder, H., Carnahan, H. (2012). The aging hand and the ergonomics of hearing aid controls. *Ear and Hearing, 22*, 1–13

Singh, G. (2009). Hearing care for adults 2009—The challenge for aging. In *Hearing care for adults.* Http://Www.Phonak.Com/Us/B2b/En/Events/Proceedings/Archive/Adult_Conference_Chicago2009.Html

Sonies, B. (2006). Swallowing. In N. Anderson & G. Shames (Eds.), *Human communication disorders* (7th ed.). Boston: Pearson

Sowers, K., & Rowe, W. (2007). Global aging. In J. Blackburn & C. Dulmus (Eds.), Handbook of gerontology: Evidence-based approaches to theory, practice, and policy. Hoboken, NJ: John Wiley

Straus, S., & Tinetti, M. (2009). Evaluation, management and decision making with the older patient. In J. Halter, J. Ouslander, M. Tinetti, S. Studenski, K. High, & S. Asthana (Eds.), *Hazzard's geriatric medicine and gerontology* (6th ed.). New York: McGraw-Hill

Supiano, M. (2009). Hypertension. In J. Halter, J. Ouslander, M. Tinetti, S. Studenski, K. High, & S. Asthana (Eds.), *Hazzard's geriatric medicine and gerontology* (6th ed.). New York: McGraw-Hill

Tabbara, K. (1989). Anatomy and embryology of the eye. In D. Vaughan, T. Asbury, & K. Tabarra (Eds.), *General ophthalmology* (12th ed.). Norwalk: Appleton & Lange

Tarawneh, R., & Galvin, J. (2010). Neurologic signs in the elderly. In H. Fillit, K. Rockwood, & K. Woodhouse (Eds.), *Brockelhurst's textbook of geriatric medicine and gerontology* (7th ed.). Philadelphia: Saunders Elsevier

Tideiksaar, R., & Silverton, R. (1989). *Falling in old age: Its prevention and treatment.* New York: Springer

Tielsch, J. M., Sommer, A., Katz, J., Royall, R. M., Quigley, H. A., & Javitt, J. (1991, Jul). Racial variations in the prevalence of primary open-angle glaucoma. The Baltimore Eye Survey. *Journal of the American Medical Association, 266*, 369–374

Tonet, A., & Nóbrega, O. (2008). Immunosenescence: The association between leukocytes, cytokines and chronic diseases. *Revista Brasileira de Geriatria Gerontologia, 11*, 259–273.

Tremblay, K., & Ross, B. (2007, Jul-Aug). Effects of age and age-related hearing loss on the brain. *Journal of Communication Disorders, 40*, 305–312

Vance, D., & Crowe, M. (2006). A proposed model of neuroplasticity and cognitive reserve in older adults. *Activities, Adaptation and Aging, 30*, 61–79

Varma, R., Choudhury, F., Klein, R., Chung, J., Torres, M., & Azen, S. (2010). Four-year incidence and progression of diabetic retinopathy and macular edema: the Los Angeles Latino Eye Study. *American Journal of Ophthalmology, 149*, 735–740

Veysey, E., & Finlay, A. (2010). Aging and the skin. In H. Fillit, K. Rockwood, & K. Woodhouse (Eds.), *Brockelhurst's textbook of geriatric medicine and gerontology* (7th ed.). Philadelphia: Saunders Elsevier

Vlassara, H., Ferrucci, L., Post, J., & Striker, G. (2009). Decline of renal function in normal aging, role of oxidants/inflammation: When does it begin: Is it inevitable, preventable, or treatable? In Geriatric Nephrology Curriculum, http://www.asn-online.org/education and meetings/distancelearning/curricula/geriatrics/OnlineGeriatricsCurriculum.pdf

Walford, R. (1969). The immunologic theory of aging. Copenhagen: Munksgaard

Warner, H., Sierra, F., & Thompson, L. (2010). Biology of aging. In H. Fillit, K. Rockwood, & K. Woodhouse (Eds.), *Brockelhurst's textbook of geriatric medicine and gerontology* (7th ed.). Philadelphia: Saunders Elsevier

Watson, G. (2009). Assessment and rehabilitation of older adults with low vision. In J. Halter, J. Ouslander, M. Tinetti, S. Studenski, K. High, & S. Asthana (Eds.), *Hazzard's geriatric medicine and gerontology* (6th ed.). New York: McGraw-Hill

Weinert, B. T., & Timiras, P. S. (2003, Oct). Invited review: Theories of aging. *Journal of Applied Physiology (Bethesda, Md.), 95*, 1706–1716

Williams, M. (1994). Clinical management of the elderly patient. In W. Hazzard, E. Bierman, J. Blass, W. Ettinger, & J. Halter (Eds.), *Principles of geriatric medicine and gerontology* (3rd ed.). New York: McGraw-Hill

Willis, S., Schaie, K., & Martin, M. (2009). Cognitive plasticity. In V. Bengtson, M. Silverstein, N. Putney, & D. Gans (Eds.), *Handbook of theories of aging* (2nd ed.). New York: Springer

Willis, S. L., Tennstedt, S. L., Marsiske, M., Ball, K., Elias, J., Koepke, K. M., et al.; ACTIVE Study Group (2006, Dec). Long-term effects of cognitive training on everyday functional outcomes in older adults. *Journal of the American Medical Association, 296*, 2805–2814[Vance]

Wingfield, A., Tun, P., McCoy, S., Steward, R., & Cox, C. (2006). Sensory and cognitive constraints in comprehension of spoken language in adult aging. *Seminars in Hearing, 27*, 273–283

Wong, T. (2002). Aging of the cerebral cortex. *McGill Journal of Medicine, 6*, 104–113

Yan, D., McPheeters, S., Johnson, G., Utzinger, U., & Vande Geest, J. (2011). Microstructural differences in the human posterior sclera as a function of age and race. *Investigative Ophthalmology & Visual Science, 52*, 821–829

Yonelinas, A. P., Widaman, K., Mungas, D., Reed, B., Weiner, M. W., & Chui, H. C. (2007). Memory in the aging brain: doubly dissociating the contribution of the hippocampus and entorhinal cortex. *Hippocampus, 17*, 1134–1140

Yorkston, K., & Garrett, K. (1997). Assistive communication with technology of elders with motor speech disability. In R. Lubinski & D. Higginbotham (Eds.), *Communication technologies.* San Diego: Singular Publishing Group

Chapter 3

Psychosocial Changes with Aging

Society in general and health care professionals in particular should be more sensitive to our plight. . . . They too will one day confront the challenge of old age.

— *M.L.S. (a 78-year-old psychiatrist)*

Lifestyle choices more than genes determine how well we age.

— *Rowe and Kahn (1998)*

◆ Learning Objectives

After reading this chapter, you should be able to

- explain the social aspects of aging;
- the psychological changes and cognitive changes associated with normal aging; and
- relate psychosocial aspects of aging to evaluative and management strategies for older hearing-impaired adults.

◆ Overview

Despite physical and cognitive decline, mounting social loss, and psychological stress, older adults enjoy high levels of affective well-being. Although individuals vary, for the most part as people age, emotional health improves, such that most older adults adjust well to their later years (Scheibe and Carstensen, 2010). The greater an individual's biological and psychological reserves, the better able he or she is to cope with life's challenges and the life course. Despite commonly held opinions, as will be discussed in this chapter, it appears that for some seniors, psychological resources are often greater because of their life experience and their acquisition of knowledge, skills, and coping strategies (Scheibe and Carstensen, 2010). It is these seniors who will more successfully cope with a hearing impairment. **Table 3.1** lists the broad domains in which change occurs. This chapter discusses the changes in these domains, the factors that influence psychosocial adjustment, and the implications of these changes for audiological practice. The premise of this chapter is that despite the onset of chronic conditions and numerous transitions, older adults have the capacity to remain functional thanks to numerous protective influences (Ryff and Singer, 2009).

Our discussion of the domains listed in **Table 3.1** will be facilitated by a preliminary overview of the interdisciplinary field of gerontology and the perspectives on which it is based (Bass, 2006). Gerontology arose as an interdisciplinary field in the mid-1940s with the establishment of the Gerontological Society of America. Late life is generally a period of transition and adjustment to a multiplicity of losses. These transitions include retirement and relocation. Bereavement is a complex phenomenon associated with loss of companionship, primarily the death of a spouse (Abrams, Beers, & Berkow, 1995). Loss triggers a decline in social interaction and often a change in social status. As would be expected, the social context of aging increases the risk of disease and the experience of illness. The literature on social gerontology posits that lifestyle is an important influence on the experience of aging and on how older adults adapt to it, and in turn such factors as sensory acuity and physical capacity are fundamental to lifestyle choices throughout life (Hendricks and Hatch, 2009).

◆ The Social Domain

Many social theories have been advanced to explain and account for the behavior of older adults in a social context. Many of the original theories of aging have been discredited, but they are discussed here because of their important role in the field of gerontology.

Pearl

The health care professional's ability to deliver timely and appropriate care depends in large part on an understanding of the social context in which illness takes place and on the care ultimately provided.

The Disengagement Theory

Constructed for and by gerontologists, and largely discredited today, the disengagement theory is the earliest, best known, and most controversial theory of American gerontology (Achenbaum, 2009). The disengagement theory was first described by Cumming and Henry (1961). It posits that normal aging is

Table 3.1 Domains of Change

1. The social domain
2. The biological domain
3. The psychological domain
   a. Personality
   b. Cognitive

an inevitable mutual withdrawal or disengagement by aging individuals and the society to which they belong. Cumming and Henry reasoned that this voluntary curtailment of involvement in social relationships arises from inner psychological changes wherein the individual comes to prefer less input and interactions with the outside world. In short, Cumming and Henry theorized that disengagement is innate, unidirectional, and universal (Achenbaum, 2009). Based on their interviews of over 200 older adults, Cumming and Henry concluded that once the disengagement process is complete, the morale of the individual will be high and the person will be satisfied with his or her niche in life and will no longer have to compete with younger rivals. For society, the withdrawal of older persons allows younger, more energetic persons to assume the functional roles necessary for society to thrive (Cox, 1988).

The validity of the contention that disengagement is a voluntary, self-imposed correlate of old age, and of Cumming and Henry's prescription of "withdrawal for happiness," has been challenged due to methodological shortcomings and because of the accumulation of empirical data that fails to support their postulates (Botwinick, 1973; Maddox, 1965). Recently, Cummings and Henry publicly disagreed with their own theory, concluding that in fact people do not normally disengage. Disengagement, if it occurs, is dependent on the lifelong personality of the individual. It can be viewed as adaptive from the perspective of the individual and society. But disengagement also can be viewed as a symptom or consequence of one or more disorders requiring professional attention (Davis, 1990). Within the disengagement theory, Cumming and Henry (1961) described three types of changes taking place in relation to their social systems, namely changes in the amount, style, and purpose of interactions (Lewis & Bottomley, 2008).

Internal factors, such as physical and mental health status, and external factors, such as social structure, socioeconomic status, and educational level, have been implicated as contributing to disengagement. With regard to health, the insults of old age (e.g., physical incapacity, mental status) preclude the maintenance of the social involvement that characterizes one's earlier years. But the quality and quantity of interpersonal contacts as well as participation in various activities bear a positive relationship to physical functional status (Maddox, 1965).

In my doctoral dissertation I reviewed the disengagement literature, and I found that none of the investigations designed to examine the contribution of physical health to social isolation considered hearing status as a possible determinant of the social withdrawal that characterizes many elderly individuals (Weinstein, 1980). I explored the relationship among hearing loss, hearing handicap, and social isolation in a sample

of older male veterans. I administered a subjective and an objective isolation scale to 80 male veterans ranging in age from 65 to 88 years. The majority (71%) of subjects had mild to moderate, bilaterally symmetrical, sensorineural hearing loss. There was a wide range in the perception of hearing handicap that was based on scores on the Hearing Measurement Scale (Noble and Atherly, 1970). Subjects were in good physical health and had no history of psychological problems. The subjective social isolation scale yielded information on the desire to interact with others, interest in engaging in various activities, feelings of loneliness, and satisfaction with the quality of interactions. The objective isolation scale quantified contacts with significant others, participation in leisure/recreational activities, and living arrangements. Scores on the isolation scales were comparable to scores obtained in a Cross-National Study of the physical, social, and mental problems confronting community-based older adults. In the latter study, hearing loss was not considered an important variable potentially contributing to social isolation.

I found that self-perceived hearing handicap, and to a lesser extent the severity of the hearing impairment, was positively associated with the magnitude of subjective social isolation reported by my sample of older adults. Interestingly, self-perceived hearing handicap accounted for more of the variability among subjects in their feeling social isolated than did the index of physical health. In contrast, an objective measure of social isolation did not bear a strong relationship to audiological measures. More in-depth analysis of responses to the objective social isolation scale revealed that the extent of participation in leisure activities and the pursuit of solitary activities such as television viewing, making telephone calls, and other activities was strongly associated with hearing loss severity. A greater proportion of individuals with moderately severe to severe hearing loss withdrew socially than did persons with lesser impairments. Further, it was possible to rank subjects as to their isolation status according to their performance on audiological tasks. In general, persons categorized as being subjectively and objectively isolated had greater hearing handicaps and hearing impairments than did nonisolates or individuals who were not classified as subjectively or objectively isolated. Further, subjective isolates were more impaired and handicapped than objective isolates.

The Lighthouse National Survey of Vision Loss (Lighthouse, 1995), a nationwide study of older adults' experiences with vision impairment, found that vision loss also has an impact on the quantity and quality of social interactions. The overriding complaint was that vision loss makes it difficult to get to places outside the home and interferes with leisure activities. Taken together, the Lighthouse study and prior studies challenging the disengagement theory lend support to the notion that disengagement is not universally natural, and very often is imposed from outside (Botwinick, 1973).

Pearl

Age-related chronic conditions, such as hearing and visual loss, are variables that may contribute to inactivity in later life.

The Activity Theory

Arising in response to the disengagement theory, the activity theory as advocated by Bernice Neugarten (1964) posited that maintenance of one's relationships and continued involvement was key to successful aging. Although having a different slant, the activity theory maintained some of the same philosophy underpinning the disengagement theory (Achenbaum, 2009; Havighurst, 1963). The activity theory poses a view of successful aging that is exactly opposite that presented by the disengagement theory. It emphasizes the importance of maintaining an active lifestyle such that for every role that an individual gives up, there should be a suitable replacement (Neugarten, 1966). It posits that older people must stay active and involved to continue to maintain their own integrity. Further, as individuals age, the nature of the activities most important to life satisfaction may change (Botwinick, 1973). Whereas formal activities (e.g., participation in voluntary activities) or solitary activities (e.g., household activities) were a priority early in life, more informal activities (e.g., interaction with friends, relatives, or neighbors) take on greater importance (Neugarten, 1975). In general, contact with friends and relatives appear not to decline until the eighties, as maintenance of social relationships is critical to life satisfaction. It is of interest that 40 to 50% of older adults with mild to moderate sensorineural hearing loss perceive that hearing impairment interferes with interactions with friends, relatives, and neighbors, leading to psychosocial handicap. The extent to which hearing loss that is handicapping in the domain of informal activities interferes with life satisfaction remains a question in need of investigation. Critics of the activity theory hold that it ignores cultural differences, health and economic disparities, and how they may contribute to curtailment of activity level (Achenbaum, 2009).

The Continuity Dialogic Theory

The continuity dialogic theory evolved as a bridge between the disengagement and activity theories. Recall that the proponents of the disengagement theory argue that disengagement is a normal, healthy, "functional" adjustment to old age. In contrast, advocates of the activity theory contend that social activity is predictive of better physical function and higher happiness/life satisfaction ratings. Sociologists disenchanted with each of these theories have proposed an alternative view of the aging process, namely the continuity theory (Atchley, 1999), which holds that in the course of the aging process, the individual tends to maintain stability in the areas established throughout life. Thus, a person's habits, associations, and lifestyle early on will predispose the person to maintain the same preferences in later years. Continuity theorists also hold that neither activity nor inactivity underly or guarantee happiness in old age. Whereas proponents of the disengagement and activity theories hold that successful adaptation to the aging process is defined by inactivity or activity, the continuity theory posits that past history and preferred lifestyle mediate the individual's adaptation (Cox, 1988). Thus, the continuity theory allows for a multiplicity of adjustment patterns and acknowledges that positive aging is an adaptive process with interactions among biological, environmental, and social factors.

Rowe and Kahn (1998) underline the importance of engagements with family and friends as critical to successful aging. According to proponents of the continuity theory, activities in old age reflect a continuation of patterns established early in life (Lewis & Bottomley, 2008). Critics of the continuity theory argue that it too ignores the importance of the variables that shape individuals as they age, namely, exogenous societal factors (Achenbaum, 2009).

> **Pearl**
>
> From the rehabilitative standpoint, a major implication of the continuity theory is that clinicians must appreciate the life activities that are important to the individual, determine the extent to which hearing loss interferes with pursuing these activities, and design an intervention program that addresses the limitations.

The Exchange Theory

Firmly rooted in rationalism, the exchange theory posits that humans choose courses of action based on the anticipated outcomes available from an array of alternatives. Exchange theorists posit that individuals choose goals that will lead to the most beneficial outcomes (Lewis & Bottomley, 2008). Further, exchange theorists hold that the goals espoused by most people include maintenance of interactions with other persons or groups. Also, people tend to be oriented toward attaining rewards for their social behavior and like to reduce their costs, with every effort being made to avoid costs that exceed the rewards (Lewis & Bottomley, 2008). The principle of reciprocity is at the heart of the exchange theory, suggesting that people tend to choose alternatives that will help those who helped them along the way. Interestingly, exchange theorists suggest that as people age they lose resources and hence they experience inequality and a loss of power. In a sense this idea is suggestive of a type of marginalization that takes place as people age, wherein policy decisions adversely affect standing in the workplace, the community, and other social institutions (Achenbaum, 2009).

Finally, it is important to note that gerontologists increasingly acknowledge that diversity is a hallmark of "late life," and that identity is as varied as the forces acting on individuals at this stage (Achenbaum, 2009). Proponents who believe older adults are marginalized in late life suggest that social factors including policy decision adversely affect older adults in the workplace, in the community, and in some social institutions. For example, recent cuts in funding for senior centers are an increasingly widespread phenomenon, as are cuts to Medicare. In contrast, gerontologists who believe that adults in later life are self-dependent and autonomous argue that older adults are empowered as they age because they enjoy resources and political access that they may not have had as younger adults (Achenbaum, 2009). In the political and social realms, this has had an impact on health care and decisions regarding end-of-life care and use of restraints in nursing homes.

In summary, theories of aging tend to swing from one extreme to the other beginning with the disengagement versus activity theory and concluding with the marginalization versus the self-dependent theory (Achenbaum, 2009). In my view this just confirms the need for theories to explain the diversity that is synonymous with individuals in later life. The dualism grows out of the multidisciplinary focus that characterizes gerontology and that should inform the work of audiologists who treat older adults. Older adults who are independent and engaged will have different needs from those who are disengaged and dependent on a caregiver. Despite the differences, however, audiological interventions can enhance the quality of life as individuals age.

<table>
<tr><td>Pearl</td></tr>
</table>

The components of successful aging include low risk of disease, high physical and mental function, and active engagement with family and friends (Rowe and Kahn, 1998).

◆ The Psychological Domain

Personality

The natural growth process of the personality from birth to late life sets the stage for understanding the psychological changes the come with aging. Human development has been described in terms of life cycle phases. Focusing on ego and personality development, the premise of Erikson's model of development is that an individual successfully overcomes or meets the challenges of each stage and emerges as a healthy, mature personality (**Table 3.2**). One of the first psychological theorists who developed a personality theory that extended from birth into old age, Erikson (1968) viewed human development as consisting of a series of eight stages (Lewis & Bottomley, 2008). Each stage represents a choice in the development the ego, and Erikson theorized that if one does not successfully complete a stage, it will be difficult to meet the demands of a subsequent stage. In fact, failure in one stage can result in psychological problems related to that stage and may predispose the individual to failure in later stages. According to Erikson, there are increasingly more chances to fail at each subsequent stage, making the final stage of life the most challenging and difficult to attain (Verwoerdt, 1976). Erikson's stages of personality and ego development help us to under-stand the emotional reactions to the physical and social changes that older adults undergo as well as the enormous individual variability so characteristic of older adults. His formulations can also be invaluable as a guide to intervening with older adults who may or may not have successfully mastered each of the stages of development (Davis, 1990). In Erikson's view, successful aging means that a person accepts his or her life, and if asked if they would want to do it over again, would resoundingly say yes (Lewis & Bottomley, 2008).

Erikson also acknowledged that family, the environment, and society influence to a large extent the ability to master the crises associated with each stage, and the ultimate move to and mastery of succeeding stages. He hypothesized that psychopathology may develop when the challenges of a stage are not met or resolved. The outcome of the final stage strongly influences the older adult's ability to cope with the losses and stresses of late adulthood. The challenge for older adults is to respond to and be aggressive about positive and negative social and physical forces that arise, with the goal being to maintain and increase self-esteem and to take responsibility for one's life (Davis, 1990). Decline in physical function and vulnerability to illness can lead to depression and psychosomatic illness, thereby interfering with the attainment of integrity (Kaplan, Sadock, & Grubb, 1994; Verwoerdt, 1976). Similarly, loss of independence and the need for physical and economic assistance can have devastating effects. The environment, including shrinkage of one's peer group; retirement; and decline of the nuclear family can also interfere with resolution of the last stage of the life cycle. Thus, biological and environmental hazards are likely to interfere with successful completion of the ultimate stage of life. Kaplan and his colleagues underline the importance of active preparation for old age as a way of offsetting some of the negative consequences that arise because of the difficulty in successfully passing through the psychosocial crisis of integrity versus despair.

Although old age historically was regarded as a time of physical, social, psychological, and economic challenges, the current thinking, paradoxically, is that older adults are very resilient and have higher rates of emotional well-being than other adult age groups (Zarit, 2009). Furthermore, to promote well-being, health care professionals must work together to create conditions so that even in the face of a multiplicity of chronic conditions and socioeconomic challenges, older adults

Table 3.2 Erikson's Stages of Development

Period in Life	Erikson's Stage	Description
0–12 months	Trust versus mistrust	Hopeful, self-confident versus mistrustful
1–3 years	Autonomy versus shame and doubt	Autonomous, proud versus self-doubt, self-conscious
3–6 years (preschool)	Initiative versus guilt	Creative, independent versus guilt and inhibition
6–12 years (school age)	Industry versus inferiority	Productive, positive learning versus inadequacy, self-doubt, and inhibited
12–18 years (adolescence)	Identity versus role/ identity confusion	Inner solidarity, knowledge of oneself versus role confusion
18–35 years (young adulthood)	Intimacy versus Isolation	Trust, sharing versus distancing from others
35–60 years (middle age)	Generativity versus Stagnation	Mentoring, guiding new generations, nurturance versus self-absorption, preoccupation
Over 60 years (late life)	Integrity versus Despair	Sense of satisfaction, acceptance with oneself and station in life versus despair, anger

Sources: Lewis, C., & Bottomley, J. (2008). *Geriatric rehabilitation: A clinical approach.* Upper Saddle River, NJ: Pearson Education; Erikson, E. (1968). *Identity: Youth and crisis.* New York: W. W. Norton; and Corey, G. (1991). *Theory and practice of counseling and psychotherapy* (4th ed.). Pacific Grove, CA: Brooks/Cole.

Table 3.3 Traits of the Five Personality Factors

Factor	Characteristics
Neuroticism	Calm, comfortable, unemotional, self-satisfied versus worrisome, self-conscious, emotional, insecure
Extraversion	Reserved, quiet, passive, task-oriented versus affectionate, talkative, active, person-oriented
Openness	Conventional, conservative, uncreative versus original, liberal, creative, curious
Agreeableness	Ruthless, suspicious, critical, manipulative, rude versus soft-hearted, trusting, lenient
Conscientiousness	Negligent, lazy, disorganized, careless, unreliable versus conscientious, hard-working, well-organized

Source: Costa, P., & McCrae, R. (1994). Personality and aging. In W. Hazzard, E. Bierman, J. Blass, W. Ettinger, & J. Halter (Eds.), *Principles of geriatric medicine and gerontology* (3rd ed.). New York: McGraw-Hill.

can be considered to be "successfully aging" (Zarit, 2009). In fact, evidence is accumulating to suggest that part of normal human development is the enhancement of emotional experience across the course of the life span (Kryla-Lighthall & Mather, 2009). Interestingly, directing one's cognitive resources toward pursuing emotionally gratifying experiences helps to promote well-being in old age.

Personality traits are highly stable and tend to remain the same throughout life, unless the social or physical stresses of old age interfere (McCrae & Costa, 2006). McCrae and Costa (2006) and Costa and McCrae (1994) described the five-factor model of personality that derives in large part from biological tendencies and unfolds over time (**Table 3.3**). Each of the five domains of personality helps to explain the four basic elements of personality: motivation, emotion, interpersonal style, and experiential style. Cross-sectional and longitudinal studies have been conducted in an effort to measure changes across each of these personality traits. In general, personality traits do not appear to change in individuals over 30 years of age (Costa & McCrae, 1994). It appears that all five of the major dimensions of personality are highly stable in adults after age 30. In short, adult personality is attained by age 30, and barring outside events, personality profiles are maintained throughout life.

The extent to which apparent changes in personality can be attributed to physical, cognitive, or social factors is constantly under investigation, yet many psychologists agree that there are individual differences in the stability of the personality traits over time. Further, cultural factors influence the evolution, development, and expression of personality, and audiologists must remain attuned to this (McCrae & Costa, 2006). It is also important to point out that personality style, such as level of neuroticism or conscientiousness, may provide insight into health behavior and may influence management decisions, and we now know that it influences outcomes with hearing aids. For example, an individual who scores high on the neuroticism scale may self-rate a mild hearing impairment as more handicapping than an individual who scores low. Similarly, an individual who scores high on the conscientiousness factor may be motivated to purchase a hearing aid and undergo audio-

logical rehabilitation, whereas an individual who scores low on this factor may require counseling to motivate him or her to seek intervention. Extraversion, which includes the components warmth, gregariousness, and assertiveness, influences the desire for social stimulation and personal interactions, and adequate reception and perception are key to fulfillment of the need for contact with family and friends (Krause, 2009). Hearing impairment and personality traits influence adjustment to hearing aid use such that individuals who score low on the agreeableness factor seem to be more variable in terms of the stability of outcome regarding self-reported benefit over time (Cox, Alexander, & Gray, 2004).

In conclusion, the evidence suggests that older adults have considerable reserve capacity or potential for change and positive growth in the cognitive domains in terms of social transactions and in terms of positive psychological functioning (Ryff & Singer, 2009). Their capacity to maintain high levels of well-being in the face of many transitions applies to their ability to cope with the multiplicity of the chronic conditions that they often face (Ryff & Singer, 2009).

Cognitive Function

Cognition is defined as the process of obtaining, organizing, and using the fund of intellectual knowledge (Kaplan et al, 1994). Cognition implies an understanding of the connection between cause and effect, between an action and the consequences of that action. It also implies calling up and processing relevant information from stored memory and making use of the fund of knowledge acquired throughout life. Cognitive changes associated with the normal aging process include decreases in attention, processing speed, working memory, cognitive flexibility, executive function, and fluid intelligence. Interestingly, as one's fund of knowledge expands throughout life, learning ability does not decline with normal aging, which bodes well for older adults who find themselves in a position to learn new skills as they adapt to sensory loss and visuospatial and perceptual changes (Tarawneh & Galvin, 2010). In light of age-related declines in cognitive performance in such domains as working memory and reasoning, it is imperative that audiologists be aware of the magnitude and rate of change in cognitive function because the changes impact on every aspect of the evaluation and management process.

The aspects of cognitive function that will be discussed here are cognitive reserve, executive function, learning capacity, memory, intelligence, attention, and processing speed (**Table 3.4**). It is noteworthy that changes in any of these domains can act as a diagnostic window into some form of medical, neurological, or psychiatric problem requiring immediate referral. The literature on cognitive plasticity and on latent cognitive potential for adaptation and change is growing, as this is a fertile area of research for audiologists (Willis, Schaie, & Martin, 2009). Cognitive plasticity also affects the older adult's ability to acquire cognitive skills. In short, it is now well accepted that cognitive plasticity takes place at the brain, behavioral, and sociocultural levels, and there are reciprocal relations among brain, experience, and behavior. Specifically, emerging data suggest that performance on tests of fluid intelligence improves as a consequence of interventions that make use of guided instruction on problem-solving tasks (Baltes & Linden-

Table 3.4 Cognitive Functions

Intelligence	Overall ability on all types of intellectual tasks, and can be divided into fluid and crystallized intelligence
Executive function	The ability to respond to a novel stimulus, to control and direct behavior, and to make reasonable judgments
Attention and processing speed	Ability to focus on one or more pieces of auditory or visual information for a prolonged period of time long and make use of the input; serves as the foundation for working memory and other cognitive processes
Memory	Learning and recall of new and learned information
Executive function	The ability to control and direct behavior, to make meaningful inferences and judgments, to plan and execute tasks, ability to complete abstract and complex tasks
Cognitive reserve	Ability to compensate once pathology interferes with the portion of the brain that underlies performance

Sources: Craft, S., Cholerton, B., & Reger, M. (2009). In J. Halter, J. Ouslander, M. Tinetti, S. Studenski, K. High, & S. Asthana (Eds.), *Hazzard's geriatric medicine and gerontology* (6th ed.). New York: McGraw-Hill; and Martin, J., & Gorenstein, M. (2010). Normal cognitive aging. In H. Fillit, K. Rockwood, & K. Woodhouse (Eds.), *Brockelhurst's textbook of geriatric medicine and gerontology* (7th ed.). Philadelphia: Saunders Elsevier.

berger, 1988). It is of interest that there is evidence that self-guided cognitive training modules that require minimal instruction and group training modules that require a tutor yield comparable results in terms of producing gains in cognitive skills and fluid intelligence (Baltes, Sowarka, & Kliegl, 1989). The contribution that restoration of audibility makes to the various levels of cognitive plasticity remains to be fully explored.

> **Pearl**
>
> Older adults display different levels of cognitive performance and different rates of cognitive decline.

Intelligence

Intelligence is a multifaceted and complex construct that can be defined as the ability to accumulate, assimilate, process, store, and retrieve information (Bienfeld, 1990). Intelligence can be viewed as having two rather different components: crystallized and fluid. Crystallized intelligence involves experience, meaning, knowledge, wisdom, and professional expertise and comprises the knowledge, skills, and information gained from experience that one brings to a situation. In short, crystallized intelligence involves experience and consists of a knowledge base acquired early in life. In contrast, fluid intelligence entails the approaches one brings to reasoning and problem solving and is not impacted by prior training (Martin & Gorenstein, 2010). To gain an appreciation of a patient's fluid intelligence, abstract problem-solving ability is assessed. Fluid intelligence can be viewed as a measure of the brain's ability to reorganize data into new pathways and is thought to be dependent on the integrity of the central nervous system (Hartke, 1991). When intelligence is measured according to this categorization scheme, profound age differences are noted, favoring younger adults. There is general agreement that fluid intelligence tends to plateau in young adulthood and eventually declines, whereas crystallized intelligence increases from childhood to late adulthood (Martin & Gorenstein, 2010).

The cornerstone of the neuropsychological assessment, intelligence is usually defined as performance on a battery of intellectual tasks. The gold standard and the most popular and widely used test to measure intellectual functioning in research

and clinical environments is the latest revision of the Wechsler Adult Intelligence Scale (WAIS-III (Martin & Gorenstein, 2010). Norms on the WAIS-III extend from 16 to 89 years of age (Swanda & Haaland, 2009). Crystallized intelligence is measured by performance on the vocabulary and general information subtests of the WAIS. Fluid intelligence is assessed using the block design and the digit symbol subtests. The WAIS uses a battery of complex verbal and visuospatial tasks to summarize Verbal, Performance, and Full-Scale IQ. Level of functioning is reported as borderline, low average, average, high average, or superior. The WAIS-III provides an estimate of premorbid ability or long-standing level of knowledge by testing overlearned activities or one's fund of general information, which is less resistant to change with age. An estimate of premorbid intelligence can help gauge the degree to which one's intellectual function has declined over time. As vocabulary, information, and picture completion tend to remain stable over time, performance on these three tests provides estimates of premorbid cognitive function. Some of the other intellectual functions assessed with the WAIS-III include auditory-verbal span of attention (Digits Forward) and cognitive manipulation of increasingly long strands of digits (Digits Backward); immediate recall and delayed retention using verbal and visual material; and performance IQ is assessed in part using block design and picture arrangement. It is critical to emphasize that there is considerable variability in performance on tests of intellectual function. The variability is most likely due to internal factors (e.g., age-related alterations in brain function) and external factors (e.g., environmental variables).

> **Special Consideration**
>
> Crystallized intelligence appears to remain stable or increase throughout adulthood, whereas fluid intelligence tends to decline with the insults of old age (Friedan, 1993; Horn & Cattell, 1967).

Executive function, which plays an important role is one's capacity to respond to novel situations, relates to an individual's ability to self-monitor, and to plan and initiate independent activities. Further, inhibition of responses that are not appropriate, problem-solving responses, control of complex motoric responses, and the ability to manipulate multiple pieces of information at one time all fall under the rubric of

Table 3.5 Components of Executive Function

Component	Definition
Volition	The ability to act intentionally
Planning	Process and steps involved in achieving a goal
Purposive Action	Productive active required to execute a plan
Effective Performance	Ability to self-correct and monitor behavior

Source: Martin, J., & Gorenstein, M. (2010). Normal cognitive aging. In H. Fillit, K. Rockwood, & K. Woodhouse (Eds.), *Brockelhurst's textbook of geriatric medicine and gerontology* (7th ed.). Philadelphia: Saunders Elsevier.

executive function (Craft, Cholerton, & Reger, 2009; Swanda & Haaland, 2009). Psychologists consider executive function to have four different components: volition, planning, purposive action, and effective performance (Martin & Gorenstein, 2010). Interestingly, as is evident from **Table 3.5**, each of these must be intact for a patient to complete an audiological evaluation, including compliance with follow-up recommendations, and is key to a successful hearing-aid fitting and to appropriate use of communication strategies. In fact, difficulty implementing strategies is a hallmark of deficits in executive function. It is noteworthy that executive functions are sometimes referred to as frontal lobe functions, as the prefrontal cortex and extensive cerebral interconnections between cortical and subcortical regions of the brain appear to underlie executive functions (Martin & Gorenstein, 2010). As was discussed in Chapter 2, the frontal lobe undergoes deterioration with age, including a loss of volume in the prefrontal cortex; hence, it is not surprising that executive function, along with memory and attention, tend to change with age. Although mental flexibility tends to decline, real-world executive functions remain amazingly intact with age. Audiologists should consider screening for executive function using the primary measures of executive function, such as the Wisconsin Card Sorting Test (WCST) and the Trail Making Test, Part B (Grant & Berg, 1948; Strauss, Sherman, & Spreen, 2006)

Pearl

Age-related reduction in working memory capacity is mediated by slowing of the processing speed with age (Salthouse, 1996)

Attention

Attention is viewed by some as the mechanism by which we identify important features or stimuli in the environment via our senses, memory, and other cognitive processes, and filter out streams of information not considered to be relevant (Pichora-Fuller & Singh, 2006). Some cognitive theorists suggest that selective attention and divided attention are related in part to inhibitory control, or the ability to restrict attention to distracting or irrelevant information. Requiring sustained concentration, attention, which is the ability to focus on one or more pieces of auditory or visual information long enough to interpret the data meaningfully, provides a foundation for most cognitive functions (Craft et al, 2009). When an individual attends to a task, several steps are involved: first filtering out stimuli from the environment, then holding and manipulating information, and finally responding appropriately to a given task. As the brain is limited in the amount it can process at a given time, attention is a complex, multistep process that includes alertness/arousal, selective attention, divided attention, and sustained attention.

Pichora-Fuller (2003) outlined three attentional processes that are essential to listening, and related each to the listening tasks required of our patients during a routine or rehabilitative evaluation. In my view this perspective is quite relevant to audiologists. The types of attention that Pichora-Fuller (2006) suggests modulate listening include vigilance and search-based attention, selective attention or filtering, and divided attention or resource allocation. Vigilance, a prolonged period of sustained awareness, comes into play when listening in quiet and the complaint that typifies the person with hearing impairment is as follows: "I can hear people talking but it is stressful and an effort to listen." Attentional strain can possibly be alleviated via auditory interventions coupled with active listening training. The complaint that "I cannot understand my family when we are speaking in a crowded room, such as a restaurant" highlights the challenges posed by deficits in selective attention. In short, when listening in noise, mental effort is expended when attending to the source or the target sound while at the same time trying to ignore the background noise and task-irrelevant stimuli (Pichora-Fuller & Souza, 2003).

Thus, auditory deficits likely compromise selective attention, which refers to the process of attending to a target while simultaneously ignoring competing inputs, and divided attention, which is the process by which one can allocate attentional resources to attend to more than one task at a time (Pichora-Fuller, 2006). The difficulty older adults experience in understanding speech in noisy environments may in part be due to a decline in the ability to filter out task-irrelevant stimuli. More specifically, when hearing-impaired individuals are asked to perform two tasks simultaneously, speech understanding becomes more difficult due to the increased listening effort and the resources being called into play. Noise-reduction algorithms, directional microphones, use of FM technology, and computer-aided auditory rehabilitation programs such as the Listening and Communication Enhancement (LACE) software (Sweetow & Sabes, 2010) are targeted at addressing the difficulty in listening and understanding in increasingly complex environments and at promoting inhibition or selective and divided attention. Finally, difficulty "multitasking" while having a conversation highlights the challenges posed by age-related deficits in divided attention. For example, when an older adult is engaged in concurrent tasks such as conversing with a family member while walking up a staircase, attentional resources are divided between listening and walking. Increased effort is required to listen and understand due to the demands posed by walking up steps, which is typically a challenge for older adults due to gait or balance disturbances.

In summary, when persons with hearing impairment move from a relatively stress-free listening environment to a more complex listening environment, it poses a considerable demand on attentional resources. Audiologists must consider ways of assessing the role of attention in speech understanding, as results will inform the hearing-aid fitting and intervention process.

Using a variety of the WAIS–III subtests, clinicians can assess each of the processes underlying attention to gain insight into an individual's ability to attend. Audiologists currently use some of these tests to screen for cognitive function. For example, the Digit Span subtest, which involves the examiner reading progressively longer strings of digits to be repeated forward and backward, is a common method for assessing attention span for immediate verbal recall of numbers. The forward and backward digit span tests require auditory attention, and, as will become apparent in a later section of this chapter, are dependent on short-term memory retention (Craft et al, 2009). In fact, the digit-span backward places considerable demand on working memory. Although the ability to perform simple tasks such as digit span is well preserved with age (i.e., after controlling for reaction time and sensory loss), divided attention or the ability to concentrate on more than one piece of information at a time, as in a dichotic task used for central auditory testing, does appear to worsen with age (Craft et al, 2009). Similarly, there is an increase in distractibility with age, which can have an impact on tests requiring selective attention. Stated differently, older adults are more susceptible to distractions and often find it difficult to divide their attention between two tasks occurring concurrently (Pichora-Fuller, 2003). Also, attention is negatively impacted by perceptual or sensory changes, depression, and anxiety; hence, when working with older adults on tasks that require attention, it would behoove audiologists to maximize audibility and visibility. A perfect example of the challenge posed by deficits in attention is the difficulty older adults experience understanding speech in noisy environments, which requires the tracking of one conversation while trying to ignore competing conversations and background noise (Pichora-Fuller & Singh, 2006). Pichora-Fuller and Singh (2006) have theorized that the difficulty in attending selectively may be due to the lack of attentional resources.

Memory

An exhaustive discussion of memory is beyond the scope of this chapter, but the principles that are most relevant to audiology practice with older adults will be highlighted. Learning and memory are related cognitive processes that must be differentiated. Although both involve a modification of behavior as a function of experience, learning is measured in relation to a change from one trial to another, whereas memory is measured in terms of the temporal interval between trials (Melton, 1963). Each process is dependent on the other. For example, if one does not learn well, then there is little to recall. Similarly, if memory is poor there is little evidence that one has learned very much. Storage is key to a good memory, as is audibility of the target message.

Memory has been defined as the product of operations that individuals perform on incoming information regardless of the intent to remember or the extent to which practice and rehearsal determine its memorability (Kausler, 1988). Memory has been likened to computer science. Common to both areas are the processes of input, throughput, and output (Bienfeld, 1990). *Input* refers to the data entry stage, *throughput* to the data manipulation and processing, and *output* to the retrieval of meaningful information or data. Sensory decline can influence memory to the extent that distorted input will negatively affect throughput and output. Similar to the way in which audiologists conceptualize the nature of auditory processing problems, memory can be conceptualized in a variety of ways. Some argue for a systems view and others for a process view. Early on, Tulving (1972) adopted a systems view, conceptualizing memory as being composed of two kinds of systems: explicit memory, which includes episodic (i.e., recollection of specific knowledge or prior experience) and semantic memory (i.e., the ability to recall concepts and general facts that are not related to a specific experience or event), and implicit or procedural memory, which is involved in learning skills and habits and in conditioning, implies remembering of procedures required for performing a particular task, and is more automatic (Craft et al, 2009; Pichora-Fuller, 2006).

In contrast, Craik and Lockhart (1972) adopted a processing view, proposing that memory can be conceptualized according to depth of processing, such that they distinguished between shallow and deep encoding (Pichora-Fuller & Singh, 2006). Baddeley and Hitch (1974), who were concerned with the relationship between short- and long-term memory, proposed a three-component model of working memory (Pichora-Fuller & Singh, 2006), and in so doing introduced the concept of working memory or short-term memory, which was later expanded to include a fourth component, namely an episodic buffer. *Working memory,* a term that bridges short- and long-term memory, allows for the storage and processing of information. According to Pichora–Fuller and Souza (2003), working memory is a "capacity-limited system that both stores recent information and provides a computational mental workspace in which the recently stored information can be manipulated and integrated with knowledge stored in long-term memory" (p. 49). The limited capacity system allows for temporary storage and manipulation of the bits of information necessary for complex tasks such as comprehension and learning (Baddeley & Hitch, 1974). In short, the concept of working memory relates to the attention and effort invested in listening and processing the input. When an older adult must expend mental energy trying to process auditory input, which is often the case due to deficits in audibility and auditory processing or due to challenging acoustic environments, less information or input will be stored in memory, and hence there will be less input to be manipulated. Models of working memory suggest that working memory capacity can be affected by the level of complexity of a particular task coupled with the presence of distracting information. Further, presentation level has a more detrimental effect on auditory working memory performance in normal hearing older adults than in younger adults, with a dramatic decline with decreasing presentation level in older adults (Baldwin & Ash, 2010). The latter was not the case for visual working memory. Hence, signal processing interventions

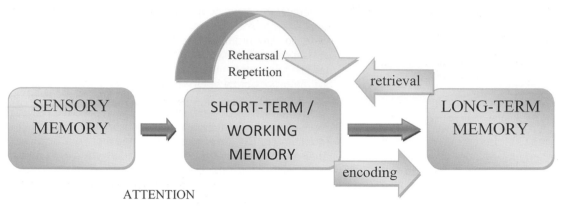

Rehearsal / Repetition

retrieval

SENSORY MEMORY

SHORT-TERM / WORKING MEMORY

LONG-TERM MEMORY

encoding

ATTENTION

Fig. 3.1 Information Processing System for Human Memory. (Based on: http://www.muskingum.edu/~cal/database/general/memory .html#BackgroundMenu)

designed to make speech understanding less effortful by increasing audibility and thereby freeing up resources for higher level processing, which demonstrate improvement in working memory capacity, should be a focus of audiological research (Pichora-Fuller & Singh, 2006).

Psychologists tend to categorize memory according to the length of time information can be stored or retained. **Figure 3.1** depicts the human memory information processing system. Sensory memory or the sensory store refers to the initial, momentary registration of information at the input stage. It is the earliest stage of information processing and relies on perceiving and attending to information (Albert, 1994). Data that are input to the system can be held there for a very brief period of time (0.25 to 0.5 seconds), so that they can be encoded and turned into a format to be relayed to the next compartment for storage. Interestingly, individuals have sensory memory for visual stimuli (e.g., iconic memory) and for auditory stimuli (e.g., echoic memory). Following this encoding, the next repository is working or short-term memory into which it is passed by attention to items of interest at a given point in time. This compartment has a slightly longer, albeit a limited, capacity. It pertains to the ability of individuals to retain a small amount of information over a brief time period (1 to 2 minutes) (Martin & Gorenstein, 2010). Short-term memory, which decays rapidly, is the compartment used to remember a phone number and then perform a mental operation such as immediately dialing a phone number that will subsequently be forgotten. Interference from distractions, for example, causes a disturbance in the ability to retain information in short-term memory. Immediate memory is the first stage of short-term memory, and it is the stage in which information is temporarily stored due to the limited capacity to store large bits of information. Through rehearsal or repetition in working memory, information is sent to secondary or long-term memory, which has a large capacity for information storage. It provides for long-term retention of unlimited amounts of information requiring analysis and organization for future storage and retrieval (Hartke, 1991; Martin & Gorenstein, 2010). It can be thought of as a file cabinet filled with several folders that hold newly learned material for retrieval or output at a later date; hence, at times it is referred to as prospective memory. The manner in which information is "filed away" will influence in-

formation storage capacity. Working memory is typically assessed by asking individuals to recall or repeat words, letters, or numbers of varying lengths.

Long-term memory, which refers to the acquisition of new information available for access at a later time, involves many more steps than short–term memory. It involves encoding, storing, and retrieving information, and is sometimes called prospective memory as it involves memory for past and future events (Martin & Gorenstein, 2010). Long-term memory requires that memory for what must be done must be maintained prior to taking action. For example, making an appointment to return to the audiologist for a hearing-aid fitting and remembering to put one's hearing aids on each morning are examples of long-term memory. Long-term memory is of two types: explicit and implicit. Explicit memory, or intentional recollection of the ability to recollect previous everyday experiences, is sometimes referred to as declarative (e.g., facts) memory. It is typically divided into episodic and semantic memory. Episodic memory, which includes memory of autobiographical information and the details of when and where events occurred, is typically assessed using free recall or retrieval tasks where information is reproduced from memory, and recognition tasks whereby presentation of information provides the evidence that the information has been seen before. It is notable that recognition tasks are less challenging than recall tasks, as they require less cognitive effort, and information is provided as a cue to the person being tested. In contrast, semantic memory, which is an individual's knowledge about the world, facts, word meaning, and concepts, is not context dependent. Tests that assess vocabulary and object naming are examples of approaches to assessing semantic memory. Tests that assess semantic memory include both delayed recall and recognition trials to determine if there is a deficit in retrieval or storage of information (Martin & Gorenstein, 2010). Implicit memory, also called procedural or nondeclarative memory, does not require conscious recollection of information, and does not afford awareness of stored knowledge, such that individuals are often unaware that remembering has taken place. Implicit memory includes motor and cognitive skill learning. Walking, dressing, riding a bicycle, and driving a car are examples of procedural memory. Interestingly, even people who cannot remember new information

Table 3.6 Examples of Stages of Information Processing and How Assessed

Stage	Examples
Sensory memory	Time necessary to identify a single letter
Short-term memory	Digit span forward, word span, recall and repeat back of words or letters
Long-term memory	Who was the third president of the United States? Among these five individuals, who was the third president?

still remember how to walk and dress, suggesting that implicit memory is a robust function. **Table 3.6** lists examples of recall and recognition tasks used to assess the various memory processes.

The aging process has a differential effect on each of the stages of memory (**Table 3.7**). Few age-related differences have been documented at the sensory phase. Storage capacity is unchanged at this stage of input; however, perceptual changes in hearing, vision, or touch can alter input into the sensory store. It is therefore imperative that clinicians verify the input into memory (i.e., information that has been seen and/or heard) to ensure that the individual can later retrieve the information in question. Older adults have minimal difficulty at the next memory repository (i.e., short-term memory). For example, absolute digit or word span is relatively unaffected by age. It is important to note that encoding at this stage is highly dependent on attention and processing speed. With increasing age, encoding becomes more and more susceptible to distracting events that tend to compromise attentional capacity and processing speed (Hartke, 1991).

When the number of items older adults are asked to recall exceeds the primary memory span, the effects of age become apparent (Robertson-Tchabo & Arenberg, 1988). In general, older adults are less proficient than young adults at tasks that test secondary memory. Each of the categories within long-term memory, that is, recall, retrieval, and recognition, is dif-

ferentially affected by age. Defects in retrieval appear to be most susceptible to aging effects. Bienfeld (1990) hypothesized that the deficits arise because of a less efficient means of classifying and placing information into long-term storage. That is, older adults use less effective strategies for organizing material. This compromises the ability to retrieve information. With regard to age decrements on recall tasks, memory for recent events can be viewed as a free recall task; for example, "What did you have for lunch yesterday?" In contrast, priming, which is a type of cued recall that implies that the examiner primes the examinee for recall (e.g., "The first thing you had was orange juice"). Age decrements are greatest on free recall rather than on cued or primed recall tasks and are most evident after age 40. Further, age decrements in delayed recall tasks have been reported in older adults as well (Albert, 1994). Recognition memory does not depend on retrieval, and older adults appear to be as successful as younger adults when asked to match or recognize a stimulus that has been stored away. At all ages recognition memory outperforms recall memory (Bienfeld, 1990). When tests of recognition memory involve storage of information over a brief time interval, there is an age effect. That is, performance on recognition tests administered 1 month after information has been learned declines with age (Botwinick, 1973). Memory for remote events in part reflects recognition memory, especially when an event or some experience triggers a memory of something similar that happened a long time ago. For example, if an older adult attends grandparents' day at their grandchild's kindergarten class, this may trigger their memory of events that took place when he or she was in kindergarten. According to Bienfeld (1990), stability of recognition memory over free recall memory most likely occurs over the entire life span. It may be more evident in the elderly because they tend to engage in active reminiscence.

In summary, memory is a very intricate form of information processing, and each aspect of memory must be understood in order to recognize the implications of age-related deficits. Further, the nature of the memory task and the assessment approach tend to interact to determine decrements due to age.

Table 3.7 Memory and Aging

Stage of Memory	Effect of Aging
Sensory memory	Unchanged by age
Short-term memory	Remains relatively stable with age, and if changes do occur with normal aging, they do not affect daily function
Procedural memory	Remains unaffected by healthy aging; few age-related changes in performance
Semantic memory (e.g., vocabulary and general information)	Remains largely unchanged by aging until very late in life; normal older adults have difficulty remembering words and names of objects and people
Explicit memory	More disadvantaged as compared with younger adults as requires active recall or recognition of information
Long-term memory	Memory deficits with age associated with storage of long-term episodic memories
Recognition tasks	Few age-related changes
Storage, recall, and retrieval tasks	Less efficient as people age

Sources: Craft, S., Cholerton, B., & Reger, M. (2009). In J. Halter, J. Ouslander, M. Tinetti, S. Studenski, K. High, & S. Asthana (Eds.), *Hazzard's geriatric medicine and gerontology* (6th ed.). New York: McGraw-Hill; and Martin, J., & Gorenstein, M. (2010). Normal cognitive aging. In H. Fillit, K. Rockwood, & K. Woodhouse (Eds.), *Brockelhurst's textbook of geriatric medicine and gerontology* (7th ed.). Philadelphia: Saunders Elsevier.

Table 3.8 Approaches to Minimizing the Influence of Age-Related Memory Deficits of Audiologic Tasks

Cognitive Process	Strategy
Sensory memory	Ensure that the new information is acquired; that is, did the individual hear, see, and /or feel the input?
Short-term memory	Allow adequate time for storage of new information.
	Provide opportunity for practicing new information.
	Have individual demonstrate his/her understanding of the instructions or new information.
	Write down information or instructions using large print.
	Provide reinforcement as a way of motivating the individual to store and later retrieve the new information.
	Share cognitive strategies to aid memory and remove distractions when working with the person with hearing impairment.
Long-term memory	Provide cues that will help the individual to remember what he/she has learned and needs to remember.
	Provide choices rather than rely on free recall.
	Provide suggestions for storage of new information into memory to facilitate later retrieval.
	Make sure that activities are relevant and meaningful, so that the new information is readily integrated into the person's knowledge base.
	Remove distractions and present one new task at a time, as older adults perform their best cognitively when their attention is not divided.
	Write down new information that the person with hearing impairment must remember.
	Have person with hearing impairment rehearse new information aloud.
	Repeat new information, instructions, or strategies on several occasions.
	Use slow rate of speaking when presenting new information, as this facilitates memory.

Finally, it is important to note that processing speed or the rate at which one can process information, which is dependent on the ability to attend to a task, is integrally related to memory. As processing speed, which is slower in older adults than in younger adults, mediates memory, it is important to acknowledge the confounding effect of this variable on tests of memory. Interestingly, Salthouse (1996) reported that after controlling statistically for processing speed, age and memory status bear a weak correlation. The data of Finkel, Reynolds, McArdle, and Pedersen (2007) confirm the findings of Salthouse (1996), as they too found that, consistent with the processing speed theory of aging, processing speed is a leading indicator of age changes in memory.

To minimize the effects of age on audiological tasks that are dependent on memory status, the audiologist should follow the steps listed in **Table 3.8**. These tips will be quite pertinent during all aspects of the audiological assessment ranging from diagnostic testing to audiological rehabilitation.

Pearl

Cognitive performance is mediated by sensory acuity in part because it interferes with information storage for later recall. Audiologists must consider the interacting effects of auditory and cognitive process, especially as pertains to speech understanding and learning and performance of new tasks (Baldwin & Ash, 2010).

Learning Capacity

Learning is defined as the change in behavior in a given situation brought about by repeated experiences in that situation, provided that the new behavior cannot be explained by the individual's native response tendencies, maturation, or some temporary state of being (Kaplan et al, 1994). Cognitive components of learning include memory and intelligence (Lewis & Bottomley, 2008). Learning can be viewed as the acquisition

of connections or associations between stimulus and response through practice and rehearsal. It is the practicing and rehearsing of information to be retained (Kausler, 1988). It is important to note that learning style and information processing are integrally related such that how older adults receive, retain, and retrieve information, and their response to the learning experience, will influence how they learn (Lewis & Bottomley, 2008). Further, working memory capacity is integral to the process of learning new information (Martin & Gorenstein, 2010). Similarly, pacing, or the speed at which material is presented and the amount of time allotted for a response, influences learning capacity as well (Lewis & Bottomley, 2008). Finally, older adults, especially, seem to learn better when material is presented with contextual details.

Contrary to common belief, older adults can learn as much as younger adults and, in the absence of pathology, have no difficulty in learning (Lewis & Bottomley, 2008). Further, the rate of forgetting what has been learned appears to be independent of age (Kausler, 1988). Although the capacity to learn does not change, the amount of effort required to learn does. Specifically, the ability to perform new tasks and flexibility of learning style undergo some decline. The fact that older adults learn more slowly than younger adults is most pronounced on tasks involving verbal skills; older adults make more errors on verbal learning tasks than do young adults. In addition to requiring more time to learn new tasks, older adults require more time to integrate new learning and to practice it before it is incorporated into their daily routine (Davis, 1990). Older adults tend to be vulnerable to distracting events that can interfere with their level of concentration. Ability to learn orally presented material (as opposed to written material) declines in persons over 70 years of age (Hayflick, 1994). **Table 3.9** lists several factors that affect an older adult's learning capacity, and **Table 3.10** lists tips for overcoming learning barriers in older adults. The information contained in these tables should help in deciding on approaches to testing and management of older adults. Sessions should be individualized such that you

Table 3.9   Strategies for Overcoming Barriers to Learning in Older Adults

Factors that Affect Learning	Strategies for Overcoming Learning Deficits
1. Hearing or visual deficits	Make sure that the hearing or visual deficit is compensated for; otherwise it may take longer to learn, and/or persons may misunderstand what has been said. Present material orally and in writing, especially to individuals over 70 years of age. Use visual aids such as magnifiers, as appropriate.
2. Poor physical health or chronic pain can interfere with concentration, stamina, and strength	Make inquiries about health status and physical comfort prior to beginning a new learning task; make adjustments in scheduling time and length of sessions.
3. Reluctance to learn new information	Build on former knowledge; present new information on a continuum with what the older adult already knows.
4. Need more time to integrate new learning	Provide ample opportunity to integrate new learning; separate new learning experiences.
5. Easily distracted by the physical environment	Minimize auditory and visual distractions.
6. Perform better with self-paced new learning, as older adults have a slowed rate of information processing	Allow adequate time for responses and for completion of forms. Do not give too much information at one sitting.
7. Experience anxiety in new learning situations	Provide an overview or summary of activities to be covered in each session so that the individual can anticipate the sequence.
8. Motivation	Information should be relevant and meaningful to maximize motivation to learn.
9. Relevance	Activities, tasks, and goals should be relevant and meaningful.

Source: Davis, C. (1990). Psychosocial aspects of aging. In C. Lewis (Ed.), *Aging: The health care challenge* (2nd ed.). Philadelphia: F. A. Davis.

introduce new information using strategies that are appropriate for the patient's learning style. Hence, it is imperative to determine whether the patient is an auditory, verbal, or kinesthetic learner, and whether the patient learns by doing or by demonstration, or by some combination (Lewis & Bottomley, 2008). Similarly, new information should be presented at a rate that corresponds to the patient's ability to understand and respond, with ample time for practice. The comfort level of the learning environment is critical; thus, comfortable chairs,

Table 3.10   Tips for Overcoming Learning Barriers

- Older adults benefit when new material is presented along a continuum with what they already know. Proceed in a slow and careful manner when resistance to new information is expected.
- Older adults need more time to integrate new learning and to rehearse it before it settles into new memory.
- Concentrate on one task at a time.
- Space new learning experiences well enough apart.
- Reduce the potential for distraction whenever possible as this interferes with concentration. Observe the person for signs of interference with concentration.
- Allow the client to set the learning pace.
- Provide an overview of the entire learning session so that the person can organize the sequence of the session.
- Learning is facilitated when the patient can hear and see the same material presented at the same time:
  - Pleasant surroundings promote learning.
  - Active involvement in the task promotes learning.
  - Learning is facilitated when older adults have more time to inspect and to respond.
  - Concrete information is easier to grasp than abstract information.
  - Practice or repeated trials promotes learning.
  - Verbal feedback regarding performance promotes learning.

Sources: Lewis, C. (1990). Aging: *The Health Care Challenge* (2nd ed.). Philadelphia: F. A. Davis; and Lewis, C., & Bottomley, J. (2008). *Geriatric rehabilitation: A clinical approach.* Upper Saddle River, NJ: Pearson Education.

adequate lighting and ventilation, the absence of background noise, and the persona of the health professional are important variables to which audiologists should attend during testing and intervention. Finally, it is noteworthy that prior learning and experience play a role in determining the range of cognitive plasticity older adults may experience.

Special Consideration

Learning capacity does not decline as one ages, but older people learn more slowly than do their younger counterparts. As a result, it takes more trials for a particular skill to be acquired (Bienfeld, 1990).

Cognitive Plasticity Versus Cognitive Reserve

Cognitive plasticity, or plastic alterations in brain and behavior, reflects a secondary change in response to a primary change in a system (Bengtsson et al, 2005). An individual's cognitive plasticity, including improved performance on cognitive tasks, is defined based on one's latent cognitive potential and one's current level of performance (Willis et al, 2009). Cognitive plasticity is an intraindividual process that is context specific and is integrally intertwined with neural plasticity. It is closely related to the concept of *cognitive reserve*, a term used in neuropsychology that refers to the ability of an individual to continue to function at an adequate cognitive level despite deficits or pathology at the neural level (Willis et al, 2009). According to Willis et al (2009), there are three different levels at which cognitive plasticity occurs: neural plasticity within the brain; cognitive plasticity at the behavioral level; and cognitive plasticity at the sociocultural level, wherein cultural resources and knowledge are preserved and transmitted.

Although cognitive plasticity is an intraindividual process, cognitive reserve proposes that there are differences across individuals in terms of their ability to compensate once a neuropathology disrupts the portion of the brain subserving a given cognitive function (Martin & Gorenstein, 2010). According to Willis et al (2009), cognitive reserve continues to exist even when neural plasticity, which contributes to cognitive plasticity, is compromised. There is a great deal of variability across individuals in their ability to compensate for age-related cognitive changes. Similar to the concept of auditory plasticity via auditory based interventions such as LACE, neuropsychologists believe that cognitive reserve can be enhanced by purposeful activity, with the person as an active agent of change. Differences across individuals in their cognitive reserve may be due to differences in innate intellectual function, environmental factors, premorbid cognitive activity level, educational pursuits, occupational status, and a variety of other considerations. According to Martin and Gorenstein (2010), the cognitive reserve model holds that cognitive impairments begin to set in when cognitive reserve is depleted via normal aging or disease-related changes.

Neural plasticity, or the capacity for neural circuits, connections between neurons, neural organization, and myelinization of axons to change in response to neural or glial activity, is closely related to cognitive plasticity, yet the directionality of the relationship remains to be determined. It is presumed that cognitive plasticity or cognitive reserve can exist despite neuropathology or a compromise in neural plasticity. In fact, it has been hypothesized that environmental stimulation and training can play a protective function against degradation of neuronal structure and function and therefore can delay cognitive decline. Interesting, there is evidence that the neurons in the hippocampal region in humans and animals may be sensitive to neurogenesis (Willis et al, 2009). The concept of cognitive-based training that focuses on processing speed, listening effort, and inhibition is implicit in the auditory training modules developed by Sweetow and Sabes (2010) and included in the LACE. In light of data demonstrating the effectiveness of interventions in improving cognitive function and ultimately improving health and overall quality of life in older individuals, audiologists are beginning to explore the potential of auditorily based interventions (Smith et al, 2009). Recognizing the significance of sensory system function, notably the auditory system, Smith and colleagues explored improvements in central system function through a cognitive training program. Specifically, their training program was designed to improve auditory system function through brain plasticity–based learning using outcome measures of attention and memory and participant-reported outcomes. Mean age of participants in the control and experimental groups was 75 years, and mean scores on the Mini-Mental State Examination (MMSE) and on intelligence tests suggested normal cognitive status and intelligence quotients, and no history of depression. Experimental interventions included computerized exercises using syllables, verbally presented stories, and instructions designed to improve the speed and accuracy of auditory information processing. Interestingly, greater improvements in digit span backwards tasks, in overall memory, and on tests of auditory memory/attention emerged in the experimental group as compared with the active control group. Self-reported improvements in systems subserving auditory-based cognition suggested that the results had implications for behavioral function. In

light of emerging data on the value of Web-based training and auditory-based training, audiologists should continue to extend the latter work into studies on the beneficial effects of hearing-assistance technologies combined with cognitive training similar to the work of Sweetow and Pichora-Fuller (Smith et al, 2009).

In summary, it is well established that cognitive and neural plasticity is a reality of aging. As will be discussed in subsequent chapters, the functional plasticity of the adult sensory system, including the tonotopic organization of the cortical region, has been established in animals and to a lesser extent in humans following hearing-aid use (Philibert, Collet, Vesson, & Veuillet, 2005). The dynamic properties of the central auditory system associated with hearing-aid use and auditory and cognitive training remain a very fruitful area of research.

Pearl

Cognitive training research has demonstrated cognitive plasticity in several cognitive domains, including processing speed, inhibition, fluid intelligence, executive functioning, episodic memory, and spatial orientation. Maintenance of treatment effects on primary mental abilities is promising as well.

Motivation: A Cognitive Factor, Not a Cognitive Function

Motivation, an intraindividual factor, is one of the most important cognitive factors that affect adaptation to chronic disease and resultant disability (Hendricks & Hatch, 2009; Kemp, 1990). An interpersonal process and the product of the interaction between people, motivation has a strong influence on mastery of various functions and hence influences lifestyle and adjustment to aging (Miller & Rollnick, 2002). Hence, it has a great impact on the well-being of older disabled adults, including those with hearing impairment (Kemp, 1990). The term *motivation* refers to self-directed behavior. It is a state of being that produces a tendency toward some type of action (Kaplan et al, 1994). Maslow's hierarchy of needs, a pyramidal framework, provides a basis for understanding motivation, especially as it pertains to need-seeking behavior or readiness to pursue interventions to overcome challenges including hearing loss. For example, the most basic of needs that individuals satisfy are the biological and physiological needs for food and clothing. The need to be safe and secure is a basic need as well, and must be satisfied before progressing to the next higher level, namely the need to be loved, followed by the need for self-esteem and self-actualization. As pertains to older adults, motivation strategies should target lower level needs, such as a sense of safety, as these are more important than the need for self-actualization (Lewis & Bottomley, 2008).

Socio-emotional selectivity theory suggests that motivation is a powerful determinant of well-being in old age. In short, the theory posits that because time is in effect running out, older adults are motivated by immediate gratification, namely achievement of emotional well-being for the short-term (Kryla-Lighthall & Mather, 2009). In fact, the role of family takes on greater importance as one ages, as older adults are motivated by the emotional gain and gratification derived from available social networks. Effort and motivation to perform are important factors to consider as they have an impact on rehabilitation potential. Motivational theorists including Freud and Lewin have stressed that motivation is a multivariate process comprising four primary variables (Kemp, 1986). Three of the variables—wants, expectations, and reinforcement—encourage or support behavior. The final variable—the cost of the behavior—discourages or deters behavior. In general, motivation is optimal when (1) the person knows what he or she wants *(W)*; (2) the person expects or believes it can be obtained *(B)*; (3) the rewards associated with it are meaningful *(R)*; and (4) the costs associated with it are minimal *(C)* (Kemp, 1990). The motive system can be expressed as the following equation:

$$Motivation = W \times B \times R/C$$

It is important to emphasize that each of these components of the motivational formula are based on the individual's perceptions rather than on what the clinician might perceive as the facts. The likelihood of success plays a critical role in motivating behavior, as does the expectancy factor, which refers to the subjective probability that, with enough effort, one's goal may be achieved (Kaplan et al, 1994).

In the audiological domain, a person's wants might include desires, wishes, needs, and goals relative to hearing status and audiological interventions (Kemp, 1990). Goals and readiness to initiate behavior are strongly related to treatment outcomes. As is discussed in Chapter 8, self-efficacy, or the belief that one can master a situation and experience positive outcomes, influences ones motivational level and desire to follow a course of action that can influence health and well-being (Antonucci, Birditt, & Akiyama, 2009). In short, higher levels of self-efficacy and motivation are likely associated with better health outcomes.

For example, a person who wants to overcome the handicapping effects of hearing loss, and is self-referred for a hearing aid, is more likely to do so than an individual who is brought in reluctantly by a family member. For audiological treatment to be successful, the clinician must identify (1) what the person wants from the intervention; (2) why the person wants the treatment; (3) how life might change if the individual receives the treatment; and (4) how the individual's goals were established. In keeping with the emotional–selectivity theory, older adults want to maintain social relationships, and as audiologists we should emphasize that integral hearing plays in maintenance of meaningful relationships (Kryla-Lighthall & Mather, 2009).

Beliefs, expectations, assumptions, and attitudes all pertain to what the client wants. Beliefs are the cognitive component of motivation and are what the person acts upon. Three areas of belief are important to fully comprehend a person's motivation: the situation or task the person is facing, the future as the person sees it, and the person him- or herself. In order to succeed, the individual must be optimistic about his or her capability to succeed at the task at hand. Belief in one's capabilities will initiate behavior. Behavior that is associated with some form of reward, reinforcement, positive feedback, or benefit will be initiated and maintained. Thus, reward is an important aspect of motivational dynamics. With regard to hearing impairment, the ability to hear birds with a new hearing aid or to

finally understand the minister at a church service with an infrared system would be considered rewarding and should be emphasized during a treatment session. It is critical that audiologists relate an intervention to rewards or successes to ensure compliance and maintenance of behavior.

Finally, the variables in the numerator of the motivational formula must be weighed against the cost of behavior for it to be initiated and maintained. Costs pertain to effort, physical pain, emotional discomfort, threats to self-esteem, money, and time. Thus, costs can be physical, psychological, and social. In general, if the denominator, the costs, is greater than the numerator, the benefits, the person will be unmotivated to pursue a behavior. In contrast, if the benefits of a particular intervention outweigh the costs, the individual will be highly motivated.

Although motivation does not decline with age, there are age-related differences in approaches to motivating older adults. Thus, fulfillment of safety and security needs is a powerful incentive for complying with a particular medical regimen (Kemp, 1986). Older adults often avoid difficult tasks because of anxiety associated with new or challenging tasks. Accordingly, the older adult should be given every reason to believe that improvement or success is possible prior to attempting a new technique or intervention. Regular corrective feedback presented in a nonthreatening, supportive manner will go a long way toward reducing anxiety about a task, sustaining continued involvement, and promoting motivation and a sense of success (Lewis, 1990). In Chapter 8, more specific suggestions for assessing and improving motivation will be presented. **Table 3.11** lists tips for motivating older adults, especially during rehabilitation sessions. Chapter 8 also discusses applying the principles of motivational dynamics to motivational interviewing and its relationship to the transtheoretical stages of change as they pertain to counseling (Miller & Rollnick, 2002). Briefly, motivational interviewing is a client-centered approach to counseling designed to promote client motivation and initiative to purchase rehabilitation services and to achieve positive outcomes from the rehabilitation encounter (Miller & Rollnick, 2002). The audiologist must be directive

Table 3.11   Tips for Overcoming Motivational Barriers

- Provide a supportive climate for learning.
- Make sure that the patient feels a part of the session.
- Appreciate and value the patient regardless of achievement. This will sustain involvement and progress.
- Materials should be meaningful and instructions clear, as this will ensure motivated involvement.
- Be directive and client centered.
- Show and express empathy and acceptance.
- Ask open questions when engaging with the person with hearing impairment or the communication partner.
- Believe in the ability of the person with hearing impairment to overcome the hearing deficit and make sure the person is aware of this.
- The person with hearing loss and the communication partner should be the individuals to come up with the solutions and strategies necessary to successful outcomes.

Sources: Lewis, C. (1990). *Aging: The Health Care Challenge* (2nd ed.). Philadelphia: F. A. Davis; and Miller, W., & Rollnick, S. (2002). *Motivational interviewing: Preparing people for change* (2nd ed.). New York: Guilford.

during motivational interviewing, with the goal being to lead the patient to engage in the treatment process from the outset.

Pearl

Older adults require more and different reinforcement. They respond better to concrete goals that are immediate and affect daily functioning.

Miscellaneous Cognitive Variables

In the aging literature, a good deal of attention has been focused on the changes in reaction time or speed of response associated with age. The term *reaction time* refers to the time that elapses between a signal being given and a required motor response being undertaken. It appears that portions of the peripheral and central nervous systems mediate this cognitive phenomenon, specifically the circuits that lie between the perception of the signal and activation of the intention to respond. The extent to which the aging process is associated with changes in the time required for peripheral and central processing dictates when and if reaction time will be prolonged. In general, one might conclude that as signal pathways deteriorate with age, there is a corresponding decline in reaction time.

Special Consideration

To compensate for possible declines in reaction time, the clinician should routinely allow time for the older adult to fully process information prior to demanding a response.

Using the computer analogy put forth earlier, when working with the elderly, one should allow sufficient time between data input, data processing, and data output in the event that there is a slowing of reaction time. Clinically, it is a rather simple matter to gain an informal appreciation for a person's reaction time. For example, during the audiological evaluation, upon presentation of the pure-tone stimulus, one should monitor the time it takes for the person to respond to the presence of the signal. The stimulus response time should dictate the time interval between stimulus presentations. In a sense, the stimulus response time is an index of reaction time for that particular procedure.

Finally, coping ability is an important cognitive variable in older adults because it influences the response to stress, disability, and similar factors. In general, coping is a highly individualized process that appears to evolve with age, rather than changing with increasing years of life. Premorbid personality influences to a great extent an older adult's coping strategies. Further, the type of stressor interacts with the lifelong coping ability. For example, as pertains to health stressors, illness severity and expectations regarding health affect the coping ability. Specifically, aging attribution has been shown to undercut the ability to cope with mild as well as severe medical conditions. There is a suggestion in the literature that at any age more effective coping responses are associated with (1) a

higher socioeconomic status; (2) the availability of a wide repertoire of coping strategies; (3) high self-esteem; (4) a good supply of internal resources, (5) assumption of personal responsibility for one's health whenever feasible; and (6) perceptions of disability, health, and aging (Hartke, 1991). Accordingly, clinicians, especially those engaged in audiological rehabilitation, have a responsibility to understand the older adult's coping ability and introduce strategies for facilitating coping and adaptation to acquired hearing impairment. This is an important aspect of assertiveness and strategies training used during audiological rehabilitation.

Special Consideration

Hartke (1991) suggests that promoting patient involvement in the rehabilitation process, enhancing a sense of realistic mastery or control, and addressing and dispelling age attribution are effective mechanisms for promoting the coping process.

◆ Conclusion

Psychosocial theories of aging emphasize the individualized nature of the aging process and the complex interaction between internal and external factors as determining the way in which one ages in each domain. The external forces are primarily social and include loss of income, loss of role/status, and bereavement. Along with physical stressors, the internal forces are psychological, including isolated changes in cognitive status and intellectual functioning. Declines in specific areas of cognition, personality, and coping have been demonstrated in older adults. However, the safest conclusion one can draw from the literature review is that people age in a highly individualized manner, and psychological development tends to proceed in such a way as to magnify the diversity of individuals within an aging cohort (Bienfeld, 1990). Life stressors such as illness, loss of job, and loss of loved ones interact with psychological variables to determine age-related declines in the psychological domain. In general, it appears that the core personality tends to remain stable throughout life, as does one's coping mechanisms. Similarly, capacity for new learning remains unaffected by age, as does the capacity for registration and storage of information. In contrast, the speed of learning tends to decline with aging, and strategies for retrieval of information tend to become less efficient (Bienfeld, 1990).

Given the multiple stresses associated with aging, the clinician must consider the total person when conducting an evaluation and instituting any form of intervention. Audiologists should operate from the perspective that many older persons have complex problems of a physical, psychological, and social nature that will influence one's diagnostic and treatment approach. More importantly, it is critical to keep in mind that older adults are purposeful and accommodating, and modify their behaviors throughout their life span to adapt to the transitions and physical changes they undergo. It is impossible to predict the biopsychosocial stressors one will encounter because of the individual variability characterizing older adults, which underscores the importance of a patient-centered approach to work with older adults. It is imperative that audiologists adopt a life course perspective, given the important role lifestyle choices play in response to life changes (Hendricks & Hatch, 2009). The fact that with advancing age, much of the cognitive reserve and control older adults have is devoted to enhancing their well-being is an important perspective that should guide work with older adults (Kryla-Lighthall & Mather, 2009).

References

Abrams, W., Beers, M., & Berkow, R. (1995). *The Merck manual of geriatrics* (2nd ed.). Whitehouse Station, NJ: Merck

Achenbaum, W. A. (2009). A metahistorical perspective on theories of aging. In V. Bengtson, D. Gans, N. Putney, & M. Silverstein (Eds.), *Handbook of theories of aging* (2nd ed.). New York: Springer

Albert, M. (1994). Cognition and aging. In W. Hazzard, E. Bierman, J. Blass, W. Ettinger, & J. Halter (Eds.), *Principles of geriatric medicine and gerontology* (3rd ed.). New York: McGraw-Hill

Antonucci, T., Birditt, K., & Akiyama, H. (2009). Convoys of social relations: An interdisciplinary approach. In V. Bengtson, D. Gans, N. Putney, & M. Silverstein (Eds.), *Handbook of theories of aging* (2nd ed.). New York: Springer

Atchley, R. (1999). *Continuity and adaptation in old age*. Baltimore: Johns Hopkins University Press

Baddeley, A., & Hitch, G. (1974). Working memory. In G. A. Bower (Ed.), *Recent advances in learning and motivation* (vol. 8, pp. 47–89). New York: Academic Press

Baldwin, C., & Ash, I. (2010) Impact of sensory acuity on auditory working memory span in young and older adults. *Psychology and Aging,* August 16, Advanced online publication 10.1037/a0020360

Baltes, P., & Lindenberger, U. (1988). On the range of cognitive plasticity in old age as a function of experience: 15 years of intervention research. *Behavior Therapy, 19,* 283–300

Baltes, P. B., Sowarka, D., & Kliegl, R. (1989, Jun). Cognitive training research on fluid intelligence in old age: what can older adults achieve by themselves? *Psychology and Aging, 4,* 217–221

Bass, S. (2006). Gerontological theory: The search for the Holy Grail. *The Gerontologist, 46,* 139–144

Bengtsson, S. L., Nagy, Z., Skare, S., Forsman, L., Forssberg, H., & Ullén, F. (2005, Sep). Extensive piano practicing has regionally specific effects on white matter development. *Nature Neuroscience, 8,* 1148–1150

Bienfeld, D. (1990). Psychology of aging. In D. Bienfeld (Ed.), *Clinical geropsychiatry* (3rd ed.). Baltimore: Williams & Wilkins

Botwinick, J. (1973). *Aging and behavior.* New York: Springer

Corey, G. (1991). *Theory and practice of counseling and psychotherapy* (4th ed.). Pacific Grove, CA: Brooks/Cole

Costa, P., & McCrae, R. (1994). Personality and aging. In W. Hazzard, E. Bierman, J. Blass, W. Ettinger, & J. Halter (Eds.), *Principles of geriatric medicine and gerontology* (3rd ed.). New York: McGraw-Hill

Cox, H. (1988). Social realities of aging. In B. Shadden (Ed.), *Communication behavior and aging: A sourcebook for clinicians.* Baltimore: Williams & Wilkins

Cox, R. M., Alexander, G. C., & Gray, G. (2004). *Hearing aid fitting: Self report outcomes over six months.* Paper presented at the American Auditory Society 2004 meeting, Scottsdale, AZ, March 7–9

Craft, S., Cholerton, B., & Reger, M. (2009). In J. Halter, J. Ouslander, M. Tinetti, S. Studenski, K. High, & S. Asthana (Eds.), *Hazzard's geriatric medicine and gerontology* (6th ed.). New York: McGraw-Hill

Craik, F., & Lockhart, R. (1972). Levels of processing: A framework for memory research. *Journal of Verbal Learning and Verbal Behavior, 11,* 671–684

Cumming, E., & Henry, W. (1961). *Growing old: The process of disengagement.* New York: Basic Books

Davis, C. (1990). Psychosocial aspects of aging. In C. Lewis (Ed.), *Aging: The health care challenge* (2nd ed.). Philadelphia: F. A. Davis

Erikson, E. (1968). *Identity: Youth and crisis.* New York: W. W. Norton

Finkel, D., Reynolds, C. A., McArdle, J. J., & Pedersen, N. L. (2007, Sep). Age changes in processing speed as a leading indicator of cognitive aging. *Psychology and Aging, 22,* 558–568

Friedan, B. (1993). *The fountain of age.* New York: Simon & Schuster

Grant, D. A., & Berg, E. A. (1948, Aug). A behavioral analysis of degree of reinforcement and ease of shifting to new responses in a Weigl-type card-sorting problem. *Journal of Experimental Psychology, 38,* 404–411

Hartke, R. (1991). The aging process: Cognition, personality, and coping. In R. Hartke (Ed.), *Psychological aspects of geriatric rehabilitation.* Gaithersburg, MD: Aspen Publishers

Havighurst, R. (1963). Successful aging. In R. Williams, C. Tibbit, & W. Donahue (Eds.), *Process of aging.* New York: Lieber-Atherton

Hayflick, L. (1994). *How and why we age.* New York: Ballantine Books

Hendricks, J., & Hatch, L. (2009). Theorizing the life course: New twists in the paths. In V. Bengtson, D. Gans, N. Putney, & M. Silverstein (Eds.), *Handbook of theories of aging* (2nd ed.). New York: Springer

Horn, J. L., & Cattell, R. B. (1967). Age differences in fluid and crystallized intelligence. *Acta Psychologica, 26,* 107–129

Kaplan, H., Sadock, B., & Grubb, J. (1994). *Synopsis of psychiatry* (7th ed.). Baltimore: Williams & Wilkins

Kausler, D. (1988). Cognition and aging. In B. Shadden (Ed.), *Communication behavior and aging: A sourcebook for clinicians.* Baltimore: Williams & Wilkins

Kemp, B. (1986). Psychosocial and mental health issues in rehabilitation of older persons. In S. Brody & G. Ruff (Eds.), *Aging and rehabilitation.* New York: Springer

Kemp, B. (1990). Motivational dynamics in geriatric rehabilitation: Toward a therapeutic model. In B. Kemp, J. Brummel-Smith, & J. Ramsdell (Eds.), *Geriatric rehabilitation.* Boston: College-Hill

Krause, N. (2009). Deriving a sense of meaning in late life: An overlooked forum for the development of interdisciplinary theory. In V. Bengtson, D. Gans, N. Putney, & M. Silverstein (Eds.), *Handbook of theories of aging* (2nd ed.). New York: Springer

Kryla-Lighthall, N., & Mather, M. (2009). The role of cognitive control in older adults' emotional well-being. In V. Bengtson, D. Gans, N. Putney, & M. Silverstein (Eds.), *Handbook of theories of aging* (2nd ed.). New York: Springer

Lewis, C. (1990). *Aging: The Health Care Challenge* (2nd ed.). Philadelphia: F. A. Davis

Lewis, C., & Bottomley, J. (2008). *Geriatric rehabilitation: A clinical approach.* Upper Saddle River, NJ: Pearson Education

Lighthouse. (1995). *The Lighthouse national survey of vision loss: The experience, attitudes, and knowledge of middle aged and older Americans.* New York: The Lighthouse

Maddox, G. L. (1965). Fact and artifact: Evidence bearing on disengagement theory from the Duke geriatrics project. *Human Development, 8,* 117–130

Martin, J., & Gorenstein, M. (2010). Normal cognitive aging. In H. Fillit, K. Rockwood, & K. Woodhouse (Eds.), *Brockelhurst's textbook of geriatric medicine and gerontology* (7th ed.). Philadelphia: Saunders Elsevier

McCrae, R., & Costa, P. (2006). Perspectives de la theorie des cinq facteurs (TCF): traits and culture. (A five-factor theory perspective on traits and culture). *Psychologie Française, 51,* 227–244

Melton, A. (1963). Implications of short-term memory for a general theory of memory. *Journal of Verbal Learning and Verbal Behavior, 2,* 1–21

Miller, W., & Rollnick, S. (2002). *Motivational interviewing: Preparing people for change* (2nd ed.). New York: Guilford

Neugarten, B. (1964). *Personality in middle and late life.* New York: Atherton Press

Neugarten, B. (1966). Adult personality: A developmental view. *Human Development, 9,* 61–73

Neugarten, B. (1975). *Middle age and aging.* Chicago: University of Chicago Press

Noble, W., & Atherly, G. (1970). The hearing measurement scale: A questionnaire for the assessment of auditory disability. *The Journal of Auditory Research, 10,* 229–250

Philibert, B., Collet, L., Vesson, J. F., & Veuillet, E. (2005, Jul). The auditory acclimatization effect in sensorineural hearing-impaired listeners: evidence for functional plasticity. *Hearing Research, 205,* 131–142

Pichora-Fuller, M. K. (2003). Cognitive aging and auditory information processing. *International Journal of Audiology, 42,* 2S26–2S32

Pichora-Fuller, M. K. (2006). Perceptual effort and apparent cognitive decline: Implications for audiologic rehabilitation. In Palmer, C. (Ed.), *The aging auditory system: Considerations for rehabilitation. Seminars in Hearing.* New York: Thieme

Pichora-Fuller, M. K., & Singh, G. (2006, Mar). Effects of age on auditory and cognitive processing: implications for hearing aid fitting and audiologic rehabilitation. *Trends in Amplification, 10,* 29–59

Pichora-Fuller, M. K. & Souza, P. (2003). Effects of aging on auditory processing of speech. *International Journal of Audiology, 42,* 2S11–2S16.

Robertson-Tchabo, E., & Arenberg, D. (1988). Cognitive performance. In G. Mueller & V. Geoffrey (Eds.), *Communication disorders in aging: Assessment and management.* Washington, DC: Gallaudet University Press

Rowe, J., & Kahn, R. (1998). *Successful aging.* New York: Random House

Ryff, C., & Singer, B. (2009). Understanding healthy aging: Key components and their integration. In V. Bengtson, D. Gans, N. Putney, & M. Silverstein (Eds.), *Handbook of theories of aging* (2nd ed.). New York: Springer

Salthouse, T. A. (1996, Jul). The processing-speed theory of adult age differences in cognition. *Psychological Review, 103,* 403–428

Scheibe, S., & Carstensen, L. L. (2010, Mar). Emotional aging: recent findings and future trends. *Journals of Gerontology, Series B, Psychological Sciences and Social Sciences, 65B*, 135–144

Smith, G. E., Housen, P., Yaffe, K., Ruff, R., Kennison, R. F., Mahncke, H. W., et al. (2009, Apr). A cognitive training program based on principles of brain plasticity: results from the Improvement in Memory with Plasticity-based Adaptive Cognitive Training (IMPACT) study. *Journal of the American Geriatrics Society, 57*, 594–603

Strauss, E., Sherman, E. M. S., & Spreen, O. (2006). *A compendium of neuropsychological tests: Administration, norms, and commentary.* New York: Oxford University Press

Swanda, R., & Haaland, K. (2009). Clinical neuropsychology and intellectual assessment of adults. In B. Sadock, V. Sadock & P. Ruiz (Eds.), *Kaplan and Sadock's comprehensive textbook of psychiatry* (9th ed.). Philadelphia: Wolters Kluwer/Lippincott, Williams & Wilkins

Sweetow, R. W., & Sabes, J. H. (2010, Oct). Auditory training and challenges associated with participation and compliance. *Journal of the American Academy of Audiology, 21*, 586–593

Tarawneh, R., & Galvin, J. (2010). Neurologic signs in the elderly. In H. Fillit, K. Rockwood, & K. Woodhouse (Eds.), *Brockelhurst's textbook of geriatric medicine and gerontology* (7th ed.). Philadelphia: Saunders Elsevier

Tulving, E. (1972). Episodic and semantic memory. In E. Tulving & W. Donaldson (Eds.), *Organization of memory.* New York: Academic Press

Verwoerdt, A. (1976). *Clinical geropsychiatry.* Baltimore: Williams & Wilkins

Weinstein, B. (1980). *Hearing impairment and social isolation in the elderly.* Doctoral dissertation. New York: Columbia University

Willis, S., Schaie, K., & Martin, M. (2009). Cognitive plasticity. In V. Bengtson, D. Gans, N. Putney, & M. Silverstein (Eds.), *Handbook of theories of aging* (2nd ed.). New York: Springer

Zarit, S. (2009). A good old age: Theories of mental health and aging. In V. Bengtson, D. Gans, N. Putney, & M. Silverstein (Eds.), *Handbook of theories of aging* (2nd ed.). New York: Springer

Chapter 4

The Aging Auditory System

I feel so bad for Uncle Ted,
There's not much hair upon his head,
And what is worse, he barely hears,
There's too much hair in his ears.

—Lansky, 1996

Every morning, the first thing I do is put my hearing aids on; this way I can communicate with my husband, as despite the many changes in my body associated with age, my priority is understanding my husband when he speaks to me.

—M.W., age 66

◆ Learning Objectives

After reading this chapter, you should be able to

◆ explain the age-related changes in the outer ear, middle ear, cochlea, eighth nerve, central auditory pathways, and auditory cortex;
◆ understand why the inner ear is susceptible to age effects; and
◆ describe the disorders of the outer ear, middle ear, inner ear, eighth nerve, and auditory cortex to which older adults are most susceptible.

◆ Overview

The entire auditory system undergoes changes with age. In addition, certain otological conditions are more prevalent in older than in younger adults. This chapter discusses the changes that occur in the peripheral and central auditory systems of the older adult, and describes some of the ear pathologies prevalent in this population. Sixty-five years of age was adopted by President Franklin D. Roosevelt as the definition of *old* for Social Security purposes. He used German Chancellor Otto von Bismarck's legal criterion for retirement age. Bismarck had adopted 65 in 1889 because his actuaries advised him that hardly anyone at that time lived to 65 in Germany, and thus the plan would rarely have to pay retirement benefits (Nielsen, 1998).

Pearl

Age 65 is an arbitrary criterion for defining someone as old.

Over the past decade, a considerable amount of research and evidence-based speculation has accumulated documenting the age-related changes in the peripheral and central auditory systems. Current thinking is that the auditory system is an integrated one involving an interplay between the many components including both the ear and the brain. In short, impoverished output from the peripheral auditory system due in part to age-related changes has implications for the integrity of the input to the central auditory system. It now appears that a central locus underlies the age-related declines in auditory temporal processing key to speech understanding, and that cognitive changes associated with age-related changes in portions of the brain help to explain individual differences in language comprehension in challenging acoustic environments. Thanks to scientific advances, our understanding of age-related changes in the auditory system has advanced considerably since the first edition of this text. The traditional way in which the subtypes of presbycusis have been described has been revisited, with acknowledgment of the link between environmental stressors and genetic factors in age-related hearing loss. This chapter provides an update on the state of the science that can assist audiologists in understanding the functional effects of the age-related changes in the auditory system and in approaching management in a way that can help to take advantage of the new information to promote improved function.

◆ Anatomical and Physiological Changes in the Outer Ear

The outer ear comprises the auricle (pinna) and the external auditory meatus or external auditory canal. The auricle, which is an irregular ovoid structure, is the external extension of the cartilaginous ear canal and as such is formed of elastic cartilage. Skin covers the auricle, with hairs present primarily in

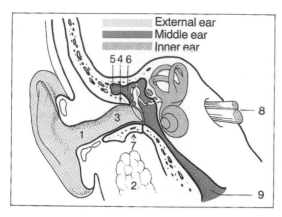

Fig. 4.1 Cartilaginous and osseous portions of the external auditory meatus relative to middle and inner portions of the ear. 1, cartilaginous part; 2, parotid gland; 3, bony meatus; 4, lateral attic wall; 5, mastoid antrum; 6, attic; 7, temporomandibular joint; 8, facial vestibular, and auditory nerves; 9, eustachian tube. [From Becker, W., Naumann, H., & Pfaltz, C. (1994). *Ear, nose, and throat diseases* (2nd ed., p. 4). New York: Thieme. Reprinted by permission.]

the tragal and anti-tragal regions (Senturia, Marcus, & Lucente, 1980). The epidermal skin, which is the skin covering the external part of the ear, is continuous with the skin covering the body, and it has evolved to serve numerous protective functions to minimize infection from the external environment (Johnson, Hawke, & Jahn, 2001). The external auditory canal is a skin lined S-shaped cul-de-sac approximately 25 mm in length (Osguthorpe & Nielsen, 2006). The anterior wall of the canal is adjacent medially to the temporomandibular joint and laterally to the parotid gland. Also, the inferior wall is closely related to the parotid gland. The external auditory canal is composed of elastic cartilage laterally and bone medially (**Fig. 4.1**). The cartilage of the outer portion of the canal is continuous with that of the pinna, whereas the skin of the osseous canal is continuous with the skin covering the lateral surface of the tympanic membrane (Ballachanda, 1995). **Figure 4.1** shows the anatomical distinctions between the cartilaginous and osseous parts of the ear canal and the canal's relation to the middle and inner parts of the ear.

The skin covering the ear canal is thinner in the osseous canal compared with the cartilaginous portion. Specifically, the skin lining the cartilaginous canal consists of epidermis with papillae, a well-developed dermis, and a subcutaneous layer. The cartilaginous infrastructure contains sebaceous and apocrine glands and hair follicles. The epidermis is composed of four layers: basal cell, prickle or squamous cell, granular cell, and cornified layers. As will be shown later, these layers give rise to tumor cells prevalent in older adults. The skin lining the osseous canal is devoid of papillae and has no subcutaneous layer. The osseous canal does not contain glands or hair follicles, whereas the skin of the fibrocartilaginous portion of the canal contains hair follicles and apocrine (ceruminous) and sebaceous glands. The skin of the osseous canal is quite thin (0.2 mm in thickness); it is susceptible to trauma during any type of manipulation, such as cerumen removal and deep insertion of hearing aids (Ballachanda, 1995).

Cerumen, or "earwax," is a naturally occurring substance that cleans, protects, and lubricates the ear canal. It consists of a mixture of secretions from sebaceous and apocrine sweat glands, such as lipids, protein-free amino acids, and several minerals, and it includes dust particles and desquamated epithelial cells (Ballachanda, 1995; Roland et al, 2008). As the cerumen migrates laterally, it mixes with hair follicles and other matter in the external auditory meatus. The secretory glands in the external auditory canal, namely the sebaceous and ceruminous glands, are responsible for secreting lipids and peptides into the cerumen (Guest, Greener, Robinson, & Smith, 2004). The sebaceous glands are closely associated with the hair follicles and are not capable of active secretion, so they form their secretions from passive breakdown of cells. The ceruminous glands are a type of apocrine gland, and they secrete their contents (i.e., cerumen) (Johnson et al, 2001). Further, the hairs in the outer third of the ear canal also produce glandular secretions that contribute to the composition of cerumen. It is normally eliminated by a self-cleaning mechanism, which leads to epithelial migration out of the ear canal, assisted by movement of the jaw (Roland et al, 2008). One of the most common reasons for physician visits is accumulation of cerumen because of failure of the self-cleaning mechanism. Accumulation of excessive cerumen, also called cerumen impaction, is present in approximately one third of older adults, with estimates ranging from 19 to 65% (Guest et al, 2004). It is more common in the elderly, in developmentally delayed adult populations, in nursing home residents, and in persons with cognitive impairments (Roland et al, 2008).

The outer ear subserves several important functions, some auditory and some nonauditory (Johnson et al, 2001). The primary auditory function of the external ear is to act as an "acoustic resonator" to intensify sound in the range of 2 to 5 KHz, the frequencies most important in speech (Howarth & Shone, 2006). In general, the role of the pinna and ear canal is to couple airborne sound waves to the middle ear. The ear canal, in combination with the concha, alters the spectral content of the signal reaching the tympanic membrane. Specifically, it modifies incoming sound by acting as a resonator or generator of additional sound (Staab, 1995). It is integral to success with hearing aids, in that it serves as the location where any style of hearing aid is placed. The ear canal is an important site for behavioral and electrophysiological tests, and its status often influences the outcomes achieved on these measures as well as the ability to administer selected tests. The audiologist therefore should be familiar with how aging may affect the structure and function of the outer ear. The nonauditory function of the ear canal is protection of the tympanic membrane and more medial structures, and maintenance of a clear, debris- and disease-free passage through which sound is transmitted to the middle ear (Johnson et al, 2001). Specifically, the outward facing hair follicles and ceruminous glands assist in preventing foreign bodies from entering the ear canal.

The primary age-related changes that occur in this structure include degeneration of elastic fibers and decreased collagen, which lead to a loss of elasticity and strength. As such, there is a thinning of surface epithelium and atrophy of the subcutaneous tissue. Further, the glandular structure within the ear canal, most notably the sebaceous and cerumen glands, lose some of their secretory ability. There is also a decrease in the fat present in the canal and an increase in the thickness and length of hair follicles in the fibrocartilaginous portion. As a result, the skin becomes dry and prone to trauma and breakdown, and cerumen becomes more concentrated, hard, and impacted (Ballachanda, 1995). The bony canal is especially susceptible to trauma that may result from manipulations associated with cerumen removal because the skin covering is so thin. This is also a concern when making ear impressions for completely in-the-canal hearing aids (Ballachanda, 1995). Associated with the changes in the ear canal is a decrease in tolerance for hard materials.

Cerumen production and extrusion go uninterrupted in most individuals by virtue of normal epithelial migration from deeper parts of the ear canal. Cerumen impaction can occur for several reasons, notably excessive production of cerumen due to increased activity of cerumen glands. Nonphysiological variables accounting for cerumen impaction include physical obstruction due to a hearing aid, frequent use of cotton-tipped swabs, or abnormalities in the shape and size of the ear canal. Older adults are more susceptible to a higher frequency of impaction for still another reason: there is a reduction in the number of active cerumen glands, which leads to the production of drier and less viscous cerumen. Combined with the presence of thicker and longer hair follicles that are oriented toward the tympanic membrane, this leads to a higher frequency of impaction (Ruby, 1986). As cerumen impaction is prevalent in persons with cognitive impairment, residents of nursing homes tend to be prone to cerumen accumulation, with a prevalence as high as 40 to 57% (Guest et al, 2004). Gleitman, Ballachanda, and Goldstein (1992) conducted a study of 892 adults to determine the prevalence of impaction in individuals of varying age groups. It was notable that the highest prevalence, 34%, was for persons 65 to 75 years, with 22% of adults 75 to 84 years having impacted cerumen. Mahoney (1987) reported the prevalence of cerumen impaction to be as high as 34% in her sample.

◆ Common Disorders of the External Ear

Disorders of the external ear are common in older adults, as discussed in the following subsections.

The Pinna

The most common changes in the pinna associated with the aging process are excessive hair growth on the tragus and on the lower portions of the helix, primarily in males; enlargement of the pinna; and changes in the physical properties of the skin, including loss of elasticity, dryness, thinning, and, on occasion, atrophy (Johnson & Hadley, 1964). For the most part, these changes do not affect hearing; however, they may interfere with hearing-aid impressions and hearing-aid use.

Chondrodermatitis, a painful or tender pink ulceration, may appear on the helix or antihelix of the ear. It results from degeneration of the epidermis, dermis, or cartilage from chronic sun exposure, pressure, or trauma (Young, Newcomer, & Kligman, 1993). If, during audiometry, cerumen management, or the making of an earmold impression, the audiologist notes

the presence of a lesion on the ear, the patient should be referred to a physician, preferably a dermatologist.

The pinna is a potential site for squamous cell carcinoma, a red-brown–appearing nodule associated with chronic sun or radiation exposure (Young et al, 1993). A large proportion of squamous cell carcinomas in fair-skinned individuals occur on the face or ears, primarily in older adults (Steigleder & Maibach, 1993). The posterosuperior aspect of the pinna is most frequently involved in men, whereas these tumors tend to occur closer to the ear canal in women (Abrams et al, 1995). Basal cell carcinomas are a common malignant tumor of the pinna, occurring more often in men, and, like squamous cell carcinomas, occur secondary to sun exposure. Basal cell carcinomas appear as nodules with pearly, heaped-up borders (Abrams et al, 1995).

> **Pearl**
>
> If the audiologist notices an unusual-looking growth when examining the pinna, appropriate referral should be made because these tumors have metastatic potential.

The External Auditory Meatus

In light of age-related changes in the structure of the ear canal, which include thinning of the surface epithelium, atrophy of the subcutaneous tissue, and decline in the secretory abilities of the glands, older adults are susceptible to the development of dry skin, which is prone to trauma and breakdown, and to hard and impacted cerumen (Ballachanda, 1995). Also, older adults are susceptible to selected functional and pathological conditions.

The most commonly reported functional condition of the ear canal is referred to as collapsed canal. In this condition, pressure from earphones applied during audiometric tests may cause the ear canal to collapse, which may occur because of atrophy of the supporting cartilage and resulting decreased skin elasticity in the cartilaginous portion of the ear canal. As a result, air conduction threshold shifts may emerge, primarily in the high frequencies leading to the presence of "artificial air–bone gaps." However, threshold shifts of 15 dB or more have been reported at all frequencies by several investigators (Ballachanda, 1995). The prevalence of collapsed ear canals in older adults varies depending primarily on the population studied, but has been reported to be as high as 30 to 40%. Although in the past the presence of collapsed canals was a major source of measurement error, the use of insert rather than supra-aural earphones during testing helps to alleviate the problem.

> **Pearl**
>
> During audiometric testing, the presence of a high-frequency air–bone gap, poor test-retest reliability, or disagreement between pure-tone and immittance test results should alert the clinician to the potential of a collapsed ear canal.

Techniques such as use of sound-field testing, insert earphones, and holding the pinna up and back prior to earphone placement can effectively alleviate the problem of a collapsed ear canal (Silman & Silverman, 1991).

Cerumen impaction, a prevalent condition in older adults, can have significant medical and audiological consequences, which for the most part are temporary, resolving upon removal of the cerumen. Common medical sequelae of impaction include tinnitus, itching, pain, fullness of the ear, external otitis, otalgia, and, less frequently, vertigo (Ballachanda, 1995; Guest et al, 2004). Occasionally, cerumen impaction is associated with discharge, odor, or cough. An audiological consequence of gradual cerumen buildup is hearing loss, which is typically high frequency and conductive, often presenting as a conductive component on an already existing sensorineural hearing loss. Hearing loss occurs because the cerumen creates a constriction of the ear canal. The presence of cerumen impaction can restrict audiologists from performing selected diagnostic tests, hearing-aid fittings, and rehabilitative procedures. For example, blockage can interfere with otoacoustic emissions, immittance measures, electrocochleography, and videonystagmography. Interference with audiological test procedures can create patient inconvenience because of the necessity to postpone testing until the cerumen has been removed. Further, impacted cerumen can preclude real ear hearing-aid measurements, render a hearing aid ineffectual, especially the Lyric hearing system, or cause hearing aids to malfunction.

It is incumbent on audiologists to thoroughly review protocols for checking for wax and to ensure that hearing-aid users know how to remove and replace wax guards, given the likelihood of blockage from cerumen, as it is a frequent complaint and occurrence among older hearing-aid users. In light of the problems posed by cerumen buildup or impaction, the American Speech-Language-Hearing Association (ASHA), the American Academy of Audiology, and licensing boards of most states officially recognize cerumen management as being within the scope of audiology practice. Audiologists engaged in cerumen management should check state licensure laws, professional insurance policies, and institutional insurance coverage, as well. In addition, universal precautions specified by the Centers for Disease Control and Prevention should be followed for those audiologists engaged in cerumen management. When performing cerumen management in older adults, exercise extreme caution in individuals prone to infection such as persons with diabetes mellitus, AIDS infection, autoimmune disease, cancer, or external otitis. With the elderly especially, excessive care should be taken when removing cerumen from the bony portion of the canal to avoid unnecessary abrasion. If external lesions are present in and around the ear canal, referral to a physician should be made. Further, patients should be instructed not to use Q-tips to clean the ear canal because the use of these cotton-tipped swabs can lead to impacted cerumen (Guest et al, 2004). As traumatic perforation of the tympanic membrane can arise when cerumen removal is not done correctly, audiologists should be selective in the patients on whom they perform this procedure. Finally, audiologists engaged in cerumen management should be familiar with the advantages and disadvantages of the various therapeutic options including irrigation, cerumenolytics, and manual removal. I recommend the clinical practice guidelines on cerumen impaction promulgated by Roland et al (2008), especially for the increasing number of audiologists dispensing Lyric hearing aids.

The external ear canal may be the site of benign, malignant, or premalignant neoplastic changes. These include keratosis obturans, exostosis and osteoma, and squamous or basal cell carcinoma. Further, radiation therapy can affect the ear as well (Roland et al, 2008). Any unusual-appearing outgrowth in the cartilaginous or bony ear canal, bleeding from the ear canal, or otorrhea may signify the presence of a neoplasm in the ear, indicating the necessity for a medical referral.

Contact dermatitis, an inflammatory process produced by contact of an irritant with the skin, may arise in the ear canal of older adults, often from hearing aids or ear molds. The length of exposure to the agent, combined with individual susceptibility, determines whether skin irritation will arise (Senturia et al, 1980). Symptoms of dermatitis might include itchiness or erythema. When dermatitis from hearing-aid use is suspected, the patient should be instructed to remove the etiological agent and contact the physician for proper treatment.

Pruritus, or itching, is the most common dermatological complaint of older adults, and the external auditory meatus is a common site. Dryness of the skin resulting from atrophy of the epithelial sebaceous glands tends to contribute to the development of pruritus. In view of age-related skin atrophy, the skin lining the canal is vulnerable to trauma. Older adults should be advised against using cotton applicators to remove debris because this can induce further itching, trauma, and potential infection (Rees & Duckert, 1995).

Otitis externa is an inflammatory process of the external ear that is typically bacterial in origin yet is occasionally fungal (Miyamoto & Miyamoto, 1995; Sander, 2001). It is more prevalent in in persons 7 to 12 years of age declining in those over 50 years (Osguthorpe & Nielsen, 2006). According to Sander (2001), the unique structure of the ear canal (i.e., it is the only skin-lined cul-de-sac in the human body) contributes to the development of otitis externa; the cul-de-sac is warm and dark, and prone to becoming moist, making it an excellent host for bacterial and fungal growth. The following conditions increase susceptibility of the ear to development of otitis externa: moisture from swimming, perspiration, or high humidity; high environmental temperatures; and insertion of foreign objects (Osguthorpe & Nielsen, 2006; Sander, 2001). Further, chronic dermatological diseases, including eczema and psoriasis, place people at risk for development of otitis externa (Sander, 2001). The symptoms can range from primarily itching to otorrhea, redness, swelling, a blocked feeling within the ear, and tenderness. The severity of the symptoms depends on the duration of the condition and on the pathogen. The most severe form, malignant necrotizing otitis externa, may develop in elderly diabetics and patients whose condition is out of control or in immunocompromised patients (Miyamoto & Miyamoto, 1995). If examination of the ear canal reveals any of the above symptoms, referral to a physician is indicated. When otitis externa is other than mild, it is typically treated with analgesics including nonsteroidal antiinflammatory agents or topicals. The topicals tend to be aminoglycosides (e.g., neomycin or gentamicin), and ototoxicity from the latter is associated with open middle ear spaces or prolonged use, so they are typically avoided when the eardrum is not intact (Osguthorpe & Nielsen, 2006). When older patients suffer from moderate acute otitis media, oral antibiotics are often prescribed, especially in persons with diabetes or in older adults who are immunocompromised.

Management of Patients

The outer ear is of considerable import to audiologists because of the emergence of interventions (e.g., Lyric hearing aids) and diagnostic procedures that directly involve its visualization and manipulation. In the diagnostic realm, the ear canal is critical to immittance measurements, otoacoustic emissions, videonystagmography, electrocochleography, and auditory brainstem responses. Further, cerumen management is now part of the scope of practice of audiologists, necessitating thorough knowledge of its anatomy and potential disorders. In the rehabilitative arena, the pinna and ear canal serve as the anchor for hearing aids of all shapes and sizes, with the bony portion becoming increasingly important with the advent of completely in-the-canal hearing aids. Precise ear canal impressions are critical for the manufacturing and dispensing of custom-molded products such as in the ear and completely in-the-canal hearing aids and for persons with moderately severe to severe hearing loss who require occluding ear molds. The Lyric hearing system, which is placed completely inside the ear canal, brings patients in more frequently for some form of cerumen management to prevent blockage of the sound port. Finally, the ear canal is critical for performing verification with real-ear systems during hearing-aid fitting and post-fittings. The audiologist working with older adults must be able to identify medical conditions involving the external ear for referral to physicians. At any time during a rehabilitative or diagnostic procedure that any unusual growth or irritation appears, it is incumbent on the audiologist to make the appropriate referral.

◆ Anatomical and Physiological Changes in the Middle Ear

The middle ear and eustachian tube are located deep in the temporal bone (Bernstein, 2001). The middle ear cleft consists of the tympanic membrane, the middle ear air-filled space containing a chain of three ossicles that mechanically connect the tympanic membrane to the oval window of the cochlea, the mastoid cavity, the attic, and the eustachian tube (Bernstein, 2001). The tympanic membrane, a multilayer fiber structure, is composed of three layers: an outer epithelial layer that is continuous with the skin of the osseous portion of the ear canal; a fibrous tissue layer; and an inner mucosal layer that is continuous with the lining of the middle ear space, mastoid system, and eustachian tube. The ossicles, within the middle ear cleft, articulate with one another at the incudomalleal (IM) and incudostapedial (IS) joints, which are lined by articular cartilages. The tensor tympani muscle attaches to the malleus via the tendon of the tensor tympani, and the stapedius muscle attaches to the head of the stapes via the stapedial tendon. The ossicles are suspended within the cavity via a system of ligaments and tendons. The eustachian tube connects the middle ear to the airways in the nasopharynx, thereby ventilating the middle ear space. Prerequisites for normal transmission of sound to the inner ear are a tympanic membrane of normal position and mobility, a continuous ossicular chain, and adequate ventilation of the middle ear via an intact eustachian tube.

The sound transmission apparatus undergoes changes with the aging process that resemble arthritic changes and loss of elasticity typically occurring in other parts of the body (Wiley, Nondahl, Cruickshanks, & Tweed, 2005). For the most part, the changes do not appear to impact dramatically on hearing sensitivity. The changes are discussed in the following paragraphs. In addition, the diseases prevalent among older adults that affect middle ear status are discussed.

The tympanic membrane, ossicular chain, articular cartilage at the surfaces of the IM and IS joints, and middle ear muscles and ligaments are susceptible to minor age-related changes. Covell (1952), Rosenwasser (1964), and Etholm and Belal (1974) have performed histological studies of the middle ear structures and have observed a series of age-related changes. The tympanic membrane appears to become stiffer and less elastic, thinner, and less vascular with increased age (Wiley et al, 2005). Some have speculated that the middle ear system may become more lax with age due to changes associated with rheumatoid arthritis in the lenticular process of the incus (Rawool & Harrington, 2007). In becoming more translucent with age, selected landmarks appear more visible during the otoscopic examination. Older adults with a history of chronic otitis media (COM) may have sclerotic changes on the eardrum that on visual inspection may present as chalky white plaques (White & Regan, 1987). The presence of the white scale-like plaques on the tympanic membrane following COM is a hallmark of tympanosclerosis. This condition typically creates a stiffening effect on the tympanic membrane. Tympanic membrane hysteresis (i.e., viscous properties of the system) is significantly reduced in older adults relative to younger adults (Gaihede and Koefoed-Nielsen, 2000). In their longitudinal study of 5-year changes in middle ear function over time, Wiley and colleagues (2005) confirmed that there are few functionally significant changes.

Arthritic changes in the middle ear have been observed in individuals over 30 years of age, increasing in frequency and severity with age. In fact, rheumatoid arthritis is known to affect the joints of the middle ear, which in some is associated with an increase in middle ear resonance (Rawool & Harrington, 2007). Rawool and Harrington (2007) reported that 93% of older adults with arthritis in their sample had abnormal admittance findings on tympanometry, and that individuals with osteoarthritis had a higher prevalence of middle ear abnormalities based on static admittance values. The arthritic changes include thinning and calcification of the cartilaginous IM and IS joints (Covell, 1952; Rosenwasser, 1964). Etholm and Belal (1974) reported that, according to their histological studies, the arthritic changes were moderate to severe in persons over 70 years of age. Because the IM and IS joints are synovial in nature, lined by articular cartilage and surrounded by an elastic tissue capsule, these arthritic and degenerative changes in joint structure are not surprising, given the modifications occurring in the articular surfaces of other joints throughout the body. Individuals with osteoarthritis and a negative family history of hearing loss, noise exposure, or chronic middle ear effusion have a higher prevalence of middle ear abnormalities than does an age-matched control group without arthritis (Rawool & Harrington, 2007). Additional age-related changes include atrophy and degeneration of the fibers of the middle ear muscles and the ossicular ligaments and ossification of the ossicles (Covell, 1952; Rosenwasser, 1964). Finally, calcification of the cartilaginous support of the eustachian tube and atrophy of the musculature have been reported in older adults. The age-related decline in muscle function may interfere with the opening of the eustachian tube especially during swallowing. Although these changes do not appear to impact on pure-tone air and bone conduction thresholds, they may account for age effects appearing in selected studies on eustachian tube function, the acoustic reflex, and acoustic immittance results in older adults.

Pearl

The middle ear structures undergo anatomical change with age, though they have little effect on the physiology of the middle ear and on behavioral tests. There is little evidence of substantial stiffening of the middle ear transmission system with age (Wiley, Cruickshanks, Nondahl, & Tweed, 1999).

◆ Common Disorders of the Middle Ear

Older adults are susceptible to developing all of the diseases that arise in the middle ear, yet some diseases are more likely than others to occur early rather than late in adult life. **Table 4.1** lists common diseases of the middle ear. Older adults are susceptible to middle ear disease associated with trauma and to neoplastic tumors, including squamous cell carcinoma and vascular tumors such as glomus tumors. Otosclerosis, a focal disease of the otic capsule, is generally associated with an early age of onset (i.e., adolescence and young adulthood); however, Farrior (1963) reported that nearly 40% of patients in his sample developed hearing loss from otosclerosis in their fifth, sixth, or seventh decade of life. Ayache, Corre, Van Prooyen, and Elbaz (2003) reviewed stapedectomy results in a sample

Table 4.1   Common Diseases of the Middle Ear

Infectious diseases of the middle ear
    Acute or chronic otitis media
    Otitis media with effusion
    Acute mastoiditis
    Tympanosclerosis
Trauma to the middle ear
    Temporal bone injury
    Tympanic membrane or ossicular damage
Neoplastic tumors and diseases of the middle ear
    Polyps
    Cholesteatoma
    Osteomas
    Glomus tumors
    Squamous cell carcinoma
Congenital diseases of the middle ear
    Ossicular anomalies
    Vascular anomalies
    Facial nerve anomalies
Idiopathic diseases of the middle ear
    Otosclerosis

Source: Northern, J. (1996). *Hearing disorders* (3rd ed.). Boston: Allyn & Bacon.

of older adults undergoing surgery for otosclerosis. Notably, improvement in hearing and closure of the air–bone gaps (of 20 dB) occurred in all cases and closure of the air–bone gap to less than 10 dB occurred in 87% of the cases. Hearing results were similar in older and younger adults, and the researchers concluded that stapes surgery is effective in older adults. Further, Vartiainen (1995) found that there was not a significant increase in surgical complications from surgery for otosclerosis in a sample of older adults.

When acute otitis media occurs after age 60, the relative incidence of mastoiditis and associated complications is higher in older adults because of the diminished responsiveness of their immune system (White & Regan, 1987). Symptoms include, but are not limited to, facial nerve paralysis and labyrinthitis, whereas complications may include meningitis and brain abscess. It is noteworthy that otitis media caused by infection with *Mycobacterium tuberculosis* may result from spread associated with pulmonary infection or from an ascending infection through the eustachian tube from the nasopharynx. Tuberculosis otitis media is generally painless, with multiple small perforations that may ultimately lead to total tympanic membrane perforation (Schleuning & Andersen, 1993).

Of all middle ear disorders, persons over 65 years of age are most prone to developing one of the many infectious diseases of the middle ear. Their susceptibility grows out of changes in the musculature of the eustachian tube with age, a less efficient immune system, and tendency toward development of complications from diseases or interventions that may terminate in middle ear infection. Data summarizing the epidemiology of middle ear problems among the elderly are imprecise; however, data from the National Hospital Discharge Survey are somewhat revealing. Among persons over 65 years of age, the most common otolaryngological diagnoses were (1) otitis media and upper respiratory infection (URI) with complication or comorbidity; (2) otitis media and URI without complication or comorbidity; (3) dysequilibrium; and (4) ear, nose, and throat (ENT) malignancy. The most common procedures were sinus and mastoid procedures, major head and neck procedures, and rhinoplasty. It is likely that conditions afflicting the elderly such as nasopharyngeal pathology, including malignancy, and radiation therapy for ENT malignancy, also place older adults at risk for otitis media. Similarly, nasotracheal intubation or prolonged nasogastric (NG) tube placement may cause edema of the eustachian tube and nasopharynx, possibly leading to development of otitis media (Kenna, 1993).

Special Consideration

Because an older person's immune system may become less effective in its primary function of protecting against infection and neoplastic disease, the case history and audiometric testing should routinely include tests of middle ear status to facilitate early diagnosis and management of middle ear disease.

◆ Aging of the Inner Ear and Neural Pathways

The site of conversion of mechanical energy to an electrophysiological signal, the inner ear is composed of several functional components that are vulnerable to the effects of aging. These components are sensory, neural, vascular, supporting, synaptic, and mechanical (Willott, 1991). The organ of Corti, which is the site of transduction of mechanical to neural energy, houses the sense organ of hearing. It extends spirally from the basal convolution to the cupula or apex of the cochlea. The organ of Corti rests atop the basilar membrane and is composed of sensory cells (outer and inner hair cells along with their stereocilia), supporting cells, Reissner's membrane, tectorial membrane, and stria vascularis, among other structures. The inner hair cells act to transduce mechanical movements into neural activity, and in fact most information about sounds is conveyed in inner hair cells (Moore, 2003), which are considered passive detectors of basilar membrane motion (Schmiedt, 2010). Hence, the inner hair cells with which the majority of eighth nerve fibers form their afferent synapses are primarily responsible for eighth nerve activity and therefore for perception of acoustic stimuli (Santos-Sacchi, 2001). They are responsible for exciting afferent fibers. In contrast, outer hair cells influence cochlear mechanics, and hence drugs or other agents selectively affect the operation of outer hair cells, leading to a loss of sharp tuning and sensitivity of the basilar membrane (Moore, 2003). Inner hair cells are more resilient than outer hair cells, often appearing normal even in the absence of all three rows of outer hair cells (Harrison & Mount, 2001). Deflection of the stereocilia, which protrude from the hair cells, leads to a flow of potassium ions into the hair cells, altering the voltage difference between the inside and outside of the hair cells (Moore, 2003). This leads to release of neurotransmitters, which initiates action potentials in the neurons of the auditory nerve.

The stria vascularis is considered the "cochlea amplifier" responsible for producing and maintaining the endocochlear potential (EP) between scala media and scala tympani (Dubno, 2009). The endolymph within scala media resembles intracellular fluid with an ion composition high in K^+ and low in Na^+, and this space exhibits a positive electrical potential relative to the perilymphatic tissues (Santi & Tsuprun, 2001). It is important to note that aerobic metabolism is high in the lateral stria vascularis, as this is necessary for maintenance of the K^+ gradient between the endolymph and perilymph and for generation of the endocochlear potential (Schmiedt, 2010). Produced largely by the stria in the basal turn where it is highest, the positive EP is approximately –90 mV within the scala media and is present across the outer hair cells. The EP, which serves as the cochlear battery, varies along the length of the basilar membrane such that the EP at the apical end is lower than at the cochlear base. Specifically, the maximum gain ranges from approximately 20 dB at the apex to 50 to 70 dB at the basal end (Schmiedt, 2010). Stria vascularis is highly vascularized and has a high metabolic rate.

> **Pearl**
>
> When the cochlear amplifier is not functioning either due to loss of outer hair cells or a low EP, the greatest effect is on high-frequency hearing (Schmiedt, 2010).

The normal auditory system is tonotopically organized, and the tonotopic organization depends on the existence of ana-

tomic connections from the cochlea to regions within the central auditory system (Willott, 1996). This tonotopic organization is the mechanism by which frequencies within the periphery are represented within the central auditory system. From the cochlea to the brain, numerous structural and chemical changes occur with age, and it is precisely the physiological changes described below that alter the way in which frequency and timing information are encoded in the peripheral and central auditory systems (Tremblay & Ross, 2007). Interestingly, melanin containing melanocytes is distributed throughout much of the cochlea, and the density of melanin within the cochlea corresponds to general pigmentation as reflected in eye and skin color (Pratt et al, 2009). Further, as melanin is considered to be otoprotective, it may be involved in the structural, metabolic, and vascular health of the cochlea and likely plays a role in the long-term health of the cochlea. The presence of melanin in the cochlea is a likely explanation for the better hearing older black males and females experience as contrasted to older Caucasians. Finally, melanin may be a factor that increases susceptibility to ototoxic medications in older adults, because many toxins and pharmacological agents tend to bind with melanin. The latter results in an accumulation of the chemicals in melanin-rich tissues, potentiating their actions.

> **Pearl**
>
> The inner ear undergoes dramatic changes with age, with corresponding effects on pure-tone thresholds and word recognition tests. Age-related peripheral hearing loss results in a deterioration of the input to auditory regions of the brain (Turner & Caspary, 2005).

> **Special Consideration**
>
> The most critical risk factor for the auditory system is age.

Degeneration of the Organ of Corti

Presbycusis is the term applied to age-related hearing loss, and it has come to encompass the conditions and insults contributing to hearing loss in older people (Gates & Mills, 2005). The most critical risk factor for the auditory sense organ is age, yet genetic susceptibility and noise exposure play a role as well (Lin, Thorpe, Gordon-Salant, & Ferrucci, 2011). The organ of Corti is the structure most susceptible to age-related histopathological changes; however, structural and chemical changes occur throughout the peripheral and central auditory systems (Tremblay & Ross, 2007). Age-related atrophy ultimately interferes with the transduction process that is integral to the reception of sound. The cells of the inner ear and neural pathways are of the nonmitotic variety (Schuknecht, 1993). They are highly differentiated cells such that once their specialized functions have been established, they can no longer reproduce. The length of cell life depends on the ability to maintain their characteristic structural organization while adapting to changes in their fluid environment (Schuknecht, 1993). Our knowledge of changes in the aging cochlea is based primarily on histopathological studies of human temporal bones and more recently on animal models using a variety of animals including Mongolian gerbils, squirrel monkeys, and mice (Frisina, Zhu, & Souza, 2009; Mills, Schmiedt, Schulte, & Dubno, 2006; Schuknecht, 1955, 1964; Schuknecht & Gacek, 1993). Prior to outlining the classic findings from the work of Schuknecht and his colleagues, some general age-related histopathological changes within the organ of Corti and spiral ganglion cells will be discussed.

The primary histopathological changes in the organ of Corti include sensory cell degeneration along with loss of supporting cells, including Deiters' cells, pillar cells, and Hensen cells (Chisolm, Willott, & Lister, 2003). In general, loss of hair cells begins in the extreme basal end, where it is most severe, with the outer hair cells degenerating first. Further, degeneration of the outer row of outer hair cells is often more severe than in the other rows (Willott, 1991). Decrease in hair cell population is greatest in persons over 70 years of age and is most pronounced for outer hair cells. That is, the hair cell population is less in older adults, especially for outer hair cells. It is important to note that outer and inner hair cells tend to degenerate independently.

In contrast to the effect the loss of hair cells in the basal turn of the cochlea has on cochlear mechanics, hair cell loss in the most apical portions of the cochlea may have little effect on audiometric thresholds. Thus, older adults who experience hair cell damage in selected regions of the cochlea do not necessarily sustain a hearing loss, whereas hair cell loss near the cochlea base is associated with hearing loss. According to Willott (1991), a loss of 20% of hair cells throughout the cochlea may result in minimal sensorineural hearing loss, whereas more severe loss of hair cells extending 10 mm or more from the base of the cochlea is associated with more significant hearing loss in the high frequencies. It is now well accepted, however, that the degeneration of outer hair cells may in fact be due in large part to noise trauma in addition to age.

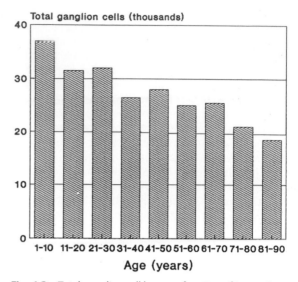

Fig. 4.2 Total ganglion cell loss as a function of increasing age. [Data from Otte, J., Schuknecht, H. F., & Kerr, A. G. (1978, Aug). Ganglion cell populations in normal and pathological human cochleae. Implications for cochlear implantation. *Laryngoscope, 88*(8 Pt 1), 1231–1246. Reprinted by permission.]

Pearl

The spectral resolving capacity of the inner ear changes with age (Frisina et al, 2001).

Degeneration of Spiral Ganglion Cells

Approximately 30,000 neurons join together to form the afferent auditory portion of the eighth nerve. In turn, the auditory nerve connects the sensory cells in the periphery to the auditory brainstem beginning at the level of the cochlear nucleus (Gates & Mills, 2005). The dendrites of the neurons are located under the hair cells, the cell bodies of the cochlear neurons (spiral ganglion cells) are found in the central core of the cochlea (modiolus), and the axons course centrally to the nuclei in the auditory brainstem. Thus, the auditory nerve comprises first-order neurons that link the sensory hair cells of the cochlea to the brainstem. The auditory nerve contains two types of fibers: 90 to 95% are type I and the remaining 5% are of the type II variety. Type I cells are large bipolar neurons composing the vast majority of the spiral ganglion cell population.

These myelinated fibers synapse with inner hair cells. The remaining 5 to 10% of the spiral ganglion neurons are type II cells (Becker, Naumann, & Pfaltz, 1994). The latter fibers are small and unmyelinated and provide efferent synapses with outer hair cells (Gates & Mills, 2005). The axons of type I and type II spiral ganglion cells project centrally in the auditory nerve as a spiraling bundle that is tonotopically organized. The center contains axons from spiral ganglion cells innervating the apical part of the cochlea, whereas the periphery of the bundle contains axons from spiral ganglion cells innervating the base (Becker et al, 1994). The nerve emerges from the internal auditory meatus and enters the ipsilateral cochlear nucleus, where each axon bifurcates to form ascending and descending branches. The centrally directed axons of the ganglion cells transmit sensory information from the periphery, via the eighth nerve, to the central auditory system for processing (Willott, 1991).

The data of Otte, Schuknecht, and Kerr (1978) and Suzuka and Schuknecht (1988) clearly demonstrate a relation between age and loss of ganglion cells. **Figure 4.2** depicts total ganglion cell loss as a function of age. The total number of ganglion cells in the cochleas of young adults ranges between 30,000 and 40,000, declining to less than 20,000 for persons between 81 and 90 years of age (Otte et al, 1978). Close analysis of the data in **Fig. 4.2** reveals progressive loss of about 2000 neurons per decade. As would be expected, neural histopathological studies suggest that age-related loss in ganglion cells is greatest near the base of the cochlea. The aging process is also associated with a decrease in the average number of fibers in the cochlear nerve. The data of Crowe, Guild, and Polvogt (1934) dramatically demonstrate that nerve fiber loss is greatest within the basal 10 mm of the cochlea. Several histopathological studies have revealed that neural degeneration can occur before and/or independently of sensory cell loss. That is to say, loss of nerve fibers in one turn of the cochlea or in all turns has

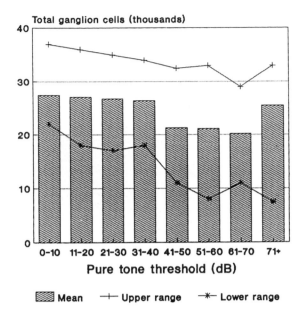

Total ganglion cells (thousands)

Pure tone threshold (dB)

▨ Mean —+— Upper range —✳— Lower range

PTA for 500, 1000, 2000 Hz

Fig. 4.3 Spiral ganglion cell loss as a function of pure-tone average. [Data from Otte, J., Schuknecht, H. F., & Kerr, A. G. (1978, Aug). Ganglion cell populations in normal and pathological human cochleae. Implications for cochlear implantation. *Laryngoscope, 88*(8 Pt 1), 1231–1246. Reprinted by permission.]

been noted without severe hair cell loss (Willott, 1991). Stated differently, loss of inner or outer hair cells "is not a prerequisite for age-related pathology of ganglion cells" (Willott, 1991, p. 28); however, inner hair cell loss is almost always associated with ganglion cell loss. Hence, shrinkage of afferent nerve fibers and their cell bodies, even with inner hair cells present, is a classic finding associated with aging.

There appears to be a relation, albeit imperfect, between amount and location of ganglion cell loss and pure-tone thresholds. Suzuka and Schuknecht (1988) reported that hearing status in their subjects was unaffected when ganglion cell loss was less than 20%. Otte et al, (1978) demonstrated that the most dramatic elevation in pure-tone thresholds occurred when the total ganglion cell population fell below 20,000. **Figure 4.3** demonstrates the relation between ganglion cell loss and pure-tone thresholds. Thus, interpolating from **Figs. 4.2 and 4.3**, persons with a ganglion cell population of about 25,000 (e.g., 30 to 60 year olds) may be predicted to have mean hearing levels within the mild range. Nadol (1981) demonstrated that ganglion cell loss restricted to the basal 3 to 5 mm of the cochlea is not associated with high-frequency hearing loss, whereas ganglion cell loss in excess of 50% in the basal 10 mm of the cochlea is associated with high-frequency loss. Several investigators have reported that speech recognition scores are poor in older adults with significant ganglion cell loss. However, cases have been reported where speech recognition performance is good in the face of significant spiral ganglion cell loss (Belal, 1975; Otte et al, 1978; Pauler, Schuknecht, & Thornton, 1986).

Recently, several additional neuronal changes have been documented with increasing age. Specifically, neural synchrony tends to be disrupted, which is associated with reduced amplitude of the action potential; neural inhibition is decreased (Caspary, Schatterman, & Hughes, 2005); neural recovery time tends to be longer (Walton, Frisina, & O'Neill, 1998); there is a decrease in the number of neurons in the auditory nuclei; there are changes in synapses between inner hair cells and the auditory nerve; and age-related changes occur in the level of inhibitory neurotransmitters (Caspary et al, 2005; Clinard, Tremblay, & Krishnan, 2010). Finally, the neural representation of sounds is altered in the aged central auditory nervous system (CANS), and there is an age-related loss of acoustic nerve activity, with both changes contributing to the processing problems experienced by many older adults especially in the temporal domain (Frisina & Walton, 2006). It is now well accepted that the consequences of the changes in the peripheral auditory system are seen throughout the central auditory system including the cochlear nucleus, the inferior colliculus, and the primary auditory cortex. Specifically, auditory deprivation in the periphery disrupts the tonotopic organization in the midbrain and in the cortex. As will be discussed later in more depth, there is central auditory reorganization due to plasticity such that intact regions of the tonotopic map adjacent to the impaired regions tend to become responsive, confirming an auditory reorganization (Tremblay & Kraus, 2002).

Pearl

Hearing loss resulting from sensory cell loss (e.g., due to noise) is characterized by a steeply sloping high-frequency hearing loss, whereas loss of cochlear nonlinearities and secondary neural degeneration are typically associated with inner hair cell loss (Dubno, 2009). There is not a one-to-one relationship between damage to auditory structures and perceptual deficits (Pichora-Fuller, 2009).

◆ Schuknecht's Subtypes of Presbycusis Revisited

Schuknecht and Gacek (1993) examined the temporal bones of 21 cases from the collection at the Massachusetts Eye and Ear Infirmary in an attempt to validate the four pathological types of presbycusis and to determine the extent to which other varieties exist. The temporal bones were prepared using the standard method of that time, the cochleas were graphically reconstructed, the inner and outer hair cells were plotted separately as being present or absent, and the neuronal population was counted and separated into four segments according to a specific formula. The stria vascularis was plotted in terms of estimated loss of volume of strial tissue. The data on the hair cells, neurons, and the stria vascularis of the 21 cochlea were transferred to histograms in which black filling indicated the percent loss as a function of distance measured from the basal end along the cochlear duct (Schuknecht & Gacek, 1993). The audiogram for each case was placed on a parallel coordinate of equal length to the cytocochleogram, with frequency on an anatomical frequency scale that expresses the spatial distribution of frequency; that is, frequencies of the audiogram are located on the abscissa in accordance with the spatial distribution of their points of maximum excitation along the

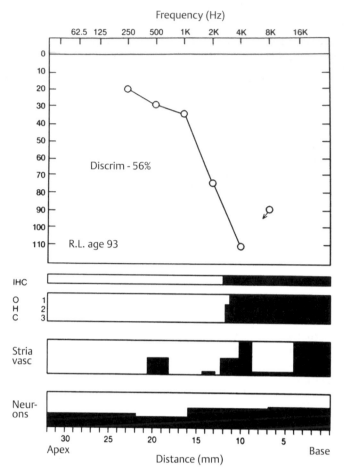

Fig. 4.4 Audiogram and cytohistogram for individual with sensory presbycusis. [From Schuknecht, H. F. (1993). *Pathology of the ear* (2nd ed.). Philadelphia: Lea & Febiger. Reprinted by permission.]

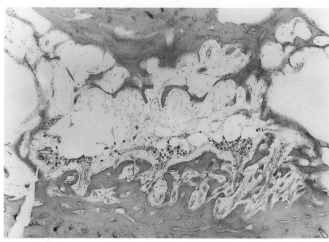

Fig. 4.5 View of the cochlea in sensory presbycusis for the individual in Fig. 4.4. The organ of Corti is totally missing in the 5.25- and 8.25-mm regions. Neurons supplying these regions of the cochlea are reduced in number. [From Schuknecht, H. F. (1993). *Pathology of the ear* (2nd ed.). Philadelphia: Lea & Febiger. Reprinted by permission.]

length of the cochlear duct (Schuknecht, 1993). As is shown in **Figs. 4.4 and 4.5,** the final product for each cochlea contained a cochlear chart consisting of both a matching audiogram and a cytocochleogram.

It is important to underscore that Schuknecht's histological technique was crude by today's standards, and in light of the primitive technology, the cellular loss in his samples had to be very advanced to be detectable. Hence, early lesions associated with subtle dysfunction could not be detected at the light microscope level. But his findings are important for historical purposes, and are currently viewed as merely a beginning in the study of the pathology of presbycusis (Gates & Mills, 2005). The development of scanning electron microscopes and laser confocal microscopes today permits improved visualization of the cochlea (Harrison & Mount, 2001). Further, over the past 30 years, use of animal models, wherein diet, genetics, and environmental toxicities are controlled, has greatly expanded the knowledge base in terms of age-related changes in the peripheral and central auditory systems (Schmiedt, 2010).

Table 4.2 summarizes the criteria and the six distinct archetypal types of presbycusis that emerged according to Schuknecht's classification system.

Sensory Presbycusis

Sensory presbycusis appears to be the least important cause of hearing loss in older adults. The sensory cell loss of sensory presbycusis is at the extreme basal end of the cochlea (8- to 12-mm region), and the section of involvement rarely includes the speech frequency area of the cochlea. The involved basal end of the cochlea shows a loss of both hair cells and sustentacular cells (Schuknecht, 1989). As is shown in the audiogram summarized in **Fig. 4.4**, the hearing loss for this 93-year-old man who worked as a shoemaker is concentrated in the higher frequencies (above 1000 Hz) and is characterized by an abrupt slope (between 1000 and 4000 Hz) and poor word recognition ability. Tonotopically, it is evident that the abrupt high-tone loss is related to a loss of hair cells in the basal 12-mm region of the cochlea. Total neuronal population is 18,315, representing a loss of 49%. This individual likely suffered from acoustic trauma as well. **Figure 4.5** shows that in this case, the organ of Corti is totally missing in selected regions (8.25 and 5.25 mm). The neurons supplying this region are diminished in number, and those that remain have lost their dendritic fibers. In sensory presbycusis, the loss of speech discrimination is inversely related to the pure-tone loss.

It was originally speculated that the cell death characterizing sensory presbycusis resulted from the accumulation of lipofuscin granules, a waste product of enzyme activity, in hair and supporting cells of the inner ear (Schuknecht, 1993). An indicator of age-associated cell damage, lipofuscin is a nondegradable substance that is produced during aging (Shankar, 2010). It is present to a greater extent in old rather than young cells (Davies, 1998). However, current thinking today is that the audiometric pattern associated with sensory presbycusis is typical of noise-induced hearing loss, and indeed most of the cases Schuknecht studied for sensory presbycusis were men with a history of noise exposure. Based on data accumulated using distortion product otoacoustic emissions and audio-

Table 4.2 Criterion for Classification of Types of Presbycusis

Type of Presbycusis	Criterion
Sensory	The presence of any total loss of hair cells beginning at the basal end of the cochlea that is at least 10 mm in length so as to involve the region of the speech frequencies on the cochlea.
Neural	Loss of 50% or more of the cochlear neurons as compared with the mean number of cochlear neurons for neonates (i.e., 35,500).
Strial	Loss of 30% or more of strial tissue.
Cochlear conductive	The criterion set for significant pathological change in the sensory cells, neurons, or stria vascularis cannot be met, and the functional criterion that must be present is a gradual descending audiogram over at least five octaves, no more than a 25-dB difference between any two adjacent frequencies, and a difference of at least 50 dB between the best and the poorest thresholds.
Mixed presbycusis	Presence of significant pathological change in more than one structure.
Intermediate presbycusis	Cochlear changes do not reach significant levels in any structure, and the audiometric profile of cochlear conductive presbycusis is not met.

Source: Schuknecht, H. F., & Gacek, M. R. (1993, Jan). Cochlear pathology in presbycusis. *Annals of Otology, Rhinology, and Laryngology, 102*(1 Pt 2), 1–16.

grams, Gates, Mills, Nam, D'Agostino, and Rubel (2002) suggested that sensory loss is not as prevalent in older adults as once theorized. The current thinking is that inner hair cells are more resistant to noise and trauma from ototoxic agents than are outer hair cells, and that aging alone does not cause outer hair cell loss, whereas noise exposure does (Schmiedt, 2010). Hence, sensory presbycusis appears to have little to do with age and more to do with environmental toxicities such as noise exposure. In summary, outer hair cell loss previously associated with sensory presbycusis is likely due to long-term exposure to noise and other environmental toxins.

Pearl

Wear and tear leads to atrophy of outer hair cells likely associated with accumulated environmental noise toxicity. Acoustic insults, such as long-term exposure to noise and ototoxic substances, "have a specific affinity for peripheral locations in the auditory system" (Frisina et al, 2001, p. 578).

Neural Presbycusis

The classic finding associated with neural lesions, which are the hallmark of neural presbycusis, is reduced word recognition ability. The most consistent pathological change in the aging inner ear is shrinkage of spiral ganglion cells, especially in Rosenthal's canal, out of proportion to organ of Corti degeneration (Chisolm et al, 2003). Further, the number of ganglion cells tends to decrease by about 15 to 25% along the entire cochlear duct (Mills, Schmiedt, & Dubno, 2006). Neural presbycusis may begin at any age, although hearing loss does not set in until the population of neural units falls below the level required for processing acoustic input (Schuknecht, 1989). Schuknecht and Gacek (1993) reported that, although puretone thresholds are variable in persons with neural presbycusis, they are not affected by neuronal loss until 90% have disappeared. The neuronal loss tends to be diffuse, involving all three turns of the cochlea and completely involving the soma, axon, and dendrites (Chisolm et al, 2003; Schuknecht, 1989). Arnesen (1982) reported that the neuronal loss in the periph-

ery is often accompanied by loss of neurons in the ventral and dorsal cochlear nuclei.

According to Otte et al (1978), loss in the ganglion cell population is much greater in persons with neural presbycusis than in adults over age 80 with no known otological disease. The relation among ganglion cell loss, otological disease, and age is depicted in **Fig. 4.6**. Here again, it is clear that the neuronal population is more than 30,000 for younger persons, declining to less than 20,000 in adults over 80 years with no known otological disease affecting the neurons. Persons diagnosed with neural presbycusis have by far the lowest population of ganglion cells—less than 15,000. The extent of neuronal loss in the 15- to 22-mm region of the cochlea where the speech frequencies lie is correlated with word recognition ability, whereas loss in the remaining regions of the cochlea is not (Pauler et al, 1986). According to Ison, Tremblay, and Allen (2010) auditory

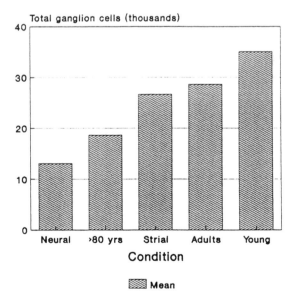

Fig. 4.6 Total ganglion cell loss for different conditions within the cochlea. [Data from Otte, J., Schuknecht, H. F., & Kerr, A. G. (1978, Aug). Ganglion cell populations in normal and pathological human cochleae. Implications for cochlear implantation. *Laryngoscope, 88*(8 Pt 1), 1231–1246. Reprinted by permission.]

evoked potentials (AEPs) are sensitive to age-related loss of audibility due to changes in the periphery, in that there tends to be a slowing of wave I (generated at the level of the auditory nerve) and subsequent waves, especially wave V. Ison et al emphasize that age-related changes in auditory brainstem response (ABR) (e.g., delay in both waves I and V) are most noticeable when high repetition rates are used, thereby stressing the system.

Strial Presbycusis

Interestingly, the deleterious effects of aging are typically first seen in highly metabolic tissue in the body, and the ear is no different. Hence, the stria vascularis, or the lateral wall of the cochlea in which metabolism is quite high, is the site of most age-related changes in the periphery (Schmiedt, 2010). Age-related degeneration of stria vascularis is the most common feature of age-related hearing loss based on recent work using animal models (Gates & Mills, 2005). It was identified by Schuknecht (1964) in his early work as the site of degenerative change as well. In fact, it is the reduction in the endocochlear potential associated with degenerative changes in the stria or lateral wall in the basal turn that likely accounts for the characteristic high-frequency hearing loss associated with the aging process (Gates & Mills, 2005). Strial presbycusis is characterized by atrophy of the stria vascularis, including loss of strial tissue and loss of strial cells, which begins in the apical and basal turns of the cochlea and extends to the midcochlear regions with aging (Gates & Mills, 2005).

Schuknecht (1993) speculated that the loss of strial tissue in aging ears affects some quality of endolymph, which in turn has a detrimental effect on the physical and chemical processes by which energy necessary to support cochlear function is made available. Studies using animals raised in quiet environments and using immunohistochemical techniques have expanded on the work of Schuknecht. Recent studies suggest that in addition to systematic degeneration of the marginal and intermediate cells of stria vascularis, there is a loss of Na+K adenosine triphosphatase (ATPase) enzyme. Further, histopathological studies of aging gerbils have shown that there are vascular changes in the stria, and areas in which there is complete capillary loss tend to correlate with regions of strial atrophy (Gates & Mills, 2005). Involvement of strial microvasculature in age-related degeneration of stria vascularis has been confirmed in laboratory studies of animals and in histopathological studies of human temporal bones. The degenerative changes in stria vascularis have a major effect on the endolymphatic potential, and hence on cochlear physiology. Specifically, the endolymphatic potential tends to decline with age, which significantly changes the voltage of the cochlear amplifier along the length of the cochlea. Using animal models, it is clear that there is a direct correlation between strial degeneration and endolymphatic potential voltage such that when strial degeneration exceeds 50%, endolymphatic potential values drop rather substantially (Gates & Mills, 2005). According to Gates and Mills (2005) the change in the endolymphatic potential with age has given rise to the dead-battery theory of presbycusis. The hearing loss that has been found to ensue tends to be flat and mild (10 to 40 dB) in the low frequencies (below 1500 Hz), gradually sloping to a moderate

level in the high-frequency region. Word recognition ability tends to be adequate in persons with pure strial presbycusis. Low frequency hearing loss is very typical of persons with strial presbycusis, and interestingly there is a hereditability factor associated with strial presbycusis that is more pronounced in women than in men.

> **Pearl**
>
> Basal atrophy is highly correlated with a reduced endolymphatic potential (Schmiedt, 2010).

Cochlear Conductive or Mechanical Presbycusis

According to Schuknecht (1964), mechanical presbycusis is associated with a stiffening of the basilar membrane and organ of Corti. A classification of cochlear conductive presbycusis ensues when the other varieties of presbycusis are histologically excluded and when linear decrements in hearing function appear. There is marked variability in the cytocochleograms. Overall, the cytocochleograms show neuronal loss, degeneration in parts of the stria vascularis, and slight loss of inner and outer hair cells. A decrease in elasticity from the basal to apical end of the basilar membrane has been implicated as a factor in cochlear conductive presbycusis (Schuknecht & Gacek, 1993). Schuknecht (1993) hypothesized that the sharpened thickening of the basilar membrane in cases of cochlear conductive presbycusis is linked to an increase in the number of its fibrillar layers. The cytocochleograms are classic, showing some neuronal loss, slight loss of hair cells, and degeneration in parts of the stria vascularis. Gates and Mills (2005) believe that this subtype of presbycusis is theoretical, but for historical purposes it is included. In fact, there is little evidence that the mechanical structure of the organ of Corti actually stiffens with age (Schmiedt, 2010). Schmiedt (2010) suggested that mechanical presbycusis may merely be an extreme case of metabolic presbycusis, because in using animal models we know that a very low endolymphatic potential is associated with a mild, flat audiogram with hearing loss greater in the low frequencies. Schuknecht and Gacek (1993) added two additional subtypes of presbycusis, namely mixed and intermediate, which may account for 25% of cases of presbycusis. In this report they also noted that sensory cell loss was the least important cause of hearing loss in older adults, with strial atrophy being the predominant change with age.

Mixed Presbycusis

Mixed presbycusis is characterized by the presence of significant pathological changes in more than one cochlear structure. Stated differently, it is characterized by involvement of two or more of the four classic types of presbycusis. As the types appear to be additive, performance on pure-tone and word recognition tests is variable. For example, the combination of sensory and strial presbycusis might present as an abrupt high-frequency hearing loss superimposed on a flat audiogram, whereas a sensory and cochlear conductive presbycusis might emerge as an abrupt high-tone loss superimposed on a descending pure-tone audiogram (Schuknecht & Gacek, 1993).

Intermediate Presbycusis

Finally, intermediate presbycusis, first described by Schuknecht and Gacek in 1993, is characterized by the absence of pathological changes on light microscopy but the presence of submicroscopic alterations in the cochlea. The latter might include alterations in the intracellular organelles that impair cell metabolism, diminished number of synapses on the hair cells, and chemical alterations in the endolymph. The audiograms are primarily flat or mildly descending, without a consistent or distinct pathological correlate.

In summary, three age-related structural changes have been observed histologically in the inner ear and auditory nerves of older adults: atrophy; degeneration of the hair cells, numerous supporting cells, and the stria vascularis; and a reduction in the number of functional spiral ganglia and nerve fibers that are of the eighth nerve. Current thinking is that age-related strial degeneration reduces the endolymphatic potential, which in turn is responsible for reduced activity in the inner hair cells. The latter change translates into reduced activity in the auditory nerve (Ison et al, (2010). For historical purposes I include **Fig. 4.7,** which provides a cross section of the human cochlea that illustrates four of the six types of presbycusis and the locus of pathology. We now know that presbycusis has variable forms of clinical expression and is not necessarily represented by a single pattern. The evaluation of hearing status in older adults must be comprehensive and individualized to ensure that intervention strategies are effective in remediating the functional sequelae of the atrophic changes within the auditory periphery. Use of distortion product otoacoustic emissions (DPOAEs) to measure outer hair cell function in combination with ABR testing to document inner hair cell and auditory nerve function is helpful in understanding the age-related hearing loss experienced by an increasing number of our clients. According to Tremblay and Burkard (2007) age-related changes in peak amplitude, latencies, and interpeak intervals are sensitive to age-related differences in peripheral sensitivity and efficiency of central auditory processing (Ison et al, 2010).

◆ Age-Related Changes in the Brainstem and Cortical Areas

Overview of the Central Auditory Nervous System

Hearing is made possible by the brain's ability to take the electrical impulses from the auditory nerve fibers and transform them into auditory sensations and perceptions (Willott, 1996). Thus, hearing cannot take place without appropriate neural activity within the central auditory system (CAS). Specifically, coding of environmental acoustic signals occurs at all levels of the ascending CAS (Caspary, Ling, Turner, & Hughes, 2008). The CAS consists of various nuclei that relay information from the cochlea and eighth nerve to other nuclei in the auditory system depicted in **Fig. 4.8** (Becker et al, 1994; Weinstein, 1998). The auditory nerve fiber system projects into centers having progressively larger populations of neurons as it ascends from the cochlea to the cortex. Coding of acoustic signals takes place throughout all levels of the CAS. Located on the lateral surface of the brain between the pons and the medulla, the cochlear nucleus (CN) complex, which consists of dorsal and ventral divisions, is the site of an obligatory synapse for all auditory nerve fibers and is the major site of projections from the auditory portion of the eighth nerve (Canlon, Illing, & Walton, 2010; Caspary et al, 2008; Frisina &

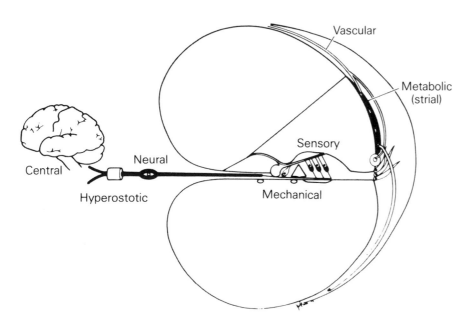

Fig. 4.7 Cross section of the cochlea showing pathological changes associated with various types of presbycusis. [From Johnsson, L., & Hawkins, J. (1979). Age-related degeneration of the inner ear. In S. Han & D. Coons (Eds.), *Special senses in aging.* Ann Arbor, MI: Institute of Gerontology, University of Michigan. Reprinted by permission.]

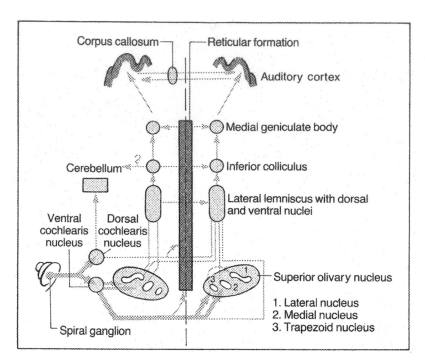

Fig. 4.8 Schematic of central auditory pathways susceptible to age-related changes. [From Roeser, R. (1996). *Roeser's audiology desk reference* (p. 17). New York: Thieme. Reprinted by permission.]

Walton, 2006). It is the first location in the central nervous system (CNS) to process and relay acoustic information from the periphery. The ventral cochlear nucleus is primarily responsible for relaying information about time and intensity cues (Caspary et al, 2008). Upon reaching the CN, about 75% of the nerve fibers cross over to the contralateral part of the brain, with the remaining 25% traveling along the ipsilateral pathway. There are two principal ascending pathways emanating from the CN. That is to say, the neurons in the cochlear nuclei send their axons to different targets. These two pathways are a bilateral projection from the ventral cochlear nucleus to the nuclei of the superior olivary complex (SOC), and projections from the dorsal (DCN) and ventral cochlear nucleus (VCN) to the contralateral inferior colliculus (IC) and nuclei of the lateral lemniscus (LL). Further, there are different morphological types of neurons within the cochlear nucleus subserving different functions.

The time, frequency, intensity, and duration features analyzed in the cochlear nuclei are relayed to the SOC, which is a major binaural processing, relay, and reflex center containing three nuclei: the lateral superior olive, the medial superior olive, and the medial nucleus of the trapezoid body. The SOC receives information from both ears through direct and indirect pathways from the respective cochlear nuclei, and along with the inferior colliculus its neurons process binaural signals critical for sound localization (Canlon et al, 2010). The SOC and CN are part of the lower brainstem. The IC comprises the auditory midbrain and houses the terminal synapse for the vast majority of incoming fibers from the CN, the SOC, and the lateral lemniscus. Virtually all ascending auditory pathways make a synapse in the IC. For example, it receives contralateral input from the DCN and VCN, ipsilateral input from the medial superior olive, and bilateral input ascending from the lateral superior olive. In short, it provides a summation of lower auditory

brainstem processing. Additionally, the VCN primarily relays information about the timing and intensity of sounds from the acoustic environment (Young & Oeretel, 2004). These VCN cells extract salient temporal features communicating the cues from both sides of the head to the SOC. At the level of the inferior colliculus, which is a mandatory relay station in the midbrain, neurons are involved with refining information regarding the location of signals in the acoustic environment (Caspary et al, 2008). According to Willott (1996), the brainstem is tonotopically organized such that, for example, neurons in the dorsal portion of the IC respond to low frequencies, and neurons at progressively more ventral locations respond to progressively higher frequencies. The inferior colliculus mediates the integration of auditory information from the brainstem nuclei. The medial geniculate body is the auditory thalamic relay to the auditory cortex. It contains a dorsal, ventral, and medial division. There are major age-related pre- and postsynaptic changes and age-related functional changes in the CN, SOC, IC, and primary auditory cortex (Caspary et al, 2008). Specifically, age-related changes of inhibitory neurotransmission occur in the ascending auditory pathways.

Pearl

Changes in temporal resolution with age are associated with degenerative changes within the brainstem pathways.

The auditory system relies on temporal coding, and a prerequisite for this is well-balanced neuronal interactions (Canlon et al, 2010). Hair cells influence neural activity via chemical synapses relying on glutametergic and cholinergic signaling to generate depolarization of the hair cell membrane and glycinergic and GAAergic interactions to generate hyperpolerization (Canlon et al, 2010). Glycine and γ-aminobutyric acid (GABA) receptors are present in the cochlear nucleus and other parts of the auditory brainstem and cortex. Glycine is a major inhibitory neurotransmitter for the neural circuitry of the auditory brainstem, and is very prominent in the cochlear nucleus (Frisina & Walton, 2006). GABA is another primary inhibitory neurotransmitter prominent in the auditory brainstem. A primary inhibitory neurotransmitter in the mammalian brain, GABA receptors are present pre- and postsynaptically (Rissman & Mobley, 2011). GABA is important to the health of hair cells and their innervations (Canlon et al, 2010). Although classified as an inhibitory neurotransmitter, it is responsible for balancing the brain by inhibiting overexcitation, and it contributes to motor control, vision, aspects of hearing, and many other cortical functions. Glutamate is an excitatory neurotransmitter. Throughout life, excitatory input from the lateral SOC releases the amino acid and excitatory neurotransmitter glutamate, and in adulthood the inhibitory input pathway secretes glycine (Alamilla & Gillespie, 2011). Both of these neurotransmitters are essential for complex sound processing (Frisina & Walton, 2006). The inferior colliculus receives excitatory glutamatergic inputs from the DCN and from the ascending projection of the SOC, and extrinsic GABAergic projections arrive at the IC from the dorsal nuclei of the lateral lemniscus, and glycinergic inputs originate from the lateral lemniscus and the SOC (Caspary et al, 2008). In addition, intrinsic GABAergic neurons are located throughout both the central nucleus and the shell nuclei of the IC. IC neurons also receive a major excitatory descending projection from the auditory cortex.

> **Pearl**
>
> Functional and neurochemical studies using animal models suggest that auditory aging may begin as a slow peripheral deafferentation, which ultimately triggers decrements in inhibitory neurotransmission (Caspary et al, , 2005). Further, age-related changes in neural recovery may be attributable to an imbalance in inhibition and excitation critical for normal cellular function (Canlon et al, 2010; Eddins & Hall, 2010).

Neuronal age-related atrophy is characterized by an overall loss of neurons; a change in neuron size (i.e., shrinkage); a decrease in size of the cell body, nucleus, or nucleolus; and a decrease in dendritic arborization along with a diminution or disappearance of dendrites and a lengthening of dendrites (Powers, 1994; Shankar, 2010; Willott, 1991). Additional functional changes in the auditory nerve system include changes in dendritic morphology, alterations in neurotransmitter receptors, and electrophysiological properties (Shankar, 2010). The frequency of spontaneous excitatory postsynaptic currents is reduced, and there is interference with the electrical firing pattern characteristic of neurons involved in information processing (Shankar, 2010). The loss of auditory nerve function with age is evident in the changes in the action potential of the auditory nerve such that the input-output function of the compound action potential (CAP) is shallow in older animals as compared with younger animals (Gates & Mills, 2005). It is now well accepted that the reduced amplitude of the action potential recording in aging ears (i.e., abnormal output of the auditory nerve) is indicative of poorly synchronized neural activity in the auditory nerve, which translates into abnormal function in the auditory brainstem as reflected in auditory brainstem studies. According to Gates and Mills (2005), the asynchronous activity in the auditory nerve associated with aging may derive from a combination of factors, including the nature of the synapse between the inner hair cells and individual auditory nerve fibers, primary degeneration of spiral ganglion cells, and a reduced endolymphatic potential. It appears that the age-related change in asynchronous activity of the auditory nerve combined with age-related changes in the CANS explain the decline in temporal resolving abilities so prevalent in older adults.

> **Pearl**
>
> Alterations in synaptic processing, decline in inhibitory neurotransmitters such as GABA, and age-related disruptions in temporal processing associated with changes in the auditory nerve and central auditory pathways likely cause the speech understanding difficulties in background noise that are the hallmarks of presbycusis (Frisina & Walton, 2006).

During normal aging, there are synaptic alterations including synaptic degeneration and change in the size of synapses in response to environmental stimuli. It is noteworthy that the greatest changes occur in persons with Alzheimer's disease in anatomical areas that underlie memory and learning (Shankar, 2010). Another hallmark of the aging CNS is that while neurons do not replicate themselves in the mature brain, they may reorganize synapses and dendritic arborizations. Several age-related changes have been reported in the CANS from the CN up to and including the auditory cortex. In general, the age-related changes in the nervous system are not uniform across the nuclei within the CANS and vary greatly among individuals. There is an increase in lipofuscin content of neurons, especially in the thalamic and cortical neurons (Shankar, 2010). Another invariant feature of aging is the formation of neurofibrillary tangles (NFTs) and senile plaques, both being a hallmark of Alzheimer's disease especially in the hippocampal regions and the frontal cortex. Interestingly, accumulation of NFTs and senile plaques occurs independent of one another.

Kirikae, Sato, and Shitara (1964) and Hansen and Reske-Nielsen (1965) were among the first investigators to perform histological studies of aging brains. Although their histopathological descriptions are limited somewhat by the methodology, it seems safe to conclude that the auditory brainstem regions do undergo some age-related changes, which include a decrease in number, size, and density of neurons; reduced cell density in selected nuclei; and an increase in pigmentation. Subsequently, Konigsmark and Murphy (1970, 1972), Arnesen (1982), and Crace (1970) evaluated portions of the auditory brainstem and expanded upon some of the findings noted above. Konigsmark and Murphy (1970, 1972) found evidence of a decrease in the volume of neurons in the VCN beginning at about 60 years of age; a decrease in the number of well-myelinated fibers in the VCN in older adults; a decrease in the number of small vessels and capillaries per unit area with increasing age; and an increase in lipofuscin accumulation with age. Crace (1970) also noted a slight decrease in neuron size and density with age, as well as a striking increase in the proportion of neurons containing pigment within the CN. Crace as well as Konigsmark and Murphy found that many neurons within the CN appear to degenerate with age.

Based on animal models, it appears that the primary aging changes in the dorsal cochlear nucleus are driven by the rapid loss of cochlear input, which is a peripherally induced central effect (Frisina & Walton, 2006). Further, there appear to be disruptions of synapses from ascending auditory nerve fibers in old animals as they contact cochlear nucleus neuron in old animals. As for the other brainstem fiber tracts, it appears that there is a slight decrease in the number of nerve fibers within the lateral lemniscus and the IC with aging (Willott, 1991). Recent auditory brainstem research has found age-related changes in the cochlear nuclei, suggesting that there may be a compensatory downregulation of inhibition following an age-related loss of peripheral input (Turner & Caspary, 2005).

There appears to be an age-related downregulation of GABAergic inhibition throughout the auditory central nervous system, which may account for the age-related changes in the strength of central synapses (Caspary et al, 2008). According to Caspary et al (2008), recent studies confirm that there is a selective loss of normal adult inhibitory neurotransmission with age, which likely subserves the loss of sensory function typical of older adults. Similarly, there are age-related declines in glycine in the cochlear nucleus (Frisina & Walton, 2006). Based on animal models, it appears that there is deterioration in glycine receptors in the cochlear nucleus, which hampers glycinergic transmission critical to auditory processing (Canlon et al, 2010). Similarly, there are age-related changes in glutamate receptors, which affect synaptic transmission in the cochlear nucleus. In contrast, there do not appear to be age-related changes in the GABA receptors in the cochlear nucleus (neurons in the CN and SOC contain GABA). There is a reduction in glycine levels in the cochlear nucleus with increasing age, which alters the response properties of cells within the CN (Caspary et al, 2008). Interestingly, SOC studies in animals show age-related changes in potassium channels and calcium-binding proteins in cells of origin in the descending pathway from the SOC to the cochlea (Zettel, Zhu, O'Neill, & Frisina, 2007). According to Gleich, Weiss, & Strutz (2004), the size of glycine and GABA neurons in the high-frequency limb of the lateral superior olive is significantly reduced in older gerbils.

The IC shows significant age-related changes in GABA neurotransmission (Caspary et al, 2005). It appears that decreased acoustic input associated with age-related changes in the auditory periphery is associated with a selective downregulation of normal adult inhibitory GABAergic function in the IC (Caspary, et al, 2008). Notably, there is a decrease in the number of GABA immunoreactive neurons, a decrease in GABA release, and a decreased concentration of GABA in the IC (Canlon et al, 2010). Further, decreased acoustic input from the auditory periphery is associated with significant changes in GABA neurotransmission in the normal adult IC (Caspary et al, 2008). In rats the IC shows significant age-related changes related to GABA neurotransmission and a loss of GABA-immunoreactive

synaptic endings as well (Turner & Caspary, 2005). The effects of age on the IC include reductions in the number of GABA-immunoreactive neurons, the concentration of GABA, GABA release, and GABA receptor binding (Leventhal, Wang, Pu, Zhou, & Ma, 2003). Similarly, there are deficiencies in glutamate function with age (Canlon et al, 2010). Reductions in the latter neurotransmitter have implications for neurotransmitter function in the IC likely affecting auditory processing. Finally, animal studies suggest that aging may be associated with a deficit in neural recovery at the level of the IC. According to Canlon et al, (2010), some of the above changes in the IC are typical of those seen in neural presbycusis and may explain deficits in intensity and temporal coding in older adults.

Pearl

"Age-related loss of acoustic nerve activity results in downregulation in the function of the glycinergic system of the cochlear nucleus leading to altered output from the cochlear nucleus" (Caspary et al, 2005). Loss in neural synchrony is responsible in large part for speech comprehension difficulties, especially in noise. Aging is associated with a selective downregulation of GABA inhibition and GABAergic function (Caspary et al, 2008).

The *primary auditory cortex* consists of areas located within the dorsal and lateral parts of the superior temporal gyrus along with areas in the inferior parietal lobe (Morosan, Rademacher, Palomero-Gallagher, & Zilles, 2005). Receptors of a variety of transmitters, including cholinergic, glutamatergic, GABAergic, and serotoninergic, are visible in the auditory cortex. The auditory cortex, which receives its major ascending projections from the medial geniculate body, is necessary for perception and interpretation of the stimulus (Caspary et al, 2008). The auditory cortex has a tonotopic map of the cochlea (Purves et al, 2007). The corpus callosum, the most important commissural tract in the brain, is responsible for connecting areas of like function in the right and left hemispheres of the brain; hence, it is the site of interhemispheric transfer. With age there is a change in the efficiency of interhemispheric transfer of auditory information across the corpus callosum (Martin & Jerger, 2005). Dichotic listening tasks are used to probe interhemispheric transfer (Ackerman, Hertrich, Lutzenberger, & Mathiak, 2005). Functionally, these age-related changes are seen in performance on dichotic tests where there appears to be an increasing right ear advantage or left ear disadvantage in processing in older adults (Eddins & Hall, 2010).

The aging process impacts on the CNS in general and on the CANS in particular. The volume and weight of the brain declines with age, and the decrease in volume is relatively diffuse and uniform in the cerebral white matter (Shankar, 2010). Consistent with cognitive changes observed in older adults, the prefrontal cortex is most affected and the occipital lobe is least affected by aging (Shankar, 2010). In fact, the prefrontal cortex is subject to considerable atrophy with age, with the lateral prefrontal region subject to the most atrophic changes (Kryla-Lighthall & Mather, 2009). These changes have implications for speech understanding in that this region is responsible for coordinating sensory inputs, executive function, and working memory (Kryla-Lighthall & Mather, 2009). It is well established that despite age-related declines in such cognitive-control structures as the prefrontal cortex, older adults recruit neighboring neural regions, and neural activation enables older adults to compensate (Kryla-Lighthall & Mather, 2009). The age-related decline in inhibitory control that occurs at various levels in the ascending auditory pathways takes place in the higher cortical areas such as in the prefrontal cortex, as well. Age-related changes in the GABA enzyme levels have been found in the primary auditory cortex of rats, and it is likely that in humans a loss of normal GABA transmission contributes to difficulties in temporal coding underlying loss of speech understanding with age (Canlon et al, 2010). Similarly, there are subtle age-related changes in the neurotransmitters in the dopaminergic, serotoninergic, cholinergic, and adrenergic systems (Ison et al, 2010)

Special Consideration

Clinically observed central sensory processing deficits that occur with age are attributable in part to decrements in inhibitory neurotransmission (Turner & Caspary, 2005).

Using a limited number of brains and in a two-dimensional space, Brody (1955) conducted a study of the brains of individuals ranging in age from newborn to 95 years (Shankar, 2010). Specifically, he studied age-related changes in the auditory cortex, comparing them to those in the inferior temporal, striate, precentral, and postcentral cortical areas. The magnitude of cell loss was greatest in the superior temporal gyrus (auditory cortex). In fact, there was almost a one-to-one correlation between age and cell loss. Brody also noted a decrease in the thickness of the superior temporal gyrus with increasing age that was not apparent in other cortical regions. Subsequently, Scheibel, Lindsay, Tomiyasu, and Scheibel (1975) also studied the superior temporal cortex, noting a loss of dendrites and cell death in older patients. Animal studies have shown that auditory deprivation from the periphery disrupts the tonotopic organization of the central auditory system or how frequencies are mapped by the central auditory system. Similarly, changes in the central auditory system take place in response to auditory stimulation, underscoring the observation that central auditory plasticity is a fact. Further, recent research confirms that the primary auditory cortex undergoes age-related plastic changes, including downregulation of inhibitory coding, similar to that observed at lower levels of the auditory pathway (Caspary et al, 2008). Finally, it is now well accepted that changes in the central auditory system with age may be peripherally induced rather than due to changes in the brain that are a *direct result of aging* of the CNS (Frisina et al, 2001).

Pearl

The hippocampus and prefrontal cortex are particularly vulnerable to age-related changes explaining in part the age-related changes in working memory and information processing.

In summary, it is evident from histological studies of the CANS that it undergoes some age-related changes with resultant changes in human cerebral cortical function. These changes result in part from a degradation of intracortical inhibition during aging (Leventhal et al, 2003). It is also apparent that the changes are not universal across individuals or across the tracts constituting the auditory brainstem. Further, the functional significance of the anatomical and physiological changes remains the subject of considerable interest among researchers. Most importantly, the peripheral, cochlear, age-related hearing loss appears to drive some of the age-related changes that take place at the level of the cochlear nucleus such that age-related declines in the inputs to the cochlear nucleus is considered to be in part a peripherally induced central effect, as opposed to changes in the brain that are a direct result of aging of the CNS (Frisina & Walton, 2006). Stated differently, deterioration in the periphery alters the quality of the neural information transmitted to the auditory pathway and brain through the auditory nerve (Ison et al, 2010). However, although some auditory midbrain changes can be linked to peripheral presbycusis, most of the age-related changes in higher levels of the auditory brainstem (beyond the CN) are unrelated to peripheral hearing loss (Frisina & Walton, 2006). These changes contribute to deterioration in speech perception in older adults.

Pearl

Age-related changes along the central auditory pathways are highly variable, as are the behavioral consequences.

◆ Beyond Presbycusis: Medical Causes of Hearing Loss

Whereas the most fundamental cause of hearing loss among older adults is the biological aging of the cells in the inner ear and auditory pathways, several other conditions give rise to the sensorineural hearing loss often exhibited by older adults. These include ototoxicity, noise exposure, metabolic conditions, and vascular disease, to name a few of the most common comorbidities.

Ototoxicity

Older adults consume millions of doses of medication daily and the level of medication exposure is associated with adverse reactions and drug interactions. The most common types of medications used by older adults include cardiovascular, gastrointestinal, central nervous system, and analgesic agents (Guay, 2010). In light of declines in hepatic metabolism and renal elimination associated with age-related changes in physiology, drug absorption, distribution, and elimination may be impaired in older adults (Guay, 2010). For example, with advancing age renal elimination of furosemide, aminoglycosides, and vancomycin is impaired, and there is a diminished maximal response to furosemide. Prescription of medications that are ototoxic for conditions ranging from cardiovascular disease and hypertension to diabetes mellitus appears to be somewhat higher in the elderly, predisposing them to drug-induced sensorineural hearing loss.

The term *pharmacokinetics* refers to the time course of absorption, distribution, metabolism, and excretion of drugs and their metabolites from the body (Vestal, 1990). The most important pharmacokinetic age-related changes (Guay, 2010) are (1) alterations in the physiology of the gastrointestinal system, which affect the absorption of drugs administered orally; (2) alterations in body composition and physiology coupled with a decline in cardiac output, which produce changes in drug distribution; (3) alterations in liver blood flow and a decrease in liver mass, which result in a decline in hepatic drug metabolism; and (4) reduction in renal mass and number and size of nephrons, which result in decreased renal elimination and excretion of drugs and metabolites. Another variable that influences drug response is pharmacodynamics or responsiveness to a given drug concentration. In short, aging is associated with alterations in drug sensitivity and impairment of physiological and homeostatic mechanisms. Finally, due to polypharmacy in older adults, adverse reactions from ototoxic agents may result from drug–disease interactions or drug–drug interactions (Guay, 2010).

Classes of drugs differ in terms of which age-related change in pharmacokinetics will pose the greatest threat to the onset of toxic effects. For example, the main route for elimination of antibiotics, including aminoglycosides (e.g., gentamicin, tobramycin), selected cardiovascular drugs, diuretics including furosemide, and psychoactive drugs, is the kidney. Renal elimination of these drugs can be reduced in the elderly. In light of this, the standard dosage regimen should be reduced in older adults. Similarly, the hepatic metabolism of cardiovascular drugs such as quinidine, psychoactive drugs such as diazepam, and selected analgesics may be reduced in older adults. There are data to indicate that clearance of analgesics such as salicylates may be reduced in older patients as well (Abrams et al, 1995). Drug toxicity can be associated with some or all of the following: nausea, vomiting, dizziness, fatigue, hearing loss, and tinnitus.

Several classes of drugs are particularly toxic to the auditory and vestibular systems, the effects of which are exacerbated by the aging process. **Table 4.3** displays the drugs reported to produce oto- or vestibulotoxic effects. The site of predilection of the drugs within a particular class differs such that, for example, streptomycin is mainly vestibulotoxic, neomycin and kanamycin are particularly toxic to the ear, and gentamicin is both oto- and vestibulotoxic. Neomycin is used topically for

Table 4.3 Categories of Ototoxic Medications (Modified from pamphlet created by the League for the Hard of Hearing (2000)*

Salicylates: aspirin and aspirin-containing products	Toxic effects usually appear after consuming an average of 6 to 8 pills per day. Toxic effects are almost always reversible once medications are discontinued.
Nonsteroidal antiinflammatory drugs (NSAIDs): Advil, Aleve, Anaprox, Clinoril, Feldene, Indocin, Lodine, Motrin, Nalfon, Naprosyn, Nuprin, Poradol, Voltaren	Toxic effects usually appear after consuming an average of 6–8 pills per day. Toxic effects are usually reversible once medications are discontinued.
Antibiotics: aminoglycosides, erythromycin, vancomycin	a. Aminoglycosides: kanamycin, neomycin, amikacin, dihydrostreptomycin, streptomycin, gentamicin, tobramycin, netilmicin—ototoxic or vestibulotoxic when used intravenously in serious life-threatening situations. b. Erythromycin: EES, Eryc, E-mycin, Ilosone, Pediazole, and new derivatives of erythromycin, Biaxin, Zithromax. Erythromycin is usually ototoxic when given intravenously in dosages of 2 to 4 g per 24 hours, especially if there is underlying kidney insufficiency. c. Vancomycin: Vancocin. Used in a similar manner to the aminoglycosides; when given intravenously in serious life-threatening infections, it is potentially ototoxic. Usually used in conjunction with the aminoglycosides, which enhances the possibility of ototoxicity.
Loop diuretics: Lasix (furosemide), Edecrin, Bumex	Usually ototoxic when given intravenously for acute kidney failure or acute hypertension. Rare cases of ototoxicity have been reported when these medications are taken orally in high doses in people with chronic kidney disease
Chemotherapeutic agents: cisplatin (Platinol), nitrogen mustard (Mustargen), vincristine, carboplatinum (Carboplatin)	Ototoxic when given for treatment of cancer. Ototoxic effects of these medications are enhanced in patients who are already taking other ototoxic medications (e.g., aminoglycoside antibiotics or loop diuretics).
Quinine: Aralen, Atabrine (for treatment of malaria), Legatrin, Q-Vel muscle relaxant (for treatment of night cramps)	Ototoxic effects are very similar to aspirin, and the toxic effects are usually reversible once medication is discontinued.
Cardiac medications: Lopressor, lidocaine	May cause tinnitus

*Ototoxic Medications Drugs that can cause hearing loss and tinnitus.

some eye, ear, and skin infections or orally before colorectal surgery (Abrams et al, 1995). Streptomycin may be used to treat tuberculosis and occasionally endocarditis.

The pathogenesis of ototoxicity from aminoglycosides relates to the fact that this class of antibiotics is retained for a longer period and in a higher concentration in the inner ear fluids than in any other body tissue or fluid (Becker, Naumann, & Pfaltz, 1989). This, in combination with the potential for reduced renal output, may predispose older adults to the development of toxic concentrations of the drug within the inner ear, leading to end-organ damage. Aminoglycosides appear to damage the outer hair cells in the basal end of the cochlea first and then the inner hair cells if a high enough concentration of the drug is reached. Ototoxicity is related to sustained peak serum levels varying considerably across the family of aminoglycosides. The damage tends to be concentrated in the high-frequency regions, extending into the lower frequencies with prolonged treatment. Audiometrically, the hearing loss manifests itself in the high frequencies and is often occasioned by tinnitus and dizziness. The hearing loss tends to be sensorineural, bilateral, and severe to profound in degree. The severity and time of onset are directly related to the time of onset of drug use, often progressing for several months after cessation of the medication. When aminoglycoside antibiotics are administered with loop diuretics, the ototoxic effect is quite powerful, resulting in a profound, permanent hearing loss (Lonsbury-Martin & Martin, 2001).

Pearl

Older adults are at particular risk for aminoglycoside ototoxicity when they have an underlying loss of auditory function associated with the aging process.

The ototoxic effects of aminoglycosides are directly related to serum levels at the end of treatment, so that serum concentration monitoring is strongly recommended. The risk of ototoxicity is increased from aminoglycosides in patients receiving cisplatin.

Cisplatin, a chemotherapeutic agent that acts against squamous cell carcinoma of the head, neck, and genitourinary systems, is primarily ototoxic and can lead in some cases to permanent hearing loss. The damage associated with cisplatin ingestion is at the level of the hair cell. It causes damage to outer hair cells, inner hair cells, supporting cells of the organ of Corti, and the stria vascularis, reducing the endolymphatic potential (Lonsbury-Martin & Martin, 2001). Of course, loss of inner hair cells may affect survival of ganglion cells. Onset of hearing loss can be detected initially in the ultra-high frequencies soon after the first or second course of chemotherapy (Boettcher, Gratton, Bancroft, & Spongr, 1992). The degree of hearing loss and frequencies affected are directly related to dosing and duration of cisplatin administration. Older adults with hearing loss prior to chemotherapy with cisplatin are more likely to experience threshold shift following administration of the drug, and thus close monitoring and counseling are recommended for these individuals (Dorr & Dalton, 1993).

Pearl

It is incumbent on audiologists to educate oncologists and the entire chemotherapy team about assistive devices cancer patients can use to facilitate communication should a patient's hearing status deteriorate during and after chemotherapy.

Loop diuretics, including furosemide and ethacrynic acid, are used in the treatment of kidney failure. These medications act directly on the stria vascularis, producing a reduction of the endolymphatic potential, with decreases in the sound-evoked responses from the cochlea (Lonsbury-Martin & Martin, 2001). The hearing loss tends to be temporary.

Salicylate ototoxicity is not uncommon, given the high prevalence of the various forms of arthritis and the wide use of this class of drugs in older adults. Salicylate ototoxicity affects the morphology and ultrastructure of outer hair cells and the cochlear vascular system as well (Lonsbury-Martin & Martin, 2001). Salicylate ototoxicity is associated with tinnitus and mild to moderate sensorineural hearing loss that is gradual in onset. The hearing loss reportedly tends to reverse itself when the drug is discontinued as early as 3 days following the final administration (Boettcher et al, 1992). Otoacoustic emissions tend to be reduced by ingestion of salicylates. Helzner et al (2005) reported that the odds of hearing loss increased in those participants who had taken salicylates; in particular, black men were most susceptible.

In summary, it is important to note that the hearing loss associated with ototoxicity from any of the aforementioned ototoxins may interact with that of presbycusis, leading to a more severe hearing loss than that associated with age alone. Risk factors for ototoxicity include age, renal insufficiency, preexisting hearing loss, family history, and use of loop diuretics or other nephrotoxic medications. Signs of ototoxicity to look out for in older adults include development of or intensification of tinnitus in one or both ears, appearance of a new sound in the ear different from already existing tinnitus, fullness or pressure in the ears (i.e., different from that caused by infection), progression of an already existing hearing loss, and development of a spinning sensation aggravated by motion, which may or may not be accompanied by nausea. Audiologists are often called upon to administer pretreatment audiograms, to conduct otoacoustic emission studies to provide baseline information about hearing status prior to the onset of drug use, and to provide midtreatment and posttreatment monitoring with audiograms and otoacoustic emissions. Results of studies conducted by audiologists should be viewed in the context of laboratory studies of serum levels to assist in maintenance of appropriate dosing and to help monitor potential ototoxic damage. With regard to management, for example, older adults sustaining a profound hearing loss from drug ingestion may require a cochlear implant, hearing aids, or assistive technology to facilitate the communication process. Given their role in evaluating and managing older adults who develop ototoxic hearing loss, audiologists must have some familiarity with clinical pharmacology including knowledge of pharmacokinetics and the prescribing practices of physicians.

Noise-Induced Hearing Loss

Hearing loss in adults can also be attributed to exposure to noise, and to the interaction of noise and aging effects. Hearing loss associated with the aging process is often difficult to distinguish audiometrically from hearing loss associated with prolonged noise exposure. The severity and location of the lesion to the inner ear, and corresponding hearing loss, depend on the acoustic characteristics of the sound including its sound pressure level and frequency content, exposure time, and the individual's susceptibility or sensitivity to the effect of the particular type of noise. Noise is associated with irreversible damage to the sensory cells of the inner ear, with outer hair cells degenerating first, followed by the inner hair cells. The lesion tends to be concentrated in the region of the cochlea associated with 4000-Hz hearing, namely, the lower basal turn of the cochlea. Unlike presbycusis, there is rarely involvement of the auditory nerve fibers and the brainstem auditory pathways. The audiometric configuration associated with noise exposure is difficult to separate from the patterns typically associated with age (Committee on Hearing, Bioacoustics, and Biomechanics, 1988). Although early on the pure-tone audiogram shows a notch at 3000, 4000, or 6000 Hz, prolonged exposure leads to involvement of higher and lower frequency regions. The loss tends to be bilateral and symmetrical. Tinnitus is a common complaint of persons with a long-term history of noise exposure.

Cruickshanks et al (2010) conducted a longitudinal study (10-year time frame) of the incidence of hearing impairment and its association with noise exposure, education, and occupation using the Beaver Dam sample. They found that a positive history of occupational noise exposure was not associated with the cumulative incidence of hearing impairment, nor was it associated with progression of hearing loss. Due to their pattern of findings Cruickshanks et al concluded that over a 10-year time frame, there is little evidence that prior occupational noise exposure plays an important role in the onset or progression of hearing impairment in older adults. Similarly, Lee, Matthews, Dubno, and Mills (2005) found that there was no difference in the rate of change in hearing levels between adults with and without positive noise histories.

Agrawal, Platz, and Niparko (2009) used data from the National Health and Nutrition Examination Survey (NHANES; 1999–2002) to explore the contribution of risk factors, including noise exposure, smoking, and cardiovascular disease (CVD), to hearing loss in a sample of adults with an upper age limit of 69 years. Participants with firearm noise exposure had significantly poorer hearing levels at 4, 6, and 8 kHz than did those without exposure to firearms. Agrawal et al found that noise exposure and history of cardiovascular disease had a synergistic effect, elevating hearing thresholds. Dubno et al (2008) explored changes in speech recognition ability in older adults

(>55 years) who were part of the Medical University of South Carolina longitudinal study. They found that rates of threshold change for subjects with a positive noise history did not differ significantly from those with a negative noise history. In contrast, Gates, Schmid, Kujawa, Nam, and D'Agostino (2000) found that age-related increases in thresholds for older subjects having an audiogram with a noise "notch" were faster at the frequencies adjacent to the noise notch than for older participants whose audiograms did not have a notch. Gates et al hypothesized that persons having audiograms with the notch had prior noise exposure, and concluded that the effect of noise on pure-tone thresholds could continue after the noise exposure had stopped. Using a random sample of Medicare beneficiaries enrolled in the Health ABC study, Helzner et al (2005) found that in their sample of older adults with essentially mild to moderately severe hearing loss, occupational noise exposure was associated with a 55% greater risk of hearing loss. Finally, exposure to loud noise appears to accelerate age-related hearing loss (Ison et al, 2010).

Rosen, Bergman, Plester, El-Mofty, and Satti (1962) reported that environmental factors such as living in a noise-free versus an industrialized society can affect the extent of the high-frequency hearing loss that emerges in older persons. In fact, individuals living in a noise-free environment reportedly have better hearing in the high frequencies than persons living in industrialized societies (Rosen et al, 1962). Earlier studies also provide support for the observation that age and exposure to noise can have a synergistic effect (Mościcki, Elkins, Baum, & McNamara, 1985). Gilad and Glorig (1979) speculated that hearing loss among the elderly is a culmination of multiple damaging processes that occur over the life span. In fact, some investigators contend that presbycusis is a multifactorial process in which expression of each factor varies greatly from individual to individual (Gates, Cobb, D'Agostino, & Wolf, 1993). It is the sum of a variety of insults to the auditory system that occur over time, and include age-related degeneration, the effects of environmental noise (sociocusis), and disease of the auditory systems (nosocusis), plus other endogenous factors such as genetics and diet (Gates et al, 1993; Kryter, 1983).

At the present time, isolating the histopathology of presbycusis, nosocusis, and sociocusis and correlating it to audiometric findings continues to be an important yet challenging research goal. The difficulty arises because the variables that interact to determine hearing status of older adults are uncontrolled, making it difficult to decide which of the visualized changes on geriatric human temporal bones are solely the results of aging (Gulya, 1991).

Cardiovascular Disease

A leading cause of death globally, CVD is a multistep process. Impaired cardiovascular function is widespread among older adults. By definition, cardiovascular insufficiency compromises the blood supply to organs throughout the body including the cochlea, which is richly supplied with blood vessels. *Atherosclerosis,* a generic term for thickening or hardening of the arterial wall, plays a major role in CVD. Several investigators have studied the relationship between hearing loss and cardiovascular disease. Findings from the Framingham and Health ABC studies suggest that hearing loss and CVD are correlated (Gates et al, 1993; Helzner et al, 2005). Helzner et al (2005) found that individuals with CVD had a 56% higher risk of hearing loss, and that low-frequency thresholds were more closely correlated with CVD than were high-frequency thresholds, suggesting a possible vascular or metabolic link. Although the association between CVD and hearing loss was impressive, the authors cautioned that a cause-and-effect relation cannot be deduced from their findings. The possible link between CVD and hearing loss is not surprising given the rich capillary supply to the stria vascularis within the cochlea. Gates, Cobb, D'Agostino, and Wolf (1993) reported that men with a history of coronary heart disease and heart attack were twice as likely to have low-frequency hearing losses as were men with negative histories of CVD. Agrawal et al (2009) also found, using the NHANES sample, that a history of diabetes was associated with increased odds of hearing loss. People with diabetes had significantly poorer hearing in the lower and higher frequencies than did those without diabetes. Gates et al (1993) found that the risk of low-frequency hearing loss was double for women with history of stroke or coronary heart disease as compared with women with negative histories of CVD. Similarly, women with history of stroke and overall CVD also were twice as likely to have high-frequency hearing loss as women without CVD.

Special Consideration

There is a substantial amount of evidence linking CVD to cochlear pathology in older adults.

Early on, Brant et al (1996) examined the relationship among cardiovascular-related risk factors and hearing loss in older adults. Participants in the Baltimore Longitudinal Study of Aging served as subjects in their study. They, too, found a relation between CVD and hearing loss in their large sample of older adults who were free of noise-induced hearing loss and other hearing-related disorders. Specifically, their data demonstrated a significant relation between systolic blood pressure and sensorineural hearing impairment. They reported that men who are borderline hypertensive with a systolic pressure of 140 have a 32% greater risk of developing hearing loss than normotensive men. Further, men who are hypertensive with a systolic pressure of 160 have a 74% greater risk of hearing than the borderline hypertensive group.

Pearl

Audiologists should query their clients regarding CVD, and closely monitor audiometrically those who are borderline or definite hypertensives.

Metabolic Disease

A variety of metabolic deficits that develop as individuals age may have a deleterious effect on hearing (Willott, 1991). These include, but are not limited to, (1) impaired glucose metabolism, which is a hallmark of diabetes mellitus; (2) selected kidney disorders, which tend to alter fluid and electrolyte metabolism; (3) hyperlipoproteinemia (HLP), a condition that accompanies high serum cholesterol and triglyceride levels and is closely linked to atherosclerosis; and (4) selected thyroid conditions, which may interfere with the production of thyroid hormone. The first two conditions have received the most attention from investigators.

Diabetes Mellitus

The prevalence rate of diabetes is 25% in persons over age 60, and interestingly the incidence rate of diabetes increases with age. Diabetes places individuals at risk for significant microvascular complications and also for declines in cognitive function (Halter, 2011). Diabetes mellitus is a syndrome characterized by generalized metabolic dysfunction and a variety of clinical disorders. There is an age-related increase in the prevalence of diabetes mellitus, undiagnosed diabetes, and impaired glucose tolerance. Diabetes mellitus is primarily characterized by abnormal glucose metabolism, and is associated with abnormal regulation of lipid and protein metabolism. Secondary to diminished insulin secretion and hyperglycemia, persons with diabetes mellitus may undergo vascular changes in small and large vessels. Peripheral neuropathy is not uncommon among diabetic persons. Because diabetes can affect the body's neurochemical balance, fluctuations in communication behavior, including degree of sensorineural hearing loss, have been reported (Groher, 1988). Although in the Framingham and Beaver Dam studies (Dalton, Cruickshanks, Klein, Klein, & Wiley, 1998; Gates, et al, 1993) diabetes was not found to be associated with hearing loss, in the majority of other studies the link is clear (Helzner et al, 2005). In the Blue Mountains Study, a history of diabetes was significantly associated with increased odds of hearing loss (McMahon, Kifley, Rochtchina, Newall, & Mitchell, 2008). Helzner et al (2005) found that diabetes mellitus was be positively associated with hearing loss in the Health ABC study. Further, it appears that hearing impairment is more prevalent among adults with diabetes, and the association is independent of such risk factors for hearing loss as noise exposure, ototoxic medication use, and smoking (Disogra, 2008). Further, the prevalence of hearing impairment is higher among persons with diabetes (21%) than those adults who do not have diabetes (9%) (Bainbridge, Hoffman, & Cowie, 2008).

Pearl

Along with these data, clinical experience suggests that diabetes that is not properly controlled places older adults at risk for sudden declines in hearing levels that may not be reversible.

I personally witnessed a diabetic uncle's hearing decline from a mild to moderate sensorineural hearing loss to the level of a moderately severe to severe loss within one day. The suddenness of the change was devastating and, while the diabetes was brought back into control, hearing levels never returned to their milder levels. Word recognition ability declined as well, to the point that hearing aids became ineffective. Subsequent speech testing revealed the presence of a central auditory processing component superimposed on the peripheral hearing loss.

Kidney Disorders

The kidney undergoes anatomical, histological, and functional changes as people age. The anatomical changes are primarily vascular, interstitial, and tubular. These changes often leave the older adult vulnerable to a variety of environmental, disease-related, and drug-induced stresses. The major clinical consequences of age-related changes include disorders of salt metabolism, disorders of water metabolism, and disorders of potassium metabolism. The total body content of sodium is the principal determinant of extracellular and intravascular fluid volume. Sodium deficiency results in hypovolemia, whereas excess sodium results in edema with or without circulatory congestion (Beck & Burkart, 1994). Potassium levels may be altered in older adults because of the use of drugs that alter potassium excretion or because of declines in glomerular filtration rates. Disturbance in water metabolism is associated with either excessive or defective water conservation. Together the above changes lead to alterations in fluid and electrolyte metabolism. The high level of metabolic activity of the stria vascularis and the high degree of vascularity would make it susceptible to the impairments in sodium, water, and potassium metabolism that attend the age-related decline in renal function. As such, cochlear pathology and primarily high-frequency sensorineural hearing loss have been reported in older adults with renal disease. Patients with Alport's syndrome (a hereditary nephropathy), chronic renal failure and kidney transplants, or persons undergoing kidney dialysis may have increased susceptibility to hearing impairment. Often it is difficult to isolate the cause of hearing loss in persons with kidney disease due to the deleterious effects of ototoxic medications conventionally used in the management of individuals with renal disease.

Genetic Factors

Although estimates of the hereditability of age-related hearing loss range from 25 to 75%, there is a paucity of information regarding the genetic basis for age-related hearing loss (McMahon et al, 2008). Using participants from the Blue Mountain Hearing Study, McMahon et al (2008) investigated the association between magnitudes of hearing loss and self-report of family history of hearing loss among residents living in Sydney, Australia, in a defined location. Of all participants with bilateral hearing impairment, 48% reported a positive family history. Of the participants reporting a family history, 62.7% were women. Further, 63.8% of participants with moderate to severe hearing loss reported a positive family history, as compared with 52.6% with mild hearing loss and 44.5% without hearing loss. The magnitude of the association between family history and hearing loss was greater with increasing severity

of hearing loss, such that the adjusted odds ratio (OR) was 1.46 (confidence interval [CI] 1.18–1.82) for mild loss and 2.40 (CI 1.76–3.28) for moderate loss. Finally, there was a strong association between a positive maternal family history and moderate to severe hearing loss in women and a significant, though slightly weaker, association between a positive paternal family history and moderate to severe hearing loss in men. Data from the Framingham Heart Study showed a similar pattern of heritability (Gates, Couropmitree, & Myers, 1999). Gates et al, too, found that mother–daughter and sister–sister pairs had stronger familial associations than father–son or brother–brother pairs.

Senile Dementia

Dementia is a syndrome that describes a pattern of symptoms than can result from different brain diseases (Lemke, 2011). Currently afflicting as many as 5.2 million people, Alzheimer's disease is the most common cause of senile dementia in older adults. Senile dementia is defined in the *Diagnostic and Statistical Manual of Mental Disorders* (DSM-IV-TR) of the American Psychiatric Association as being based on common clinical criteria including multiple cognitive deficits, memory impairment, and decline in ability to carry out daily activities, accompanied by personality and behavior changes (Bayer, 2010). The deficits must show a decline from a previous level of function, and be irreversible, progressive, and chronic in duration. The prevalence of dementia is projected to double every 20 years, so that by 2050, more than 100 million people will be affected worldwide. The devastating impact of dementia on affected individuals and the burden imposed on their families and society has made the prevention and treatment of dementia a public health priority (Ferri et al, 2005). Lin et al (2011) conducted a prospective study of hearing loss and incident cases of all-cause dementia. Participants were part of the Baltimore Longitudinal Study of Aging. Lin et al found that the risk of incident Alzheimer's disease increased with the severity of baseline hearing loss. Further, hearing loss was independently associated with incident all-cause dementia after adjusting for sex, age, race, education, diabetes, smoking, and hypertension. The risk of all-cause dementia increased log linearly with hearing loss severity. Interestingly, for individuals 60 years of age or older, more than one third of the risk of incident all-cause dementia was associated with hearing loss (Lin, 2011). Results of a large-scale longitudinal study by Gates, Beiser, Rees, D'Agostino, & Wolf, (2002) revealed that measures of central auditory function are predictive of developing Alzheimer's disease even after taking pure-tone sensitivity into account. More specifically, Gates et al demonstrated that poor performance on the Synthetic Sentence Identification with Ipsilateral Competing Message (SSI-ICM) is common in people with probable Alzheimer's disease, and in fact very poor performance in either ear may precede the clinical onset of dementia of the Alzheimer's type by several years. The authors speculated that age-related degenerative changes in the prefrontal cortex may be at play as this part of the brain and may be responsible for executive control function, and that lesions of the central auditory pathway in Alzheimer's disease are uncommon in early cases.

Individuals with hearing loss are more likely to have a diagnosis of dementia and poorer cognitive function (Uhlmann,

Larson, Rees, Koepsell, & Duckert, 1989). Some investigators have speculated that hearing loss and cognitive decline coexist incidentally as a function of age; others have suggested that the auditory system is preferentially involved in Alzheimer's disease, and several investigators have demonstrated a strong positive relationship between hearing impairment and cognitive status (Gates et al, 1996). Further, hearing impairment is reportedly more common and more severe in demented versus nondemented subjects. Specifically, Uhlmann et al (1989), Uhlmann, Rees, Psaty, and Duckert (1989), and Weinstein and Amsel (1986) reported the prevalence of hearing impairment to be higher in a sample of adults with a diagnosis of dementia than in a comparable sample free of the diagnosis. The discrepancy in prevalence is apparent among older adults living in the community and in institutions. They also reported the severity of hearing loss to be greater in subjects with a diagnosis of dementia than in an age-matched group free of cognitive impairment. Finally, Ives, Bonino, Traven, & Kuller (1995) reported that in their sample of rural older adults, persons with hearing impairment had higher rates of dementia and depression.

Pearl

Dementia is more than just memory impairment; it involves impairment in multiple areas of cognition (Lemke, 2011).

Strouse, Hall, and Burger (1995) performed tests of peripheral and central auditory processing ability on a sample of age-matched older adults with mean hearing levels between 500 and 8000 Hz of better than 30 dB HL. One group was diagnosed with probable senile dementia of the Alzheimer's type, whereas the second group was free of cognitive or neurological deficits. Peripheral testing consisted of an immittance test battery, pure-tone and speech testing, and distortion-product otoacoustic emissions. The central auditory test battery consisted of the synthetic sentence identification test, the dichotic sentence identification test, the dichotic digits test, the pitch pattern sequence, and the duration pattern test. The screening version of the Hearing Handicap Inventory for the Elderly (HHIE-S) was completed by all subjects as well.

Special Consideration

It is not clear whether hearing loss and cognitive decline coexist as a function of age or whether the auditory system is preferentially involved in Alzheimer's disease.

Given the subject selection criteria (i.e., hearing levels better than 30 dB HL), it is not surprising that the groups did not differ significantly in their performance on the peripheral auditory measures, with one exception. The Alzheimer's group showed slightly poorer low-frequency pure-tone thresholds than the matched control group. HHIE-S scores were comparable as well. The comparability of HHIE-S scores was to be expected because subjects were selected on the basis of being free of peripheral hearing loss and hearing-related difficulties (Strouse et al, 1995).

In contrast to performance on peripheral auditory measures, percent correct performance on the majority of tests of central auditory processing was significantly lower in the Alzheimer's group than in the matched controls. Six of 10 subjects scored below normal on all five tests of central auditory function, three of 10 were deficient on four measures, and one of the subjects failed three of the five tests. On the dichotic digits test and on the dichotic sentence identification test, left ear performance was poorer than right ear performance in more than 50% of subjects with a diagnosis of Alzheimer's disease. In contrast, the majority (70%) of subjects in the control group scored normally on all five central auditory tests. Further, no differences in ear performance were noted among members of the control group. These data attest to the presence of a central auditory processing problem in older adults diagnosed with Alzheimer's disease along with the presence of peripheral hearing loss in this population. Weinstein and Amsel (1986) did find that scores on tests of cognitive status improved when people with a diagnosis of dementia were able to hear the questions on the test of cognitive function. They also reported that the correlation between severity of pure-tone hearing loss and scores on a test of mental status is obliterated when persons with a diagnosis of dementia were able to hear the questions with the assistance of an auditory trainer or hand-held amplifier. As inability to hear questions on orally administered tests of cognitive function can result in lower test scores that confound the interpretation of test results, hand-held amplifiers or desk-top auditory trainers should be used in the diagnostic process to ensure reception of the questions. It is incumbent on audiologists to acquaint members of the assessment team with assistive devices that are inexpensive and can be easily incorporated into the diagnostic protocol.

Pearl

The behavioral consequences of senile dementia are similar to those associated with moderately severe to severe sensorineural hearing loss. Audiologists must determine the extent to which hearing loss contributes to the symptomology of dementia.

◆ Conclusion

This chapter has outlined many of the structural and functional changes that occur within the peripheral and central auditory systems as a result of aging or disease. Although several subtypes of presbycusis have been described, the term *presbycusis* refers to hearing loss in older adults with no specific cause such as noise exposure or ototoxicity (Schneider, Pichora-Fuller, & Daneman, 2010). It is evident that each part of the ear undergoes changes with age, with the most dramatic changes occurring in the inner ear, neural structures, and the auditory brainstem pathways and auditory cortex. Understanding the changes in the peripheral and central auditory system can help clinicians isolate the functional and behavioral effects. It is important to emphasize that age-related changes in the brain and resulting slowing of brain function has dramatic implications for complex cognitive function, especially language comprehension and speech understanding in complex situations (e.g., in the presence of multiple talkers) (Schneider et al, 2010). Flexibility in the reconfiguration of cortical networks is reduced with aging due to degradation of neural structures, including brain atrophy, decrease in the number of neurons, and changes in synaptic density (Willis, Schaie, & Martin, 2009). However, the fact that adult brains and neural circuitry retain the capacity for plasticity, thereby potentially impacting frequency representation within the auditory cortex, is critical for speech understanding in complex situations. Further, despite age-related changes in the brain, it does appear that top-down control is preserved with aging, which helps to compensate for the age-related declines in the periphery (bottom–up processing), thereby promoting comprehension of spoken language (Schneider et al, 2010).

These changes have dramatic effects that are readily tapped using traditional behavioral tests. In light of the high prevalence of hearing loss among older adults and the variety of medical conditions that give rise to hearing loss, audiologists should make every attempt to become part of the extended geriatric health care team. As a member of the team, the role of the audiologist should be to impress upon others the importance of identifying hearing loss and its etiology in older adults undergoing a comprehensive assessment of their health status. Further, controlling for hearing loss in older adults suffering from a multitude of acute or chronic conditions can promote the quality of life, which may be compromised.

Pearl

Audiologists must convince physicians of the importance of including a hearing screen in the routine physical.

References

Abrams, W., Beers, M., & Berkow, R. (1995). *Merck manual of geriatrics* (2nd ed.). Whitehouse Station, NJ: Merck

Ackerman, H., Hertrich, I., Lutzenberger, W., & Mathiak, K. (2005). Cerebral organization of speech sound perception: Hemispheric lateralization effects at the level of the supratemporal plane, the inferior dorsolateral frontal lobe and the cerebellum. In R. Konig, P. Heil, E. Budinger, & H. Scheich (Eds.), *The auditory cortex: A synthesis of human and animal research*. Mahwah, NJ: Lawrence Erlbaum

Agrawal, Y., Platz, E. A., & Niparko, J. K. (2009, Feb). Risk factors for hearing loss in US adults: Data from the National Health and Nutrition Examination Survey, 1999 to 2002. *Otology and Neurotology, 30*, 139–145

Alamilla, J., & Gillespie, D. C. (2011, Nov). Glutamatergic inputs and glutamate-releasing immature inhibitory inputs activate a shared postsynaptic receptor population in lateral superior olive. *Neuroscience, 196*, 285–296 [Epub ahead of print]

Arnesen, A. R. (1982, Jun). Presbyacusis—loss of neurons in the human cochlear nuclei. *Journal of Laryngology and Otology, 96*, 503–511

Ayache, D., Corre, A., Van Prooyen, S., & Elbaz, P. (2003, Dec). Surgical treatment of otosclerosis in elderly patients. *Otolaryngology–Head and Neck Surgery, 129*, 674–677

Bainbridge, K. E., Hoffman, H. J., & Cowie, C. C. (2008, Jul). Diabetes and hearing impairment in the United States: Audiometric evidence from the National Health and Nutrition Examination Survey, 1999 to 2004. *Annals of Internal Medicine, 149*, 1–10

Ballachanda, B. (1995). Cerumen and the ear canal secretory system. In B. Ballachanda (Ed.), *Introduction to the human ear canal*. San Diego: Singular

Bayer, A. (2010). Presentation and clinical management of dementia. In H. Fillit, K. Rockwood, & K. Woodhouse (Eds.), *Brockelhurst's textbook of geriatric medicine and gerontology* (7th ed.). Philadelphia: Saunders Elsevier

Beck, L., & Burkart, J. (1994). The renal system and urinary tract. In W. Hazzard, E. Bierman, J. Blass, W. Ettinger, & J. Halter (Eds.), *Principles of geriatric medicine and gerontology* (3rd ed). New York: McGraw-Hill

Becker, W., Naumann, H., & Pfaltz, C. (1989). *Ear, nose, and throat diseases*. New York: Thieme

Becker, W., Naumann, H., & Pfaltz, C. (1994). *Ear, nose, and throat diseases* (2nd ed.). New York: Thieme

Belal, A., Jr. (1975, Oct). Prebycusis: Physiological or pathological. *Journal of Laryngology and Otology, 89*, 1011–1025

Bernstein, J. (2001). The middle ear mucosa. In A. Jahn & J. Santos-Sacchi (Eds.), *Physiology of the ear* (2nd ed.). San Diego: Singular

Boettcher, F., Gratton, M., Bancroft, B., & Spongr, V. (1992). Interaction of noise and other agents: Recent advances. In A. Dancer, D. Henderson, R. Salvi, & R. Hamernik (Eds.), *Noise induced hearing loss*. St. Louis: Mosby

Brant, L. J., Gordon-Salant, S., Pearson, J. D., Klein, L. L., Morrell, C. H., Metter, E. J., et al. (1996, Jun). Risk factors related to age-associated hearing loss in the speech frequencies. *Ear and Hearing, 7*, 152–160

Brody, H. (1955, Apr). Organization of the cerebral cortex. III. A study of aging in the human cerebral cortex. *Journal of Comparative Neurology, 102*, 511–516

Canlon, B., Illing, R., & Walton, J. (2010). Cell biology and physiology of the aging central auditory pathway. In S. Gordon-Salant, R. Frisina, A. Popper, & R. Fay (Eds.), *The aging auditory system*. New York: Springer

Caspary, D. M., Ling, L., Turner, J. G., & Hughes, L. F. (2008, Jun). Inhibitory neurotransmission, plasticity and aging in the mammalian central auditory system. *Journal of Experimental Biology, 211*(Pt 11), 1781–1791

Caspary, D., Schatterman, T., Hughes, L. (2005). Age-related changes in the inhibitory response properties of dorsal cochlear nucleus output neurons: Role of inhibitory inputs. *Journal of Neuroscience, 25*, 10952–10959

Committee on Hearing, Bioacoustics, and Biomechanics (CHABA). (1988). Chaba working group on speech understanding and aging. *Journal of the Acoustical Society of America, 83*, 859–895

Chisolm, T., Willott, J., & Lister, J. (2003). The aging auditory system: Anatomic and physiological changes and implications for rehabilitation. *International Journal of Audiology, 42*, 2S3–2S10

Clinard, C. G., Tremblay, K. L., & Krishnan, A. R. (2010, Jun). Aging alters the perception and physiological representation of frequency: Evidence from human frequency-following response recordings. *Hearing Research, 264*, 48–55

Covell, W. P. (1952, Apr). Histologic changes in the aging cochlea. *Journal of Gerontology, 7*, 173–177

Crace, R. (1970). *Morphologic alterations with age in the human cochlear nuclear complex*. Ph.D. Dissertation, Ohio University

Crowe, S., Guild, S., & Polvogt, L. (1934). Observations on the pathology of high-tone deafness. *Johns Hopkins Hospital Bulletin, 54*, 315–380

Cruickshanks, K. J., Nondahl, D. M., Tweed, T. S., Wiley, T. L., Klein, B. E., Klein, R., et al. (2010, Jun). Education, occupation, noise exposure history and the 10-year cumulative incidence of hearing impairment in older adults. *Hearing Research, 264*, 3–9

Dalton, D. S., Cruickshanks, K. J., Klein, R., Klein, B. E., & Wiley, T. L. (1998, Sep). Association of NIDDM and hearing loss. *Diabetes Care, 21*, 1540–1544

Davies, J. (1998). Cellular mechanisms of aging. In R. Tallis, H. Fillit, & J. Brockelhurst (Eds.), *Brockelhurst's textbook of geriatric medicine and gerontology*. London: Churchill Livingstone

Disogra, R. (2008). Adverse drug reactions and audiology practice. *Audiology Today, 20*, 60–70

Dorr, R., & Dalton, W. (1993). Cancer chemotherapy. In R. Bressler & M. Katz (Eds.), *Geriatric pharmacology*. New York: McGraw-Hill

Dubno, J. (2009). Longitudinal changes in hearing and speech perception in older adults. In *Hearing care for adults*. file:///Users/bweinstein/Desktop/book%20chapters/adult_conference_chicago2009.html

Dubno, J., Lee, F., Matthews, L., Ahlstrom, J., Horwitz, A., & Mills, J. (2008). Longitudinal changes in speech recognition in older persons. *Journal of the Acoustical Society of America, 123*, 462–475

Eddins, D., & Hall, J. (2010). Binaural processing and auditory asymmetries. In S. Gordon-Salant, R. Frisina, A. Popper, & R. Fay (Eds.), *The aging auditory system*. New York: Springer

Etholm, B., & Belal, A., Jr. (1974, Jan-Feb). Senile changes in the middle ear joints. *Annals of Otology, Rhinology, and Laryngology, 83*, 49–54

Farrior, J. B. (1963, Aug). Stapes surgery in geriatrics: Surgery in the nerve deaf otosclerotic. *Laryngoscope, 73*, 1084–1098

Ferri, C. P., Prince, M., Brayne, C., Brodaty, H., Fratiglioni, L., Ganguli, M., et al.; Alzheimer's Disease International. (2005, Dec). Global prevalence of dementia: A Delphi consensus study. *Lancet, 366*, 2112–2117

Frisina, R., Zhu, X., & Souza, P. (2009). Biological bases of age related hearing loss. In *Proceedings of the Phonak hearing care for adults: The challenge of aging*. Chicago. http://www.phonakpro.com/com/b2b/en/events/proceedings/archive/adult_conference_chicago2009.html.html

Frisina, R. D., Frisina, R. D., Snell, K. B., Burkard, R., Walton, J. P., & Ison, J. R. (2001). Auditory temporal processing during aging. In P. R. Hof & C. V. Mobbs (Eds.), *Functional neurobiology of aging* (pp. 565–579). San Diego: Academic Press

Frisina, R. D., & Walton, J. P. (2006, Jun-Jul). Age-related structural and functional changes in the cochlear nucleus. *Hearing Research, 216-217*, 216–223

Gaihede, M., & Koefoed-Nielsen, B. (2000, Mar-Apr). Mechanics of the middle ear system: Age-related changes in viscoelastic properties. *Audiology and Neuro-Otology, 5*, 53–58

Gates, G. A., Beiser, A., Rees, T. S., D'Agostino, R. B., & Wolf, P. A. (2002, Mar). Central auditory dysfunction may precede the onset of clinical dementia in people with probable Alzheimer's disease. *Journal of the American Geriatrics Society, 50*, 482–488

Gates, G. A., Couropmitree, N. N., & Myers, R. H. (1999, Jun). Genetic associations in age-related hearing thresholds. *Archives of Otolaryngology–Head and Neck Surgery, 125*, 654–659

Gates, G. A., Cobb, J. L., D'Agostino, R. B., & Wolf, P. A. (1993, Feb). The relation of hearing in the elderly to the presence of cardiovascular disease and cardiovascular risk factors. *Archives of Otolaryngology–Head and Neck Surgery, 119*, 156–161

Gates, G. A., Cobb, J. L., Linn, R. T., Rees, T., Wolf, P. A., & D'Agostino, R. B. (1996, Feb). Central auditory dysfunction, cognitive dysfunction, and dementia in older people. *Archives of Otolaryngology–Head and Neck Surgery, 122*, 161–167

Gates, G. A., Mills, D., Nam, B. H., D'Agostino, R., & Rubel, E. W. (2002, Jan). Effects of age on the distortion product otoacoustic emission growth functions. *Hearing Research, 163*, 53–60

Gates, G. A., & Mills, J. H. (2005, Sep). Presbycusis. *Lancet, 366*, 1111–1120

Gates, G. A., Schmid, P., Kujawa, S. G., Nam, B., & D'Agostino, R. (2000, Mar). Longitudinal threshold changes in older men with audiometric notches. *Hearing Research, 141*, 220–228

Gilad, O., & Glorig, A. (1979, Mar-Apr). Presbycusis: The aging ear. Part I. *Journal of the American Auditory Society, 4*, 195–206

Gleich, O., Weiss, M., & Strutz, J. (2004, Aug). Age-dependent changes in the lateral superior olive of the gerbil (Meriones unguiculatus). *Hearing Research, 194*, 47–59

Gleitman, R., Ballachanda, B., & Goldstein, D. (1992). Incidence of cerumen impaction in general adult population. *Hearing Journal, 45*, 28–32

Groher, M. (1988). Modifications in speech-language assessment procedures for the older adult. In B. Shadden (Ed.), *Communication behavior and aging*. Baltimore: Williams & Wilkins

Guest, J. F., Greener, M. J., Robinson, A. C., & Smith, A. F. (2004, Aug). Impacted cerumen: Composition, production, epidemiology and management. *QJM, 97*, 477–488

Guay, D. (2010). The pharmacology of aging. In H. Fillit, K. Rockwood, & K. Woodhouse (Eds.), *Brocklehurst's textbook of geriatric medicine and gerontology* (7th ed.). Philadelphia: Saunders Elsevier

Gulya, J. (1991). Structural and physiological changes of the auditory and vestibular mechanisms with aging. In D. Ripich (Ed.), *Handbook of geriatric communication disorders*. Austin: Pro-Ed.

Halter, J. (2011). Aging and insulin secretion. In E. Masoro & S. Austral (Eds.), *Handbook of the biology of aging* (7th ed.). London: Academic Press

Hansen, C. C., & Reske-Nielsen, E. (1965, Aug). Pathological studies in presbycusis. *Archives of Otolaryngology, 82*, 115–132

Harrison, R., & Mount, R. (2001). The sensory epithelium of the normal and pathological cochlea. In A. Jahn & J. Santos-Sacchi (Eds.), *Physiology of the ear* (2nd ed.). San Diego: Singular

Helzner, E. P., Cauley, J. A., Pratt, S. R., Wisniewski, S. R., Zmuda, J. M., Talbott, E. O., et al. (2005, Dec). Race and sex differences in age-related hearing loss: The Health, Aging and Body Composition Study. *Journal of the American Geriatrics Society, 53*, 2119–2127

Howarth, A., & Shone, G. R. (2006, Mar). Ageing and the auditory system. *Postgraduate Medical Journal, 82*, 166–171

Ison, J., Tremblay, K., & Allen, P. (2010). Closing the gap between neurobiology and human presbycusis: Behavioral and evoked potential studies of age-related hearing loss in animal models and in humans. In S. Gordon-Salant, R. Frisina, A. Popper, & R. Fay (Eds.), *The aging auditory system*. New York: Springer

Ives, D. G., Bonino, P., Traven, N. D., & Kuller, L. H. (1995, Jul). Characteristics and comorbidities of rural older adults with hearing impairment. *Journal of the American Geriatrics Society, 43*, 803–806

Johnson, A., Hawke, M., & Jahn, A. (2001). The nonauditory physiology of the external ear canal. In A. Jahn & J. Santos-Sacchi (Eds.), *Physiology of the ear* (2nd ed.). San Diego: Singular

Johnson, J., & Hadley, R. (1964). The aging pinna. In J. Converse (Ed.), *Reconstructive and plastic surgery* (pp. 1306–1346). Philadelphia: W. B. Saunders

Johnsson, L., & Hawkins, J. (1979). Age-related degeneration of the inner ear. In S. Han & D. Coons (Eds.), *Special senses in aging*. Ann Arbor, MI: Institute of Gerontology, University of Michigan

Kenna, M. (1993). Otitis media with effusion. In B. Bailey (Ed.), *Head and neck surgery–Otolaryngology*. Philadelphia: Lippincott

Kirikae, I., Sato, T., & Shitara, T. (1964, Feb). A study of hearing in advanced age. *Laryngoscope, 74*, 205–220

Konigsmark, B. W., & Murphy, E. A. (1970, Dec). Neuronal populations in the human brain. *Nature, 228*, 1335–1336

Konigsmark, B. W., & Murphy, E. A. (1972, Apr). Volume of the ventral cochlear nucleus in man: Its relationship to neuronal population and age. *Journal of Neuropathology and Experimental Neurology, 31*, 304–316

Kryla-Lighthall, N., & Mather, M. (2009). The role of cognitive control in older adults' emotional well-being. In V. Bengtson, D. Gans, N. Putney, & M. Silverstein (Eds.), *Handbook of theories of aging* (2nd ed.). New York: Springer

Kryter, K. D. (1983, Dec). Addendum and erratum: "Presbycusis, sociocusis, and nosocusis" [J. Acoust. Soc. Am. 73, 1897-1919]. *Journal of the Acoustical Society of America, 74*, 1907–1909

Lansky, B. (Ed.). (1996). *Age happens: The best quotes about growing older*. New York: Meadowbrook Press

Lee, F. S., Matthews, L. J., Dubno, J. R., & Mills, J. H. (2005, Feb). Longitudinal study of pure-tone thresholds in older persons. *Ear and Hearing, 26*, 1–11

Lemke, U. (2011). Hearing impairment in dementia—How to reconcile two intertwined challenges in diagnostic screening. *Audiology Research, 1*, 58–60

Leventhal, A., Wang, Y., Pu, M., Zhou, Y., & Ma, Y. (2003). Gaba and its agonists improved visual cortical function in senescent monkeys. *Science, 2*, 812–815

Lin, F. R. (2011, Oct). Hearing loss and cognition among older adults in the United States. *Journals of Gerontology, Series A, Biological Sciences and Medical Sciences, 66*, 1131–1136

Lin, F. R., Metter, E. J., O'Brien, R. J., Resnick, S. M., Zonderman, A. B., & Ferrucci, L. (2011, Feb). Hearing loss and incident dementia. *Archives of Neurology, 68*, 214–220

Lin, F. R., Thorpe, R., Gordon-Salant, S., & Ferrucci, L. (2011, May). Hearing loss prevalence and risk factors among older adults in the United States. *Journals of Gerontology, Series A, Biological Sciences and Medical Sciences, 66* 582–590

Lonsbury-Martin, B., & Martin, G. (2001). Otoacoustic emissions. In A. Jahn & J. Santos-Sacchi (Eds.), *Physiology of the ear* (2nd ed.). San Diego: Singular

Mahoney, D. F. (1987, Sep-Oct). One simple solution to hearing impairment. *Geriatric Nursing, 8*, 242–245

Martin, J. S., & Jerger, J. F. (2005, Jul-Aug). Some effects of aging on central auditory processing. *Journal of Rehabilitation Research and Development, 42*(4, Suppl 2), 25–44

McMahon, C. M., Kifley, A., Rochtchina, E., Newall, P., & Mitchell, P. (2008, Aug). The contribution of family history to hearing loss in an older population. *Ear and Hearing, 29*, 578–584

Mills, J., Schmiedt, R., & Dubno, J. (2006). Older and wiser but losing hearing nonetheless. *Hearing Health, Summer*, 12–17

Mills, J. H., Schmiedt, R. A., Schulte, B. A., & Dubno, J. R. (2006). Age-related hearing loss: A loss of voltage, not hair cells. *Seminars in Hearing, 27*, 228–236

Miyamoto, R., & Miyamoto, R. (1995). Anatomy of the ear canal. In B. Ballachanda (Ed.), *Introduction to the human ear canal*. San Diego: Singular

Moore, B. (2003). *An introduction to the psychology of hearing* (5th ed.). Boston: Academic Press

Morosan, P., Rademacher, J., Palomero-Gallagher, N., & Zilles, K. (2005). Anatomical organization of the human auditory cortex: Cytoarchitecture and transmitter receptors. In R. Konig, P. Heil, E. Budinger, E., & H. Scheich (Eds.), *The auditory cortex: A synthesis of human and animal research*. Mahwah, NJ: Lawrence Erlbaum

Mościcki, E. K., Elkins, E. F., Baum, H. M., & McNamara, P. M. (1985, Jul-Aug). Hearing loss in the elderly: An epidemiologic study of the Framingham Heart Study Cohort. *Ear and Hearing, 6*, 184–190

Nadol, J. (1981). The aging peripheral hearing mechanism. In D. Beasley & G. Davis (Eds.), *Aging: Communication processes and disorders*. New York: Grune & Stratton. *Statement, 8*(1). Bethesda: Office of Medical Applications of Research

Nielsen, N. (1998). Who said 65 was old? *New York Times*, June 30, p. 22

Northern, J. (1996). *Hearing disorders* (3rd ed.). Boston: Allyn & Bacon

Osguthorpe, J. D., & Nielsen, D. R. (2006, Nov). Otitis externa: Review and clinical update. *American Family Physician, 74*, 1510–1516

Otte, J., Schuknecht, H. F., & Kerr, A. G. (1978, Aug). Ganglion cell populations in normal and pathological human cochleae. Implications for cochlear implantation. *Laryngoscope, 88*(8 Pt 1), 1231–1246

Pauler, M., Schuknecht, H. F., & Thornton, A. R. (1986). Correlative studies of cochlear neuronal loss with speech discrimination and pure-tone thresholds. *Archives of Otolaryngology, 243*, 200–206

Pichora-Fuller, K. (2009). Using the brain when the ears are challenged helps healthy older listeners compensate and preserve communication function. In: *Phonak adult conference: The challenge of aging*. Chicago. http://www.phonakpro.com/com/b2b/en/events/proceedings/archive/adult_conference_chicago2009.html.html

Powers, R. (1994). Neurobiology of aging. In *Textbook of geriatric neuropsychiatry*. Washington, DC: American Psychiatric Press

Pratt, S. R., Kuller, L., Talbott, E. O., McHugh Pemu, K., Buhari, A. M., & Xu, X. (2009, Aug). Prevalence of hearing loss in black and white elders: Results of the Cardiovascular Health Study. *Journal of Speech, Language, and Hearing Research, 52,* 973–989

Purves, D., Augustine, G. J., Fitzpatrick, D., Katz, L. C., Lamantia, A.-S., Mcnamara, J, O., & Williams, S. M. (2007). The auditory system. In D. Purves, G. J. Augustine, D. Fitzpatrick, W. C. Hall, A.-S. Lamantia, J. O. Mcnamara, & L. E. White (Eds.), *Neuroscience* (4th ed., pp. 283–314). Sunderland, MA: Sinauer

Rawool, V. W., & Harrington, B. T. (2007). Middle ear admittance and hearing abnormalities in individuals with osteoarthritis. *Audiology and Neuro-Otology, 12,* 127–136

Rees, T., & Duckert, L. (1995). Auditory and vestibular dysfunction in aging. In W. Hazzard, R. Andres, E. Bierman, & J. Blass (Eds.), *Principles of geriatric medicine and gerontology* (2nd ed.). New York: McGraw-Hill

Rissman, R. A., & Mobley, W. C. (2011, May). Implications for treatment: GABAA receptors in aging, Down syndrome and Alzheimer's disease. *Journal of Neurochemistry, 117,* 613–622

Roeser, R. (1996). *Roeser's audiology desk reference.* New York: Thieme

Roland, P. S., Smith, T. L., Schwartz, S. R., Rosenfeld, R. M., Ballachanda, B., Earll, J. M., et al. (2008, Sep). Clinical practice guideline: cerumen impaction. *Otolaryngology–Head and Neck Surgery, 139*(3, Suppl 2), S1–S21

Rosen, S., Bergman, M., Plester, D., El-Mofty, A., & Satti, M. (1962). Presbycusis study of a relatively noise free population in the Sudan. *Transactions of the American Otological Society, 50,* 135–151

Rosenwasser, H. (1964, Jan). Otitic problems in the aged. *Geriatrics, 19,* 11–17

Ruby, R. R. (1986, Aug). Conductive hearing loss in the elderly. *Journal of Otolaryngology, 15,* 245–247

Sander, R. (2001, Mar). Otitis externa: A practical guide to treatment and prevention. *American Family Physician, 63,* 927–936, 941–942

Santi, P., & Tsuprun, V. (2001) Cochlear microanatomy and ultrastructure. In A. Jahn & J. Santos-Sacchi (Eds.), *Physiology of the ear* (2nd ed.). San Diego: Singular

Santos-Sacchi, J. (2001). Cochlear physiology. In A. Jahn & J. Santos-Sacchi (Eds.), *Physiology of the ear* (2nd ed.). San Diego: Singular

Scheibel, M. E., Lindsay, R. D., Tomiyasu, U., & Scheibel, A. B. (1975, Jun). Progressive dendritic changes in aging human cortex. *Experimental Neurology, 47,* 392–403

Schleuning, A., & Andersen, P. (1993). Otologic manifestations of systemic disease. In B. Bailey (Ed.), *Head and neck surgery–otolaryngology.* Philadelphia: Lippincott

Schmiedt, R. A. (2010). The physiology of cochlear presbyacusis. In S. Gordon-Salant, R. Frisina, A. Popper, & R. Fay (Eds.), *The aging auditory system.* New York: Springer

Schneider, B., Pichora-Fuller, K., & Daneman, M. (2010). Effects of senescent changes in audition and cognition on spoken language comprehension. In S. Gordon-Salant, R. Frisina, A. Popper, & R. Fay (Eds.), *The aging auditory system.* New York: Springer

Schuknecht, H. F. (1955, Jun). Presbycusis. *Laryngoscope, 65,* 402–419

Schuknecht, H. F. (1964, Oct). Further observations on the pathology of presbycusis. *Archives of Otolaryngology, 80,* 369–382

Schuknecht, H. F. (1989). Pathology of presbycusis. In J. Goldstein, H. Kashima, & C. Koopman (Eds.), *Geriatric otorhinolaryngology.* Toronto: B. C. Decker

Schuknecht, H. F. (1993). *Pathology of the ear* (2nd ed.). Philadelphia: Lea & Febiger

Schuknecht, H. F., & Gacek, M. R. (1993, Jan). Cochlear pathology in presbycusis. *Annals of Otology, Rhinology, and Laryngology, 102*(1 Pt 2), 1–16

Senturia, B., Marcus, M., & Lucente, F. (1980). *Diseases of the external ear.* New York: Grune & Stratton

Shankar, S. K. (2010, Oct-Dec). Biology of aging brain. *Indian Journal of Pathology and Microbiology, 53,* 595–604

Silman, S., & Silverman, C. (1991). *Auditory diagnosis: Principles and applications.* San Diego: Academic Press

Staab, W. (1995). Deep canal hearing aids. In B. Ballachanda (Ed.), *Introduction to the human ear canal.* San Diego: Singular

Steigleder, G., & Maibach, H. (1993). *Pocket atlas of dermatology.* New York: Thieme

Strouse, A. L., Hall, J. W., III, & Burger, M. C. (1995, Apr). Central auditory processing in Alzheimer's disease. *Ear and Hearing, 16,* 230–238

Suzuka, Y., & Schuknecht, H. F. (1988). Retrograde cochlear neuronal degeneration in human subjects. *Acta Oto-Laryngologica Supplementum, 450,* 1–20

Tremblay, K., & Burkard, R. (2007). The aging auditory system: Confounding effects of hearing loss on AEPs. In R. Burkard, M. Don, & J. Eggermont (Eds.), *Auditory evoked potentials: Basic principles and clinic applications.* Baltimore: Lippincott Williams & Wilkins

Tremblay, K., & Kraus, N. (2002). Beyond the ear: Central auditory plasticity. *Otorrinolaringologia, 52,* 93–100

Tremblay, K., & Ross, B. (2007, Jul-Aug). Effects of age and age-related hearing loss on the brain. *Journal of Communication Disorders, 40,* 305–312

Turner, J. G., & Caspary, D. (2005). Comparison of two rat models of aging. In J. Syka & M. M. Merzenich (Eds.), *Plasticity and signal representation in the auditory system.* New York: Springer

Uhlmann, R. F., Larson, E. B., Rees, T. S., Koepsell, T. D., & Duckert, L. G. (1989, Apr). Relationship of hearing impairment to dementia and cognitive dysfunction in older adults. *Journal of the American Medical Association, 261,* 1916–1919

Uhlmann, R. F., Rees, T. S., Psaty, B. M., & Duckert, L. G. (1989, Mar-Apr). Validity and reliability of auditory screening tests in demented and non-demented older adults. *Journal of General Internal Medicine, 4,* 90–96

Vartiainen, E. (1995, Jul). Surgery in elderly patients with otosclerosis. *American Journal of Otology, 16,* 536–538

Vestal, R. (1990). Clinical pharmacology. In W. Hazzard, R. Andres, E. Bierman, & J. Blass (Eds.), *Principles of geriatric medicine and gerontology* (2nd ed.). New York: McGraw-Hill

Walton, J., Frisina, R., & O'Neill, W. (1998). Age-related alteration in processing of temporal sound features in the auditory midbrain of the CBA mouse. *Journal of Neuroscience, 18,* 2764–2776

Weinstein, B. (1998). Disorders of hearing. In R. Tallis, H. Fillit, & J. Brockelhurst (Eds.), *Brockelhurst's textbook of geriatric medicine.* London: Churchill Livingstone

Weinstein, B., & Amsel, L. (1986). Hearing loss and senile dementia in the institutionalized elderly. *Clinical Gerontologist, 4,* 3–15

White, J., & Regan, M. (1987). Otologic considerations. In G. Mueller & V. Geoffrey (Eds.), *Communication disorders in aging: Assessment and management.* Washington, DC: Gallaudet University Press

Wiley, T. L., Cruickshanks, K. J., Nondahl, D. M., & Tweed, T. S. (1999, Apr). Aging and middle ear resonance. *Ear and Hearing, 10,* 173–179

Wiley, T. L., Nondahl, D. M., Cruickshanks, K. J., & Tweed, T. S. (2005, Mar). Five-year changes in middle ear function for older adults. *Journal of the American Academy of Audiology, 16,* 129–139

Willis, S., Schaie, K., & Martin, M. (2009). Cognitive plasticity. In V. Bengtson, D. Gans, N. Putney, & M. Silverstein (Eds.), *Handbook of theories of aging* (2nd ed.). New York: Springer

Willott, J. F. (1991). *Aging and the auditory system.* San Diego: Singular

Willott, J. F. (1996, Jun). Anatomic and physiologic aging: A behavioral neuroscience perspective. *Journal of the American Academy of Audiology, 7,* 141–151

Young, E., Newcomer, V., & Kligman, A. (1993). *Geriatric dermatology.* Philadelphia: Lea & Febiger

Young, E., & Oeretel, D. (2004). Cochlear nucleus. In G. M. Shepherd (Ed.), *The synaptic organization of the brain.* New York: Oxford University Press

Zettel, M. L., Zhu, X., O'Neill, W. E., & Frisina, R. D. (2007, Jun). Age-related decline in Kv3.1b expression in the mouse auditory brainstem correlates with functional deficits in the medial olivocochlear efferent system. *Journal of the Association for Research in Otolaryngology, 8,* 280–293

II

Age-Related Changes in Hearing

Chapter 5

Pure-Tone Data, Otoacoustic Emissions, and Immittance Findings

As they finished listening, Mrs. M. looked up at me and asked, "What does it sound like?" Taking her cue, I put my stethoscope in her ears. And then it happened. Almost exactly as I placed the stethoscope on her left sternal border, my phone rang with one of those classic cell phone tunes. I saw Mrs. M.'s eyebrows rise way above her eyeglass frames. "I hear music!" she exclaimed without skipping a beat.

—Ouslander, 2010, p. 1875

They say that I am legally deaf, and all I can hear is some background noise, such as the refrigerator humming. I can still hear a whole lifetime of sounds, people and places—all the details, even if the audiometer says I can't hear anything now.

—N.B., born 1897

◆ Learning Objectives

After reading this chapter, you should be able to

- explain the behavioral correlates of the anatomical and physiological age-related changes within the auditory system;
- appreciate the potential medical covariates of hearing impairment in older adults; and
- discuss the prevalence estimates of hearing loss by age, gender, and race.

◆ Overview

Presbycusis, the hearing loss associated with aging, is a multifactorial condition. Age-related changes in the periphery include hair cell loss, strial atrophy, and spiral ganglion cell degeneration. An understanding of the prevalence and pure-tone data along with information on comorbidities is essential to the diagnostic process. The most appropriate test protocols need to be selected so that intervention strategies are appropriately targeted. This chapter highlights the results of recent studies that describe the audiological manifestations of age-related changes in the periphery.

◆ Prevalence Data

According to estimates from the World Health Organization (WHO), worldwide 278 million people experience moderate to profound hearing loss bilaterally (WHO, 2010). In fact, adult-onset hearing loss is the second leading cause, after depression, of years living with a disability (YLD) (Mathers et al, 2003). In the United States, it consistently emerges as one of the most prevalent chronic conditions afflicting older adults. Over the last generation, the hearing loss population has grown at a rate 1.6 times that of U.S. population growth, due in large part to the growth of the aging population, including the growth in the percentage of supercentenarians (individuals at least 110 years old) (Kochkin, 2009). Approximately 34 to 36 million Americans report suffering from some degree of hearing impairment and it is projected that this number will rise to 52.9 million by the year 2050 (Kochkin, 2009; Pleis & Lethbridge-Cejku, 2006). Hearing impairment is considered the number one communication disorder among older adults, yet over 22 million adults with hearing impairment do not seek solutions for this chronic condition (Kochkin, 2007). According to the Marke Trak VIII survey, the prevalence of self-reported hearing problems increases dramatically with age, more so in men than in women. In addition, there has been a considerable increase in self-reported hearing problems from the Marke Trak III survey reported in 1991. According to the Marke Trak VIII survey, conducted by Kochkin (2009), 20.6 million men and 14 million women reported hearing loss in contrast to 15.7 million men and 10 million women in the 1991 survey. This represents an increase in prevalence of between 31% and 35%. Hearing-aid use also differed by gender, with fewer older women (11%) than older men (18%) reporting having worn a hearing aid.

Within the various age groups, it is notable that while the prevalence of self-reported hearing loss has declined among those between 18 and 44 years, the increase in prevalence since 1991 has been dramatic among individuals 45 years of age or older (Kochkin, 2009). If current hearing loss rates are applied to the 2030 population estimates, the number of individuals with hearing loss will be 7 million in the 65- to 75-year age category, and 13.3 million in the 75 or older category. Given the proportion of women relative to men over 65 years of age, by 2030 nearly 13 million women may present with hearing loss.

Hearing problems are not manifest conditions; hence, they are often unrecognized and untreated (Crews & Campbell, 2004). Thus, prevalence estimates may underrepresent the true magnitude of the "epidemic of hearing impairment" (Agrawal,

Table 5.1 Likelihood of Comorbid Condition in Those with Hearing Loss and Dual Sensory Impairment

Condition	Likelihood of presenting with co-morbid condition among those with hearing loss as compared with those without hearing loss	Likelihood of presenting with co-morbid condition among those with vision and hearing loss as compared with those without dual sensory loss
Experienced falls in past 12 months	1.7 times more likely to have experienced falls (statistically significant)	3 times more likely to have fallen in past 12 months (significant)
Heart Disease	1.7 times more likely to report heart disease (significant)	2.4 times more likely to report heart disease (significant)
Hypertension	Significantly higher rates of hypertension	1.5 times more likely to report hypertension (significant)
Broken Hip	Significantly higher rates of broken hips	2 times more likely to have broken a hip (significant)

Source: Data from Crews, J. E., & Campbell, V. A. (2004, May). Vision impairment and hearing loss among community-dwelling older Americans: Implications for health and functioning. *American Journal of Public Health, 94*, 823–829. (SOURCE)

Platz, & Niparko, 2008). The tendency to overlook hearing impairment in older adults is problematic, given data that suggest that older adults with hearing loss report higher rates of comorbid and secondary conditions than do those who do not have hearing loss (Crews & Campbell, 2004). According to **Table 5.1**, compiled from the work of Crews and Campbell (2004), individuals with hearing loss, vision loss, and dual sensory loss have an increased likelihood of presenting with comorbid conditions ranging from falls to cardiovascular disease. The latter data underscore the burden posed by untreated sensory loss.

Several large-scale studies have been conducted to determine prevalence and progression of hearing loss among U.S. adults. These include the Epidemiology of Hearing Loss Study (EHLS) (Cruickshanks et al, 2003), the Framingham Heart Study (Gates and Cooper, 1991; Gates, Cooper, Kannel, & Miller, 1990), the Baltimore Longitudinal Study of Aging (BLSA; Brant and Fozard, 1990; Brant et al, 1996; Pearson et al, 1995), and the Blue Mountains Hearing Study (BMHS), a companion to the EHLS. The large-scale population-based studies are unique in that they have considered hearing loss prevalence in the context of conditions that affect large proportions of older adults, including smokers and those with diabetes, heart disease, or vision impairment. These data along with data from the more traditional studies on hearing loss are included below. The EHLS and the BMHS, both population-based studies of hearing loss in adults, grew out of the population-based studies of ocular disorders in Beaver Dam, Wisconsin. The Framingham Heart Study (FHS) included a population-based cohort that has been studied biennially beginning with the first group in 1948 to 1950. The FHS has collaborated with other research projects including hearing studies and studies with a dementia cohort (Gates, Beiser, Rees, D'Agostino, & Wolf, 2002). Finally, the National Health and Nutritional Examination Survey (NHANES) is an ongoing program of studies designed to assess the health and functional and nutritional status of the civilian noninstitutionalized U.S. population. Each cross-sectional study on which data are reported from the NHANES uses a complex sampling design to survey a sample of the population, representative of low-income individuals, racial minorities, and older adults. Because of the sampling-weighting techniques, the results are generalizable to the U.S. population (Lin, Thorpe, Gordon-Salant, & Ferrucci, 2011).

◆ Audiometric Studies: Cross-Sectional Data

Within the past several decades several large-scale studies have been conducted using an epidemiological approach to gathering and analyzing data on hearing status of a large, essentially unscreened sample of older adults. Cross-sectional data of average thresholds have been reported using the NHANES cross-sectional survey of the civilian noninstitutionalized population of the U.S., and data from the Framingham Cohort Study, the Beaver Dam EHLS, and the Health Interview Study (Cooper, 1994; Gates et al, 1990; Moscicki, Elkins, Baum, & McNamara, 1985). **Table 5.2** summarizes the prevalence estimates from selected population-based studies, and in older subjects the prevalence ranges from 45 to 47%. As would be expected, the incidence is higher in older age groups as well, such that the incidence of hearing impairment in the EHLS rose from 20% in those 48 to 59 years of age to 98% in those between 80 and 92 years of age, with the 5-year incidence in men being 100% among those between 80 and 92 years of age (Cruickshanks et al, 2003). According to Cruickshanks (2010), older Caucasian men are at the greatest risk of developing hearing loss.

Agrawal et al (2008) assessed the prevalence of hearing loss among adults of ages 20 to 69 years using data from the NHANES 1999 to 2004 cohort. In addition to prevalence, the authors explored the role of noise exposure and cardiovascular factors on hearing levels. The 3527 participants in the study were free of otalgia, and some were hearing-aid users, but the number of hearing-aid users was not included in the description of the sample. The sample was diverse in terms of ethnic-

Table 5.2 Prevalence and Incidence of Hearing Impairment in Selected Population Based Studies.

Study	Age of Sample	Prevalence of Hearing Impairment
EHLS	48–92 years	46%
FHS	57–89 years	47%
BMHS	49–80+	45%
NHANES	20–69 years	16%

Abbreviations: BMHS, Blue Mountains Hearing Study; EHLS, Epidemiology of Hearing Loss Study; FHS, Framingham Heart Study; NHANES, National Health and Nutrition Examination Survey.

ity, as white non-Hispanics, black non-Hispanics, and Mexican Americans were included. Forty-seven percent were men and 53% were women; 46% of the sample was between 20 and 39 years of age, and the rest were between 40 and 69 years of age. With regard to comorbidities, 9.5% reported a diagnosis of diabetes mellitus, and 32% reported a diagnosis of hypertension. Half of the subjects were nonsmokers and half were smokers. Approximately one third reported excessive exposure to occupational or recreational noise. Hearing loss was defined as four frequency pure-tone averages (500, 1000, 2000, and 4000 Hz) poorer than 25 dB HL in either ear, and high-frequency hearing loss was defined as mean pure-tone average (3000, 4000 and 6000 Hz) in excess of 25 dB HL in one or both ears. Although the sample was relatively young (66% were younger than 50), 31% of participants had high-frequency hearing loss, which was bilateral in most cases (the equivalent of 55 million Americans), and defined as mean thresholds 25 dB HL or greater at 3000, 4000, and 6000 Hz in one or both ears. Age, race, and gender were factors for the risk of hearing loss; the prevalence of hearing loss was higher among older white men; and the odds of hearing loss was 5.5 fold higher in men than women and significantly lower in blacks than whites. The data of Lin et al (2011) confirm that black race may be a protective factor against developing hearing loss, in that prevalence among black women and men over 70 years of age is dramatically lower (i.e., 45%) than in white (67%) participants. Although the prevalence of hearing loss was higher among black men (43%) than among black women (40%), white men had the highest prevalence (72%). Lin et al speculated that the lower prevalence in blacks may be due to the protective effect of melanin in the stria vascularis.

Hearing loss prevalence was higher among smokers, those with diabetes mellitus, hypertensives, and those with higher exposure to noise. In terms of age and gender as risk factors, white men between 60 and 69 years of age had a 93% prevalence of high-frequency hearing loss. Interestingly, prevalence of hearing loss among men with comorbidities including noise exposure and cardiovascular disease was high for those between 40 and 49 years of age. In fact, prevalence of hearing loss was higher among men between 40 and 49 years of age who smoked and who had comorbidities than it was among participants 60 to 69 years of age. After adjusting for noise exposure and cardiovascular risk, older white men had significantly higher odds of bilateral high-frequency hearing loss. One particularly noteworthy finding is that comparisons between self-reported hearing difficulties and measured hearing impairment revealed that the former underestimated true prevalence of hearing loss in this sample. The data also suggest that the prevalence of hearing loss is increasing among younger age groups, occurring as early as the third decade of life. The findings of Agrawal and colleagues (2008) confirm that decrements in hearing begin first in the higher frequencies but is not as obvious to those afflicted unless it is bilateral. Further, hearing loss prevalence increases with age across both genders and all races, but prevalence progresses at an earlier age among individuals who smoke or suffer from diabetes mellitus, cardiovascular disease, or noise exposure. The authors projected that cessation of smoking, reduction of noise exposure, and treatment of comorbidities might delay the onset of hearing loss.

The data of Zhan et al (2010) confirm that controlling modifiable risk factors may in fact delay the onset of hearing loss or slow down the progression, as suggested by Agrawal and colleagues (2008). Zhan and colleagues used data from the population-based EHLS and the study of those subjects' adult children, namely the Beaver Dam Offspring Study (BOSS; participants in the BOSS were adults born to participants in the EHLS), to evaluate the effect of birth cohort on hearing loss prevalence in these two samples, albeit nonrepresentative, of adults throughout the U.S. and globally. EHLS participants ranged in age from 48 to 92 years, and the majority of BOSS participants were between 45 and 64 years, with only 10% of the sample 65 years of age or older. In the BOSS sample, hearing loss was defined as pure-tone average at 500, 1000, 2000, and 4000 Hz in excess of 25 dB HL in either ear. The 5275 participants, representing 2661 families, were born between 1902 and 1962. The authors compared prevalence of hearing impairment in the parent generation and the child generation by age group. Trends were comparable to previous cross-sectional studies in that hearing loss prevalence increased in both samples with increasing age, with the prevalence in the oldest group (70 to 74 years) dramatically higher than in the 55- and 59-year group. The prevalence of hearing loss was 60% in the oldest group in the ELHS versus 50% in the BOSS, but the sample size was drastically different (ELHS, 510; BOSS, 28) in this age group. Across all age groups, hearing loss prevalence was higher in the parent generation than in the child generation, which may in fact speak to the contribution of modifiable risk factors to hearing loss and the possibility that risk factor reduction may be an important approach to reducing the prevalence and progression of hearing loss. In short, the authors speculated that reduction of modifiable risk factors early may in fact postpone the onset of hearing loss or reduce its prevalence overall. This is speculative, as data on risk exposure were not included in their study, and their sample drawn from a single Midwestern town may not be representative (Zhan and colleagues, 2010).

Gates, Feeney, and Mills (2008) conducted a cross-sectional cohort study of changes in hearing level in the elderly over time. Participants were volunteer enrollees in the Adult Changes in Thought (ACT) population-based study. Mean age of the men was 79.3 years and of the women was 78.8 years; 35% of the women and 8% of the men were hearing-aid users, and 54% of the women and 68% of the men complained of hearing loss. Thirty-three percent of the men had a history of noise exposure through the years. Eighty-seven percent of participants presented with high-frequency hearing loss, typically of presbycusis with symmetrical hearing levels in the higher frequencies. Pure-tone averages were significantly correlated with increasing age in both the men and the women. The most compelling finding was that the rate of change in performance on various audiometric tests was not uniform among participants in their seventh and eighth decades. Specifically, performance on central auditory tests (e.g., Synthetic Sentence Identification, Dichotic Sentence Identification, Dichotic Digit Test) declined the most, followed by pure-tone thresholds. Distortion product otoacoustic emissions appeared to be relatively stable over time.

Moscicki et al (1985) conducted one of the first of these large-scale cross-sectional studies on the nature of hearing loss in the elderly by using data from the Framingham Heart Study, a prospective investigation of risk factors leading to the development of cardiovascular disease. The study was initiated in 1950 and included biennial physical examinations and histories of all subjects. During the 15th cycle of examinations (1977 to 1979), a hearing study was conducted under the auspices of the National Institute of Neurological and Communicative Disorders and Stroke. Of the 2634 individuals undergoing complete physical examinations, 2293 community-based individuals (87%) received a hearing examination. The age range of subjects was comparable for the men and women, as were the mean ages (men, 68 years; women, 69 years). Participants included 935 men and 1358 women. All subjects underwent pure-tone air and bone conduction testing in a sound-treated booth. Sensorineural hearing loss was defined as a hearing level greater/poorer than 20 dB HL at any one frequency from 500 to 4000 Hz and no air–bone gap.

Using a traditional definition of hearing loss (pure-tone average [PTA] >25 dB HL), 31% of subjects presented with hearing impairment. According to subjective reports, many of the subjects did not feel they had a problem at the time of the study, despite the presence of decrements in pure-tone thresholds. Further, many subjects did not have a "pure-presbycusic" hearing loss. A significant proportion of subjects attributed their hearing loss to noise exposure and illness, among other potential etiologies. Overall, 59% of the cohort had sensorineural hearing loss, 24% had a mixed loss, and the remainder had a conductive loss.

The authors generated threshold values as a function of frequency for men and women and for those with a pure-presbycusic loss and those with a history of noise exposure, illness, and so on. Interestingly, the audiometric configuration for the entire cohort was comparable to that obtained for the pure presbycusics, confirming that it is difficult to conclude from the audiogram whether a hearing loss is due to age or exogenous factors such as noise or illness. Several trends from their data remain sustainable in 2011. First, the configuration of hearing loss tends to differ for men and women. The audiogram for women shows a gradually sloping high-frequency configuration, whereas for the men it is abruptly falling and high frequency, suggesting a possible noise component (Moscicki et al, 1985). Further, mean pure-tone averages in both ears were poorer for men than for women and tended to increase with age most prominently in the frequencies above 1000 Hz. Pure-tone thresholds for the women revealed average hearing levels to be within normal limits through 2000 Hz, gradually sloping to the level of a mild hearing loss thereafter. In the men, hearing was within normal limits through 1000 Hz, sloping to the level of a mild to moderate hearing loss thereafter. In general, women tended to have better thresholds than men for thresholds above 2000 Hz. The apparent relation between pure-tone threshold and age was borne out upon statistical analysis of the data. According to a logistic regression model used to determine risk factors for hearing loss, age emerged as the most important risk factor.

Special Consideration

Persons 70 years of age and older are more likely than younger persons to have pure-tone hearing loss for the speech frequencies.

Gates et al (1990) tested a subsample of subjects from the FHS 6 years later as part of examination cycle 18. In total, 1739 subjects reported for their biennial examination, and 1662 persons, or 96% of the cohort, volunteered for follow-up hearing tests, which included pure-tone thresholds, word recognition testing, and immittance measures. The mean age of subjects was 72.7 years for men and 73 years for women. Using a criterion of PTA >26 dB HL in the better ear, 29% of the cohort had a hearing impairment, with 32.5% of the men and 26.7% of the women having reduced thresholds. On the basis of their self-reports, most subjects ascribed their hearing loss to age, noise exposure, infection, injury, or other unknown causes. Their data corroborated the gender and age effects noted by Moscicki and her colleagues. Mean pure-tone thresholds worsened with age, with the effects being most pronounced in the higher frequencies and for men. Further, among the men, left ear pure-tone thresholds were slightly poorer than right ear thresholds. Finally, the majority of men had gradually or sharply sloping pure-tone audiograms, whereas the majority of women had flat or gradually sloping configurations.

Cooper (1994), reported on hearing data extracted from the Health and Nutrition Examination Survey (HANES) of 1971 to 1975. HANES was a multistage, stratified probability sample of 65 geographic areas. As part of the design of the survey, audiograms were obtained from 6913 persons ranging in age from 25 to 74 years. Both air- and bone-conduction thresholds were gathered on the subjects in the sample. The trends emerging from the data corroborate the studies described above. Age and frequency effects emerged such that air-conduction thresholds became poorer as age or frequency increased. Similarly, gender and race effects emerged as well. Overall, the men's thresholds were poorer, especially in the higher frequencies. At selected frequencies, most notably 500 Hz, the women tended to have poorer frequencies than the men. There was a trend toward poorer hearing in the black subjects. However, this did not occur in the majority of comparisons.

Cruickshanks et al (1998b) conducted a population-based study on the prevalence of hearing loss in older adults residing in Beaver Dam, Wisconsin, as part of the EHLS. In total, 3753 adults with an average age of 65.8 years participated in their study. The prevalence of hearing loss was 45.9%, with the odds of hearing loss increasing with age (odds ratio = 1.88 for every 5 years) being greater for men than for women. The authors concluded, as did previous investigators, that hearing loss is a very common disorder affecting older adults.

◆ Hearing Loss Among Nursing Home Residents

According to the National Nursing Home Survey, of the 1.5 million residents of nursing homes, the majority (88.3%) are aged 65 years or older and 45.2% are 85 years or older. The typical nursing home resident is over 85 years of age and presents with a multiplicity of chronic conditions including hearing loss. Further, the majority of residents suffer from intellectual impairments and have several functional impairments necessitating assistance in the nursing facility. Specifically, 63% of elderly nursing home residents exhibit disorientation or memory impairment, with nearly half being diagnosed with some form of senile dementia. The potential for hearing loss is great, further complicating the picture of those already-compromised individuals. The number of people residing in nursing homes is projected to double by the year 2020. Interestingly, at the time of admission, 14% of nursing home residents had a primary admission diagnosis of disease of the nervous system and sense organs (Jones, Dwyer, Bercovitz, & Strahan, 2009); 33.9% of all residents reported at least one fall in the 180 days prior to the interview for the National Nursing Home Survey, 46% had some form of dementia, and 8.9% reported having fallen in the 30 days prior to the interview. There have been very few studies of hearing loss among nursing home residents since the cross-sectional study conducted by Schow and Nerbonne (1980). Cohen-Mansfield and Taylor (2004) conducted a cross-sectional interview survey of 279 nursing home resident and caregiver dyads, and based on the interviews and a review of medical records drew some general conclusions about the hearing status of nursing home residents. The questions about hearing status and hearing-aid use from the Minimum Data Set (MDS) were the basis for many of the conclusions about hearing. The survey found that 39% of the residents were treated for cerumen impaction, yet 81% of residents had not had their hearing tested; hence, hearing loss went undetected in the majority of residents. The vast majority of the nursing home residents who had hearing aids required assistance in taking care of the devices, yet close to half of the staff members had no training in the operation and care of hearing aids. Further, among those with hearing aids, 69% reportedly had problems with their devices.

In light of the fact that 46% of nursing home residents have some form of dementia and an even higher percentage have cognitive deficits, Burkhalter, Allen, Skaar, Crittenden, and Burgio (2009) explored the feasibility of testing the hearing of nursing home residents using traditional methods. Of the 307 residents they studied, 76% were considered compliant for the testing process, and 74% (*n* = 228) tolerated putting on headphones. Yet air conduction testing could be completed in both ears on only 32% of the residents, and only 5% of the 307 residents were able to complete a full traditional audiometric assessment. The fact that the majority of residents are over 80 years of age, and the fact that the data of Cruickshanks (2010) indicates an incidence of hearing loss of close to 100% for adults in their 80s followed over a 10-year time frame, would suggest that to optimize function, the use of personal amplifiers by staff should be routinized, and in-service training should focus on strategies for communicating with residents, with the presumption that most will have hearing impairment. Behavioral testing should always be attempted, and the cost-effectiveness and diagnostic utility of otoacoustic emissions explored, but if hearing tests cannot be completed, hearing status cannot be ignored. The data of Schow and Nerbonne (1980) are the most complete for this population and should be reviewed to provide perspective on the hearing status of typical residents by age.

Schow and Nerbonne (1980) sampled the hearing levels of residents of five nursing facilities in three cities in Idaho. The mean age of subjects in their sample was 81 years, versus 73 years for the Gates et al (1990) sample and 68 years for subjects in the Moscicki et al (1985) study. Approximately 58% of their subjects were 80 years of age or older. Approximately 70 to 80% of subjects sampled had a hearing loss far exceeding the prevalence within the noninstitutionalized population of older adults. Average hearing level ranged from moderate to moderately severe. As residents age, a greater proportion have more severe hearing loss. Approximately 50% of the subjects in their sample had a mild hearing loss and 50% had a moderate to profound hearing loss, after correcting for contamination attributable to collapsed ear canals. Women had slightly poorer high-frequency thresholds than men. Subsequent studies have verified the finding that nursing home residents have a higher prevalence of hearing loss and more severe hearing loss than older adults residing in the community. This finding has implications for hearing screening protocols and the more widespread use of hearing assistance technologies to facilitate communication in this setting.

Special Consideration

The prevalence and severity of hearing loss among nursing home residents is higher than in the community-based population. Overall, nursing home residents have a higher prevalence of hearing loss and more severe hearing loss than the elderly living in the community, most likely because of their advanced age.

Cross-Sectional Studies: Summary

The majority of cross-sectional studies on hearing loss suggest that 45 to 47% of individuals over 65 years of age present with a hearing impairment for pure tones. Available data confirm that hearing loss tends to decline with increasing age in both men and women. Further, the decline in high-frequency sensitivity appears to be greatest in men, whereas low-frequency thresholds are poorer in women of comparable age. The average hearing loss in men can be described as mild to moderately severe, with a sharply sloping configuration, whereas women tend to present with a mild to moderate gradually sloping hearing loss. It appears that there may be a trend for high-frequency hearing threshold levels to be slightly better as compared with those obtained nearly 40 years ago (Hoffman, Dobie, Ko, Themann, & Murphy, 2010). **Figure 5.1** summarizes the mean thresholds on three distinct samples of older adults drawn from the FHS, EHLS, and Medical University of South Carolina (MUSC) longitudinal studies (Cruickshanks et al, 1998b; Dubno et al, 2008; Gates et al, 1990). Despite, differences in sample characteristics, geography, and protocols, pure-tone thresholds appear to be comparable. Hearing levels differ by gender in the high frequencies, with men having significantly poorer hearing in the high frequencies than do women.

◆ Audiometric Studies: Longitudinal Data

Several longitudinal studies of hearing have been conducted including the Baltimore Longitudinal Study of Aging (Brant & Fozard, 1990; Pearson et al, 1995), the Framingham Heart Study (Gates & Cooper, 1991), the Beaver Dam Epidemiology of Hearing Loss Study (Cruickshanks et al, 2003), and most recently the Medical University of South Carolina (Lee, Matthews, Dubno, & Mills, 2005). For the most part, these studies reported rates of change in hearing thresholds over time. Repeated measurements were conducted between two to six

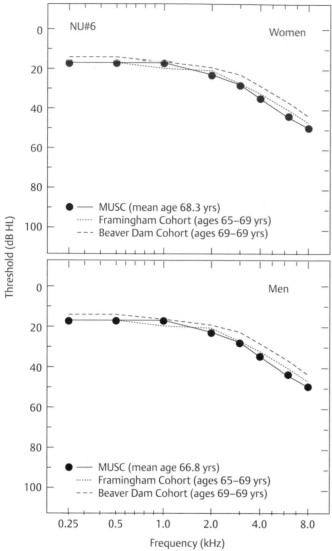

Fig. 5.1 Mean initial pure-tone thresholds (in dB HL) for women and men enrolled in the Medical University of South Carolina (MUSC) longitudinal study of age-related hearing loss. For comparison, thresholds in samples from the Framingham Heart Study and the Beaver Dam, Wisconsin, Epidemiology of Hearing Loss Study EHLS are included. [From Dubno, et al. 2008. Reprinted with permission]

fect in that hearing loss was greater in the high than the low frequencies. There also appeared to be an interaction effect, wherein the frequencies at which threshold changes were greatest was dependent on the age of participants and on baseline hearing threshold levels. Only small threshold changes were observed at the frequencies that had the poorer baseline hearing levels, which tended to be in the higher frequencies. Interestingly, but in keeping with the latter trend, there was a greater change in thresholds with increasing age at 2000 and 3000 Hz in women than in men, most likely because men had poorer baseline thresholds at these frequencies. In addition, the percentage of ears with baseline thresholds poorer than 60 dB HL increased as a function of both age and frequency.

Nearly 60% of persons between 80 and 92 years had ears with thresholds greater than 60 dB HL at 4000 Hz versus 40% of persons between 70 and 79 and 10% of persons between 48 and 59 years. It appeared that younger age groups demonstrated faster rates of threshold changes for higher frequencies, and older groups demonstrated faster rates of threshold changes for lower frequencies. Specifically, for both men and women, subjects in the younger age groups evidenced greater rates of threshold change in the higher frequencies. Of note is the fact that the difference in rate of change for lower and higher frequencies decreased with increasing age. The fact that for men and women in the oldest groups the rate of change in threshold was greatest for lower frequencies suggests a possible central effect that typically becomes more pronounced with age. A previous study conducted by Wiley and colleagues (1998) confirmed a gender effect in older adults in ultra-high frequency hearing levels as well. Older men had poorer hearing than older women for frequencies between 9000 Hz and 14,000 Hz, with no gender differences beyond 14,000 Hz, most likely due to difficulty measuring thresholds in those frequencies. In summary, the data of Wiley and colleagues (2008) revealed that age was a significant risk factor for decrements in hearing and was a determinant of the frequencies at which the greatest threshold changes emerged. A finding of considerable clinical significance is the observation that the best predictor of hearing threshold level after 10 years of follow-up was the baseline threshold at the same frequency, and the next best predictor was the baseline threshold at the next highest test.

Lee et al (2005) reported on the results of a longitudinal study of hearing levels on a sample of 188 adults who were 60 years of age or older. Subjects were in good health and had no history of otological or neurological disease; however, almost half of the subjects reported a positive history of noise exposure. All subjects were tested at conventional (250 to 8000 Hz) and extended high frequencies (9000, 10,000, 11,000, 12,000, 14,000, 16,000, and 18,000 Hz). Participants had between two and 21 threshold measurements over a period of 3 to 11.5 years. Some interesting trends emerged that were consistent with earlier studies. Men had significantly poorer thresholds than women from 2000 to 8000 Hz, whereas thresholds at 250 through 1000 Hz were comparable for men and women. Overall, the average rate of change across frequencies was quite small, ranging from 0.7 dB at 250 Hz to 1 dB at 1000 Hz to 1.23 dB at 12,000 Hz. The average rate of change in pure-tone thresholds varied with gender, age, frequency, and baseline threshold. Women had a slower rate of change at 1000 Hz but a significantly faster rate of change at 6000 through 12,000

times on participants (Dubno et al, 2008). Wiley, Chappell, Carmichael, Nondahl, and Cruickshanks (2008) examined changes in hearing thresholds at specific frequencies over a 10-year period in an unscreened population of 3625 older adults participating in the EHLS study who ranged in age from 48 to 92 years. Progression of hearing loss was defined as a change greater than 5 dB HL in the pure-tone average (500, 1000, 2000, and 4000 Hz). Participants underwent air- and bone-conduction threshold testing at baseline and at intervals of 2.5, 5, and 10 years. Overall, hearing thresholds increased with advancing age, with the slope of the curve becoming steeper in the high frequencies with advancing age. There appeared to be an age effect on the rate of change in the higher frequencies. There was a gender effect, as hearing levels of men were poorer than those of women, and there was a frequency ef-

Hz than did men. Men had a slightly faster rate of change in threshold at 1000 Hz than did women, yet at the higher frequencies (6000 to 12,000 Hz) women had a faster rate of change in threshold. Further, women 70 years of age and over had a significantly faster rate of change in threshold at 250 to 3000 Hz and a slower rate of change at 10,000 and 11,000 Hz than did women less than 70 years of age. In contrast, men 70 years of age or older showed a faster rate of change at 250 to 1000 Hz than did men under 70 years of age, but the differences did not reach statistical significance. In general, subjects with more hearing loss at 3000 to 8000 Hz at baseline had less of a threshold change at these frequencies, whereas subjects with more hearing loss at high frequencies at baseline had a faster rate of threshold change at 250 to 2000 Hz.

Mitchell et al (2011) examined the prevalence, 5-year incidence, and progression of hearing loss in a cohort of adults participating in the Blue Mountains Hearing Study. Mean age of participants was 68 years; 52% of participant had hypertension and 8% were smokers. Prevalence data were based on a sample of 2956 individuals with hearing loss defined as four frequency PTAs (500, 1000, 2000, and 4000 Hz) poorer than 25 dB HL in the better ear. Based on the latter definition, the prevalence of hearing loss was 33% at baseline, with 22% having a mild hearing loss, 9% having a moderate hearing loss, and 2% having a severe hearing loss. Above 2000 Hz, hearing levels for men were poorer than for women, and below 2000 Hz hearing levels were slightly poorer for women than for men. Hearing levels decreased with age, as in most other longitudinal studies. Incidence data were noteworthy. The 5-year incidence of mild hearing loss was 17.9% and of moderate to severe hearing loss was 5.9%. For each decade of age over 60 years, the risk of incident hearing loss increased threefold. Regarding hearing loss progression, 15.7% of participants demonstrated a progression in terms of hearing loss severity, with women having a slightly higher but not significant progression of hearing loss than men. It was noteworthy that the highest rate of progression (22%) was observed among adults aged 80 years or older. Interestingly, 31.7% of participants with bilateral hearing loss reported using a hearing aid at baseline, and most of these individuals were using their hearing aids at follow-up. Hearing-aid use was more frequent among those subjects with a severe hearing impairment than among those with a mild impairment, which is consistent with hearing loss data across studies and populations. The authors concluded that age was the strongest risk factor for incident hearing loss. Mitchell and colleagues also concluded that there was a nonsignificant association between self-reported history of noise exposure and incident hearing loss. Interestingly, 14.9% and 12.8% of incident cases of hearing loss were attributable to family history and history of occupational noise exposure, respectively.

Cruickshanks et al (2003) reported on the results of a population-based study of hearing in Beaver Dam, Wisconsin. Participants in the EHLS were followed for a 5-year period. The sample included people able to travel to the clinic site and those unable to travel, including nursing home residents, homebound elderly, and people residing in remote areas. For the latter group, testing was conducted at their place of residence using a portable audiometer calibrated according to American National Standards Institute (ANSI) standards, and the testing

environment in the home complied with ANSI S3.1 1991 standards. Of the 3753 individuals tested at baseline, 1925 (51%) had no hearing loss and 1631 (43%) had a hearing loss defined as hearing levels greater than 25 dB HL in either ear. The mean four-frequency pure-tone average of the group with hearing loss at follow-up was 46.3 dB HL versus 39.5 dB HL at baseline. Approximately 53% of individuals in this group showed an overall progression of hearing loss that exceeded 5 dB HL. Interestingly, the risk of hearing loss was comparable for men and women and it increased with age. Further, 20% of the sample developed impaired hearing during the 5-year follow-up, and interestingly men were more likely than women to develop a hearing loss. The variable most associated with the likelihood of developing hearing loss over the 5-year period was having a job that entailed exposure to damaging levels of noise. Consistent with previous longitudinal studies, those with hearing loss at baseline were more likely to have their hearing loss progress, and age was the factor most strongly associated with the risk of worsening hearing loss. The authors concluded that, overall, the 5-year incidence of hearing impairment was 21% in their sample. **Figure 5.2** shows the 5- and 10-year incidence of hearing impairment by age in the Beaver Dam study, with the incidence increasing dramatically with age and it is greater after 10 years (Cruickshanks, 2010). Of interest in this study and confirmed in a study conducted by Agrawal et al (2008) is the young age at which participants first presented with hearing loss—66 years for men and 73 years for women. It appears that hearing loss is setting in earlier and hence it is likely that adults will spend many years of life with hearing loss.

Divenyi, Stark, and Haupt (2005) conducted a longitudinal study over a span of 5 years on a small sample of older adults with a baseline mean age of 69.6 years (range of 60 to 83.7 years) and the mean age at follow-up of 74.9 years (range of 65.2 to 88.6 years). Participants were free of tinnitus and noise exposure and were in good general health. At the time of the initial testing, participants self-assessed their hearing as being good to excellent. Pure-tone thresholds in this sample were consistent with normal hearing at baseline and at the follow-up at 500 through 2000 Hz, with an essentially mild to moderate hearing loss thereafter. Hearing threshold levels were symmetrical at each frequency at each test session. The hearing loss in the high frequencies was sensorineural. Over time, the most dramatic change in hearing was at 4000 and 8000 Hz with thresholds declining approximately 14 dB/decade at 4000 Hz and approximately 11 dB/decade at 8000 Hz. There was considerable variability, however, in terms of the threshold changes in the high frequencies based on the large standard deviations at the latter frequencies. As will be discussed in a later section, performance on speech measures declined more rapidly than did pure-tone thresholds. The fact that declines in pure-tone thresholds were observed over a 5-year span in healthy older adults with relatively good hearing has implications for the timing of follow-up testing and for health promotion activities.

Brant and Fozard (1990) and Pearson et al (1995) conducted a longitudinal study of changes in hearing thresholds in a sample of adults participating in the Baltimore Longitudinal Study of Aging, a multidisciplinary study of normal human aging that began in 1958. Subjects participating in the study reported on in 1990 were 813 men between the ages of 20 and

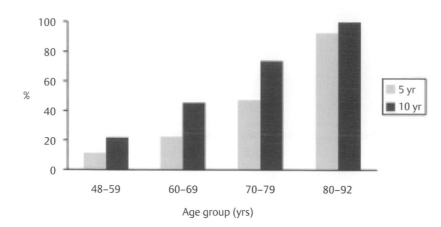

Fig. 5.2 Five- and 10-year incidence of hearing impairment by age. [From Cruickshanks, K. (2010). Age related hearing loss: Demographics and risk factors. Presented at the ARC meeting in San Diego, California, April 14. http://www.audiologynow.org/pdf/Aging/2010_ARC_Cruickshanks.pdf. Reprinted by permission].

95 years. They were generally well educated, white, and financially comfortable, with the majority residing in the Baltimore–Washington metropolitan area. Hearing tests on all participants were gathered on two or more occasions from 1968 to 1987. Subjects were divided into seven age groups. Test results suggested longitudinal and cross-sectional age-related changes in mean hearing thresholds over the range of frequencies tested in all age groups over the 15-year follow-up period. However, the cross-sectional data gathered on a subset of subjects underestimated the rate of hearing loss among the older adults as compared with the longitudinal data. Their data suggest a marked increase in the rate of hearing loss at 500, 1000, 2000, and 3000 Hz starting at between 40 and 50 years of age. Further, by 70 years of age, the rate of change in mean hearing thresholds was greater at these frequencies than it was at higher frequencies. Finally, large individual differences in mean pure-tone thresholds emerged across age groups, suggesting that hearing threshold levels cannot accurately be predicted from age data alone. The data of Brant and Fozard (1990) confirm that hearing threshold levels at all frequencies change over time, with the rate of change greatest in the high frequencies and for those over 70 years of age.

In the next phase of data collection by Pearson et al (1995), a sample of women was added to allow for exploration of gender differences in hearing loss as a function of age. A total of 681 men and 416 women underwent a series of audiometric tests over a 10-year period. Of the women, 48% had at least 5 years of follow-up data, as did 60% of the men. **Table 5.3** summarizes several interesting trends that emerged from the study. Overall, the findings agree with those of previous studies in that there is an age-associated reduction in hearing sensitivity that is particularly pronounced at higher frequencies. The change in hearing level with age tended to be gradual and progressive. At most ages and frequencies, the longitudinal change in hearing level over a 10-year period was more than twice as fast in men than in women, with the rate of change converging somewhat after age 60. Among men, decline in hearing sensitivity first became apparent as early as age 30, whereas in women the age of onset tends to be frequency dependent, occurring for the most part when they are somewhat older than the men. The largest gender differences in longitudinal rates of hearing loss occurred at the frequencies most affected by noise, namely 3000 to 4000 Hz, with the rate of dB change per decade considerably greater in men than women. Finally, the study found that in adults over age 80, the rate of hearing loss was comparable for men and women.

Gates and Cooper (1991) performed a longitudinal study of changes in hearing over a 6-year period in a large cohort of older adults. Pure-tone data were gathered on 1475 individuals as part of the FHS biennial examinations. Pure-tone thresholds at 250 to 8000 Hz obtained in 1978 to 1979 were compared with those obtained in 1983 to 1985. Subjects ranged in age from 58 to 94 years. Mean pure-tone thresholds for men and women at each biennial examination revealed trends similar to those reported by Moscicki and colleagues (1985) using the same cohort. Hearing loss was primarily confined to the high frequencies, men had poorer thresholds than women at frequencies above 2000 Hz and better thresholds at 250 and 500 Hz, and the hearing loss tended to be bilateral and symmetrical. Differences in mean pure-tone thresholds in the right and left ears over the 6-year time interval were rather small for both men and women. In women, the mean differences in PTA were 3.6 ± 0.21 dB and 5.3 ± 0.22 dB for the right and left ears, respectively, whereas in men the mean differences were 2.9 ± 0.25 dB and 4.7 ± 0.26 dB. For men and women, the greatest threshold change occurred at 6000 and 8000 Hz. The magnitude of the change at each of these frequencies was slightly greater in women than in men. An interesting finding was the relation between initial age at time of testing and the proportion of subjects whose PTAs changed dramatically over time. Overall, only 18% of subjects experienced a significant (>10 dB) change in the PTA over time, whereas 48% of subjects evidenced a change in the mean high-frequency pure-tone average (PTA_H) over time. For both genders, the 6-year rate of hearing loss increased with age in the frequencies below 2000 Hz, yet at 4000 and 6000 Hz men's threshold change slowed with age whereas the women's increased with age.

In summary, it is clear that mean high frequency pure-tone averages increase over time in older adults, with changes ranging from 15.5 dB (500, 1000, 2000, and 4000 Hz) over a 14-year time frame in the MUSC study to a 5-dB change over a period of 4 years. Initial pure-tone thresholds at baseline tend to be higher for men than for women, and this difference tends to remain over time.

Table 5.3 Selected Characteristics by Hearing Loss Category

Characteristic	Entire Cohort (N = 2052)	Normal Hearing (n = 411)	Hearing Loss (n = 1230)[1]	High-Frequency Hearing Loss Only (n = 411)[2]	P-value[3]
Demographic					
Age, mean ± standard deviation	77.5 ± 2.8	76.4 ± 2.6	77.9 ± 2.9	77.2 ± 2.8	<.001
Sex, n (%)					
Male	970 (47.3)	117 (12.1)	608 (62.7)	245 (25.3)	<.001
Female	1082 (52.7)	294 (27.2)	622 (57.5)	166 (15.3)	
Race, n (%)					
White	1291 (62.9)	192 (14.9)	802 (62.1)	297 (23.0)	<.001
Black	761 (37.1)	219 (28.8)	428 (56.2)	114 (15.0)	
< High School education, n (%)	446 (21.7)	91 (20.4)	289 (64.8)	66 (14.8)	.007
Annual household income <$25,000, n (%)	700 (34.1)	164 (23.4)	409 (58.4)	127 (18.1)	.02
Lifestyle factors, n (%)					
Current smoker	126 (6.1)	21 (16.7)	83 (65.9)	22 (17.5)	.37
Previous smoker	982 (47.9)	172 (17.5)	597 (60.8)	213 (21.7)	.01
Alcohol use (≥4 drinks/wk)	309 (15.1)	55 (17.8)	179 (57.9)	75 (24.3)	.15
Occupational noise exposure	536 (26.1)	58 (10.8)	370 (69.0)	108 (20.1)	<.001
Medical history, n (%)					
Cardiovascular disease	172 (8.4)	33 (19.2)	114 (66.3)	25 (14.5)	.13
Hypertension	1371 (66.8)	278 (20.3)	830 (60.5)	263 (19.2)	.40
Diabetes mellitus	371 (16.1)	77 (20.8)	248 (66.8)	46 (12.4)	<.001
Cerebrovascular disease	208 (10.1)	34 (16.3)	145 (69.7)	29 (13.9)	.009
History of ear surgery	99 (4.8)	6 (6.0)	82 (82.9)	11 (11.1)	<.001
Ototoxic medications (current use), n (%)					
Salicylates	902 (44.0)	176 (19.5)	528 (58.5)	198 (22.0)	.16
Loop diuretics	199 (9.7)	37 (18.6)	125 (62.8)	37 (18.6)	.68
Quinine derivatives	24 (1.2)	4 (16.7)	19 (79.2)	1 (4.1)	.10

[1]Pure-tone average of 500, 1000, and 2000 Hz >25 dB HL in the worse ear.
[2]Pure-tone average of 2000, 4000, and 8000 Hz >40 dB HL in the worse ear.
[3]Difference across all hearing categories.
Source: Helzner, E. P., Cauley, J. A., Pratt, S. R., Wisniewski, S. R., Zmuda, J. M., Talbott, E. O., et al. (2005, Dec). Race and sex differences in age-related hearing loss: the Health, Aging and Body Composition Study. *Journal of the American Geriatrics Society, 53,* 2119–2127. Reprinted by permission

◆ Comorbidities

Over 10 million U.S. residents aged 65+ years live with four or more chronic health conditions, yet primary care physicians tend to treat one chronic condition at a time, rather than treat the whole person. Given the increase in the number of chronically ill older adults, there is a trend toward comprehensive assessment of all of the patient's diseases, disabilities, cognitive abilities, medications, health-related devices, health-related lifestyle habits, and environmental risks (Boult & Wieland, 2010). The global prevalence of diabetes is rising, and cardiovascular disease is the leading cause of death among those with diabetes. Individuals with diabetes and cardiovascular disease are at high risk for falls; they take several prescription medications and also have hearing loss. In fact, the likelihood of hearing loss is higher in older adults with a diagnosis of type 2 diabetes than in those without the diagnosis, and progression of hearing loss is higher in those with a diagnosis of diabetes than in those without diabetes (70% versus 48%) (Mitchell et al, 2009). One of our roles as professionals is to work with primary care physicians to help promote attain-

ment of and compliance with therapeutic goals (Katz & Gilbert, 2008). Hence, we must begin by knowing the prevalence of hearing loss in the many chronic conditions affecting older adults. Based on this perspective and on the important role hearing plays in promoting the patient's clinical status and in ensuring adherence to a care plan and engagement in health care, this section discusses the many chronic conditions with which hearing impairment tends to co-occur.

The extent to which race, gender, and medical factors such as cardiovascular disease play a role in the development of hearing loss in older adults was explored in a population-based study by Helzner et al (2005). The subjects were Medicare beneficiaries recruited from a random sample of participants in the Health, Aging, and Body Composition (Health ABC) study that began in 1997. Participants were cancer free for 3 years, free of middle ear obstruction, and free of walking difficulty. At the 5-year clinical follow-up visit, 78% of survivors from the start of the Health ABC study underwent air-conduction testing. The composition of the sample was as follows: 32% white men, 31% white women, 15% black men, and 22% black women. The age range of participants was 73 to 84 years with a mean age of

77.5. Hearing loss was defined as PTA >25 dB HL in the poorer ear or high-frequency (2000-, 4000-, and 8000-Hz) PTA greater than 40 dB HL in the poorer ear. In addition to pure-tone testing, data on demographic factors including sex, race, lifestyle, noise exposure, and medical history was gathered via in-clinic interviews and examinations. Cognitive status was assessed using the modified Mini-Mental State Examination (MMSE), with a score less than 80 being indicative of dementia.

The results were of interest in terms of demographic correlates, risk factors, and prevalence. The overall prevalence of hearing loss (PTA >25 dB HL in the poorer ear) in the sample was 59.9%, with the prevalence for white men (64.9%) and the prevalence for black men (58%) being relatively comparable. Interestingly, the prevalence of high-frequency hearing loss was 91.8% in white men and 76% in black men, suggesting a race effect for the high frequencies. With regard to women, 59% of white women and 55% of black women had a hearing loss in the poorer ear in excess of 25 dB HL, whereas 74% of white women and 59% of black women presented with a high-frequency hearing loss in the poorer ear, suggesting a race effect once again. Mean hearing thresholds for air conduction were consistent with previous studies in that hearing levels suggested a mild hearing loss in the frequency range between 250 and 2000 Hz, with a moderate to moderately severe high-frequency hearing loss thereafter, with the exception of white men and women whose threshold at 8000 Hz was suggestive of a severe hearing loss. In fact, a race/sex difference emerged at 4000 and 8000 Hz, with men of both races having poorer hearing, whites having poorer hearing than blacks, irrespective of gender, and whites having a 63% greater likelihood than blacks of having a hearing loss. **Figure 5.3** displays hearing threshold levels by race and the poorer threshold levels in the high frequencies among whites is evident.

Consistent with the work of earlier investigators, age emerged as a consistent risk factor for hearing loss, such that for each 5-year increase in age, the prevalence of hearing loss doubled. Further, white men were three times more likely than black men to have a hearing loss, but there was no such race effect for women. Cerebrovascular disease was associated with a higher risk of hearing loss in white men, and diabetes mellitus was associated with a higher risk of hearing loss in white men and women. Interestingly, black men with cardiovascular disease had three times as great a risk of hearing loss, and white men with high diastolic pressure were more likely to have hearing loss. Consistent with the findings above, occupational noise exposure was linked to hearing loss in white men. Salicylate use was associated with a modest decrease in risk of hearing loss in the overall sample and in black men (Helzner et al, 2005).

Cognitive status was associated with hearing loss in the cohort such that the poorer the score on the test of mental status, the greater the likelihood of a hearing loss. The data as to risk factors are listed in **Table 5.3** and summarized in **Table 5.4**. In terms of lifestyle variables, smoking was a risk factor for hearing loss, with black men who smoked being three times as likely to have hearing loss, Drinking emerged as a possible protective factor against developing hearing loss. There seems to be agreement that damage to the microvasculature in the cochlea and neuronal damage through toxicity or infection are

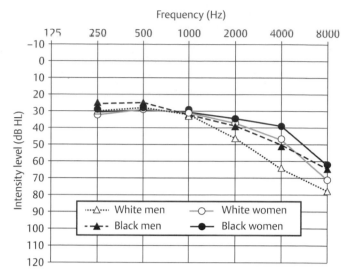

Fig. 5.3 Mean hearing threshold levels by sex and race for the worse ear of participants in the Health, Aging and Body Composition Study 2001/2002. [From Helzner, E. P., Cauley, J. A., Pratt, S. R., Wisniewski, S. R., Zmuda, J. M., Talbott, E. O., et al. (2005, Dec). Race and sex differences in age-related hearing loss: the Health, Aging and Body Composition Study. *Journal of the American Geriatrics Society, 53,* 2119–2127. Reprinted by permission]

likely explanations for the association between smoking and hearing loss (Nondahl et al, 2010).

Using a cross-sectional design, Gates, Cobb, D'Agostino, and Wolf (1993) explored the relation between hearing loss and risk factors for cardiovascular disease using participants from the FHS cohort (1983 to 1985). The majority of participants (n = 1662) were women, and the mean age of the women (73 years) was comparable to that of the men (72.7 years). Low-frequency (250-, 500-, and 1000-Hz) PTA in excess of 40 dB HL was defined as a hearing loss at the lower frequencies for the odds ratio (OR) analysis, and a high-frequency (4000-, 6000-, and 8000-Hz) PTA in excess of 40 dB HL was used for the OR analysis. The 18 subjects confirmed by a panel of three physicians to have had a cardiovascular event prior to the biennial

Table 5.4 Risk Factors for Hearing Loss in Older Adults

Demographic factors
 Age
 Gender
 Race
 Familial factors
Lifestyle factors
 Smoking
Medical conditions
 Cerebrovascular disease (white men)
 Diabetes mellitus (white men and women)
 Cardiovascular disease (black men)
 High diastolic pressure (white men)
 Cognitive status
 Dementia
Protective factors
 Alcohol consumption
 Salicylates

examination that was part of the FHS, which included coronary heart disease, heart attack, transient ischemic attack, and stroke, were classified as having cardiovascular disease (CVD). In addition to the presence or absence of the CVD, risk factors including high blood pressure and hypertension, diabetes mellitus, smoking, elevated cholesterol levels, and obesity were examined in relation to hearing status.

The prevalence of CVD in this sample was higher for men (33%) than for women (22%). The mean high-frequency (4000-, 6000-, and 8000-Hz) PTA in the better ear of men in the sample was 60.9 dB HL and for women 45.6 dB HL, whereas the mean low-frequency (250-, 500-, and 1000-Hz) PTA in the better ear was 18.5 dB HL for men and 19 dB HL for women. The mean age of men was 72.7 and of women was 73 years. Interestingly, the relation between CVD and hearing status was mediated by gender. The OR for a prevalent CVD in women with a mean low-frequency PTA in excess of 40 dB HL was 3.06, and the OR for an intermittent claudication defined as cramping in one or both claves provoked by walking and relieved by bed rest was 4.39. In contrast, for men the OR for stroke was 3.46. There was no relation between CVD and high pure-tone hearing levels in men, whereas in women the OR for CVD was 1.68. Hence, the data suggest a significant albeit modest relation between hearing level and CVD in women that did not emerge in men, with low-frequency hearing level emerging as having the strongest relationship. The risk factors that Gates and colleagues explored did not change the relation between hearing status and CVD; however, hypertension and systolic blood pressure were related to hearing levels in both men and women. It must be cautioned that participants in this study were required to have no evidence of coronary heart disease when first recruited to participate.

According to Helzner et al (2011), given the rich capillary supply to the stria vascularis it is logical that CVD or its precursors could influence hearing. Using a sex-stratified sample from the Health ABC study, Helzner et al explored the relationship among CVD, subclinical measures of CVD including ankle–arm blood pressure index, a surrogate measure of peripheral occlusion, and arterial pulse-wave velocity, which is an indicator of arterial stiffness. The mean age of men and women was comparable (73 years). Men were more likely than women to have smoked in the past, to have had exposure to occupational noise, and to have had a history of CVD. Interestingly, the authors found that risk factors for hearing loss among men differed from those of women. Risk factors for men included a positive history, high resting heart rate, and high triglyceride levels, whereas high body mass index (BMI), high resting heart rate, fast aortic pulse wave velocity (PWV), and low ankle–arm index (AAI) placed women at risk for hearing loss. The associations were dependent on the PTA of the better or poorer ear on some measures. Specifically, in the poorer ear faster resting heart rate was associated with poorer low-frequency hearing, history of smoking was associated with poorer hearing in the high frequencies, and high triglyceride levels were associated with poorer low- and mid-frequency hearing levels in men. In women, a faster resting heart rate was the only risk factor associated with poorer hearing sensitivity in the poorer ear. In men, high triglyceride levels were associated with poorer mid-frequency hearing sensitivity in the better ear, and smok-

ing history was associated with poorer high-frequency hearing sensitivity in the better ear. In women, higher BMI was associated with poorer low- and mid-frequency hearing sensitivity, faster resting heart rate and low AAI were associated with poorer hearing in the better ear at all frequencies, and a faster PWV was associated with poorer high-frequency hearing. Interestingly, race played a role in the findings, in that black women with a history of stroke had higher high-frequency hearing thresholds than did black women without a history of stroke.

The fact that insufficient cochlear blood supply can disrupt the chemical balance of endolymph, which in turn affects the electrical activity of the hair cells and, subsequently, activation of the auditory nerve, may account for the relationships that emerged in this study (Helzner et al, 2011). As with other investigators, Helzner et al speculated that the link between hearing loss and cigarette smoking may be due to the antioxidative effect of smoking on the auditory system or because of the effect of smoking on the vasculature of the inner ear. Once again, the above findings suggest that there are modifiable risk factors for hearing loss, and it is the responsibility of audiologists to caution accordingly.

> **Pearl**
>
> Smokers with higher noise exposure have much worse hearing than smokers with limited noise exposure, such that women who are not exposed to occupational noise may be less affected by the synergistic effect of noise and smoking (Ferrite & Santana, 2005; Helzner et al, 2011).

Using data from the NHANES, Bainbridge, Hoffman, and Cowie (2008) explored the relation between self-reported diagnosis of diabetes and hearing loss in adults ranging in age from 20 to 69 years. The mean age of the hearing-impaired subjects in the sample was relatively young, 53 years, with 76% of subjects considered to be non-Hispanic whites. One third of the sample reported occupational noise exposure, one fifth had taken ototoxic medications, and 16% of the sample with hearing loss (*n* = 587) had diabetes as compared with 4.9% (*n* = 4553) without hearing loss. With the exception of participants in the oldest group (60 to 69 years of age), the prevalence of hearing impairment among those with diabetes exceeded the prevalence among those without the diagnosis, and this trend was not affected by race, gender, or ethnicity. In addition to contrasting prevalence levels, Bainbridge and colleagues compared hearing levels of those with and without a diagnosis of diabetes. Interestingly, at all decades (20s through 60s) individuals with diabetes presented with poorer hearing threshold levels across frequencies than did those without diabetes, and the difference appeared to be greatest in the higher frequencies. Their data compare favorably with the data of Helzner and colleagues (2005), who also noted a higher prevalence of diabetes in those with hearing impairment in the poorer ear (PTA poorer than 25 dB HL), and it is noteworthy that their sample was considerably older than were the participants in the Bainbridge sample.

Smoking

There has been an accumulation of evidence regarding the relationship between smoking and hearing loss and the interaction between risk factors such as cardiovascular disease, noise exposure, and smoking. The rationale for exploring the possible link between smoking and hearing loss is smoking's antioxidative mechanisms or its effects on the vascular supply to the inner ear. As part of the EHLS, Cruickshanks et al (1998a) conducted a cross-sectional, population-based study of the relationship between smoking and hearing loss. The average age of participants was 65.8 years; 58% were women and 42% were men. Hearing loss in this sample was defined as PTA (500, 1000, 2000, and 4000 Hz) greater than 25 dB HL in the poorer ear; 45.9% of participants had hearing levels consistent with a hearing loss. As for smoking, 14.7% were current smokers and 39% were ex-smokers. Interestingly, smoking pattern varied by age such that older participants were less likely to be current smokers. As many of the participants also reported a history of occupational noise exposure, the association between hearing loss and smoking was considered in persons with and without a history of noise exposure. The relation between smoking and hearing loss was statistically significant in those with a history of occupational noise exposure and in those without a history of noise exposure but with adult-onset hearing loss. Number of pack-years was a contributing factor to the relationship, such that those with more than 40 pack-years were 1.3 times as likely to have a hearing loss as those with no pack-years of exposure. In addition to the dose-related effect, age was a variable, as prevalence of hearing loss was highest in the older age groups with the greatest number of pack years. **Table 5.5** depicts the relation between hearing loss prevalence and smoking. Cruickshanks and colleagues explored the effect of passive smoking on hearing loss, and they noted that after adjusting for age, sex, and CVD, those living with a smoker were more likely to have a hearing loss. Fransen et al (2008) conducted a cross-sectional study that confirmed the deleterious effect of smoking on high-frequency hearing thresholds.

Pearl

The prevention of CVD and factors that contribute to the onset of CVD has the potential to slow the progression of age-related hearing loss (Helzner et al, 2011).

Smoking and Alcohol Consumption

As part of the 10-year follow-up to the BMHS, Gopinath et al (2010) examined the extent to which smoking and/or alcohol consumption impacts hearing levels in a population-based sample of older adults living in Australia. Specifically, they explored the temporal association between smoking or alcohol consumption and hearing loss, and whether smoking or alcohol consumption influenced the prevalence and incidence of age-related hearing loss in their sample. All participants completed an interviewer-administered questionnaire designed to gather information on risk factors for hearing loss, including alcohol consumption, smoking status, history of diabetes, and cardiovascular risk. All participants underwent air conduction testing, with hearing impairment defined by the PTA of thresholds at 500, 1000, 2000, and 4000 Hz in each ear. Hearing loss was classified as mild, moderate, or severe according to thresholds in the better of the two ears. Incidence of hearing loss was defined as the proportion of participants with hearing levels in the excess of 25 dB HL in the better ear at the 5-year follow-up examination among those without any hearing loss at the baseline hearing study (1997 to 1999) or at the 5-year follow-up from the original study. The total number of participants in the baseline study was 2815, of which 43% were male, 36.9% experienced exposure to noise at work, 11% had a diagnosis of diabetes, 43% had a family history of hearing loss, and 9.8% were current smokers. The hearing loss prevalence was 33%.

As with data from the NHANES and EHLS studies, an association between smoking and hearing loss prevalence emerged, and this association was independent of such conditions as CVD, diabetes, and stroke. Interestingly, current smokers who did not report exposure to occupational noise were 63% more likely to have a hearing impairment. Alcohol consumption appeared to have a protective association with hearing loss, and moderate consumption of alcohol was associated with a reduced likelihood of severe hearing loss. The joint effect of alcohol consumption and smoking on prevalence of hearing loss was noteworthy. Among smokers and nonsmokers, drinkers had a higher likelihood of hearing loss than nondrinkers, with nonsmokers having a slightly higher prevalence of hearing loss than smokers. The authors speculated that effects of alcohol and tobacco exposure may be additive. The 5-year incidence of hearing loss was 17.9%, yet combined smoking status and alcohol consumption were not risk factors for developing hearing loss. In summary, the cross-sectional

Table 5.5 Relation Between Hearing Loss and Smoking

Age	Nonsmokers		Current Smokers	
	Number of Participants	Percent with Hearing Loss	Number of Participants	Percent with Hearing Loss
60–69 years	417	36%	179	56%
70–79 years	429	60%	66	71%
80–92 years	220	89%	13	92%

Source: Data from Cruickshanks, K. J., Klein, R., Klein, B. E., Wiley, T. L., Nondahl, D. M., & Tweed, T. S. (1998, Jun). Cigarette smoking and hearing loss: the epidemiology of hearing loss study. *Journal of the American Medical Association, 279,* 1715–1719. Data from SOURCE)

data confirmed that current smoking is a risk factor for hearing loss and that moderate alcohol consumption may have a protective association with hearing status. The temporal data emerging from this study did not confirm an association among smoking, alcohol consumption, and hearing loss. Confirming the data of Gopinath et al (2010), evidence emerged regarding the protective function of alcohol in terms of forestalling hearing loss onset.

Smoking, Occupational Noise Exposure, and Cardiovascular Risk Factors

Agrawal, Niparko, and Dobie (2010) used data from the 1999–2002 NHANES, a cross-sectional study, to explore the contribution of occupational noise exposure, smoking, and cardiovascular risk factors to hearing threshold levels in a sample of adults aged 20 to 69 years. Individuals selected to participate in the audiometry component of the study were excluded if they were unable to remove their hearing aids and if otalgia was so severe that it precluded positioning of the headphones. Hearing loss was defined as a PTA of 25 dB HL or greater at 500, 1000, 2000, and 4000 Hz in both ears. Data were collected on smoking history (e.g., number of years of smoking and pack-years). History of diabetes and hypertension was recorded on all participants using subjective reports and objective data such as medication use, fasting glucose levels in the case of the former, and diastolic/systolic blood pressure in the case of the latter. Of the 3319 participants, 33% reported a history of occupational noise exposure based on responses to a question about exposure in the workplace; another question addressed exposure to recreational noise. Interestingly, those individuals reporting exposure to noise in the workplace were more likely to be male, white, and heavy smokers, and to have had exposure to noise outside of the workplace. Although only a small proportion of participants with and without a reported occupational noise exposure were between the ages of 60 and 69, the findings are noteworthy. In addition to the significant association among exposure to occupational noise, hearing threshold levels, age, gender, and ethnicity, occupational noise exposure is also related to smoking, exposure to recreational noise, and educational level, which also influence hearing threshold levels. The multivariate analysis was of interest in that after controlling for the numerous demographic factors associated with hearing loss, the effect of occupational noise exposure on hearing loss was dramatically reduced. The fact that preexisting medical conditions such as CVD can potentiate the effect of noise exposure on hearing levels sheds light on "cochlear vulnerability due to microvascular insufficiency" (Agrawal, Platz, & Niparko, 2009, p. 139). Previous investigators including Wild, Brewster, and Banerjee (2005) and Ferrite and Santana (2005) found an interaction between noise exposure and smoking, wherein the adverse effects of occupational noise are in fact exacerbated by smoking. Finally, in their BMHS sample, McMahon, Kifley, Rochtchina, Newall, and Mitchell (2008) found that smoking and diabetes were significantly associated with an increased odds of hearing loss, confirming a probable link to age-related hearing loss. Hence, it is clear that a multitude of environmental and physical factors interact with and contribute to age-related hearing loss.

Tinnitus

Tinnitus is often associated with auditory system disorders. Tinnitus prevalence and incidence estimates vary with age, the presence or absence of hearing loss, and definition. Hence, prevalence estimates range from 7 to 20%. Nondahl et al (2002) reported the 5-year incidence of tinnitus in their population-based sample of older adults to be 5.7%, suggesting that within their sample, of those older adults free of tinnitus at baseline, 5.7% developed it over a 5-year period with risk factors including hearing loss, serum total cholesterol, history of head trauma, and otosclerosis. Determination of significant tinnitus was made based on the subject's self-report of having buzzing, ringing, or other noise in the ears in the past year of at least moderate severity, or of having difficulty falling asleep because of tinnitus. Mild tinnitus was described as not affecting falling asleep. Notably, a potential risk factor for the 5-year incidence was found to be hearing loss at the baseline examination, which entailed an 83% higher risk of developing tinnitus. As part of their population-based study in Beaver-Dam, Wisconsin, Nondahl et al (2010) reported that the 10-year incidence rate of tinnitus in their sample overall was 12.7%; the incidence rate was higher in men than women. The authors explored baseline factors associated with the development of tinnitus over time and noted that a history of arthritis, a head injury, hearing loss (in women), and a history of smoking each increased the risk of developing tinnitus over time. The authors conducted a multivariate analysis and found an association between hearing loss severity and risk of developing tinnitus when controlling for such risk factors as arthritis, age, alcohol consumption, smoking, and head trauma in women. They found that the longer participants had refrained from smoking, the greater the likelihood that the tinnitus subsided. Interestingly, moderate alcohol consumption reduced the hazard of developing tinnitus over a 10-year period, suggesting a protective effect that may be due to findings that moderate alcohol consumption has some cardiovascular benefits as well (Nondahl et al, 2010).

These data suggest that modifiable factors, such as smoking, and head injury do increase the risk of developing tinnitus, which is important in terms of counseling, given the contribution of smoking and head trauma to hearing loss incidence as well. Although age does not appear to influence the incidence of tinnitus, the prevalence of tinnitus is somewhat higher in older than younger adults, suggesting that "accumulated exposures, rather than biological aging" (Nondahl et al, 2010, p. 584) may be a factor.

Gopinath, McMahon, Rochtchina, Karpa, and Mitchell (2010) explored the incidence, persistence, and progression of tinnitus over a 5-year period using over 2000 older adults participating in the BMHS. The presence of tinnitus was based on response to the following question: "Have you experienced any prolonged ringing, buzzing, or other sounds in your ears or head within the past year … that are lasting for five minutes or longer?" If the patient answered yes, additional questions were asked regarding the qualitative aspects of the tinnitus. Approximately 37% of participants reported experiencing tinnitus. The 5-year incidence of tinnitus was 18%. The incidence of tinnitus decreased with increasing age, such that it was lowest among persons 75+ years of age, with women in that age group having the lowest incidence. The presence of hearing loss was also associated with incidence of tinnitus. Interestingly, in this sample, tinnitus was a persistent symptom; 82% of the persons reporting tinnitus at baseline also had tinnitus at the 5-year follow-up. The incidence of tinnitus in the age group of 55 to 64 years was slightly higher among men than among women. It was noteworthy that less than 10% of participants sought treatment for their tinnitus, and among those seeking treatment the tinnitus reportedly persisted. The finding that hearing loss present at baseline was associated with an increased risk of tinnitus is in agreement with the findings of Nondahl et al (2002).

Sindhusake et al (2003) conducted a large cross-sectional population-based study on risk factors for tinnitus in a sample of older adults participating in the BMHS; 88% of participants were over 60 years of age, and 42% were 80 years of age or older. Hearing loss was a major predictor of tinnitus, such that for each 10-dB increase in hearing loss, there was a 10% increased likelihood of reporting tinnitus. Similarly, better cochlear function based on auditory brainstem response (ABR) and transient-evoked otoacoustic emission (TEOAE) resulted in lower tinnitus prevalence rates. Work-related noise exposure was a risk factor for tinnitus in this sample as well. Nonaudiological risk factors included a history of neck injury, a history of migraine, and middle ear or sinus infections.

In summary, one of the more interesting findings from the variety of studies on tinnitus is that tinnitus is most prevalent in individuals between 51 and 70 years of age, with the prevalence seeming to plateau in the age groups over 75 years of age (Hoffman & Reed, 2004). Further, race appears to be a factor, with tinnitus more often reported in Caucasians than in African Americans (9% versus 5.5%). Finally, tinnitus prevalence estimates differ globally as well, most likely due to the definition of the condition (e.g., buzzing, lasting 5 minutes, severe enough to interfere with sleep) and the characteristics of participants in the study. For example, Nondahl et al (2002), in their non–case-controlled cohort study of adults in Beaver Dam, Wisconsin, which based prevalence estimates on the severity and extent to which it interfered with sleeping, found a prevalence of 8.2%, whereas in Rosenhall and Karlsson's (1991) non–case-controlled cohort study of Swedes aged 70 years or older age it was 29%, and the prevalence of prolonged tinnitus in the non–case-controlled cohort study of adults between 55 and 99 years of age participating in the BMHS in Australia was 30% (Sindhusake et al, 2003).

Pearl

The more severe the hearing loss, the higher the risk of developing tinnitus in women. Age does not bear a relationship to tinnitus incidence; however, hearing loss appears to be a risk factor.

Vision Impairment

Vision impairment is very common among older adults, and age is the most common risk factor for vision impairment in older adults. Because age is also the most common risk factor for hearing loss, it follows that many older adults present with dual sensory impairments. Regarding visual impairment, 18% of adults 70 years of age or older report blindness in one or both eyes or difficulty seeing, and 8.6% report having difficulty seeing and hearing (Campbell, Crews, Moriarity, Zack, & Blackman, 1999).

Caban, Lee, Gómez-Marín, Lam, and Zheng (2005) and Crews and Campbell (2004) have looked at the prevalence and effects of dual sensory impairment among older adults. Using data from the National Health Interview Survey (1997–2002), Caban and colleagues (2005) analyzed the prevalence of hearing and visual impairment in adults 18 years of age and older living in the community. Interestingly, the overall prevalence of hearing impairment was twice that of visual impairment, with the overall prevalence of dual sensory impairment related significantly to advancing age. Although 9% of individuals 80 years of age or older reported visual impairment and 37% reported hearing impairment, the overall prevalence of hearing and visual impairment was 16.6% in the participants in this age group. Further, age-adjusted rates of hearing and visual impairment were significantly higher in men than in women. In addition to a gender effect, there were cultural differences as well, such that Aleut, Eskimo, and American Indians reported more than three times the rate of concurrent visual impairments of Asian/Pacific Islanders.

Using data from the 1994 Second Supplement of Aging (SOA-II) coproduced by the National Institute on Aging, Crews and Campbell (2004) reported on health, activity level, and social participation rates of adults 70 years of age or older with vision impairment, hearing loss, or both. The SOA-II data build on data from the 1984 SOA study. Data from the SOA-II study are obtained from four databases that are part of various National Health Interview Surveys. The sample consists of individuals 70 years of age or older who provided self-reported information on hearing and visual impairment. A visual problem was defined as blindness in one or both eyes or trouble seeing with glasses, whereas hearing impairment was defined as deafness in one or both ears or any other trouble hearing. Although 58% of respondents reported no sensory impairment, 24% reported a hearing impairment and 9% reported a vision impairment. The prevalence of concurrent impairments was relatively low, at 8.2%. Interestingly, those with vision and hearing impairment were less likely to report their health to be good than were those with hearing impairment alone. Similarly, individuals with no sensory impairment were the most likely to report their health to be excellent. The authors examined health conditions, activity limitations, and social participation across individuals with and without sensory impairments. Individuals reporting both vision and hearing impairment were most likely to report a history of arthritis, hypertension, injury from falls, heart disease, and confusion. A similar trend emerged when exploring the link among hearing impairment, vision impairment, and activities of daily living. Older adults with both vision and hearing impairment were more likely to report difficulty with such activities as going outside, ambulating, and preparing meals. The differences in social participation that emerged were notable as well. Although 74% of those without sensory loss reported visiting friends in the past 2 weeks, only 63% of those with both vision and hearing impairment reported visiting friends. Older adults with concurrent sensory impairments reported difficulty sustaining social participation activities and were less likely to speak to friends on the phone or attend religious services (Crews & Campbell, 2004). These data convincingly suggest that the prevalence of dual sensory impairment in older adults is high and increasing, and that the effect on social participation, activity level, and health is dramatic.

Data from the National Health Interview Survey, a continuous, multistage, probability survey of the U.S. civilian noninstitutionalized population, revealed some interesting trends on concurrent hearing and visual impairment and mortality in older adults (Lee et al, 2007). The data revealed that severity of concurrent hearing and visual impairment was associated with mortality in women more so than in men; specifically, moderate to severe concurrent sensory impairment had stronger associations with the risk of mortality. In summary, the health consequences for individuals with multiple chronic conditions, including hearing loss, visual impairment, diabetes, and cerebrovascular disease, are complex, presenting an increasing challenge to individuals and the health care system.

Multiple Comorbid Conditions: Visual Status, Balance, Diabetes, and Cognitive Ability

Lindenberger and Baltes (1994) conducted a classic study of the relationship between sensory function, namely visual acuity and hearing status, and intellectual function, to determine the extent to which sensory loss may underlie intellectual changes with age. They used a stratified probability sample of community-dwelling adults in Berlin, Germany, ranging in age from 70 to 103 years. The mean age of subjects in the age group between 70 and 84 years was 77 years, and the mean age of those in the group between 85 and 103 years was 92.6 years. Mean three-frequency PTA of the better ear of the former group was 41 dB HL and of the latter group was 51 dB HL. Corrected visual acuity in decimal units on the Snellen Eye Chart was 0.42 in the younger age group and 0.25 in the oldest age group; 16.7% of the subjects were hearing-aid users. In this sample, pure-tone thresholds decreased with increasing age, women had somewhat better hearing than men, and the configuration and severity of hearing loss was comparable to that in other studies of hearing and aging. As would be expected, pure-tone thresholds of men and women in the 70- to 84-year age group were dramatically better than thresholds of those 85 years of age or older with thresholds for women somewhat better. Interestingly, men and women in the 70- to 84-year group had essentially comparable distance vision and close right and close left vision. Not surprisingly, there was a strong negative correlation between age and hearing status (–0.54) and an even stronger negative correlation between age and visual acuity (–0.75). The correlation between hearing status and visual acuity was moderate (0.53), and the correlations between hearing status and intelligence and visual status and intelligence were moderate. Similarly, age was moderately correlated with each of the cognitive functions assessed. Assessment of intelligence or general cognitive ability was based on performance on tests of memory, speed of processing, reasoning, knowledge, and fluency. The authors concluded that the interrelationship between vision and hearing was in large part due to the variance they both shared with age. Interestingly, age had a greater effect on visual acuity.

The authors regressed intelligence on several predictor variables including age, vision, and hearing, and found that 40% of the variance in intelligence was accounted for by age, 41% by corrected visual status, and 34.5% by hearing status. Together, hearing, vision and age, accounted for 52% of the variance in intelligence. Interestingly, the authors also assessed balance-gait in their sample and found that it accounted for an additional 3.6% of the variance in intelligence after age, vision, and hearing, and together these sensory functions explained 55.6% of the variance. In contrast, when somatic health was added to the equation, it did not account for any of the additional variance in cognitive ability. The authors concluded that sensory functioning is a major predictor of intelligence later in life, and the contribution of sensory functions to the variance in intelligence is comparable in those 70 to 84 years of age and in those 85 to 103 years of age. In summary, taken together, vision and hearing accounted for 93% of the age-related variance in intellectual function. In fact, Lindenberger and Baltes (1994) concluded that age differences in intellectual function are mediated by vision and hearing, and that sensory factors are important correlates of individual differences in intellectual functioning in old age. Similarly, sensorimotor bodily efficacy, as measured with indices of balance and gain, was also predictive of individual differences in intellectual function. These data support a common cause hypothesis wherein the significant correlations are due to the fact that the sensory functions and cognition reflect the same changes in the brain (Baltes & Lindenberger, 1997; Lindenberger & Baltes, 1994).

As part of the BMHS, Chia and colleagues (2006) conducted a population-based study exploring the association between age-related vision and hearing impairment along with identifying risk factors for these chronic conditions. Vision impairment was defined as visual acuity less than 20/40 in the better eye, and hearing impairment was defined as a four-frequency PTA poorer than 25 dB HL in the better ear. The majority of participants also completed the Short Form Health Survey (SF-36), the gold-standard measure of physical functional status. The mean age of their sample was 69.8 years. Approximately 9% of participants had visual impairment and 40% had hearing impairment. The prevalence of each impairment and of dual sensory loss increased with age. Interestingly, smoking, diabetes, and noise exposure were significant risk factors for hearing loss in this sample, with the risk posed by each decreasing with increasing age. Hearing loss was present in 65% of participants presenting with visual impairment. Moderate hearing loss was present in 22% of those with vision impairment. Participants with hearing impairment had a high likelihood or presenting with vision impairment, yet the odds ratio of the two co-occurring was greatest in those with moderate to severe hearing impairment. Participants with cataracts or age-related maculopathy (ARM) were more likely to have hearing loss. It is noteworthy that individuals with dual sensory impairment had poorer scores on the SF-36, specifically on the physical and mental component scales, which suggests that sensory impairments contribute to deficits in functional status and well-being. The authors found that the relation between hearing impairment and visual impairment remained after controlling for the effects of age. As has been noted in previous chapters, these data confirm that similar biological and environmental factors may underlie these sensory changes.

Pearl

Sensory functioning is a major predictor of intelligence later in life.

Family History

McMahon et al (2008) explored the role of family history in hearing loss as part of the population-based BMHS. The prevalence of hearing loss in their sample of 2669 adults was higher in men (39%) than in women (29%). The majority (68%) of participants had mild hearing loss, and 47% reported a family history of hearing loss. Most notable was that the majority (63%) of people reporting a family history of hearing loss were women. Severity of hearing loss was linked to family history such that 64% of participants with moderate to severe hearing loss reported a positive family history as compared with 53% of those with mild hearing loss and 45% of those without hearing loss. Among those with moderate hearing loss, the family history was on the mother's side, and siblings in this cohort were also more likely to have a hearing loss. The work of McMahon et al suggests a strong association between presbycusis and family history, with the relationship greater among women and their mothers than that found in men. This pattern of heritability emerged in the Framingham Heart Study cohort as well (Gates, Couropmitree, & Myers, 1999).

Dementia

As cognitive decline associated with dementia is a major cause of death and disability in the elderly, efforts are underway in the general population to identify risk factors or correlates. Using participants in the Baltimore Longitudinal Study, Lin et al (2011) attempted to determine the degree to which hearing impairment is associated with incident all-cause senile dementia and Alzheimer's disease. In their prospective study, 639 adults ranging in age from 36 to 90 years underwent audiometric testing and cognitive testing over time. At baseline, participants were dementia free, and when tested close to 12 years later 58 cases of all-cause dementia were identified, of which 37 were dementia of the Alzheimer's type. The risk of incident dementia increased with severity of hearing loss, such that adults with moderate hearing loss were more likely than those with normal hearing to develop dementia, and adults with severe hearing loss were at greatest risk for developing dementia. These data corroborate the work of earlier investigators who suggested that older adults with senile dementia have more significant hearing loss than those without dementia. The degree to which hearing loss is a modifiable risk factor for dementia and the contribution of amplification to forestalling the onset of dementia are exciting areas worthy of investigation.

Pearl

Because many of the identified hearing loss risk factors, including smoking and cardiovascular disease, are modifiable, some of the burden associated with hearing loss in older people may be preventable (Helzner et al, 2005).

Prevalence, Ethnicity, Comorbidities, and Hearing-Aid Use

Lin et al (2011) analyzed data from the 2005–2006 cycle of the NHANES to study the epidemiology of hearing loss in adults aged 70 years or older living in the United States. Overall, 717 older adults were interviewed, had a medical examination, and completed audiometric studies. Pure-tone thresholds at 500 to 8000 Hz were obtained, and the severity of hearing loss was based on three-frequency (500, 1000, and 2000 Hz) and four-frequency (500, 1000, 2000, and 4000 Hz) PTAs. Traditional categorizations by severity were employed, with thresholds poorer than 25 dB HL indicative of hearing impairment. Lin and colleagues estimated the prevalence levels in adults 70 years of age or older based on thresholds in the poorer ear, using various cutoff levels. Prevalence varied such that the lower/better the cutoff level (e.g., 15 dB HL versus 25 dB HL) the higher the prevalence. Using a cutoff of 25 dB HL, the prevalence of hearing loss in their sample of adults 70 years of age or older was 61%, dropping to 28% using a cutoff of 40 dB HL. Approximately 37% of the sample had mild hearing loss and 26% had moderate hearing loss. Hearing loss prevalence also varied with age, such that the majority (81%) of people over 85 years had hearing loss, whereas only 46% of persons between 70 and 74 years had hearing impairment. Prevalence was higher in men (70%) than in women (58%) and in non-Hispanic whites (64%) and Mexican or other Hispanics (65%) than in non-Hispanic blacks (43%). Approximately 35% of the white men, 39% of the black men, 36% of the white women, and 24% of the black women had mild hearing loss. As expected, those with occupational or leisure-time exposure to noise and those who used firearms had a higher prevalence of hearing loss than did those reporting no noise exposure. Medical covariates such as a history of diabetes, hypertension, and stroke were not factors relating to prevalence. Overall, only 19% of the sample reportedly used hearing aids for more than 5 hours per week. Although it is surprising that only 3% of those with mild hearing impairment used hearing aids, 40 and 77%, respectively, of those with moderate and severe hearing loss used hearing aids. Individuals with higher education and leisure-time noise exposure were more likely to use hearing aids. Interestingly, the low rate of hearing-aid use emerging from this study is comparable to data on usage rates in England, suggesting that the potential impact of hearing aids on function may be undervalued cross-nationally.

Utilizing participants in the prospective population-based Cardiovascular Health Study (CHS), Pratt et al (2009) looked at the impact of gender, age, and race on hearing levels in a cohort of 548 older adults ranging in age from 72 to 96 years. Participants included 227 men and 321 women. Overall, 22% of participants were black—21% of the men and 23% of the women. An age, gender, and ethnicity effect emerged. Fifty-five percent of participants had PTAs indicative of hearing loss based on thresholds in the worse ear, with 71% of participants over 80 years having a hearing loss. Overall, the white men had the poorest thresholds and the black women had the most sensitive hearing threshold levels. Among participants less than 80 years of age, 46% of white women and 43% of white men had a hearing loss as compared with 39% of black men and 34% of black women. The trend that emerged for those

80 years of age or older was noteworthy, with 66% of white men and 75% of white women have a hearing loss as compared with 61% of black women and 73% of black men. Interestingly, in this sample a history of cardiovascular disease and smoking did not influence the pattern of findings. Hearing-aid use patterns differed slightly by gender and race; 21% of white men 80 years of age or older had hearing aids as compared with 27% of black men and 26% of white women. Black women in this age group were least likely to use hearing aids (5.6%) as were black women under 80 years of age (1.8%). White women and black and white men under 80 years of age were equally as likely to use hearing aids. These health disparities are noteworthy; however, caution must be used in interpreting the data given the small number of black participants in each group relative to the white participants, especially those 80 years of age or older.

◆ **Objective Tests: Immittance and Otoacoustic Emissions Testing**

Immittance testing and otoacoustic emissions are an important part of the routine test battery, and it is important for the clinician to be aware of any age effects on test results. As these tests provide important diagnostic information, it is imperative that audiologists consider the effects of age when they interpret the test results to ensure a valid conclusion about middle ear function, the status of the acoustic stapedial reflex, and outer hair cell status.

Age-related changes in the middle ear rarely affect hearing status, but of note are the changes in the joints and cartilage joining the ossicular chain. The cartilage within the incudostapedial and incudomalleolar joints undergoes the degenerative changes commonly associated with osteoarthritis, which, in selected individuals, can lead to middle ear abnormalities and possible conductive hearing loss (Rawool & Harrington, 2007). A recent report by Rawool and Harrington (2007) found that subjects with osteoarthritis and no family history of hearing loss, noise exposure, or chronic middle ear effusion sustained a higher prevalence of middle ear abnormalities and of sensorineural hearing loss than did an age-matched control group without arthritis. It is recommended that individuals suffering from osteoarthritis undergo tympanometric studies as part of the routine test battery.

Although structural changes in the middle ear mechanism occur, including loss of tympanic membrane elasticity, thinning of the tympanic membrane, a less static eardrum, increased stiffening of the ossicular chain, arthritic changes in the joints of the ossicular chain, and atrophy of intra-aural muscles, the data on the functional effect of these age-related changes are equivocal. Wiley et al (1996) found that in a sample of adults with normal otic history ranging in age from 48 to 90 years, statistically significant but very small differences in the distribution of peak compensated static acoustic admittance measures (peak Y_{tm} [peak compensated static acoustic admittance]) emerged. In addition, there were no differences between young and older adults in mean peak Y_{tm} values or across older age groups.

There is a dearth of data on the effect of age on the tympanometric pressure peak (TPP). Accordingly, TTP values used for adults can comfortably be used with older adults. Holte (1996) reported that median resonant frequency did not change significantly as a function of age, ranging between 800 and 1000 Hz depending on age and on where the pressure peak was compensated (e.g., +250 or –300 daPa). Wiley, Cruickshanks, Nondahl, and Tweed (1999) reported that there were no significant age-related trends for middle ear resonant frequency. Their findings support the data of Holte (1996). Holte did note a statistically significant correlation between age and tympanometric width. However, the correlation was slight, rendering the finding clinically insignificant.

More recently, Wiley, Nondahl, Cruickshanks, and Tweed (2005) conducted a longitudinal study of changes with age in the following tympanometric measures: peak compensated static acoustic admittance (peak Y_{tm}; in acoustic mmho [mllimhos]); equivalent ear canal volume (Vea; in cubic centimeters [cm^3]); tympanogram width (TW; in daPa); and tympanogram peak pressure (TPP; daPa). Subjects were drawn from the EHLS and ranged in age from 48 to 92 years. Subjects were tested at baseline and at a 5-year follow-up, with the mean length of follow-up being 5.3 years. Tympanometric data were obtained on 2366 adults; 39% were men and 61% were women. All subjects were free of otological problems and had air–bone gaps of <15 dB. Across all age groups and both genders, there was a small but statistically significant increase in mean peak compensated static acoustic admittance. As the magnitude of the mean changes was slight relative to the standard error of measurement, they are considered to be clinically insignificant. Similarly, there was a slight but statistically significant increase in equivalent ear-canal volume in men and women across the majority of age groups. The mean change, measured in cubic centimeters, was so small that again Wiley and colleagues (2005) concluded that the changes were not of clinical significance. A similar trend with a slight increase in tympanogram width measured in daPA emerged across most gender/age combinations. Again, these changes were too small to be considered clinically significant. Finally, the mean changes in tympanogram peak pressure that emerged in the oldest age group were considered clinically insignificant. In general, the authors concluded that changes in middle ear function over 5 years are minimal; however, they cautioned that perhaps this time interval was too brief to detect changes of clinical significance. Given the above findings, normative values used for adults can be applied to older adults during routine tympanometric testing.

In their cross-sectional study of the effect of age on otoacoustic emissions and tympanometry, Johansson and Arlinger (2003) did not find an age, gender, or ear effect on middle ear compliance in their cross-sectional sample of adults. Similarly, age did not appear to impact middle ear pressure in their sample.

Pearl

A robust age effect on acoustic admittance values, tympanometric peak pressure, middle ear resonance, and tympanometric width has not been documented.

Routine acoustic reflex testing (ART) includes establishing thresholds to tonal stimuli and determining whether a reflex contraction can be maintained during continuous stimulation (i.e., acoustic reflex decay). There is some disagreement among investigators as to the effect of age on acoustic reflex thresholds, depending for the most part on stimulus frequency, hearing level, and the nature of the stimulus. For normal-hearing older adults, there appears to be little change in the ART for frequencies between 500 and 2000 Hz (Jepson, 1963; Osterhammel & Osterhammel, 1979; Thompson, Sills, Recke, & Bui, 1979). Jerger, Jerger, and Mauldin (1972) found that for subjects with sensorineural hearing loss, ARTs for high frequencies were slightly higher than those for normals; however, this trend was apparent across age groups. In their comprehensive discussion of age and the acoustic reflex, Wilson and Margolis (1991) concluded that the changes in acoustic reflex thresholds to tonal activators of 2000 Hz are too small to be considered statistically significant. Data on reflex thresholds at 4000 Hz are conflicting, most likely due to the difficulty associated with eliciting reflexes for higher frequency stimuli. For example, Wilson (1981) reported a notable increase in ART with age for an activator signal of 4000 Hz, whereas Jerger, Jerger, and Mauldin (1972) reported a decrease in the ART at 4000 Hz for older adults. To further complicate the picture, several investigators have reported that the activator signal affects the reflex threshold, such that ARTs for broadband noise (BBN) stimuli are elevated for normal-hearing older adults (Silman, 1979; Wilson & Margolis, 1991). As would be expected, ARTs are elicited at reduced sensation levels but at normal-hearing levels relative to the 90th percentile values generated by Silman and Gelfand (1981). In contrast, it appears that thresholds for BBN activators are slightly elevated in older adults relative to younger adults, and acoustic-reflex latencies for both tonal and BBN appear to be prolonged in older adults relative to younger adults (Bosatra, Russolo, & Silverman, 1984; Gelfand & Piper, 1981). Further, the growth of the acoustic reflex amplitudes tends to be decreased in the elderly, and the acoustic reflex growth function appears to saturate more frequently in older adults (Rawool, 1996).

More recently, Emmer, Silman, Silverman, and Levitt (2006) explored aging effects on temporal integration of the contralateral acoustic reflex using a BBN activating signal. Young and older adults (mean age = 67.5 years) were comparable with regard to hearing threshold levels at 250 through 8000 Hz. That is, all subjects had normal hearing, although higher frequency thresholds were poorer for the older subjects, but not dramatically so. The data suggested that as the duration of the activator signal increased, the acoustic reflex threshold for BBN decreased in young and older participants. When the activator signal duration was longer (>200 milliseconds), the ART for BBN was higher in older than younger adults. At 1000 milliseconds the threshold difference between young and older participants was greatest, namely, 10 dB. This difference was not attributable to peripheral hearing sensitivity, as the threshold levels were comparable. These results should not affect routine testing of the ART in older adults. In summary, aging effects for tonal activators appear to be negligible. Hence, the values generated by Silman and Gelfand (1981) should be used in interpreting ARTs.

Pearl

ARTs for tonal stimuli (500 to 2000 Hz) are similar across age groups. Age-related increases in thresholds for BBN are of statistical and clinical significance and should be considered in drawing conclusions about the status of the auditory system in older individuals (Wilson & Margolis, 1991).

Otoacoustic Emission Tests

Otoacoustic emission tests provide a unique window into the cochlear amplifier, most particularly outer hair cell function, which helps in the differential diagnosis of hearing loss. Although outer hair cell loss is commonly observed in persons with presbycusis, more recently evidence is accumulating that suggests that cochlear aging is due in large part to strial atrophy (Gates, Mills, Nam, D'Agostino, & Rubel, 2002). The controversy surrounding the etiology of presbycusis has raised discussions regarding the role of otoacoustic emissions (OAEs) in the evaluation of older adults. Although OAE tests may not add relevant information to the routine clinical evaluation of elderly individuals with hearing impairment, the effects of age on emissions should be understood by clinicians, primarily because they have excellent sensitivity to cochlear dysfunction.

A few studies have been conducted on the effects of aging on the measurement of OAEs to help tease out the physiological factors underlying the elevated hearing threshold levels associated with the aging process. In short, is outer hair cell loss to blame, or are decreases in endocochlear potential (EP) due to changes in the stria vascularis, the source of the EP, the primary cause of hearing loss in older adults (Gates et al, 2002)? The goal of research in this area has also been to determine the affect of age on OAEs and to determine the extent to which possible age-related changes can be explained by hearing threshold levels. The earliest studies focused on spontaneous emissions, which are known to be present in 40 to 60% of ears with normal hearing threshold levels. According to Bright (1997), the prevalence of spontaneous otoacoustic emissions (SOAEs) decreases for subjects over 60 years of age, even when hearing thresholds are within normal limits. In addition, the total number of SOAEs observed decreases in aged ears, although other SOAE features (e.g., frequency and amplitude characteristics) remain unchanged and are not affected by age (Bonfils, 1989; Lonsbury-Martin, Cutler, & Martin, 1991). The variability in their appearance and their presence at discrete and unpredictable frequencies, coupled with the fact that SOAEs tend to be present in some but not all persons with normal hearing, limit their validity in the diagnosis of peripheral hearing loss. Probst, Lonsbury-Martin, and Martin (1991) found the prevalence of SOAEs to decline after age 50, as did Stover and Norton (1993).

Johansson and Arlinger (2003) conducted a cross-sectional study of otoacoustic emissions in an adult sample living in Sweden. The subjects were free of excessive noise exposure and were not otologically screened. The authors did not present mean hearing levels of their sample, which makes the data difficult to interpret. However, it was noteworthy that the majority of subjects did not have SOAEs, and age did not have an impact on prevalence. In those with normal hearing the prevalence of SOAEs was 48%. There was a gender effect, with more women than men having SOAEs. Most SOAEs were present at 1000 to 2000 Hz. Hence, these data differ from those of previous investigators, but this could be due to several variables, such as the instrumentation, and to the fact that the characteristics of the sample were loosely defined.

Elicited by a broadband click of short duration, TEOAEs can typically be recorded in nearly all persons with normal hearing irrespective of gender. The prevalence of TEOAEs tends to be higher in women than in men, and the amplitude tend to be larger. Typically, TEOAEs are not elicited when hearing levels exceed 30 to 40 dB HL (Bertoli & Probst, 1997). They are considered a feature of the human peripheral auditory system (Johansson & Arlinger, 2003).

The effect of age on the prevalence and characteristics of TEOAEs has been explored in a variety of samples. Bertoli and Probst (1997) gathered click-evoked otoacoustic emissions (CEOAEs) on a sample of 201 older adults with sensorineural hearing loss. CEOAEs were not detectable in ears with a PTA greater than 30 dB HL, and only 60% of ears with PTAs better than 30 dB HL had CEOAEs. As would be expected, the prevalence of CEOAEs increased with improved hearing level, rising to 77% for older adults with PTAs better than 15 dB HL. When comparing subjects with and without CEOAEs, age was not a distinguishing variable, but hearing level was. Similarly, amplitude or response level of the OAE did not appear to correlate with age. Bertoli and Probst concluded that TEOAEs do not substantially contribute to the audiometric test battery for the typical presbycusic who presents with hearing levels in excess of 30 dB HL. The authors reported a prevalence of 60% among older adults with three-frequency PTAs better than 30 dB HL.

Stenklev and Laukli (2003) explored the prevalence of TEOAEs in individuals over 60 years of age and the effect of age on TEOAEs independent of peripheral hearing loss. The prevalence of TEOAEs was 55.6%, and it was slightly higher in women than in men. As one might expect, the proportion of individuals with TEOAEs decreased with increasing age, such that the majority of participants between 60 and 64 years had TEOAEs; however, very few people over 90 years had TEOAEs. When plotted against hearing threshold level at the best frequency, emissions were essentially not detectable when hearing levels exceeded 40 dB HL. The distribution of TEOAEs by age, five-frequency (1000, 1500, 2000, 3000, and 4000 Hz) PTAs and gender is shown in **Table 5.6**. The interaction among hearing level, age, and prevalence of TEOAEs is clear, as is the gender effect. A separate analysis revealed that the amplitude of TEOAEs did not vary with age, but there was a statistically significant but not clinically significant relation between age and wave reproducibility, with reproducibility decreasing with age. The overall mean five-frequency PTA of the sample was 40 dB HL, and 56% of the sample had TEOAEs. In comparing normal-hearing young participants with normal-hearing older participants, the elderly had lower overall mean wave reproducibility and response levels; however, although normal, the pure-tone thresholds were poorer in the older adults.

Table 5.6 Prevalence of Transient-Evoked Otoacoustic Emissions (TEOAEs) by Median Age, Five Frequency Pure-Tone Average, and Gender

Median Age in Years	Gender	Pure-Tone Average	% TEOAEs present	Number of Participants
63	Male	28.8	73.7	19
62.5	Female	22.4	95.8	24
66.5	Male	40.9	60.0	30
67	Female	23.7	90.9	22
73	Male	38.5	61.9	21
72.5	Female	34.2	75.0	12
76	Male	43.7	55.0	20
75	Female	45.3	54.5	11
82	Male	56.1	11	18
82	Female	44.8	35.3	17
85	Male	51.4	40	5
87	Female	40.9	44.4	9
92.5	Male	67.8	0.0	10
92.5	Female	59.2	7.1	14

Special Consideration

TEOAE measurements are highly sensitive to hearing loss greater than 30 dB HL.

Prieve and Falter (1995) compared the status of click-evoked otoacoustic emissions (CEOAEs) in a sample of older adults with normal hearing to those of a group of younger adults. They failed to find a significant difference in CEOAE levels between the two groups, corroborating the results of Robinette (1992), who also sampled adults with normal hearing. Although age did not appear to account for a significant proportion of the variance in CEOAE level or threshold, the presence of synchronized spontaneous otoacoustic emissions (SSOAEs) did. Harris and Probst (1997) reviewed the literature and concluded that when controlling for hearing level, age does not have a strong effect on the morphology of the TEOAE. In light of the findings described above, age-adjusted norms may not be necessary for clinical applications. The results to date suggest that TEOAEs do not help the audiologist gain specific information about factors in the cochlea that may underlie sensorineural loss (Harris & Probst, 1997). Hence, I do not believe this testing should be a routine part of the test battery for older adults.

Distortion-product otoacoustic emissions (DPOAEs), an intermodulation distortion response produced by the ear in response to primary tones, tend to be correlated with hearing threshold levels (i.e., two simultaneous pure-tone stimuli) (Lonsbury-Martin, Martin, & Whitehead, 1997). There appears to be a gender effect, with the response stronger in women than in men especially at 4000 Hz. DPOAEs accurately identify hearing status for frequencies ranging from 1500 to 6000 Hz, falling off in accuracy for frequencies above and below this range (Gorga et al, 1997). Although DPOAEs reflect the underlying nonlinear response properties of the human cochlea that are associated with the outer hair cell system, the data on age effects on DPOAEs are inconclusive (Gorga et al, 1997). According to Gorga et al (1997) DPOAEs are an inversely graded response of hearing loss over the 50- to 60-dB range especially in the higher frequencies. For hearing levels above 60 dB, ears did not produce measurable emissions, minimizing their contribution to the prediction of severe to profound hearing loss. Gorga et al's large-scale study did not consider age to be a significant variable when gathering normative data on DPOAE. Their philosophy is in keeping with the conclusions of Karzon, Garcia, Peterein, and Gates (1994), that when compensating for differences in audiometric threshold, there are no significant changes in DPOAEs that can be attributed to age. Stover and Norton (1993) also examined the effects of age on DPOAE amplitude and concluded that age did not affect the OAE in their sample of normal-hearing individuals.

Lonsbury et al (1997) demonstrated an age effect on the amplitude of the DPOAE. In their sample, older adults had poorer hearing thresholds than did the younger adults. They found that DPOAE amplitudes decreased with increasing age at most frequencies, with differences achieving statistical significance. Kimberley, Brown, and Allen (1997) also provided evidence of a significant, albeit weak, relation between DPOAE level in dB sound pressure level (SPL) and age. In their study of individuals with normal hearing, response amplitude appears to decrease with increasing age, with the relation varying only slightly with increasing frequency.

Uchida et al (2008) attempted to determine whether deterioration in cochlear function, as evaluated by DPOAEs, exists before the elevation of audiometric thresholds occurs during the aging process. As part of their population-based sample, participants included adults ranging in age from 40 to 82 years with hearing thresholds better than 15 dB HL. Mean age was 48 years in men and 49 years in women. The authors found that, at selected middle to high frequencies, DPOAEs deteriorate with age irrespective of the hearing threshold levels being normal. These findings suggest that DPOAEs possibly can be used for early detection of hearing loss before it actually can be detected via pure-tone threshold testing, especially in women. The fact that DPOAEs deteriorate with age, even in normal-hearing older adults, confirms their potential for detecting cochlear damage from ototoxicity or noise exposure.

Cilento, Norton, and Gates (2003) explored the effect of age and gender on DPOAE amplitude in a sample of adults participating in the Framingham Heart Study. The 445 participants had presbycusis or noise-induced hearing loss. Specifically, pure-tone thresholds were normal at 1000 and 2000 Hz and reflected a mild hearing loss for men at 4000 and 8000 Hz and for women only at 8000 Hz. In all, 44% of the participants had normal pure-tone thresholds (53% of the women and 33% of the men). Hearing levels declines with age, such that the oldest participants had significantly poorer thresholds than the younger irrespective of gender. Mean age of the women in the sample was 59.4 years and of the men was 57.8 years, with ages ranging from 30 to 82 years. Distortion-product (DP)-grams were obtained on participants at presentation levels of 65 dB for the lowest primary tone (L1) and 50 dB SPL for intensity level of second primary tone (L2) using an f2/f1 ratio of 1.22 with f2 frequencies of 500, 750, 1000, 1500, 2000, 3000, 4000, 6000, and 8000 Hz. A gender difference emerged on DPOAE amplitude in that it was significantly lower for men than for women. Further, across age groups, the amplitude of the DPOAE decreased in men and in women. Multivariate re-

gression analysis revealed that there was no effect of age on DPOAE amplitude at any frequency; for men the decline was attributable to elevated hearing threshold levels. The age effect for women was evident from 2000 to 8000 Hz. The rate of decrease in amplitude for women was on the order of 1 or 2 dB/decade. The decline in DPOAE amplitude appears to mirror the change in high-frequency thresholds that occurs with advancing age; however, the rate of decline in amplitude with age is less than the decrement in pure-tone thresholds. The data suggest that in women there is a slight decrease in DPOAE amplitude at the higher frequencies with increasing age. This change is unrelated to change in hearing threshold levels with age. In light of the findings, Cilento et al theorized that the locus of age-related atrophy in the cochlea may be the stria rather than the outer hair cells.

Johansson and Arlinger (2003) found the overall prevalence of broadband TEOAEs was 41%, with the prevalence quite low in the 500- to 1000-Hz frequency band and in the 2000- to 4000-Hz frequency band. There was a definite age effect in the broadband and in the frequency band between 2000 and 4000 Hz, and a pure-tone hearing threshold level effect as well. The correlation between TEOAE signal level at the various frequency bands and pure-tone thresholds was statistically significant at 1000 to 2000 Hz, 2000 to 4000 Hz, and 500 to 4000 Hz, with the strength of the correlation being stronger in the right ear with a range from −0.38 to −0.45. A gender effect emerged, with women having higher response levels; this finding remained even after controlling for hearing level. With regard to age, the signal level decreased slightly (approximately 5 dB) from age 20 to 29 years to age 70 to 79 years; however, the effect for the right ear was due to changes in hearing threshold level. For the left ear, the age effect remained after adjusting for hearing level, but the change was most pronounced from age 20 to 29 years through age 30 to 39 years. With regard to DPOAEs, an age effect emerged at 4000 Hz after adjusting for hearing level, with the signal level decreasing by approximately 8 dB in the age group of 20 to 29 years to those 70 to 79 years of age. The rate of decrease was most pronounced between age groups 20 to 29 years and 30 to 39 years. Similarly, there was an age effect at 6000 Hz, the decrement being approximately 8 dB, but this effect was highest before age 40 to 49 years. Thus, for both TEOAEs and DPOAEs, an age effect emerged even after controlling for hearing threshold level. However, the critical age for the decrease in signal level was rather young, namely 30 years of age. In contrast, and as noted above, Gates et al (2008) noted that relative to hearing levels, DPOAEs are relatively stable over time. Similarly, Oeken, Lenk, and Bootz (2000) reported that DPOAEs decreased in the older age groups with an increase in pure-tone thresholds. Using partial correlations and multiple regressions, they concluded that pure-tone thresholds have a greater influence on DPOAEs than age alone.

Thus, given the evidence that DPOAE levels may be reduced before the manifestation of shifts in hearing threshold levels, DPOAEs hold promise as indices of changes in the cochlea due to ingestion of ototoxic drugs or exposure to excessive noise. Hence, in my view their greatest promise in older adults is in the possible detection of incipient cochlear damage in noise- or drug-exposed older adults. As Jupiter (2009) noted, DPOAEs have the potential for use as part of health promotion to detect individuals at risk for hearing loss and also for monitoring older adults with acute conditions who are ingesting ototoxic agents.

◆ Conclusion

The data emerging from longitudinal and cross-sectional studies are quite comparable, confirming that women and men are at risk for age-associated hearing loss. The rate of decay is approximately 5.5 to 8 dB per decade in the better ear, with the worse ear tending to deteriorate more quickly than the better ear (Divenyi et al, 2005). There is a gender difference in the rate of decline and the frequency at which the decline takes place that tends to equalize in the eighth and ninth decades of life (Gates et al, 1990). Auditory thresholds in each ear are not completely symmetrical, and, according to Gates and Cooper (1991), the left ear tends to be poorer than the right ear and as will be seen in Chapter 6, the left ear disadvantage is evident on speech recognition tasks. The risk of developing a hearing impairment is about 1 in 25 people per year, with the risk perhaps slightly lower with more recent generations due to healthier lifestyles and increased attention to modifiable risk factors (Cruickshanks, 2010). In terms of healthier lifestyles, as vascular health improves, hearing status appears to be preserved (Cruickshanks, 2010). According to Divenyi et al (2005), the decline in hearing sensitivity is not comparable between ears, as the left ear tends to have poorer thresholds than the right throughout the aging process; hence, there is a right ear advantage for peripheral hearing sensitivity that is evident in performance on speech tests as well. There is large individual variability in absolute hearing thresholds and in the amount of change with age. In addition to age, although the data are equivocal, there is the suggestion that smoking, cardiovascular disease, noise exposure, and diabetes mellitus are modifiable risk factors for hearing loss. Hearing loss is most common in Caucasian men and least common in black women (Helzner et al, 2005). Finally, effects of age on otoacoustic emissions and routine immittance tests suggests that the tests are robust enough that age effects on these electrophysiological tests are minimal.

Data from the BMHS suggested the following trends: (1) using a four-frequency PTA, 39% of adults aged 55 or older have hearing impairment; (2) the frequency of hearing loss almost doubles by decade, rising from 10.5% in those aged less than 60 years to close to 80% in those aged 80 or older; (3) hearing loss is significantly more frequent in men; (4) the majority of persons with hearing loss do not seek help or use hearing aids; and (5) risk factors for hearing loss include age, male gender, diabetes, noise exposure, smoking, and impaired visual status. It seems safe to conclude from the studies above that (1) hearing level declines gradually and progressively with age; (2) the amount of threshold change appears greatest in the highs; (3) there are gender differences in rate of decline in hearing level and in frequencies at which declines take place; and (4) risk factors other than age contribute to the individual variability in decline in hearing level after age 50. Finally, aging does not appear to have an appreciable effect on tympanometric, acoustic stapedial reflex, and otoacoustic emission test results.

References

Agrawal, Y., Niparko, J. K., & Dobie, R. A. (2010, Apr). Estimating the effect of occupational noise exposure on hearing thresholds: The importance of adjusting for confounding variables. *Ear and Hearing, 31*, 234–237

Agrawal, Y., Platz, E., & Niparko, J. (2009). Risk factors for hearing loss in US adults: Data from the National Health and Nutrition Examination Survey, 1999 to 2002. *Otology & Neurotology, 30*, 139–145

Agrawal, Y., Platz, E. A., & Niparko, J. K. (2008, Jul). Prevalence of hearing loss and differences by demographic characteristics among US adults: Data from the National Health and Nutrition Examination Survey, 1999–2004. *Archives of Internal Medicine, 168*, 1522–1530

Bainbridge, K. E., Hoffman, H. J., & Cowie, C. C. (2008, Jul). Diabetes and hearing impairment in the United States: audiometric evidence from the National Health and Nutrition Examination Survey, 1999 to 2004. *Annals of Internal Medicine, 149*, 1–10

Baltes, P. B., & Lindenberger, U. (1997, Mar). Emergence of a powerful connection between sensory and cognitive functions across the adult life span: A new window to the study of cognitive aging? *Psychology and Aging, 12*, 12–21

Bertoli, S., & Probst, R. (1997, Aug). The role of transient-evoked otoacoustic emission testing in the evaluation of elderly persons. *Ear and Hearing, 18*, 286–293

Bonfils, P. (1989, Jul). Spontaneous otoacoustic emissions: Clinical interest. *Laryngoscope, 99*(7 Pt 1), 752–756

Bosatra, A., Russolo, M., & Silverman, C. A. (1984). Acoustic-reflex latency: State of the art. In S. Silman (Ed.), *The acoustic reflex: Basic principles and clinical applications* (pp. 301–328). New York: Academic Press

Boult, C., & Wieland, G. D. (2010, Nov). Comprehensive primary care for older patients with multiple chronic conditions: "Nobody rushes you through". *Journal of the American Medical Association, 304*, 1936–1943

Brant, L. J., & Fozard, J. L. (1990, Aug). Age changes in pure-tone hearing thresholds in a longitudinal study of normal human aging. *Journal of the Acoustical Society of America, 88*, 813–820.

Brant, L. J., Gordon-Salant, S., Pearson, J. D., Klein, L. L., Morrell, C. H., Metter, E. J., et al. (1996, Jun). Risk factors related to age-associated hearing loss in the speech frequencies. *Journal of the American Academy of Audiology, 7*(3), 152–160.

Bright, K. (1997). Spontaneous otoacoustic emissions. In M. Robinette & T. Glattke (Eds.), *Otoacoustic emissions: Clinical applications*. New York: Thieme

Burkhalter, C. L., Allen, R. S., Skaar, D. C., Crittenden, J., & Burgio, L. D. (2009, Oct). Examining the effectiveness of traditional audiological assessments for nursing home residents with dementia-related behaviors. *Journal of the American Academy of Audiology, 20*, 529–538

Caban, A. J., Lee, D. J., Gómez-Marín, O., Lam, B. L., & Zheng, D. D. (2005, Nov). Prevalence of concurrent hearing and visual impairment in US adults: The National Health Interview Survey, 1997–2002. *American Journal of Public Health, 95*, 1940–1942

Campbell, V., Crews, J., Moriarity, D., Zack, M., & Blackman, D. (1999). Surveillance for sensory impairment, activity limitations, and health-related quality of life among older adults. Surveillance for selected public health indicators affecting older adults-United States, 1993–1997. *MMWR CDC Surveillance Sumary, 48*, 131–146

Chia, E. M., Mitchell, P., Rochtchina, E., Foran, S., Golding, M., & Wang, J. J. (2006, Oct). Association between vision and hearing impairments and their combined effects on quality of life. *Archives of Ophthalmology, 124*, 1465–1470

Cilento, B., Norton, S., & Gates, G. (2003). The effects of aging and hearing loss on distortion product otoacoustic emissions. *Otolaryngology–Head and Neck Surgery, 129*, 382–389 PMID: 14574293

Cohen-Mansfield, J., & Taylor, J. W. (2004, Sep-Oct). Hearing aid use in nursing homes. Part 1: Prevalence rates of hearing impairment and hearing aid use. *Journal of the American Medical Directors Association, 5*, 283–288

Cooper, J. C., Jr. (1994, Jan). Health and Nutrition Examination Survey of 1971-75: Part I. Ear and race effects in hearing. *Journal of the American Academy of Audiology, 5*, 30–36

Crews, J. E., & Campbell, V. A. (2004, May). Vision impairment and hearing loss among community-dwelling older Americans: Implications for health and functioning. *American Journal of Public Health, 94*, 823–829

Cruickshanks, K. (2010). *Age related hearing loss: Demographics and risk factors.* Presented at the ARC meeting in San Diego, California, April 14. http://www.audiologynow.org/pdf/Aging/2010_ARC_Cruickshanks.pdf

Cruickshanks, K. J., Klein, R., Klein, B. E., Wiley, T. L., Nondahl, D. M., & Tweed, T. S. (1998a, Jun). Cigarette smoking and hearing loss: The epidemiology of hearing loss study. *Journal of the American Medical Association, 279,* 1715–1719

Cruickshanks, K. J., Tweed, T. S., Wiley, T. L., Klein, B. E., Klein, R., Chappell, R., et al. (2003, Oct). The 5-year incidence and progression of hearing loss: The epidemiology of hearing loss study. *Archives of Otolaryngology–Head and Neck Surgery, 129,* 1041–1046

Cruickshanks, K. J., Wiley, T. L., Tweed, T. S., Klein, B. E., Klein, R., Mares-Perlman, J. A., et al. The Epidemiology of Hearing Loss Study (1998b, Nov). Prevalence of hearing loss in older adults in Beaver Dam, Wisconsin. *American Journal of Epidemiology, 148,* 879–886

Divenyi, P. L., Stark, P. B., & Haupt, K. M. (2005, Aug). Decline of speech understanding and auditory thresholds in the elderly. *Journal of the Acoustical Society of America, 118,* 1089–1100

Dubno, J. R., Lee, F. S., Matthews, L. J., Ahlstrom, J. B., Horwitz, A. R., & Mills, J. H. (2008, Jan). Longitudinal changes in speech recognition in older persons. *Journal of the Acoustical Society of America, 123,* 462–475

Emmer, M. B., Silman, S., Silverman, C. A., & Levitt, H. (2006, Sep). Temporal integration of the contralateral acoustic-reflex threshold and its age-related changes. *Journal of the Acoustical Society of America, 120,* 1467–1473

Ferrite, S., & Santana, V. (2005, Jan). Joint effects of smoking, noise exposure and age on hearing loss. *Occupational Medicine (Oxford, England), 55,* 48–53

Fransen, E., Topsakal, V., Hendrickx, J. J., Van Laer, L., Huyghe, J. R., Van Eyken, E., et al. (2008, Sep). Occupational noise, smoking, and a high body mass index are risk factors for age-related hearing impairment and moderate alcohol consumption is protective: a European population-based multicenter study. *Journal of the Association for Research in Otolaryngology, 9,* 264–276, discussion 261–263

Gates, G. A., Beiser, A., Rees, T. S., D'Agostino, R. B., & Wolf, P. A. (2002, Mar). Central auditory dysfunction may precede the onset of clinical dementia in people with probable Alzheimer's disease. *Journal of the American Geriatrics Society, 50,* 482–488

Gates, G. A., Cobb, J. L., D'Agostino, R. B., & Wolf, P. A. (1993, Feb). The relation of hearing in the elderly to the presence of cardiovascular disease and cardiovascular risk factors. *Archives of Otolaryngology–Head and Neck Surgery, 119,* 156–161

Gates, G. A., & Cooper, J. C. (1991). Incidence of hearing decline in the elderly. *Acta Oto-Laryngologica, 111,* 240–248 [Stockholm]

Gates, G. A., Cooper, J. C., Jr, Kannel, W. B., & Miller, N. J. (1990, Aug). Hearing in the elderly: The Framingham cohort, 1983–1985. Part I. Basic audiometric test results. *Ear and Hearing, 11,* 247–256

Gates, G. A., Couropmitree, N. N., & Myers, R. H. (1999). Genetic associations in age-related hearing thresholds. *Archives of Otolaryngology–Head and Neck Surgery, 125,* 654–659

Gates, G. A., Feeney, M. P., & Mills, D. (2008, Dec). Cross-sectional age-changes of hearing in the elderly. *Ear and Hearing, 29,* 865–874

Gates, G., Mills, D., Nam, B., D'Agostino, R., & Rubel, R. (2002). Effects of age on the distortion product otoacoustic emission growth functions. *Hearing Research, 163,* 53–60

Gelfand, S. A., & Piper, N. (1981). Acoustic reflex thresholds in young and elderly subjects with normal hearing. *Journal of the Acoustical Society of America, 69,* 295–297

Gopinath, B., Flood, V. M., McMahon, C. M., Burlutsky, G., Smith, W., & Mitchell, P. (2010, Apr). The effects of smoking and alcohol consumption on age-related hearing loss: The Blue Mountains Hearing Study. *Ear and Hearing, 31,* 277–282

Gopinath, B., McMahon, C. M., Rochtchina, E., Karpa, M. J., & Mitchell, P. (2010, Jun). Incidence, persistence, and progression of tinnitus symptoms in older adults: The Blue Mountains Hearing Study. *Ear and Hearing, 31,* 407–412

Gorga, M. P., Neely, S. T., Ohlrich, B., Hoover, B., Redner, J., & Peters, J. (1997, Dec). From laboratory to clinic: A large scale study of distortion product otoacoustic emissions in ears with normal hearing and ears with hearing loss. *Ear and Hearing, 18,* 440–455

Harris, F., & Probst, R. (1997). Otoacoustic emissions and audiometric outcomes. In M. Robinette & T. Glattke (Eds.), *Otoacoustic emissions: Clinical applications.* New York: Thieme

Helzner, E. P., Cauley, J. A., Pratt, S. R., Wisniewski, S. R., Zmuda, J. M., Talbott, E. O., et al. (2005, Dec). Race and sex differences in age-related hearing loss: The Health, Aging and Body Composition Study. *Journal of the American Geriatrics Society, 53,* 2119–2127

Helzner, E. P., Patel, A. S., Pratt, S., Sutton-Tyrrell, K., Cauley, J. A., Talbott, E., et al. (2011, Jun). Hearing sensitivity in older adults: Associations with cardiovascular risk factors in the health, aging and body composition study. *Journal of the American Geriatric Society, 59,* 972–979

Hoffman, H. J., Dobie, R. A., Ko, C. W., Themann, C. L., & Murphy, W. J. (2010, Dec). Americans hear as well or better today compared with 40 years ago: Hearing threshold levels in the unscreened adult population of the United States, 1959-1962 and 1999-2004. *Ear and Hearing, 31,* 725–734

Hoffman, H. J., & Reed, G. W. (2004). Epidemiology of tinnitus. In J. B. Snow (Ed.), *Tinnitus: Theory and management* (pp. 16–41). Lewiston, NY: B. C. Decker

Holte, L. (1996, Feb). Aging effects in multifrequency tympanometry. *Ear and Hearing, 17,* 12–18

Jepson, O. (1963). Middle ear muscle reflexes in man. In J. Jerger (Ed.), *Modern developments in audiology.* New York: Academic Press

Jerger, J., Jerger, S., & Mauldin, L. (1972, Dec). Studies in impedance audiometry. I. Normal and sensorineural ears. *Archives of Otolaryngology, 96,* 513–523

Johansson, M. S., & Arlinger, S. D. (2003, Dec). Otoacoustic emissions and tympanometry in a general adult population in Sweden. *International Journal of Audiology, 42,* 448–464

Jones, A, Dwyer, L., Bercovitz, A., & Strahan, G. (2009). The National Nursing Home Survey: 2004 overview. National Center for Health Statistics. *Vital Health Stat 13.*

Jupiter, T. (2009, Dec). Screening for hearing loss in the elderly using distortion product otoacoustic emissions, pure tones, and a self-assessment tool. *Journal of the American Academy of Audiology, 18,* 99–107

Karzon, R. K., Garcia, P., Peterein, J. L., & Gates, G. A. (1994, Sep). Distortion product otoacoustic emissions in the elderly. *American Journal of Otology, 15,* 596–605

Katz, P., & Gilbert, G. (2008). Diabetes and cardiovascular disease among older adults: An update on the evidence. *Geriatrics and Aging, 11,* 509–514

Kimberley, B., Brown, D., & Allen, J. (1997). Distortion product emissions and sensorineural hearing loss. In M. Robinette & T. Glattke (Eds.), *Otoacoustic emissions: Clinical applications.* New York: Thieme

Kochkin, S. (2007, April). MarkeTrak VII: Obstacles to adult non-user adoption of hearing aids. *Hearing Journal, 60,* 27–43

Kochkin, S. (2009). MarkeTrak VIII: 25 year trends in the hearing health market. *Hearing Review, 16,* 12–31

Lee, D. J., Gómez-Marín, O., Lam, B. L., Zheng, D. D., Arheart, K. L., Christ, S. L., et al. (2007, Jun). Severity of concurrent visual and hearing impairment and mortality: The 1986–1994 National Health Interview Survey. *Journal of Aging and Health, 19,* 382–396

Lee, F. S., Matthews, L. J., Dubno, J. R., & Mills, J. H. (2005, Feb). Longitudinal study of pure-tone thresholds in older persons. *Ear and Hearing, 26,* 1–11

Lin, F. R., Metter, E. J., O'Brien, R. J., Resnick, S. M., Zonderman, A. B., & Ferrucci, L. (2011, Feb). Hearing loss and incident dementia. *Archives of Neurology, 68,* 214–220

Lin, F. R., Thorpe, R., Gordon-Salant, S., & Ferrucci, L. (2011, May). Hearing loss prevalence and risk factors among older adults in the United States. *Journal of Gerontology, Series A, Biological Sciences and Medical Sciences, 66,* 582–590

Lindenberger, U., & Baltes, P. B. 1994. Sensory functioning and intelligence in old age: A strong connection. *Psychol. Aging, 9,* 339–355

Lonsbury-Martin, B. L., Cutler, W. M., & Martin, G. K. (1991, Apr). Evidence for the influence of aging on distortion-product otoacoustic emissions in humans. *Journal of the Acoustical Society of America, 89*(4 Pt 1), 1749–1759

Lonsbury-Martin, B., Martin, G., & Whitehead, M. (1997). Distortion product otoacoustic emissions. In M. Robinette & T. Glattke (Eds.), *Otoacoustic emissions: Clinical applications.* New York: Thieme

Mathers, C., Smith, A., & Concha, M. (2003). *Global burden of hearing loss in the year 2000.* Geneva: World Health Organization. http://www/who.int/health/statistics/bod_hearingloss.pdf

McMahon, C., Kifley A., Rochtchina, E., Newall, P., Mitchell P. (2008). The contribution of family history to hearing loss in an older population. *Ear and Hearing, 29,* 578–584

Mitchell, P., Gopinath, B., McMahon, C. M., Rochtchina, E., Wang, J. J., Boyages, S. C., et al. (2009, May). Relationship of type 2 diabetes to the prevalence, incidence and progression of age-related hearing loss. *Diabetic Medicine, 26,* 483–488

Mitchell, P., Gopinath, B., Wang, J., McMahon, C., Schneider, J., Rochtchina, E., et al. (2011). Five-year incidence and progression of hearing impairment in an older population. *Ear and Hearing, 32,* 251–257

Moscicki, E. K., Elkins, E. F., Baum, H. M., & McNamara, P. M. (1985, Jul-Aug). Hearing loss in the elderly: An epidemiologic study of the Framingham Heart Study Cohort. *Ear and Hearing, 6,* 184–190

Nondahl, D. M., Cruickshanks, K. J., Wiley, T. L., Klein, B. E., Klein, R., Chappell, R., et al. (2010, Aug). The ten-year incidence of tinnitus among older adults. *International Journal of Audiology, 49,* 580–585

Nondahl, D. M., Cruickshanks, K. J., Wiley, T. L., Klein, R., Klein, B. E., & Tweed, T. S. (2002, Jun). Prevalence and 5-year incidence of tinnitus among older adults: The epidemiology of hearing loss study. *Journal of the American Academy of Audiology, 13,* 323–331

Oeken, J., Lenk, A., & Bootz, F. (2000, Mar). Influence of age and presbyacusis on DPOAE. *Acta Oto-Laryngologica, 120,* 396–403

Osterhammel, D., & Osterhammel, P. (1979). Age and sex variations for the normal stapedial reflex thresholds and tympanometric compliance values. *Scandinavian Audiology, 8,* 153–158

Ouslander, J. G. (2010, Nov). A piece of my mind. A murmur of music. *Journal of the American Medical Association, 304,* 1875

Pearson, J. D., Morrell, C. H., Gordon-Salant, S., Brant, L. J., Metter, E. J., Klein, L. L., et al. (1995, Feb). Gender differences in a longitudinal study of age-associated hearing loss. *Journal of the Acoustical Society of America, 97,* 1196–1205

Pleis, J. R., & Lethbridge-Cejku, M. (2006, Dec). Summary health statistics for U.S. adults: National Health Interview Survey, 2005. *Vital and Health Statistics, Series 10, Data from the National Health Survey, 232,* 1–153 [PMID: 18361164]

Pratt, S. R., Kuller, L., Talbott, E. O., McHugh-Pemu, K., Buhari, A. M., & Xu, X. (2009, Aug). Prevalence of hearing loss in black and white elders: Results of the Cardiovascular Health Study. *Journal of Speech, Language, and Hearing Research, 52,* 973–989

Prieve, B. A., & Falter, S. R. (1995, Oct). COAEs and SSOAEs in adults with increased age. *Ear and Hearing, 16,* 521–528

Probst, R., Lonsbury-Martin, B. L., & Martin, G. K. (1991, May). A review of otoacoustic emissions. *Journal of the Acoustical Society of America, 89,* 2027–2067

Rawool, V. (1996). Effect of aging on the click-rate induced facilitation of acoustic reflex thresholds. *Journal of Gerontology Biological Sciences. 5IA,* BI24–BI3I

Rawool, V. W., & Harrington, B. T. (2007). Middle ear admittance and hearing abnormalities in individuals with osteoarthritis. *Audiology and Neuro-Otology, 12,* 127–136

Robinette, M. (1992). Clinical observations with transient evoked otoacoustic emissions with adults. *Seminars in Hearing, 13,* 23–36

Rosenhall, U., & Karlsson, A. K. (1991). Tinnitus in old age. *Scandinavian Audiology, 20,* 165–171

Schow, R. L., & Nerbonne, M. A. (1980, Feb). Hearing levels among elderly nursing home residents. *Journal of Speech and Hearing Disorders, 45,* 124–132

Silman, S. (1979, Sep). The effects of aging on the stapedius reflex thresholds. *Journal of the Acoustical Society of America, 66,* 735–738

Silman, S., & Gelfand, S. A. (1981, Aug). The relationship between magnitude of hearing loss and acoustic reflex threshold levels. *Journal of Speech and Hearing Disorders, 46,* 312–316

Sindhusake, D., Mitchell, P., Newall, P., Golding, M., Rochtchina, E., & Rubin, G. (2003, Jul). Prevalence and characteristics of tinnitus in older adults: The Blue Mountains Hearing Study. *International Journal of Audiology, 42,* 289–294

Stenklev, N. C., & Laukli, E. (2003, Apr). Transient evoked otoacoustic emissions in the elderly. *International Journal of Audiology, 42,* 132–139

Stover, L., & Norton, S. J. (1993, Nov). The effects of aging on otoacoustic emissions. *Journal of the Acoustical Society of America, 94,* 2670–2681

Thompson, D. J., Sills, J. A., Recke, K. S., & Bui, D. M. (1979, Mar). Acoustic admittance and the aging ear. *Journal of Speech and Hearing Research, 22,* 29–36

Uchida, Y., Ando, F., Shimokata, H., Sugiura, S., Ueda, H., & Nakashima, T. (2008, Apr). The effects of aging on distortion-product otoacoustic emissions in adults with normal hearing. *Ear and Hearing, 29,* 176–184[Ear Hear]

Wild, D. C., Brewster, M. J., & Banerjee, A. R. (2005, Dec). Noise-induced hearing loss is exacerbated by long-term smoking. *Clinical Otolaryngology, 30,* 517–520

Wiley, T. L., Chappell, R., Carmichael, L., Nondahl, D. M., & Cruickshanks, K. J. (2008, Apr). Changes in hearing thresholds over 10 years in older adults. *Journal of the American Academy of Audiology, 19,* 281–292, quiz 371

Wiley, T. L., Cruickshanks, K. J., Nondahl, D. M., & Tweed, T. S. (1999, Apr). Aging and middle ear resonance. *Ear and Hearing, 10,* 173–179

Wiley, T. L., Cruickshanks, K. J., Nondahl, D. M., Tweed, T. S., Klein, R., & Klein, B. E. (1996, Aug). Tympanometric measures in older adults. *Journal of the American Academy of Audiology, 7,* 260–268

Wiley, T. L., Cruickshanks, K. J., Nondahl, D. M., Tweed, T. S., Klein, R., Klein, R., et al. (1998, Oct). Aging and high-frequency hearing sensitivity. *Journal of Speech, Language, and Hearing Research, 41,* 1061–1072

Wiley, T. L., Nondahl, D. M., Cruickshanks, K. J., & Tweed, T. S. (2005, Mar). Five-year changes in middle ear function for older adults. *Journal of the American Academy of Audiology, 16,* 129–139

Wilson, R. H. (1981, Sep). The effects of aging on the magnitude of the acoustic reflex. *Journal of Speech and Hearing Research, 24,* 406–414

Wilson, R., & Margolis, R. (1991). Acoustic-reflex measurements. In W. Rintelmann (Ed.), *Hearing assessment* (2nd ed.). Austin: Pro-Ed

World Health Organization. (2010). Deafness and hearing impairment. Factsheet No. 300. Geneva: World Health Organization. http://www.who.int/mediacenter/factsheets/fs300/en/index.htms; http://www.who.int/health info/global_burden_disease/GBD_report_2004update_part3.pdf

Zhan, W., Cruickshanks, K. J., Klein, B. E., Klein, R., Huang, G. H., Pankow, J. S., et al. (2010, Jan). Generational differences in the prevalence of hearing impairment in older adults. *American Journal of Epidemiology, 171,* 260–266

Chapter 6

Speech Recognition and Functional Deficits

If only my hearing aids were less of a nuisance; they really do help me understand my friends and family more easily and with less effort.

—N.S., 84 years of age

Sometimes I think I am forgetting everything, but it is really that I am not understanding what my friends are saying, so it is not my memory, it is the input to my ears that is deficient.

—M.S., 91 years of age

Close inspection of their complaints suggests that a portion of seniors' speech-understanding difficulties derive from age-related declines in cognitive abilities, changes in higher-order auditory processes, or a combination of the two.

—Martin and Jerger (2005, p. 25)

◆ Learning Objectives

After reading this chapter, you should be able to

- distinguish among the various theories that attempt to explain speech-understanding deficits associated with aging;
- identify the elements accounting for variability in speech understanding characteristic of older adults;
- appreciate the complexity of the speech-understanding problems associated with aging; and
- appreciate the importance of a test battery approach to assessing and understanding the auditory deficits experienced by older adults.

◆ Overview

Age-related changes in the peripheral and central auditory pathways and in associated areas contribute differentially to deficits in speech understanding. Specifically, the degraded input from the periphery hampers cognitive processing, and in turn decrements in speech understanding, especially in complex listening environments, ensue (Cruickshanks, 2010). An understanding of the behavioral consequences of the physiological effects of aging throughout the peripheral and central auditory systems can guide the audiologist in selecting the most appropriate test protocols and targeted intervention strategies. This chapter highlights the results of recent studies on speech understanding related to cognitive factors, along with peripheral and central deficits.

◆ Speech Recognition Correlates of Aging

Age-related changes in the cochlea reduce spectral and temporal resolution and impair hearing sensitivity. These losses in resolution and audibility degrade the speech signal and lead to speech-understanding difficulties (Schneider, Daneman, Murphy, & See, 2000). Difficulty understanding speech is most pronounced in challenging listening conditions, notably in the presence of extraneous noise or reverberation or when people speak too quickly. There are large individual differences in the nature and extent of complaints voiced by older adults, and the emerging literature suggests that peripheral, perceptual, cognitive, and central factors interact with and contribute to speech-understanding difficulties. This chapter discusses the hypothesized factors and mechanisms that may underlie the speech-understanding difficulties experienced by our older clients with hearing problems. The perspective here is of necessity historical, as past research has informed current thinking. Historically, studies on speech understanding in the elderly have concluded that there are large individual differences in performance among individuals over 60 years of age, and the lack of audibility does not fully account for listener differences (George et al, 2007).

Several hypotheses guided by a report of the Committee on Hearing, Bioacoustics, and Biomechanics (CHABA, 1988) emerged in the late 1980s to explain the mechanisms underlying the speech-understanding problems experienced by older adults. These include the peripheral hypothesis, the central auditory hypothesis, and the cognitive hypothesis (Humes, 2002, 2005). In the peripheral hypothesis, the auditory periphery is implicated; in the central auditory hypothesis, any level along the brainstem pathways, auditory cortex, and associated areas is implicated; and in the cognitive hypothesis, the cortex, which is responsible for information processing, labeling, and storage, are implicated (Humes, 2005). Based on the report of the Berlin Aging Study (Baltes & Lindenberger, 1997), the extent to which speech understanding is affected by bottom-up or stimulus-driven factors (i.e., ear to brain) or top-down or knowledge-driven processes (i.e., brain to ear) has received considerable attention (Goldstein, 2002). Here the discussion focuses on whether it is the ear's analysis of the acoustic signal or the brain's ability to disambiguate and use knowledge acquired over time to assign meaning to utterances that sheds light on the speech-understanding deficits of older adults (Gatehouse, Naylor, & Elberling, 2003). Pichora-Fuller and Singh (2006) and Wingfield (1996) are credited with first challenging the traditional site-of-lesion view, suggesting an information degradation hypothesis that acknowledges that changes in audition and cognition are interrelated and account for speech-understanding problems especially in complex listening situations.

Beginning with the traditional, the peripheral hypothesis holds that the speech-recognition difficulties are attributable to audiometric hearing thresholds or individual differences in the encoding of sound by the outer ear through the inner ear and eighth nerve (George et al, 2007). The peripheral component is reflected in the frequency-specific sensitivity loss revealed by the audiogram, most notably in the high frequencies. The complaint, "I can hear speech, but cannot make out the words" is literally the behavioral response consistent with the peripheral hypothesis. The peripheral hypothesis has been further subdivided into two versions. One suggests that simple changes in audibility in which sound energy falls below an individual's audible region accounts for the speech-understanding problems characterizing older adults. The other suggests that reduced physiological processing associated with age-related changes in the cochlea creates distortions beyond loss-of-hearing sensitivity. Sources of distortion may arise from individual differences in other peripheral encoding mechanisms including loss of spectral and temporal resolution or loss of intensity discrimination.

The second hypothesis, namely the central auditory hypothesis, holds that age-related changes in the central auditory system including the auditory pathways of the brainstem or portions of the auditory cortex degrade the speech signal, leading to central auditory-processing disorders (George et al, 2007). Dysfunction in the auditory pathways within the brainstem or brain tends to impair neural transmission, feature extraction, information processing, labeling, or storage resulting in an impairment commonly referred to as a central auditory processing dysfunction (CAPD) (Humes, Christopherson, & Cokely, 1992). The term *central presbycusis* implies age-related changes in the auditory portions of the central auditory system, which impacts auditory perception and speech communication performance and is typically associated with difficulty understanding speech in noise (Humes et al, 2011). Age-related changes in the central auditory system either are attributable to biological aging or are a correlate or sequela of cochlea pathology (Pichora-Fuller & Singh, 2006). Poorer speech recognition performance in older individuals on measures of speech understanding involving time-altered or fast speech is a hallmark of auditory processing difficulties, as is difficulty understanding speech in noisy or reverberant listening conditions, in a background of modulated noise (Tremblay, Piskosz, & Souza, 2003) or in the presence of competing conversations.

Helfer (2009) offered an excellent description of the steps required to understand speech in the presence of competing noise, particularly conversations, that in my view is helpful in appreciating the complexity involved in decoding a message. The steps are as follows: (1) figuring out the message or determining who is the conversational partner, (2) directing attention to the speaker once he or she is identified, (3) separating out the target message from the background of other competing speakers, (4) maintaining attention on the target message while simultaneously ignoring the background conversations, and finally (5) dividing attention to monitor other ongoing conversations so as not to ignore others or with the intention of including them in the conversation. The challenge to the listener is heightened when there are several competing voices, when the target voice is similar to the competing voice, when the signal-to-noise ratio is unfavorable, when visual cues are unavailable, when the target voice is unfamiliar to the speaker or speech is accented, and when the competing voices are understandable. The fact that the nature of the competing message, be it informational masking or energetic masking, will influence the relative difficulty one encounters is in large part due to the processes involved in decoding the message. In addition to the filtering and attenuation effect of the peripheral hearing loss, understanding a message in the presence of competing speech is cognitively demanding, as it forces the listener to allocate attention effectively, and this ability is often compromised as individuals age.

The final hypothesis, known as the cognitive hypothesis, implicates higher centers in the auditory pathways as a source of individual variations in cognitive abilities. In these individuals, listening is an "effortful act." According to the cognitive hypothesis, nonauditory factors or top-down (brain to ear) cognitive functions, such as working memory capacity (the brain's ability to hold and process information relative to events occurring at that time), executive function, use of context, attention, or the rate at which information processing takes place, account in large part for individual differences in speech understanding (Pichora Fuller & Singh, 2006). Pichora Fuller and Singh (2006) contend that the interplay between cognition and audition, referred to by some as integrated processing, helps us to appreciate the speech-understanding difficulties experienced by older adults. When the speech signal is degraded by environmental factors or biological factors such as deficits in auditory processing, cognitive factors come into play, compromising speech understanding. It is noteworthy that cognitive deficits are not confined to the auditory modality; in fact, individual differences in short-term memory may emerge on tasks involving auditory or visual presentation of stimuli (Humes et al, 1992). **Figure 6.1** is a model of bottom-up and top-down processing of auditory input.

Pearl

The hearing loss of older adults is greatest in the frequency region (≥2000 Hz) for which the amplitude of speech is the lowest (Humes, Burk, Strauser, & Kinney, 2009).

In contrast to the site-of-lesion view described above, the processing view emerging from the Berlin Aging Study holds that the link between sensory and cognitive abilities or the intersystem connections are at the heart of the speech-understanding difficulties. The four hypotheses espoused by the Berlin group regarding perception and cognition have particular

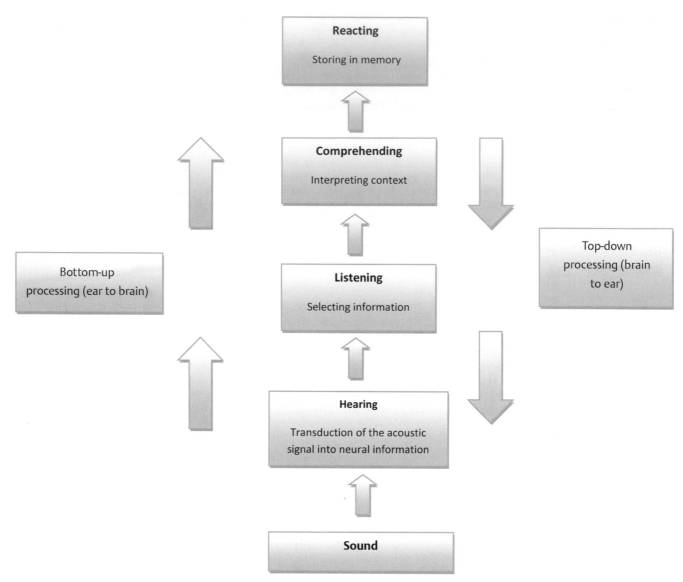

Fig. 6.1 Bottom-up versus top-down processing of auditory input. [Modified from Sweetow, R., & Sabes-Henderson, J. (2004). Components of communication. The case for LACE (listening and communication enhancement). *Hearing Journal, 57*, 32–38.]

relevance to speech understanding in terms of helping to grasp the perceptual mechanisms and the rationale for auditory-cognitive training to facilitate speech understanding (Linden-berger & Baltes, 1997; Pichora-Fuller, 2003a,b). The first hypothesis holds that the declines in perception and cognition are symptomatic of widespread neural degeneration consistent with the common cause hypothesis. Inconsistent with this hypothesis is a possible causal relationship between changes in audition and cognitive aging (Pichora-Fuller & Singh, 2006). The second hypothesis, namely the cognitive load on perception hypothesis, holds that cognitive decline hampers perceptual decline. This hypothesis is inconsistent with the findings of Wingfield (1996) that older adults are able to benefit more from contextual information than are younger adults. In contrast, the third hypothesis, the deprivation hypothesis, holds that perceptual decline leads to permanent cognitive decline,

which is supported by new evidence that amplification may reduce or forestall cognitive decline at least for the short term. The final hypothesis, namely the information degradation hypothesis, is consistent with the third hypothesis in that it holds that impoverished perceptual input results in compromised performance on cognitive tasks. This hypothesis, that degraded input hampers cognitive processing, is borne out by studies on speech understanding in complex listening environments, which because of increased listening effort and demands on cognitive processing, yield dramatic deficits in performance (Pichora-Fuller, 2003a,b).

The information degradation hypothesis has prompted a good deal of research that has shed light on how the interaction between changes in audition and cognition affect speech understanding in complex and demanding listening environments. The discussion to follow is a historical perspective of the classic articles helping to clarify the factors that explain the speech-understanding deficits of older adults. I first highlight classic studies that have paved the way for our current understanding of the complexity of speech understanding thanks to advances in the cognitive neuroscience of aging. Beginning with studies of speech in quiet conditions, we proceed to studies that conclude that compromised word recognition in acoustically challenging situations is complex due in large part to central aspects of auditory processing, especially temporal processing and cognitive declines. The important role that cognitive resources play in speech understanding, including working memory, top-down attentional mechanisms, and contextual factors, is cause for some optimism, given the volumes of literature on cognitive plasticity and its sustainability and transferability (Pichora Fuller & Singh, 2006). The discussion of cognitive aging will set the stage for the chapters on hearing aids, hearing-assistive technologies, and rehabilitation, which focus on the potential to ameliorate speech-understanding deficits by including auditory-based cognitive training.

Pearl

Because of the potential for "cognitive interference," older listeners have more difficulty than younger listeners when the target and the competing speech are similar (Helfer, 2009; Rossi-Katz & Arehart, 2009).

◆ Background History

Early studies using elderly participants found that speech-recognition scores in the elderly declined with increasing age and that performance on monosyllabic word-recognition tests was poorer than what would have been predicted from the audiogram. The term *phonemic regression* was coined by Gaeth (1948) to describe this phenomenon, in which older hearing-impaired adults experience more difficulty understanding speech than one would predict from the pure-tone audiogram. Recently, investigators have challenged Gaeth's hypothesis regarding age-related decrements in speech understanding. These investigators have speculated that earlier studies were most probably confounded by design problems, leading to erroneous conclusions regarding the contribution of age to decrements in speech understanding. More recent studies, such as those described in the following subsections, have attempted to compensate for the threats to the validity of earlier studies by employing better matching techniques and adaptive procedures for estimating word-recognition ability.

Pearl

Peripheral, central-auditory, and cognitive factors overlap, and it is therefore a challenge to disentangle and document them using behavioral measures (e.g., speech materials) (Humes et al, 2011).

The Peripheral Hypothesis

Studies attempting to explore the validity of the peripheral hypothesis have compared speech understanding of older and younger individuals with comparable hearing levels in quiet and in noise, have used spectrally shaped speech to minimize the role of audibility, and have manipulated the audibility of speech to remove this factor as a variable. One of the earliest studies, by Townsend and Bess (1980), included older participants with high-frequency hearing loss matched with a young hearing-impaired control group having a similar configuration. They found that speech-recognition ability in quiet was comparable for the two groups. Their study corroborated an earlier study, contrasting young and elderly participants with flat audiometric configurations and three-frequency pure-tone averages (PTAs) <50 dB HL. They too found that performance on monosyllabic word-recognition tasks in quiet was comparable. However, word-recognition ability did decline in older participants with hearing levels exceeding 49 dB HL, implicating audibility as a factor intertwined with age. In this study, the differences in word-recognition ability may be due to depressed hearing levels at 3000 or 4000 Hz, which was not taken into account when the groups were matched. The important contribution of high-frequency hearing to speech understanding is elucidated in the discussion that follows.

Dubno, Dirks, and Morgan (1984) employed an adaptive strategy to determine the effects of chronological age on speech-recognition ability in quiet and in noise. They noted that mean speech levels required for 50% recognition of spondee words, and of low- and high-predictability items of the speech perception in noise (SPIN) test presented without babble, were comparable for the normal and the hearing-impaired participants. That is, within each hearing-loss group, age effects were not observed for speech-recognition levels obtained in quiet at the hearing levels associated with 50% correct performance. It was of interest that the Articulation Index for 50% performance of low-predictability SPIN sentences in quiet was comparable for the young and old participants with and without hearing loss. The findings of this classic study support the conclusion that age effects are not observed for speech-recognition procedures conducted in the absence of a background of noise. Frisina and Frisina (1997) also noted that when Northwestern University (NU-6) word lists presented in quiet are used, word-recognition scores did not differ for young and older adults.

Gordon-Salant (1987a) conducted a comparative study of speech-recognition ability of young and older listeners with normal hearing and mild to moderate high-frequency sensorineural hearing loss. She compared open and closed set word-recognition scores for the NU-6 and modified rhyme test (MRT) word lists presented in quiet, at 80 dB sound pressure level (SPL) and at 90 dB SPL. In general, age effects were usually not observed for recognition of the monosyllabic word lists when presented in a quiet condition. Gordon-Salant and Fitzgibbons (1995a) confirmed these findings when they compared young and elderly listeners with normal hearing, and elderly listeners with mild to moderate sloping sensorineural hearing loss to young listeners with comparable hearing levels in their ability to recognize the low predictability SPIN sentences in quiet at 90 dB SPL. As is evident from **Table 6.1**, mean percent-correct

Table 6.1 Mean Percent-Correct Word-Recognition Scores and Standard Deviations for Young and Elderly Listeners Matched for Hearing Loss

Condition	Young Normal	Elderly Normal	Young Impaired	Elderly Impaired
SPIN-LP-Q	98.8% (1.9)	98.8% (1.9)	86.8% (10.5)	88.4% (10.7)

Abbreviation: SPIN-LP-Q, low-predictability speech perception in quiet.
Source: Data from Gordon-Salant, S., & Fitzgibbons, P. J. (1995a, Jun). Comparing recognition of distorted speech using an equivalent signal-to-noise ratio index. *Journal of Speech and Hearing Research, 38*, 706–713.

recognition scores were comparable for the young and old normal-hearing individuals and for the young and old hearing-impaired listeners. As would be expected, performance of the hearing impaired was poorer than that of the normal. This pattern emerged in the Dubno et al (1984) study as well.

Jerger and Hayes (1977) analyzed phonetically balanced–maximum (PB-max) scores obtained from performance intensity (PI) functions of 204 participants with sensorineural hearing loss associated with a cochlear site of lesion. They reported that when monosyllabic speech-recognition ability was assessed at suprathreshold levels (i.e., PB-max), performance was equivalent across hearing-impaired participants between 35 and 85 years of age. That is, mean percent-correct scores at PB-max were comparable across the age spectrum. Correlational studies using a variety of monosyllabic word-recognition materials confirmed the presence of a weak correlation between age and word-recognition ability as well.

The findings of Dubno, Lee, Matthews, and Mills (1997) are most compelling. They explored the relationship among gender, age, and word-recognition ability in a large sample of adults with sensorineural hearing loss of cochlear origin. Participants ranged in age from 55 to 84 years. Mean pure-tone thresholds were indicative of normal hearing in the low frequencies, sloping to the level of a mild to moderate hearing loss from 2000 to 8000 Hz. Word-recognition ability was assessed with a variety of materials including the NU-6 monosyllabic word lists, low- and high-predictability word lists from the SPIN test, and the Synthetic Sentence Identification (SSI) test materials. Participants in three age groups (55 to 64, 65 to 74, and 75 to 84) were selected to be closely matched for hearing level. Interestingly, mean scores on the speech-recognition tests were comparable across age groups for each of the six measures of speech recognition. Hence, the authors did not find a significant change in speech recognition with age when average pure-tone thresholds at each frequency were compared across age groups.

Special Consideration

The preponderance of evidence suggests that in good acoustic environments, when speech is presented at high enough levels to receive the weak acoustic cues inherent in the speech signal, age does not affect standard word-recognition ability in quiet for normal or hearing-impaired individuals. However, age effects are apparent when using nonsense syllables, an adaptive paradigm, and closed-set materials.

The studies of Gelfand, Piper and Silman (1986) and of Gordon-Salant (1987a) were among the first to suggest a possible cognitive overlay to the loss of audibility that might contribute to speech recognition deficits. Gelfand et al found that older adults with minimal hearing loss may experience difficulty understanding nonsense syllables presented in quiet. They assigned a sample of 64 adults with normal hearing to five age groups ranging from 20 to 69 years. Consonant recognition at the most comfortable listening (MCL) level in quiet was assessed using the nonsense syllable test (NST). Their findings suggest that consonant recognition assessed at MCL tends to decline systematically, albeit slightly, with increasing age. Gordon-Salant (1987a) employed an adaptive paradigm to compare speech-recognition performance of young (<42 years) and elderly (>65 years) normal-hearing participants. Open set (NU-6) and closed-set (MRT) monosyllabic word lists were used to gather information about speech-recognition ability. Age effects emerged and appeared to be task and condition dependent. Although mean speech-recognition percent scores of young normal-hearing participants were comparable in quiet for NU-6 and MRT word lists presented at 80 and 95 dB SPL, age effects did emerge for selected conditions in the hearing-impaired participants. Specifically, in quiet, at 95 dB SPL, mean word-recognition scores on the MRT were better for the young hearing-impaired as compared with the elderly hearing-impaired participants. Gordon-Salant concluded that although age effects for normal and hearing-impaired individuals did not emerge using the NU-6 word lists, a higher presentation level, coupled with a closed-set response task, helped to produce age effects in hearing-impaired participants, possibly due to the fact that performance on a closed-set response task such as the MRT may be confounded by cognitive status. It appears from most of the foregoing studies that age effects are not manifest for normal-hearing and elderly participants with minimal hearing loss when monosyllabic word lists are audible, of good quality, and presented in quiet, and that task complexity may influence outcomes.

Pearl

There does not appear to be a significant age effect for speech understanding when speech-recognition ability is sampled using traditional materials presented at high presentation levels in quiet. However, selected paradigms may be sensitive to uncovering cognitive age effects or factors beyond peripheral hearing status.

The Audibility Factor

In general, the preponderance of older studies on the relation between hearing level and speech perception in older adults suggest that speech-recognition performance of elderly listeners can be explained in large part by the audibility. Humes and colleagues have performed a series of studies designed to identify the correlates of speech-recognition performance among older adults. One of the first in the series was a comparative study among three groups of listeners: young normal-hearing adults, elderly hearing-impaired adults (65 to 75 years), and young normal-hearing adults with simulated sensorineural hearing loss comparable to that of the elderly sample (Humes & Roberts, 1990). Both groups had normal hearing out to 1000 Hz, sloping gradually from a mild to severe level. The full 11 subtests of the City University of New York (CUNY) NST served as the stimuli in the study. The speech materials were presented in quiet, noise, and in a reverberant environment in an attempt to sample a variety of acoustic conditions. The most striking finding was that the performance of young adults with simulated hearing loss was comparable to that of the older hearing-impaired adults across acoustic conditions. There were, however, large individual differences in performance among the older adults. Pearson product moment correlations between speech recognition performance and average hearing loss revealed that approximately 80% of the variance in speech identification scores could be accounted for by average high-frequency pure-tone hearing loss (1000, 2000, and 4000 Hz), irrespective of the listening condition. Using recordings of the MRT, Humes, Nelson, and Pisoni (1991) confirmed that much of the word-recognition difficulty experienced by older hearing-impaired adults is attributable to their hearing loss. Further, they found that older hearing-impaired adults who had difficulty with natural speech also had difficulty with synthetic speech and that the level of difficulty was similar to that in a sample of young adults with comparable simulated hearing loss. These data are consistent with the peripheral hypothesis, which ascribes individual differences in speech-recognition ability to the peripheral processing deficits accompanying sensorineural hearing loss.

Confirming the work of Humes and colleagues, van Rooij and Plomp (1992), and van Rooij, Plomp, and Orlebeke (1989) conducted a series of studies exploring the relation among auditive and cognitive factors in speech-understanding abilities of older adults. Their participants underwent a large battery of tests designed to measure several different modalities. Auditory function including sensitivity, frequency selectivity, and temporal resolution was assessed. Cognitive tests that assessed memory, processing speech, and intellectual abilities were administered. Speech understanding in quiet and noise and under varying conditions of reverberation was assessed using phonemes, spondees, and sentence materials. They found that the extent of high-frequency sensorineural hearing loss was the major factor accounting for individual differences in speech understanding among the elderly, and that cognitive status accounted for only a very small portion of additional variability.

Humes et al (1994) measured speech-recognition performance on a wide range of materials and listening conditions in a sample of 50 older adults 63 to 83 years of age. The goal of the study was to identify the variables that accounted for some of the individual differences in clinical measures of speech recognition. Participants had normal middle-ear function in the test ear as determined by results of immittance tests. Mean pure-tone thresholds were consistent with a mild to moderate sensorineural hearing loss primarily in the higher frequencies (1000 to 8000 Hz). All participants underwent a complete battery of speech tests, cognitive tests, and tests of auditory discrimination. Three sets of speech materials were used in this study: the CUNY NST, the Central Institute for the Deaf (CID) W-22 word lists, and the revised SPIN test. Selected speech tests were presented in quiet and noise, and some of the speech materials were spectrally shaped. Further, the speech tests were

Table 6.2 Mean Score in Percent on Five Speech Tests (*N* = 50)

Speech Materials	70 dB SPL		90 dB SPL	
	Quiet	Noise	Quiet	Noise
SPIN-LP	67.1	44.1	82.9	42.5
SPIN-HP	86.6	81.4	95.5	87.4
W-22S	85.5	72.0	90.1	72.1
W-22U	81.5	65.6	86.0	64.3
NST	71.4	55.3	78.9	61.1

Abbreviations: NST, nonsense syllable test; SPIN-HP, high-predictability speech perception in noise; SPIN-LP, low-predictability speech perception in noise; W-22S, Central Institute for the Deaf (CID) W-22 word lists spectrally shaped; W-22S, Central Institute for the Deaf (CID) W-22 word lists spectrally unshaped.

Source: Modified from Humes, L. E., Watson, B. U., Christensen, L. A., Cokely, C. G., Halling, D. C., & Lee, L. (1994, Apr). Factors associated with individual differences in clinical measures of speech recognition among the elderly. *Journal of Speech and Hearing Research, 37*, 465–474.

presented at two levels, 70 and 90 dB SPL. In total, 20 measures of speech recognition were administered to each of the 50 participants over four test sessions.

Table 6.2 presents mean performance for the participants on the five speech tests in quiet and noise at 70 and 90 dB SPL. Several trends emerged. First, performance in quiet was better than performance in noise on all speech tests. Next, participants performed better at the higher presentation level in quiet. However, this trend was not as clear-cut in noise. Finally, in quiet and noise, at 70 and at 90 dB SPL, participants overwhelmingly performed best on the high-predictability SPIN (SPIN-HP). A correlational analysis among the speech-recognition measures revealed a strong correlation among measures, suggesting that participants who obtained a high score on one of the speech-recognition measures likely scored high on the other tests. Similarly, participants scoring poorly on one task tended to perform poorly on all of the speech-recognition tasks. Results of the principal components analysis among the 20 speech-recognition measures and hearing loss showed that 74% of the variance in scores on the speech-recognition measures could be accounted for by the peripheral hearing status. That is, among the 50 older adults participating in the study, individual differences in average high-frequency hearing loss accounted for the bulk of the variability in performance on speech-recognition tests, across a variety of materials and conditions (Humes et al, 1994).

The findings of van Rooij et al (1989) and van Rooij and Plomp (1992) are in agreement with Humes and colleagues' findings in that they too found that high-frequency hearing loss was highly predictive of speech-understanding ability. Their findings suggest that the degree of sensorineural hearing loss is the primary factor accounting for individual differences in speech recognition in the elderly. Their participants ranged in age from 60 to 93 years and presented with symmetrical high-frequency hearing loss. Speech materials primarily consisted of tests of phoneme perception and spondee perception in noise. van Rooij and Plomp (1992) found that speech perception ability correlated with age as well. However, a large component of the latter relation was attributable to the association between progressive high-frequency hearing loss and age. Their conclusion, that hearing loss is the primary determinant

Table 6.3 Correlation Among Speech Recognition Measures and Hearing Loss Along with Percentage of Variance Explained

	DSI	SSI	SPIN-HP	SPIN-LP	PB
Correlation	−.55	−.65	−.73	−.78	−.76
% Variance explained	30	42	54	61	58

Abbreviations: DSI, dichotic sentence identification; PB, phonetically balanced; SPIN-HP, high-predictability speech perception in noise; SPIN-LP, low-predictability speech perception in noise; SSI, Synthetic Sentence Identification.

of individual differences in speech-recognition ability of older adults, has been echoed by Jerger, Jerger, and Pirozzolo (1991); Helfer and Wilber (1990); Divenyi and Haupt (1997a); Wiley et al (1998), and other investigators.

Jerger et al (1991) administered a battery of speech audiometric and neuropsychological measures to a sample of 200 older adults (mean age = 69.7 years) to determine the contribution of these factors to speech recognition performance. The average high-frequency hearing loss (average of 1000, 2000, and 4000 Hz) of participants in the sample was 32 dB HL for the right ear and 31 dB HL for the left ear. The speech materials included the phonetically balanced (PB) word test, the SSI test, SPIN test, and the dichotic sentence identification (DSI) test. Once again, across all of the test conditions, the most powerful predictor of speech-recognition performance was degree of hearing loss. Age was significantly correlated with speech-recognition performance. As will be discussed in a later section, cognitive status affected speech-recognition performance on selected measures as well. With regard to the latter, the Wechsler Adult Intelligence Scale (WAIS) digit-symbol score accounted for 13% of the variance in scores on the DSI. **Table 6.3** shows the correlations among the speech measures and hearing status.

Dubno and Schaefer (1992) confirmed the primary source for the speech-understanding difficulties of hearing-impaired adults to be reduction in audibility of important portions of the speech signal. They argued that loss of frequency selectivity is not strongly associated with deficits in consonant recognition. Using a paradigm similar to that of Humes and colleagues, Dubno and Schaefer compared frequency selectivity and speech-recognition performance of hearing-impaired listeners with that of a sample of masked normal-hearing listeners with comparable thresholds. Although frequency selectivity was poorer for the hearing-impaired listeners, their consonant-recognition scores fell within the range of scores for the masked normal-hearing participants. They concluded that their data support the hypothesis that differences in speech-spectrum audibility accounts for a significant proportion of the variance in speech-recognition scores of the hearing impaired (Dubno, Horwitz, & Ahlstrom, 2007).

Several interesting trends emerged in a study conducted by Gordon-Salant (1987b) of consonant recognition and confusion patterns among elderly participants with normal hearing and hearing impairment. Three groups of participants ranging in age from 65 to 75 years participated. The first group had normal hearing, the second had sensorineural hearing loss with gradually sloping configurations, and the third had sen-

sorineural hearing loss with sharply sloping configurations. Consonant recognition was assessed at 70 and 90 dB SPL in the presence of a +6-dB signal-to-babble ratio. Consonant recognition in noise at 75 and 90 dB HL was best among normal-hearing elderly and poorest among those with sharply sloping configurations. Consonants paired with /u/ were recognized with greater accuracy than those paired with /i/ and /a/. At the higher presentation level, normal-hearing elderly and participants with gradually sloping loss achieved higher consonant-recognition scores than did those with sharply sloping loss. Performance differences emerged as a function of hearing-loss group and presentation level. Finally, differences in consonant-recognition patterns were found between normal-hearing and hearing-impaired participants, but few differences were found between the hearing-impaired participant groups in terms of error patterns. That is, the hearing-loss configuration did not affect the pattern of errors in consonant recognition. Gordon-Salant concluded that the attenuation imposed by the hearing loss that could not be compensated for by a higher presentation level accounted for decrements in consonant recognition. Further, hearing loss experienced by older adults does not appear to affect the pattern of performance. Her data, once again, lent some support to the audibility model. Using the Articulation Index (AI) framework to explore the role of speech acoustics and audibility of the speech area to speech-understanding performance, investigators have confirmed that more than 50% of the variance on speech measures is accounted for by peripheral hearing status as measured using AI values (Humes, 2002).

More recently, Dubno et al (2008) conducted a longitudinal study of change in speech recognition for isolated monosyllabic words in quiet and for key words presented in low- and high-context sentences in babble (SPIN). Followed over a period of 3 to 15 years, participants were over 55 years of age, were free of active otological disease, and they passed a cognitive screening test. The mean age of participants undergoing monosyllabic word recognition testing at the beginning of the study was 67.6 years and the mean age at the time of the last test was 75 years. Similarly, the mean age of participants taking the low- and high-context sentences in babble (SPIN) test was 67 years at the first measurement and 77.2 years at the last measure. Pure-tone thresholds were measured annually as were scores on recognition of the NU-6 words lists. In contrast, SPIN testing was administered at 2- to 3-year intervals; thus, participants undergoing SPIN testing remained in the study for approximately 3 years longer than those who did not. The signal-to-babble ratio for the SPIN sentences presented at 50 dB above a babble threshold was +8 dB. Mean four-frequency PTAs (500, 1000, 2000, and 4000 Hz) changed 15.5 dB HL over the 14-year time span of the participants being followed; hence, the presentation level for the NU-6 word lists varied in accordance with the change in speech recognition threshold (SRT)(words were presented relative to the SRT). Further, adjusted word-recognition scores, which were calculated, took into account changes in audibility attributable to changes in pure-tone thresholds and presentation level for the NU-6 word lists. In general, word recognition scores for the NU-6 word lists declined significantly over time even when accounting for age-related changes in audibility of speech due to change in peripheral hearing levels.

Dubno and colleagues (2008) noted that the rate of decline in word-recognition scores was fastest in those with the most severe hearing loss, and the rate of decline increased as initial hearing loss increased even when hearing level–related differences in audibility were taken into account. Interestingly, the authors did not note an age effect on the initial rate of decline in word-recognition scores, leading them to conclude that underlying peripheral distortions rather than age was a variable underlying the change in word recognition. They did, however, note a gender effect, with changes in word recognition occurring more rapidly for women than for men, unrelated to age-related changes in hearing threshold levels. The authors found that initial hearing levels played a role in the change in word-recognition scores as did serum progesterone levels. Interestingly, women with higher levels of progesterone in their blood had faster decline in word recognition than did women with lower levels of progesterone. In looking at change in scores on word recognition in quiet using the NU-6 word lists over time, Dubno and colleagues found that the magnitude of change with age was greater than that predicted using the AI and pure-tone levels. Interestingly, a similar trend did not emerge with the SPIN sentence materials. That is, key word recognition for low- and high-context sentences did not change with increasing age, suggesting that when words are presented with syntactic and semantic content, they may be less susceptible to age effects.

In summary, the decline in word-recognition ability for monosyllabic words in quiet with age was greater than the decline in pure-tone thresholds over time in this sample. However, the correlational analysis did reveal that high-frequency thresholds accounted for 36 to 41% of the variability in word-recognition scores. Dubno and colleagues attributed their findings to underlying changes in auditory function resulting from peripheral rather than cognitive or central pathology. The fact the rate of decline in word-recognition ability increased as initial hearing loss increased, even after taking into account hearing level–related differences in audibility coupled with the fact that initial age did not affect the rate of decline in word recognition, underscores the thesis that age-related decline in word recognition is attributable to peripheral auditory factors rather than central variables. Dubno et al did speculate that since individuals with poorer baseline PTAs had faster rates of decline, the common cause hypothesis of Baltes and Lindenberger (1997) could be at play (**Fig. 6.2**).

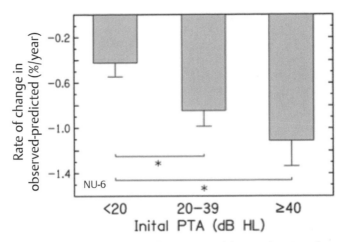

Fig. 6.2 Rate of decline in word recognition ability as a function of baseline pure-tone average (PTA; in dB HL). [From Dubno, J. R., Lee, F. S., Matthews, L. J., Ahlstrom, J. B., Horwitz, A. R., & Mills, J. H. (2008, Jan). Longitudinal changes in speech recognition in older persons. *Journal of the Acoustical Society of America, 123*, 462–475. Reprinted by permission.]

Pearl

Auditory deficits directly affect speech understanding by altering the number of words perceived correctly and indirectly because the listening effort required to understand consumes cognitive resources necessary for understanding (George et al, 2007). The audibility of speech is a primary contributor to variations in word-recognition scores in older adults (Wiley et al, 1998).

Gender Differences

In an effort to isolate the variables that might account for individual differences in word-recognition ability characterizing older adults, Wiley et al (1998) reported on data evolving from an epidemiological study of hearing in older adults living in Beaver Dam, Wisconsin. The mean age of the 3753 participants was 65.8 years; 57.5% of the participants were women and 98.9% were non-Hispanic whites. For the most part, participants presented with high-frequency sensorineural hearing loss, which overall tended to be mild to moderate in degree, with individuals over 80 years of age presenting with poorer hearing levels. Interestingly, a strong gender difference in word-recognition ability emerged in quiet and noise. In general, word-recognition ability using the NU-6 word lists presented in quiet was better for women than for men across age groups. When participants were stratified by gender and hearing-loss category, women tended to have better word-recognition ability than men of comparable age and hearing level. The latter trend emerged when word-recognition ability was assessed in the presence of a competing message (signal-to-noise ratio [SNR] = +8). After adjusting for age, Wiley and colleagues found that word-recognition scores in the presence of a competing message were better for women than for men overall and within all hearing-loss categories. As would be expected, word-recognition ability was significantly poorer when assessed in noise than in quiet. Interestingly, results of the analysis of covariance revealed that pure-tone hearing sensitivity accounted for the greatest proportion of the variance in word-recognition scores in quiet (26%) and in competing noise (48%), whereas gender accounted for a small proportion of the variance in word-recognition scores in quiet (4%) and in competing noise (9%). It is of interest that age, when entered into the equation alone, accounted for a considerable amount of the variance in speech-understanding ability when assessed in the presence of competing noise.

As previously discussed, Dubno et al (1997) were also interested in isolating factors that might account for individual differences in word-recognition ability with age. When they cast the pure-tone data as a function of gender, mean pure-tone thresholds for men were poorer than those for women, an expected finding. PTA accounted for more of the variance in speech-recognition scores for women (0.395 to 0.739) than for men (0.289 to 0.464). Interestingly, when word-recognition score and age were controlled for their mutual relation with PTA, the relation between word-recognition ability and age was reduced dramatically to a statistically insignificant level. Stated differently, in women the correlation between word-recognition ability and age is minimal when controlling for the effect of hearing level (R^2 = 0.02). The latter was not the case for men, where nearly 12% of the variance in scores on word-recognition tests was accounted for by age, after controlling for PTA. Hence, PTA and age account for some of the variance in speech-recognition scores in men. Audibility accounts for the largest proportion of the variance in speech-recognition scores for men and women, but more for women than for men.

The anatomical and physiological changes in the auditory periphery including the cochlea and the auditory nerve are associated with elevated thresholds, reduced cochlear compression, and broader tuning curves (Humes & Dubno, 2010). The resulting sensorineural hearing loss of the listener systematically emerges as the primary variable accounting for performance on measures of speech understanding. The work of Humes and his colleagues in the Audiology Research Laboratory at Indiana University and of van Rooij and Plomp (1990), van Rooij et al, (1989), Gordon-Salant and Fitzgibbons (2001) ,and Humes and colleagues (2011) is rather conclusive regarding the primacy of peripheral hearing sensitivity as a determinant of speech understanding of older adults (Humes, 2007). When listening to speech presented in quiet over a range of 60 to 90 dB SPL, 50 to 90% of the variance in performance on speech recognition tasks can be accounted for by high-frequency hearing thresholds (Humes & Dubno, 2010). Similarly, high-frequency hearing loss contributes to individual variability, albeit to a lesser extent, in performance on speech tasks that have been temporally distorted (time compression and reverberation) or when speech is presented in the presence of temporally interrupted noise (Gordon Salant & Fitzgibbons, 1997; Humes, 2005).

Pearl

Peripheral factors including elevated thresholds and broadened tuning curves account for a minimal amount of the variability in performance on challenging listening tasks (e.g., when background noise is temporally distorted) (Humes & Dubno, 2010).

Central Auditory Hypothesis

Several investigators have hypothesized that the speech-recognition deficits of elderly listeners are attributable to structural or functional changes in the auditory pathways of the brainstem or in the auditory cortex. Age-related changes in the latter structures appear to account in part for the decrements in speech-understanding performance on temporally distorted speech, dichotic speech, and speech tasks presented in a background of temporally interrupted background noise (Humes & Dubno, 2010). Underlying these problems appears to be a difficulty perceiving and extracting temporal informa-

tion from the speech signal. The principle behind central auditory processing tests using the latter measures is that stressing the auditory system by forcing the individual to understand speech in unfavorable conditions enables audiologists to uncover deficits due to changes in the central auditory processing system. Further, most of the tests require the patient to use selective attention skills, which translates into increased listening effort to understand the target speech signal while repressing a competing message presented to the nontest ear. The increased cognitive demand posed by deficits in temporal processing is emerging as a variable underlying the speech-understanding deficits in older adults. In light of the above, defining CAPD is difficult, but Gates, Anderson, Feeney, McCurry, & Larson (2008a) define CAPD as referring to persons with normal or near-normal hearing and understanding in quiet yet with substantial difficulty understanding in the presence of auditory stressors such as competing noise (selected types) and other difficult listening situations. A traditional test paradigm involves evaluating how well an individual functions in the presence of competing signals or using temporally distorted messages. We now are aware that these approaches require adequate short-term memory, processing speed, and effort, so it is increasingly difficult to separate CAPD from cognitive aging.

Pearl

The majority of studies on temporal discrimination using nonspeech stimuli, specifically gap-detection measures, have concluded that in most cases older adults perform worse than younger adults and that hearing loss is seldom a contributing factor to the findings (Humes et al, 2011).

Table 6.4 summarizes possible changes in temporal processing along with approaches to their measurement. Deficits in understanding artificially speeded speech, which have been attributed to generalized declines in speed of processing, have been most readily highlighted in older adults using time-compressed speech. The traditional thinking has been that time-compressed speech increases the rate of flow of information and degrades and distorts speech, thereby disadvantaging older adults. More recently, many have speculated that older adults have more difficulty understanding speeded speech not only because of hearing deficits but because of age-related slowing in cognitive, semantic, and linguistic functioning or processing (Pichora-Fuller, 2003a,b; Schneider, Daneman, & Murphy, 2005).

Special Consideration

The odds of demonstrating abnormality on tests of auditory processing increases dramatically by 4 to 9% per year among older participants (Golding, Taylor, Cupples, & Mitchell, 2006).

The theory that hearing loss for speech arises because sensorineural hearing impairment attenuates the auditory signal and

Table 6.4 Measures of Temporal Processing

Function Assessed	Measure	Challenge for the Older Adult
Temporal acuity: assesses the smallest silent interval or gap inserted within a continuous signal that a listener can detect	Gap detection: listeners are asked to make judgments about the presence of a silent interval to identify specific phonemes (nonspeech stimuli)	Age effects emerge when the location of the gap is not as easily detected
Perception of temporal order processing ability: assesses ability to discriminate or recall the order of different stimuli in a sequence	Temporal order recall tasks presented at fast rates	Age effects emerge when, for fast presentation rates, component tones or contiguous tones are very brief in duration
Temporal patterning or rhythm of speech	Ability to recall a message when the temporal prosody is disrupted	Older adults exhibit difficulty when asked to discriminate the patterning of a sequence for sequences that are temporally or spectrally complex
Gap threshold	Gaps-in-noise (GIN) test: estimates gap threshold in presence of broadband noise at various presentation levels	Older adults have a higher gap threshold than do younger adults

Source: From Gordon-Salant, S. (2006). Speech perception and auditory temporal processing performance by older listeners: Implications for real-world communication. *Seminars in Hearing, 27*, 264–268. (Reprinted by permission)

introduces distortion even when speech is presented within the audible range of the individual has held up throughout the decades (Humes & Dubno, 2010; Plomp & Duquesny, 1982). According to Plomp and Duquesny (1982), attenuation that results from the threshold loss causes speech and noise signals to fall below the individual's audible region. Difficulty understanding speech in noise, which is characteristic of the vast majority of elderly listeners, may be due in part to the distortion component accompanying the sensitivity loss. The distortion factor results in a reduction in the "functional" SNR. Further, distortion may be associated with deficits in frequency resolution, or temporal resolution, or frequency or intensity discrimination, and so on, even when speech is within the audible range of the individual (Crandell, Henoch, & Dunkerson, 1991).

The first series of studies below focuses on the controversy over the extent to which CAPD is a principal cause of speech-perception deficits in the elderly. Studies on prevalence of CAPD in older adults yield estimates ranging from 10 to 90%. Stach, Spretnjak, and Jerger (1990) were among the first investigators to report on the prevalence of central presbycusis as a function of age in a clinical population. Mean PTAs of their participants ranged from 15 dB HL in the youngest group (50 to 54 years of age) to 40 dB HL in the oldest group (80+ years of age). They defined central presbycusis operationally, based on the pattern of test scores that emerged when comparing results on the SSI test to those on the profile of aided loudness (PAL) PB-50 word lists. According to their definition of CAPD, 17% of persons 50 to 54 years of age, 58% of persons between 65 and 69 years, and 90 to 95% of persons 80 years or older showed evidence of central presbycusis. They concluded that in their sample, 70% of persons over the age of 60 had some degree of speech-understanding deficit that could not be explained on the basis of pure-tone hearing levels.

Using a different definition of CAPD, Jerger, Jerger, Oliver, and Pirozzolo (1989), namely PB-SSI differences of more than 20%, abnormal SPIN scores, or inter-ear differences on the DSI test that exceeded a criterion level, they reported the prevalence of CAPD to be 50% among hearing-impaired adults over

51 years of age. In their sample, cognitive deficits emerged in 54% of participants with CAPD and in 28% of those without CAPD. Cooper and Gates (1991), using a stratified random sample of the United States population, reported that the prevalence of CAPD may be less than previously believed. They administered a series of central auditory tests to a large sample of adults over 60 years of age. For the most part, mean three-frequency PTAs were within normal limits. Speech-recognition performance was assessed using CID W-22 word lists, the Synthetic Sentence Identification with Ipsilateral Competing Message (SSI-ICM), and the staggered spondaic word (SSW) test. Rollover was considered significant and indicative of the presence of CAPD if the rollover index exceeded 0.20 for the CID W-22 word lists. For the synthetic sentences presented with an ipsilateral competing message at a 0 dB message-to-competition ration (MCR), rollover was considered significant and CAPD present if the difference between the minimal and maximal level was more than 20 percentage points. On the SSW test, evidence of CAPD was based on adult norms for the test. The overall prevalence of CAPD in their sample was 22.6% based on abnormal findings on any one of the above speech tests. More recently, Golding, Carter, Mitchell, & Hood (2004) estimated the prevalence of CAPD to be close to 75% among their sample of participants over 55 years of age in their Blue Mountains Hearing Study (BMHS) based on Australian measures of speech tests used to measure central auditory processing including dichotic sentences and synthetic sentence materials. Their sample was free of cognitive deficits and had essentially normal hearing.

Cooper and Gates (1991) attempted to analyze the rate of CAPD as a function of speech test to clarify the relation between CAPD prevalence and test sensitivity. They found that prevalence rates did in fact differ according to the criterion measure. The rate of CAPD was highest, 18%, when comparing PB-max to SSI-ICM scores at a 0 dB MCR. The rate was lowest, 1.4%, using the PI-PB rollover (RO) index as the criterion measure. When the total corrected SSW error score was the criterion measure for CAPD, the prevalence rate was 10.7%. It was of interest that the prevalence rate declined when the criterion for CAPD was made more stringent, namely abnormal performance on two out of three tests of CAPD, or on all three tests of CAPD. This finding lends support to the theory that loose criterion for CAPD may inflate prevalence estimates (Humes et al, 1992). Also, although chronological age had a statistically significant effect on the rate of CAPD, it accounted for no more than 15% of the variability on the three indices of CAPD. Cooper and Gates concluded that age was not a dominant factor in the etiology of CAPD. However, age may function to increase the likelihood of exposure to events that may produce CAPD. A cautionary note is in order based on the association between scores on the SSI and peripheral hearing levels. Prevalence rates based on performance on tests of central auditory functions, especially, the SSI, may be somewhat inflated due to the confounding presence of peripheral hearing loss (Divenyi & Haupt, 1997b; Humes, 1996).

A few investigators have considered the question of prevalence using a sample of patients with confirmed Alzheimer's disease (AD). This population lends itself nicely to the question because of focal deficits in temporal areas of the brain. In addition, early studies have shown a relation between performance on tests of the central auditory nervous system and neuroanatomical, physiological, and cognitive function in a sample of patients with AD. The rationale for these inquires is the finding of a clinically significant relation between central auditory function and tests of cognition in adults with dementia (Gates et al, 1996; Grimes, Grady, Foster, Sunderland, & Patronas, 1985). Strouse, Hall, and Burger (1995) compared performance of adults with and without a diagnosis of AD on a battery of behavioral tests designed to assess central auditory processing ability. Participants in the Alzheimer's group had a mean age of 72 years, a mean high-frequency PTA of 36 dB HL, and mean monosyllabic word-recognition score of 95%. Participants in the control group had a mean age of 70 years, a mean high-frequency PTA of 28.2 dB HL, and a mean monosyllabic word-recognition score of 98%. Statistical analyses showed that the groups were comparable on the preceding measures. Distortion product otoacoustic emissions found that peripheral auditory status was equivalent for both groups. The prevalence of CAPD, defined as an abnormal score on one or more of the five CAPD measures, was 100% for the Alzheimer's group versus 30% for the control group of older adults. On the more widely used scales of central auditory processing ability, namely, the SSI and the DSI, scores for all control participants were within the normal range.

Thus, a number of studies have been conducted to determine the prevalence of CAPD in older adults. Some studies have estimated a prevalence rate of 50 to 70%, with prevalence increasing as a function of age. Other studies have reported prevalence rates of 20 to 30% among older adults with minimal peripheral-hearing loss. The more stringent the criterion for CAPD, the less likely the existence of measured CAPD. The evidence concerning CAPD as a factor in the speech-perception problems of older adults is incomplete given its interaction with cognitive function. However, even a prevalence rate as low as 20% would suggest that audiologists must measure central auditory processing ability in older adults to determine which older adults are afflicted, as this will inform decisions regarding management.

External distortions such as noise explain in part the speech-recognition deficits experienced by older adults. As discussed in an earlier section, Dubno et al (1984) used an adaptive procedure, spondee words, and the high- and low-predictability items on the SPIN test to assess speech-recognition differences between young (<44 years of age) and elderly (>65 years of age) listeners with normal hearing and mild sensorineural hearing loss. They found that elderly listeners with and without hearing loss performed more poorly than younger listeners with matched hearing sensitivity in their recognition of low-predictability items from the SPIN test presented in the presence of multi-talker babble. Similarly, irrespective of speech level (i.e., 56, 72, and 88 dB SPL), normal and hearing-impaired participants over 65 years of age required more advantageous signal-to-babble ratios to achieve a 50% criterion score on the low-predictability sentences. Pure-tone thresholds of participants could not be used to accurately predict overall performance in quiet and noise, underlining the large individual variability inherent in sentence recognition. Dubno et al's findings were noteworthy in that they suggested that even in the presence of normal hearing, older listeners require more advantageous signal-to-babble ratios for their performance to be equivalent to young normal-hearing participants. Frisina and Frisina (1997) also found that even after adjusting for audibility, older adults have greater difficulty understanding words in the presence of noise than do young adults. Dubno et al hypothesized that age effects on speech-recognition in noise may be a result of the peripheral effects of the aging process in combination with central processing dysfunction.

Pearl

Age, independent of hearing loss, is a significant variable affecting speech-recognition ability in noise.

Gordon-Salant (1987a) employed an adaptive paradigm to compare speech-recognition performance of young (<42 years) and elderly (>65 years) normal-hearing and hearing-impaired participants when speech was presented in fixed-noise conditions. Open- (NU-6) and closed-set (MRT) monosyllabic word lists presented in the presence of 12-talker babble were used to gather information about speech-recognition ability. In addition to comparing percent-correct word-recognition scores, mean signal-to-babble ratios required for 50% criterion scores on the word lists were compared. The results were noteworthy, supporting for the most part the conclusions of earlier investigators. Age effects did emerge for selected conditions in the hearing-impaired participants. Specifically, mean percent-correct recognition scores on the MRT were significantly higher for the younger hearing-impaired participants than for older hearing-impaired participants in noise at both presentation levels. Age effects were most apparent when the adaptive strategy was applied to determine mean signal-to-babble ratios necessary for 50% criterion scores. Age effects emerged for the normal and hearing-impaired participants and for the young and older participants, such that older participants consistently required more favorable signal-to-babble ratios to achieve 50% criterion scores. The conclusions to be reached from this study are as follows: (1) age effects can emerge independent of hearing loss using an adaptive noise paradigm, (2) testing in noise helps to produce age effects in both normal and hearing-impaired participants, and (3) fixed-noise paradigms are less effective than an adaptive paradigm in uncovering age effects on speech-recognition tasks.

Although there is evidence suggesting that the elderly perform more poorly than younger listeners on speech tasks presented in noise, the large individual differences among the elderly in their susceptibility to noise is a critical factor as well. Crandell (1991) examined speech-recognition performance of 26 older adults with mild to moderate high-frequency sensorineural hearing loss. Speech-recognition ability was assessed using the high-predictability sentences from the SPIN test presented in quiet and in the presence of multi-talker babble. The most notable finding was the lack of a relation between word-recognition ability in quiet and in noise. That is, speech-recognition ability in noise could not be predicted from that obtained in quiet. Similarly, participants with comparable speech-recognition scores in quiet differed dramatically in their speech-recognition performance in noise. This apparent individual susceptibility to noise underlines the importance of performing tests of speech understanding in both quiet and in noise to determine the quality of the peripheral deficit and the technology most appropriate for the older adult with hearing impairment.

Gordon-Salant and Fitzgibbons (1995b) assessed the impact of age and hearing loss on recognition of undistorted speech materials (i.e., low-predictability SPIN [SPIN-LP] sentence-materials) presented at various SNRs. Forty participants were assigned to one of four groups: normal-hearing young and elderly, and hearing-impaired young and elderly. The hearing-impaired participants presented with essentially mild to moderate sensorineural hearing loss. The SPIN-LP sentences were presented in five noise conditions at 90 dB SPL. The SNRs were as follows: –8 dB, 0 dB, +8 dB, +16 dB, and +24 dB. As would be expected, hearing level influenced recognition scores. Listeners with hearing loss performed more poorly than listeners with normal hearing at all SNRs. The impact of age on speech-recognition ability was highly dependent on the difficulty of the listening condition such that at 0 dB SNR younger listeners scored better than older listeners. However, at more favorable SNRs such as +8 dB, +16 dB, and +24 dB, age-related differences did not emerge. It was noteworthy that at all SNRs, performance of the normals was comparable irrespective of condition, whereas at 0 dB SNR the mean percent-correct scores were poorer for the elderly hearing impaired even at a relatively high presentation level. Humes et al (1994) found that even when the presentation level is increased (e.g., 70 to 90 dB SPL), speech-recognition ability in noise remains compromised in older adults with mild to moderate high-frequency sensorineural hearing loss for a range of materials, including the revised SPIN test, CUNY NST, and CID W-22 unshaped or shaped word lists. Wiley et al (1998) tested a large sample of older adults with varying degrees of sensorineural hearing loss and found, as well, that word-recognition ability in the presence of a competing message decreased with increasing age. Hence, decrements in word-recognition ability in the presence of noise are attributable in part to age, even when controlling for audibility.

Pearl

Compensating for audibility (e.g., high-presentation level) may not improve speech-recognition ability in the presence of noise.

Gordon-Salant and Fitzgibbons (1997) conducted a series of psychoacoustic studies in the late 1990s to explore the contribution of auditory temporal processing ability to speech understanding. Gordon-Salant and Fitzgibbons (1995b) examined the effects of multiple stimulus degradations on speech-recognition performance of young and old listeners with normal hearing and mild to moderate sensorineural hearing loss. Speech-recognition ability was assessed using low-predictability items from the revised speech perception in noise (SPIN-R) test presented in undistorted form, presented in the presence of reverberation, and with the temporal characteristics distorted via time compression, which merely increased the rate of speech without producing spectral distortions. A time-compression ratio of 40% and a fixed reverberation time of 0.3 seconds were used. Finally, 12-talker babble presented at an SNR of +16 dB was used as a form of degradation as well. In total, seven listening conditions of varying levels of distortion were presented in a randomized fashion to the participants at a fixed level of 90 dB SPL. Their findings support the theory that external distortions such as reverberation, noise, and fast speech may interact with even minor internal distortions (little or no peripheral hearing loss) to disadvantage older listeners (Helfer, 1991). Specifically, they found the following: (1) elderly listeners with normal hearing performed more poorly than younger listeners on time-compressed materials presented in quiet, (2) elderly listeners with normal hearing performed more poorly than young listeners with normal hearing in the time-compressed and reverberant-speech condition and the time-compressed and noise condition, (3) elderly hearing-impaired listeners performed more poorly than young listeners with comparable hearing levels in the time-compressed and noise conditions and in the time-compressed plus reverberant-speech condition, and (4) speech-recognition deficits for the young and older listeners with and without hearing loss were greatest in the condition combining time compression and reverberation. In light of the above findings, the authors concluded that age effects are pronounced even in the presence of minimal hearing loss when speech materials are subjected to multiple external distortions, most notably time compression and noise, or time compression and reverberation.

An earlier study by Gordon-Salant and Fitzgibbons (1993) also revealed age effects independent of hearing loss when speech materials are subjected to varying types of temporal distortion. Four groups of participants participated in this study: elderly adults with normal hearing, elderly adults with mild to moderate sensorineural hearing loss, young listeners with normal hearing, and young listeners with comparable hearing loss levels. The low-predictability items of the SPIN-R test were presented in undistorted form and with varying degrees of temporal distortion. The forms of distortion included time compression, reverberation, and interruption. Within each form of distortion were varying degrees or rates of distortion. For example, time-compression ratios ranged from 30 to 60%, reverberation time ranged from 0.2 to 0.6 seconds, and the interruption rate ranged from 12.5 to 100 interruptions per second. In the undistorted condition, the young and elderly normal-hearing listeners obtained comparable percent-correct scores, as did the young and older listeners with sensorineural hearing loss. Thus, recognition of the undistorted sentence materials was more affected by hearing loss than age even at a high presentation level, namely 90 dB SPL. For the most part, hearing loss affected recognition of the three types of distorted materials at a high presentation level. In the time-compressed condition, an effect of age, hearing level, and time-compression ratio emerged. Older listeners with hearing loss performed more poorly than younger listeners on time-compressed speech tasks such that they might be expected to experience difficulty understanding the speech of fast talkers. Performance scores on the reverberant speech tasks also revealed significant effects for age, reverberation time, and hearing status. The latter finding would suggest that reverberant environments may distort speech in a manner particularly difficult for older listeners. Also, significant effects of age and hearing status emerged on the interrupted speech task. Further, in light of the decrements in performance for older participants with and without hearing loss, Gordon-Salant and Fitzgibbons concluded that there were significant age effects, independent of peripheral hearing loss, in performance on the temporally distorted speech tasks. Specifically, rapid speech appears to be a source of challenge to the slowed processing system of many older adults.

Humes and Christopherson (1991) examined the contribution of auditory discrimination to speech understanding as well. They compared the auditory skills of young-old listeners and old-old listeners to those of a sample of young listeners with normal hearing for whom a hearing loss was simulated via noise masking. Auditory discrimination ability was examined using a battery of discrimination tests known as the Test of Basic Auditory Capabilities (TBAC). This battery of tests makes use of simple tonal stimuli and more complex sequences of tone bursts. Speech materials were nonsense syllables that were spectrally and temporally degraded. Temporal degrading was accomplished using reverberation, and spectral distortion was introduced by band-pass filtering materials from 500 to 4000 Hz. The authors noted that the primary factor determining performance on the NST was the sensorineural hearing loss of the listener. The greater the hearing loss, the lower the speech-identification scores. Further, simple tonal-frequency discrimination for a 1000 Hz-tone accounted for a significant, albeit small, proportion of the individual variability in performance on speech-identification tests. To better isolate the factor(s) that determined scores on the speech-identification tasks, performance of the noise-masked group was compared with that of the young normal-hearing listeners and the elderly hearing-impaired listeners. Decrements in performance emerged for the elderly participants on auditory discrimination tasks that involved pure-tone frequency discrimination, temporal-order discrimination for sequences of tones or syllables, and intensity discrimination involving complex tonal patterns. The findings of Humes and Christopherson (1991) and Gordon-Salant and Fitzgibbons (1993) suggest that older adults may experience difficulty in the processing of complex signals such as temporal rhythmic structure. These difficulties can be identified using speech materials that have been un-

naturally distorted by time compression or interruption. The conclusions of Gordon-Salant and Fitzgibbons that high-frequency hearing sensitivity was the most important variable contributing to understanding of undistorted speech materials, time-compressed speech materials (40% time compression [TC]), and reverberant materials (0.2 second reverberation time [RT]) was in agreement with the findings of Humes and Christopherson.

Pearl

Because time compression appears to remove normally available processing necessary for speech understanding, older adults do not have adequate time to process the brief acoustic cues inherent in speeded speech (Tremblay et al, 2003). This suggests a cognitive factor possibly at play.

Jerger and Chmiel (1997) conducted a multivariate analysis of variables contributing to the speech-understanding difficulties experienced by older adults. A total of 180 older adults over 60 years of age participated in their study; 100 of the participants were experienced hearing-aid users. The mean PTA was 45 dB HL in each ear, and the mean score on the Hearing Handicap Inventory for the Elderly (HHIE) was 38%, suggesting significant self-perceived hearing handicap. All participants underwent a complete audiological evaluation including comprehensive word-recognition testing. Speech understanding was tested using (1) PB-50 word lists, (2) the SSI test presented dichotically and in the presence of single-talker competition (word materials were presented at several suprathreshold levels to define a performance-intensity function), and (3) conventional immittance testing. The participants completed the HHIE and their spouse or significant other responded to the HHIE-SO (significant other) using a face-to-face administration. A factor analysis was applied to the data to determine the factor structure of conventional audiometric measures. The major trends emerging from this study have set the stage for future studies and for protocols for testing older adults. Factor 1, the average of low-frequency thresholds (250, 500, and 1000 Hz) in the right ear and 500 and 1000 Hz in the left ear accounted for 24% of the variance in the data. Factor 2, high-frequency hearing sensitivity, namely the average of 3000 and 4000 Hz in both ears, accounted for only 16% of the variance in the data. PB scores on both ears accounted for 14% of the variance in the data, and emerged as factor 5 in the factor analysis. HHIE scores as reported by the client and a significant other accounted for only 8% of the variance in the data. Of interest was the proportion of the variance accounted for by central processing, as quantified using dichotically presented sentences. Specifically, central processing of speech materials presented to the left ear and right ear, respectively, accounted for 20% and 18% of the variance and together accounting for 38% of the variance in the data. As a result of their findings, Jerger and Chmiel concluded that the degree of hearing impairment, which determines speech audibility, is the key to the speech-understanding problems characterizing older adults, that central processing of verbal input is a significant factor underlying auditory processing, and that self-perceived hearing handicap is a factor independent of pure-tone and speech audiometric data.

Summarizing to this point, the evidence from the early studies presented here suggests that speech distorted by noise or temporally may be particularly difficult for older adults beyond what one would expect from peripheral hearing level. It is clear from the above review that auditory changes at the periphery degrade the signal delivered to higher auditory centers. The role of cognitive and linguistic processing, in isolation and in combination with central processing has been the subject of extensive research in the first decade of the 21st century. Hearing loss is a key factor in understanding speech in quiet or in the presence of steady-state background noise, but age and hearing loss interact to affect understanding of speech that has been temporally distorted (Humes & Dubno, 2010). The recent findings of Peelle, Troiani, Grossman, and Wingfield (2011), who examined the effects of hearing ability on neural processes, shed light on the physiological evidence regarding the effect of peripheral changes on higher auditory function. These authors reported that a moderate decline in peripheral auditory acuity can lead to downregulation of neural activity during speech comprehension tasks and, based on preliminary findings using functional magnetic resonance imaging, may also contribute to the loss of gray matter volume in the primary auditory cortex. Their findings support the resource allocation and listening effort framework expounded upon by Pichora-Fuller (2008).

Special Consideration

The central auditory hypothesis holds that the existence of a CAPD may account for the speech-understanding problems experienced by older adults. Stimulus complexity and nature of the listening task underlie many of the speech understanding deficits characterizing older adults (Gordon-Salant, 2006).

Central Auditory Deficits and Cognitive Factors: The Interconnections

A big challenge in central auditory testing is distinguishing cognitive effects from central auditory effects, as earlier studies did not attempt to do so. For example, one factor is the extent to which performance on dichotic tasks can be attributable to age-related declines in cognitive function versus age-related changes in the central auditory pathways. As will become clear, the use of auditory stimuli to isolate central auditory deficits ignores other modalities that present day investigators have incorporated to isolate factors contributing to speech understanding (Humes & Dubno, 2010). In fact, the most recent data emerging from laboratories across the country suggest that central auditory dysfunction may be an early manifestation of cognitive impairment, and that performance on central auditory tests relies on cognitive resources (e.g., working memory), and this may be a contributor to poor performance of older adults (Gates, Feeney, & Mills, 2008b).

Having documented that CAPD is highly prevalent in persons with a diagnosis of AD and adequate peripheral hearing status, Gates et al (2008a) explored further the extent to which persons with memory impairments exhibit abnormal central auditory function. They compared performance on tests of CAPD and cognitive function across three groups: a group with memory impairment without Alzheimer's disease, a group with memory impairment with AD, and a control group. The mean age of each of the three groups ranged from 78.8 years to 84 years, and all participants had excellent word-recognition scores and mean PTAs in the poorer ear ranging from 27 to 34 dB HL. The authors found that the majority of individuals with memory impairment had abnormal scores on the CAPD tests, with performance on the DSI showing the most sensitivity to memory impairment. Interestingly, prevalence of CAPD in the control group, which had a younger mean age than the target groups with memory impairment, and had essentially normal PTAs in the better and poorer ears and essentially normal cognitive function, was 42% based on scores on the DSI, which confirms that CAPD is prevalent in older adults with normal hearing and normal cognitive function. The recent work of Lin et al (2011), suggesting an association between hearing loss and incident dementia, confirms the possibility that dementia may be overdiagnosed in individuals with hearing loss and processing problems. Lin et al agree with assertions of Gates, Beiser, Rees, D'Agostino, and Wolf (2002) that hearing loss and progressive cognitive impairment may arise from a common neuropathological process or from degenerative changes in central auditory nuclei required for performance on auditory processing tasks that may be affected by neuropathology associated with Alzheimer's disease (Baloyannis, Mauroudis, Manolides, & Manolides, 2009).

Pearl

It appears that there is an underlying central component to the auditory processing abilities of older adults, and central factors account for some of the individual differences in word-recognition ability so apparent in the elderly (Wiley et al, 1998). The high prevalence of central auditory processing disorders in people with a diagnosis of Alzheimer's disease suggests an auditory processing component that could play a role in early diagnosis of AD and must be considered when making patient-centered decisions regarding intervention (Gates et al, 2008a).

Roup, Wiley, and Wilson (2006) assessed speech recognition ability of older adults using dichotic stimuli in a sample ranging in age from 19 to 79 years. The hearing-impaired participants in the sample presented with normal hearing in the low frequencies, which gradually sloped to the level of a mild to moderately severe hearing loss beginning at 2000 Hz and beyond. The levels are representative of the sensorineural hearing loss typical of presbycusics. In addition, word-recognition scores for NU-6 words lists were 80% or better in each ear, and all participants were required to be right-handed due to the impact of handedness of dichotic speech-recognition performance. Finally, to ensure normal cognitive status, all participants passed the Mini-Mental State Examination (MMSE) with scores in excess of 25 for all participants. Word recognition for the three groups of participants, namely the young normal hearing, and the older men with sensorineural hearing loss aged 60 to 69 years and 70 to 79 years, was assessed and compared across three conditions as shown in **Table 6.5**. The most important outcome was that older adults exhibited poorer word

Table 6.5   Three Response Conditions for Dichotic Word Recognition Testing

Response Condition	Task Using Northwestern University (NU-6) Word Lists as the Dichotic Stimuli (100 Dichotic Word Trials)
Free recall presentation level = 50 dB HL	Repeat both words after the carrier phrase irrespective of order
Directed attention right presentation level = 80 dB HL	Repeat the word presented to the directed (right ear) or cued ear and then the word presented to the opposite or noncued ear (left ear)
Directed attention left presentation level = 80 dB HL	Repeat the word presented to the directed (left ear) or cued ear and then the word presented to the opposite or noncued ear (right ear)

recognition scores on a dichotic speech-recognition task when speech was presented to the left ear than when it was presented to the right ear. The study found a left ear disadvantage for dichotic stimuli presented in the presence of competition for older adults with hearing loss, supporting the hypothesis that aging appears to impact the corpus callosum and interhemispheric transfer of speech information (Martin & Jerger, 2005). Another interesting finding attributable to the left-ear disadvantage was that the right-ear advantage exhibited by the older hearing-impaired adults in the sample was larger than the right-ear advantage that emerged for the younger normal-hearing adults. Stated differently, although older adults with hearing loss in this study exhibited good to excellent word recognition ability for NU-6 word lists presented monaurally, they were disadvantaged when dichotic stimuli (the same NU-6 word lists) were presented to the left ear. With regard to dichotic speech understanding, Humes and Dubno (2010) and others speculate that cognitive factors such as attention and listening effort could account for declines in performance on these tasks.

Pearls

Older adults who use hearing aids require a more favorable speech-to-noise ratio than do younger adults especially in the presence of competing speech in large part due to cognitive factors (George et al, 2007).

The most widely used approaches to detecting the presence of CAPD in the elderly include assessment of speech understanding in the presence of competing noise, assessment of speech understanding when temporal aspects of the signal are altered (e.g., recognition of time-compressed speech), and assessment of the ability to attend to a target message while ignoring the masking messages (e.g., assessment of inhibitory mechanism). As a left-ear disadvantage (reduced ability to perceive stimuli presented to the left ear in a dichotic situation) is reportedly associated with unsuccessful use of binaural hearing aids, clinicians should consider assessing auditory processing ability prior to the hearing-aid fitting, as a deficit may affect the approach to the hearing-aid fitting (Roup et al, 2006). Dichotic speech tests are an excellent means of studying auditory processing.

Gates et al (2008b) explored the role of central auditory processing in speech understanding in a population-based sample of older adults free of cognitive impairment based on results of the Cognitive Abilities Screening Instrument (CASI). Participants were part of a population-based longitudinal study into the incidence of dementia, cognitive impairment, and other risk factors in older adults. Participants were enrolled in the Adult Changes in Thought (ACT) study, an ongoing study of aging and dementia that began in the early 1990s, with the goal being to explore the incidence of AD and cognitive impairment and to further determine risk factors for the dementias. Primarily English speakers, the mean age of participants was 78.9 years with an age range of 71 to 92 years. Of the 241 participants, 68% complained of hearing difficulty and 25% used hearing aids; 33% of the men had been exposed to noise. Cross-sectional data were used to calculate rates of aging on given tests. Mean pure-tone thresholds were consistent with normal hearing, gradually sloping to the level of a moderately severe high-frequency hearing loss bilaterally, typical of hearing levels of a sample of older adults. Behavioral central auditory tests included the SSI-ICM, the DSI in the free mode, and the dichotic digits test (DDT)—three of the most commonly used tests of CAPD. A battery of electrophysiological tests was also administered, including auditory-evoked potentials and distortion product otoacoustic emissions. The protocol for administration of each test is shown in **Table 6.6**.

The findings were of interest in that despite the fact that participants were deemed to have normal cognitive function, there was a nonuniform rate of age-related changes in performance on the central auditory tests. For participants in their seventh decade and beyond, a decline in central auditory processing was the most pronounced, more so than the decline in pure-tone threshold sensitivity. The decline in performance on the SSI-ICM test (after adjusting for hearing threshold level) was more rapid than that which occurred on the other two dichotic tests. Gates and colleagues (2008b) speculated that the decline in performance on the SSI-ICM is attributable to cognitive factors, specifically executive control function, which resides in the frontal lobe. More pronounced declines were noted in performance on test materials using competition, such as the SSI-ICM, than on tests of peripheral function (distortion product otoacoustic emissions) and tests of eighth nerve and central pathway function (i.e., auditory brainstem response wave V latency). Hence, the authors concluded that age-related changes in the auditory system are nonuniform and probably indicate which cognitive resource allocation, including memory and listening effort, may be sensitive to changes in the auditory system beyond the periphery.

As part of the BMHS, Golding et al (2006) attempted to determine the odds of demonstrating auditory processing abnormalities on seven speech-based measures of auditory processing. A total of 1192 participants were included in the study. The mean age of the 696 women who participated was 68.19 years, and the mean age of the 496 men who participated was 68.32 years. Participants had excellent pure-tone thresholds, with a mean PTA better than 20 dB HL in each ear. The vast majority of participants passed a cognitive screening test (the MMSE) with scores of 24 or greater out of a possible total of 30 points. Following completion of the central auditory test battery, participants were categorized as demonstrating cen-

Table 6.6 Central Auditory Processing Dysfunction (CAPD) Test Protocol

Test	Score Interpretation	Presentation Level	Signal-to-Noise Ratio
SSI-ICM	Normal performance is the correct identification of 80% or more of 10 to 30 sentences (abnormal performance in those with cognitive decline and Alzheimer's disease [AD])	50 dB HL above the PTA using insert earphones	0 dB
DSI	Normal scores are 80% and above (right-ear scores typically higher than left-ear scores due to age-related corpus callosum dysfunction	50 dB above the PTA	NA
DDT	Normal scores are 90% and above (depressed scores are common in individuals with a clinical diagnosis of AD)	50 dB above the PTA	NA

Abbreviations: DDT, dichotic digits test; DSI, dichotic sentence identification; NA, not applicable; PTA, pure-tone average; SSI-ICM, Synthetic Sentence Identification with Ipsilateral Competing Message.

tral auditory processing abnormalities based on performance on the Macquarie versions of the Synthetic Sentence Identification (MSSI) Test, on the DSI, and on the relationship between scores on the PB word lists and SSI maximum scores. Hence, seven central auditory processing test outcomes emerged and served as the basis for the analyses. In general, men were more likely than women to have test results suggestive of CAPD based primarily on performance on the DSI dichotic tests. Jerger, Chmiel, Allen, and Wilson (1994) also observed a gender difference on dichotic tasks, with men having higher rates of abnormality as well. In contrast, a gender difference also emerged in the longitudinal study by Dubno and colleagues (2008); however, in their study the rate of decline on monosyllabic word recognition tests was faster in women than in men, but the samples were different.

In the study by Golding et al (2006), the odds of abnormal performance on most of the central tests increased with increasing age. It was notable that the odds of demonstrating CAPD increased by 24% with every one-unit decrease in scores on the MMSE. This finding was notable, as the majority of participant scores fell within the normal range on the cognitive screening test. In addition to the predictive value of the score on the MMSE, the score on the screening version of the HHIE (HHIE-S) was predictive of CAPD on the PB-MSSI maximum test for both ears, such that the odds of CAPD increased by 5% for every point increase on the HHIE-S. Thus, in their sample of older adults with relatively normal hearing who were free of cognitive impairment, the odds of demonstrating CAPD increased with age, declining cognitive skills, and self-perceived hearing handicap based on HHIE-S scores.

Golding, Mitchell, and Cupples (2005) explored the correlates of central auditory processing disorders in 1192 participants in the BMHS. Mean PTAs were better than 25 dB HL in their sample of older adults. The majority of participants were classified as having mild to severe central auditory processing abnormalities based on performance on a range of speech measures. Of 16 predictor variables including age, cardiovascular disease, gender, cognitive status, and smoking status, only four variables emerged as predictive of the severity of CAPD: the score on the MMSE was highly predictive, and the HHIE-S scores and age were significant predictors of moderate and severe auditory processing deficits. Interestingly, the odds in favor of moderate to severe central auditory processing abnormality increased with each additional year of age and with increasing HHIE-S scores. In this sample, men were more likely than women to be classified as having severe central auditory

processing abnormality. It is notable from the perspective of a test battery that while participants had normal hearing, and the majority had moderate to severe CAPD, 44% felt they had a hearing handicap based on HHIE-S scores. The authors pointed out that risk factors for peripheral hearing loss such as cardiovascular disease, history of stroke, smoking, diabetes, and hypertension were not predictive of central auditory processing abnormalities. Also, although age, MMSE score, gender, and HHIE-S score were risk markers for CAPD, they only accounted for 29.5% of the variance in performance on tests of central auditory processing, leaving a considerable amount of variance unexplained (correlates of peripheral hearing loss such as stroke and diabetes do not account for the remaining variance).

The findings of Humes et al (1994) corroborated some of the findings of Jerger and colleagues (1991). As described in an earlier section, a total of 50 participants with essentially mild to moderate hearing loss and ages ranging from 63 to 83 years participated in this study. Scores on the CUNY NST, the CID W-22 word lists, and the SPIN-R test presented in quiet and noise were correlated with a variety of measures of cognitive function derived from the Wechsler Adult Intelligence Scale–revised (WAIS-R), the Wechsler Memory Scale–revised (WMS-R), and auditory processing ability. The authors found that the average hearing loss at 1000, 2000, or 4000 Hz, or the extent of audibility of the speech signal, correlated most strongly with speech-recognition scores, accounting for 70 to 75% of the variability in performance of speech-recognition tests. Cognitive function and auditory processing ability accounted for little of the individual variability in performance on speech tests used in this study.

Divenyi, Stark, and Haupt (2005) revisited the question of the role of aging, auditory thresholds, and speech understanding using a sample of older adults. As discussed above, participants presented with essentially normal hearing in the low frequencies, sloping gradually to the level of a mild to moderate high-frequency symmetrical sensorineural hearing loss. Speech understanding was assessed using temporally or spectrally distorted material (two conditions) and with speech interference (eight conditions) in each ear. Conditions included time compression, reverberation (modified rhyme reverberation test—0.45, 0.85, 1.25 seconds), low-pass filtered speech, competing sentences, and SPIN testing. Participants were tested on two occasions (5.27 years between initial test and retest), with each testing session lasting 8 to 10 hours spanning a period of 3 weeks. The average session lasted 1½ hours with breaks provided between tasks on an as-needed basis. As pure-tone thresholds in the high frequencies declined over time, presentation levels at follow-up visits were adjusted to ensure audibility of the signal, especially at 4000 Hz.

One interesting finding, as discussed in an earlier section, was that the rate of decline on tests of speech understanding was greater than that associated with change in audiometric thresholds. It was noteworthy that change in high-frequency pure-tone thresholds was associated with change in understanding of spectrally and spatially disturbed speech and the ability to use context to facilitate speech understanding. Overall, the decline in speech understanding over time, which emerged in the majority of tests, was statistically significant. The authors noted that there was a significant change in the individual variability in performance on the speech measures over time that did not emerge on the pure-tone tests, and they attributed this to large individual differences among older adults in cognitive function. They also noted a right-ear advantage in both phases of their study that did not increase in magnitude over time. Divenyi and colleagues noted that age and peripheral hearing sensitivity yielded different correlations with speech measures during phase 1 and phase 2. An example of this change over time in the relationship among scores on speech tests, age, and pure-tone thresholds was the finding that with age understanding of monosyllabic words in the presence of reverberation and in the presence of babble changed, as did dichotic sentence recognition. However, as hearing thresholds in the high frequencies declined, so too did perception of temporally and spectrally altered speech and the ability to use contextual cues. Based on their constellation of findings, the authors concluded that deterioration in auditory function over time is attributable to peripheral as well as nonperipheral factors, which in the case of the latter they considered to be primarily a deficit in auditory temporal processing. Hence, they consider presbycusis to include a large central component. In support of the theory posited by Jerger, Alford, Lew, Rivera, and Chmiel (1995), Divenyi et al agreed that deterioration of the fibers in the corpus callosum accounted for the right-ear advantage.

Pearl

The extent to which audibility determines speech understanding ability in older adults depends on several signal and listener variables (Souza, Boike, Witherell, & Tremblay, 2007).

Cognitive Factors

Speech processing involves the peripheral sense organ, the central auditory brainstem pathways, as well as cognitive resources, including working memory, selective attention, and speed of information processing (Hällgren, Larsby, Lyxell, & Arlinger, 2001). There is a generalized slowing in brain function with age that translates into a slowing in the speech at which selected cognitive operations can be performed (Schneider et al, 2005). The extent to which speech perception deficits are attributable to cognitive pathology has been the subject of considerable study over the past decade. The report from the Berlin Aging Study was instrumental in setting the stage for

exploring the contribution of decline in processing speed to speech understanding and the interaction between mental perceptual processing and linguistic redundancy (Pichora-Fuller, 2003a). As was discussed in an earlier section, the extent to which such age-related decline in cognitive abilities is associated with speech-understanding problems has been explored by several investigators using cognitive measures such as indices of attentional resources, processing speed, intelligence, memory span, and working memory. The theoretical basis for these studies is related in part to several considerations that have recently garnered considerable attention in terms of attempts at unraveling the speech-understanding difficulties older adults experience in noisy environments: (1) generalized slowing across a variety of perceptual, cognitive, and motor domains with aging; (2) increased cognitive demands or an increase in the number of mental operations required for selected speech tasks, potentially compromising performance of older adults; and (3) linguistic context and listening effort (Gordon-Salant & Fitzgibbons, 1997; Stewart & Wingfield, 2009).

The challenge driving researchers is a need to understand why older adults have difficulty understanding speech in challenging listening situations, including in noise, with multiple talkers, with accented speech when speech is fast paced, and, for some, even when speech is amplified (Pichora-Fuller, 2010). Pichora-Fuller (2010) aptly explained that communication in the real world is very complex. One has to be able to analyze the acoustic information that is typically degraded if one has a hearing impairment; next, attention is required as part of the listening process; and comprehension or assigning meaning to the information being transmitted is the final step necessary for communication to take place. As the amount of listening effort increases, top-down processing (brain to ear) becomes more necessary as bottom-up processing (ear to brain) becomes less efficient. This subsection discusses the role of cognitive factors, regardless of age and the audiogram, shedding light on a new look at an old problem.

Jerger et al (1991) were among the first investigators to explore the relation among speech-recognition ability, age, hearing level, and cognitive abilities. As noted earlier, 200 individuals participated in their study. For the most part, participants presented with mild to moderate sloping sensorineural hearing loss. Speech measures included PB words, the SSI test, the SPIN test, and the DSI test. Several neuropsychological measures were administered including the WAIS, the Wechsler Memory Scale (WMS), and the Boston Naming Test (BNT). Although their data suggested that degree of hearing loss was the most powerful predictor of speech-recognition performance, the authors did acknowledge that speed of mental processing as measured by the digit symbol subtest of the WAIS as well as age accounts in part for performance on speech tests. Interestingly, the nature of the speech audiometric task determined the extent to which cognitive status or age influenced performance. Whereas hearing loss influenced performance on each of the speech tests, cognitive status and age affected performance on the SSI and DSI. It was of interest that knowledge of the participant's age significantly increased the variance in scores on the SSI test beyond that already accounted for by degree of hearing loss. In contrast, on the DSI, knowledge of speed of mental processing significantly increased the variance in scores beyond that already accounted for by degree of hearing loss. This finding is not surprising, because the DSI test is a dichotic task that requires the respondent to process two speech targets presented simultaneously and to execute an appropriate response. Interestingly, peripheral-hearing loss accounted for less of the total variance in scores on the DSI than on any of the three other monotic speech-recognition tests.

Gordon-Salant and Fitzgibbons (1997) explored the role of memory, speech rate, and availability of contextual cues in recognition performance of older as compared with younger adults. They found that older adults with and without hearing loss had more difficulty recalling the low-predictability (LP) sentences of the SPIN than did young listeners, but that recall of individual words did not pose as much of a problem for older adults. Understanding of sentence material did not improve for older adults with slowing of the speech rate. The authors noted that availability of contextual cues (e.g., high-predictability sentences on the SPIN) helped older adults with and without hearing loss to achieve excellent word-recognition scores even in the presence of competition.

Wingfield (1996) reviewed a series of studies used to highlight the role of cognitive factors in auditory performance on selected speech tasks that varied in their linguistic complexity. He reported that increasing speech rate beyond the normal 140 to 180 words per minute (wpm) posed a disadvantage to older adults, with the disadvantage affected by the content and structure of the speech materials. Specifically, he reported that the percent of words correctly identified by older and younger adults tends to be comparable for speech rates ranging from 275 to 425 wpm when normal sentence materials were used. However, older adults are at a significant disadvantage (percent of words correctly identified dramatically less than by young adults) at progressively higher speech rates when random strings of words are used. This early study, along with the work of Gordon-Salant and Fitzgibbons (1997), further highlighted the role of linguistic structure as a compensatory agent for understanding speech that has been temporally degraded (i.e., time compression).

Stewart and Wingfield (2009) explored further the link among age, audibility, cognitive ability, syntactic complexity, reduced inability at inhibition, and speech understanding. Participants included young adults with normal hearing, older adults with essentially normal hearing in the low frequencies

and age-appropriate high-frequency loss, and older adults with hearing loss. The latter two groups were comparable in terms of performance on the forward and backward digit span, digital symbol substitution, and trail-making test, which measure specific cognitive functions as listed in **Table 6.7**. **Table 6.8** lists the stimuli used along with the stimuli that differed by syntactic complexity. It is important to note that at the heart of the differences that emerged between young and older adults is task complexity, such that, for example, a recall task that requires recall of an entire sentence was more difficult than recall of the final word in a sentence. Not surprisingly, the younger adults had superior scores on these tests as compared with the older groups. Further, the older participants with poorer hearing performed more poorly than the older participants with the less severe high-frequency hearing loss on the monosyllabic word lists (NU-6) and on both the subject and object relative sentences, with performance poorest on the object relative sentences.

The results of the study confirmed that although linguistic knowledge tends to be preserved as people age, syntactic complexity places older adults at a greater disadvantage than that experienced by younger adults. Hearing impairment further disadvantages older adults as the task becomes more complex with greater demands placed on working memory and synthetic or integrative ability. According to Stewart and Wingfield (2009), older adults are disadvantaged because of greater demands being placed on working memory resources that come into play during comprehension tasks using sentence materials with complex syntax plus the additional effort required in listening when audibility is impaired. Interestingly, Stewart and Wingfield speculated that when older adults are challenged to understand complex syntactic structures, they

Table 6.7 Measures of Cognitive Function in Older Adults

Test	Cognitive Function
Forward and backward digit span	Short term and working memory
Digital symbol substitution	Psychomotor speed or speed of information processing
Trail making test parts A and B	Executive control
Shipley vocabulary test	Verbal ability

Table 6.8 Classes of Stimuli Used in Word-Recognition Tasks

Stimuli	Degree of Difficulty	Task
Monosyllabic word lists: Northwestern University (NU-6) word list	Most difficult, as there is no context	Recognize each word at the softest presentation level possible (score = percent score at each presentation level)
Sentences with subject-relative center and embedded clause structures	Simpler of the two syntactic forms yet difficult because the listener must understand the first part of the clause, which is interrupted by a relative clause that modifies the subject	Repeat the full sentence correctly at the lowest possible presentation level (score = percent words correct at given presentation level)
Sentences with object-relative center and embedded clause structures	Most difficult of the two syntactic forms because the subject functions as both the subject of the main clause and the objective of the relative clause	Repeat the full sentence correctly at the lowest possible presentation level (score = percent words correct at given presentation level)

are being penalized because the resources called upon to understand (e.g., effort required) in a sense reduce the audibility of the signal. Stated differently, "for the older adult with mild to moderate hearing loss," simplifying the syntax is equivalent to "a 7.8-dB increase in sound level" (Stewart & Wingfield, 2009, p. 153).

In an attempt to unravel the link between auditory processing and cognitive status, Humes (2005) examined the relation between performance on auditory processing tasks and performance on tests of cognitive and auditory function. Participants were older adults with a mean age of 73 years with mild to moderate high-frequency sensorineural hearing loss with excellent monaural suprathreshold word-recognition scores and poor word-recognition scores in the presence of noise in each ear. Approximately one third of participants were hearing-aid users. The auditory processing tests were presented at 90 dB SPL to minimize the confounding effects of peripheral hearing loss. Some of the auditory processing tests were tonal (duration, temporal order discrimination) and others involved dichotic consonant-vowels (CVs) and time compression of NU-6 word lists. The auditory processing tasks primarily involved temporal manipulations. Some interesting trends emerged in this study. Overall, normal-hearing older adults performed better than the hearing impaired on the auditory processing measures. Age and nonverbal IQ explained the greatest proportion of the individual variability in scores on the auditory processing tasks, accounting for 11 to 14% of the variance on the processing tasks, which were also highly correlated to one another. The findings underscore the role of cognition in auditory processing and the sensitivity of measures that have been temporally distorted to uncover auditory processing; however, it is clear that the majority of the individual variability remains unknown.

As part of their effort to further understand the speech-recognition difficulties experienced by older adults, Gordon-Salant and Fitzgibbons (2001) examined the effects of age, hearing loss, and processing speed, on speech recognition. Participants included young and older listeners with normal hearing and young and older listeners with gradually sloping sensorineural hearing loss that was mild to moderate in degree. All were native speakers of English with normal cognitive function based on score on the Short Portable Mental Status Questionnaire (SPMSQ). The SPIN-R was used to measure speech understanding without time compression, with various types of time compression, and as three stimulus forms with varying amounts of syntactic redundancy. As expected, there was a main effect of hearing loss, with listeners with hearing loss doing more poorly than those without hearing loss, and of stimulus, with all listeners performing more poorly as syntactic redundancy was reduced from sentence materials to randomly ordered words. Further, older listeners did more poorly than young listeners when the speech materials were most lacking in syntactic redundancy or as the amount of syntactic cues was reduced. The effects of time compression interacted with linguistic redundancy such that older listeners did more poorly than younger listeners when the material was time compressed and the contextual information made available was limited. It was of interest that listeners with hearing loss, irrespective of age, did poorly in the condition where there was selective time compression of consonants, which naturally reduced the availability of cues necessary for intelligibility. The authors also found that the combined effect of age and hearing loss placed older adults at a disadvantage when listening to time-altered speech and speech with reduced linguistic cues. **Table 6.9** summarizes the principal findings of this study and their implications.

Pearl

Older adults are disadvantaged in terms of speech understanding when extra demands are placed on their capacity to process information.

Schneider et al (2005) explored the role of audibility and cognitive variables in older adults' ability to understand speeded speech, in an attempt to sort out the interaction among age, processing speed, and distortions created by speeded speech. They assessed speech understanding using different approaches to speeded speech and using varying backgrounds including quiet and babble. The young and old participants were matched in terms of their ability to understand low-context sentences presented in the presence of babble, but the sentences were not speeded. Speech recognition using various speeds and methods of speeding was compared across groups. Older adults had essentially normal hearing for their age. The

Table 6.9 Principal Findings of Study on Effects of Age, Speech Form, Type of Noise, and Time Compression on Speech Understanding

Finding	Implication
Speech understanding in older adults is influenced by available linguistic information	Removing linguistic redundancy in the message increases cognitive demand, which adversely effects older adults
Older adults perform more poorly with acoustic alteration of consonants than with vowels; that is, they have difficulty processing the brief limited acoustic cues for consonants typical of rapid speech	Older adults' difficulty processing rapid speech is due to their limited processing capacity for brief consonant cues
Older adults' performance is most compromised when speech is time compressed acoustically (bottom-up processing) and linguistic redundancy is reduced (top-down processing demand)	Strategies for reducing cognitive effort or demand are important for assisting older adults to understand speech
Speech understanding in noise varies with type of noise, such that when the competition is composed of meaningful words or speech and/or the masker is similar in precept to the target message, degraded performance often ensues (multi-talker babble) (Souza, et al, 2007)	Cognitive remediation interventions can help promote cognitive reserve

Source: Gordon-Salant, S., & Fitzgibbons, P. J. (2001, Aug). Sources of age-related recognition difficulty for time-compressed speech. *Journal of Speech, Language, and Hearing Research, 44,* 709–719

results were interesting in that when the low-context sentences were presented at a normal rate of speed at a 3-dB SNR for the young participants, the older participants performed comparably at an 8-dB SNR. This was considered the baseline condition at which performance was comparable. When the low-context sentences were speeded by deleting every third amplitude sample (which shifts energy in speech to higher frequencies, speeds up formant transitions, and reduces the gap in stop consonants), older adults' performance dropped significantly more dramatically than did that of the younger adults. This is predictable given the effect of this form of speeding on consonant and vowel transitions and absolute frequency.

In a related experiment, the older adults achieved correct word-recognition scores for the high-context sentences that were comparable to those of the younger sample; however, when the high-context sentences were speeded by deleting every third amplitude sample, older adults recognized significantly fewer words than did younger adults. Thus, the decline in performance associated with speeding was significantly greater for the older participants for both high- and low-context sentences. Interestingly, when speech was speeded by deleting steady-state portions of the signal (pitch and formant transitions remain), the older adults were not especially disadvantaged in their understanding of the final word of high-context sentences, most likely due to the contextual support that remained with this method of time compression. However, under this condition of speeding, older adults were more affected than younger adults for low-context information.

Schneider and colleagues (2005) conducted additional experiments with varying speeds and approaches to speeding, and the overall conclusion is that contextual benefit varies with speed. In fact, older adults benefited more, although the differences did not achieve statistical significance, from context than did younger adults at faster speeds. The ability of older adults to make better use of context has important implications for counseling regarding cognitive strategies for improving speech understanding. The authors drew some very relevant conclusions from their series of studies that have implications for assessment and treatment. In general, older and younger adults are differentially affected by the introduction of speed-induced acoustic distortions based on the nature of spectral distortion produced (e.g., shortening of gaps in stop consonants, shortening vowel duration and pauses between words, shifting the energy in speech up in frequency). If the goal is to uncover peripheral and cognitive effects, the way in which speech is speeded will affect the deficits to be uncovered, such that shifting the energy in the speech signal (be it low- or high-context sentences) up to the high frequencies by deleting every third amplitude value, for example, has dramatic perceptual effects. Conversely, speeding by deleting every third 10-millisecond segment, which shortens vowel duration, has a negative effect on understanding of low-context sentences. When speeding by deleting steady-state portions of the signal, older adults do not appear to be disadvantaged for either low- or high-context sentence materials, most likely because cues to phoneme recognition remain available to the listener.

Humes (2007) extensively explored speech understanding in the elderly in an effort to isolate the variables contributing to our understanding of this complex phenomenon. His working hypothesis was that as more speech sounds are amplified to suprathreshold levels, speech-recognition ability attributable to loss of audibility of important speech cues would improve. He conducted a series of experiments in which speech was spectrally altered in an effort to restore audibility. Further, cognitive testing was conducted on selected participants. Some very interesting trends emerged. Restoration of the audibility of high-frequency sounds through spectral shaping was imperative for adequate speech-understanding performance. The latter was the case for high presentation levels and for unaided listening, suggesting that audibility of key speech areas is integral to speech-understanding performance. It was noteworthy that when audibility was restored, individual differences in speech understanding were attributable to aging, cognitive, or central factors, suggesting an interaction among central auditory processing, cognition, and audibility. In light of the role of these residual factors, Humes speculated that even with "well-fit" hearing aids, which provide sufficient audibility, many older adults will continue to experience challenges unless the SNR is more favorable than is typical of most listening situations. As Humes and Dubno (2010) suggest, because better than normal SNRs are critical for optimizing speech understanding performance with hearing aids, technology-based approaches to improve SNR remain a priority, and auditory and cognitive retraining hold great promise.

George et al (2007) explored the role of auditory and non-auditory factors in affecting speech recognition in noise in a sample of older listeners with and without hearing loss. The auditory factors explored included speech reception in noise, and the nonauditory factors included modality-specific central, cognitive, or linguistic skills. The mean age of the hearing-impaired listeners who had a mild sloping to severe high-frequency sensorineural loss beginning at 1000 Hz was 65.5 years, and the mean age of the normal-hearing listeners was 63.5 years. All participants reported normal to corrected to normal vision, which was important as the text reception threshold was assessed using visually presented material. A major goal of the study was to determine how well listeners can restore missing phonemes or words through the visual or auditory modality when modulated noise is present and redundancies such as phonetic, phonological, or lexical cues are relied upon. How well can normal and hearing-impaired participants use context information to improve sentence readability or intelligibility in modulated noise was an additional goal.

The findings were noteworthy. As would be expected, the speech-reception threshold of the hearing-impaired participants in modulated and stationary noise differed significantly from that of the normal-hearing listeners; however, normal-hearing and hearing-impaired participants were comparable in terms of their performance on the text reception threshold (TRT) test or masked text. The groups also differed in terms of temporal acuity or temporal resolution. Hence, the results suggested that the differences between the groups were auditory based. To explore further the role of nonaudiological factors in speech-reception thresholds in noise, a stepwise regression analysis was conducted to identify the predictor variables that could explain individual differences in speech-reception thresholds in modulated noise and in the presence of stationary noise. Interestingly, in the normal-hearing sample, scores on the TRT accounted for 31% of the individual differences on the speech-reception task in the presence of stationary noise and 60% of the variance in the presence of modulated noise. In the hearing-impaired sample temporal resolution and TRT score explained 73% of the variance in the speech-reception threshold in the presence of modulated noise. However, the contribution of temporal resolution to the variance was greater than the contribution of visual factors as quantified by the TRT. These trends suggest that nonauditory factors play an important role in explaining individual differences in speech reception in normal-hearing individuals, and auditory and nonauditory factors appear to play a role in hearing-impaired individuals.

The authors also conducted a statistical manipulation of the data in an attempt to compare in absolute terms the role of nonauditory factors in speech reception in modulated noise or in nonstationary backgrounds, and found that they accounted for a comparable proportion of the variability in scores in both group of participants. From a clinical perspective, the authors concluded that a listener with poor text reception thresholds (nonauditory factor) will be less able to use context to improve readability or intelligibility, and such a person might require a more favorable SNR than someone with a better TRT score. The authors concluded that nonauditory and auditory factors are independently used to process speech in normal and hearing-impaired individuals, and deterioration in auditory processing may not alter the relative contribution of nonauditory factors (e.g., perceptual closure as measured by the TRT) to speech reception. This is a novel conclusion and perspective that has considerable clinical relevance. Examination of the modality specificity of the speech understanding deficits is an excellent way of isolating central auditory deficits from cognitive factors (Humes & Dubno, 2010). The findings of George et al (2007) may provide additional support to the common cause hypothesis, suggesting an anatomical and physiological link underlying cognitive and sensory deficits in older adults.

Special Consideration

Aging has a negative impact on peripheral, central, and cognitive processing during speech communication (Tremblay & Ross, 2007).

Hällgren et al (2001) systematically attempted to study the effect of age on dichotic speech tests and how dichotic listening ability is related to cognitive ability in a sample of older adults with symmetrical sensorineural hearing loss that was essentially mild to moderate in degree. The cognitive tests included a reading span test, which is a test of working memory; a test of verbal information processing speed; and a test of phonological processing. Dichotic CVs, digits, and sentences were the stimuli used to assess right- or left-ear advantages in their sample. Overall, older adults, although having comparable peripheral hearing levels, performed more poorly on each of the dichotic speech tasks. A significant relation between PTAs and performance on dichotic speech tasks emerged, such that peripheral hearing status was potentially a confounding variable when considering absolute performance on the tests. In their sample, an age effect emerged in the left-focusing condition, such that the younger adults reported hearing significantly more stimuli in the left ear than in the right ear, which was not the case for the older participants with comparable

hearing levels. In fact, there was no correlation between PTA and left-ear advantage.

Regarding the interaction between age and performance on cognitive and dichotic tests, a significant correlation between age and cognitive test performance and age and dichotic test performance emerged, such that the correlation between cognitive test performance and dichotic test performance was nullified when the effect of age was partialed out. The correlation between cognitive factors was stronger for the left focusing condition than for the right focusing condition. The authors concluded that the age effect on the left-ear advantage is most likely due to functional asymmetries in the central auditory system, possibly the corpus callosum and the left hemisphere, or to cognitive functions that are challenged when forced to listen to information presented to the left ear (left focusing ear). The authors suggest that good working memory is critical when information is presented to the left ear and that the correlation between dichotic tests and cognitive tests points to "true central involvement of general cognitive mechanisms" (Hällgren et al, 2001, p. 127). The interpretation offered by Humes and Dubno (2010) regarding factors beyond the periphery that contribute to deficits in speech understanding is consistent with the theory espoused by Hällgren et al. Humes and Dubno posit that "there exists a finite amount of information-processing resources, and if older adults with high-frequency hearing loss have to divert some of these resources to repair what is otherwise a nearly automatic resource free process of encoding sensory input, then fewer resources will be available for subsequent higher-level processing" (p. 237).

Pearl

Working memory requires perception, storage, processing, and interpreting of spoken information in an effort to unravel the role of memory in performance on tests of central auditory function, and to garner further support for the hypothesis implicating frontal lobe dysfunction as the contributor to decline in memory and central auditory dysfunction.

Vaughan, Storzbach, and Furukawa (2008) attempted to identify the tests most sensitive to cognitive deficits in older adults using a sample of native speakers of English ranging in age from 50 to 75 years with hearing loss typical of older adults (mild in low frequencies, sloping to moderate to severe in the high frequencies). Participants were free of depression and had normal cognitive function based on screening tests for memory (California Verbal Learning Test–II [CVLT-II]) and intellectual ability (Wechsler Abbreviated Scale of Intelligence [WASI]). **Table 6.10** displays the test of working memory, speed of processing, and attention administered to all participants. Speech-recognition ability was also assessed using low-predictability sentences that were time compressed at rates ranging from 40 to 65%.

Age and hearing loss accounted for 28% of the variance in performance on the time-compressed speech tasks, with age accounting for slightly more of the variance than did hearing level. The neurocognitive test that had the strongest associa-

Table 6.10 Neurocognitive Tests Used by Vaughan and Colleagues (2008)

Neurocognitive Function	Test and Task
Visual working memory[1]	N-back: participants are asked to identify from a series of letters each letter that had previously appeared either one or three letters before Self-ordered pointing (SOP) test: participants are asked to point to one of eight or ten abstract black and white drawings that appear simultaneously in an array on a computer screen
Verbal working memory	Wechsler Adult Intelligence Scale, 3rd edition (WAIS-III): digit span subtest forward and backward; forward: participant repeats a series of numbers in exactly the same order; backward: participant repeats a series of numbers in the reverse order
Auditory working memory	Letter-number sequencing (LNS): participants must reorder the letters and numbers they hear in ascending order for the numbers and in alphabetical order for the letters
Speed of processing tests[2]	WAIS-III: digital symbol coding test: participants are timed in their ability to copy symbols for an array of numbers to which they are exposed after seeing the numbers next to the symbols in a box Choice reaction time in visual and auditory modalities: participants are timed in the response latency necessary to identify the word they see or hear
Tests of attention	Brief test of attention (BTA): participants have to recall the number of letters they heard while ignoring the numbers, and then they are asked to say how many number they heard while ignoring the letters The Connors continuous performance test: participants are asked to press a space bar each time they see a letter (except x) on the screen presented at various interstimulus intervals

[1]Working memory or memory capacity: the processes involved in holding information in one's mind while using it to make a decision or to problem solve (Aarts, Adams, & Duncan, 2003).

[2]Processing speed: speed at which one can manage information and extract meaning from it (Aarts, Adams, & Duncan, 2003).

Source: Data from Vaughan, N., Storzbach, D., & Furukawa, I. (2008, Jul–Aug). Investigation of potential cognitive tests for use with older adults in audiology clinics. *Journal of the American Academy of Audiology, 19,* 533–541, quiz 579–580.

tion with scores on the time-compressed speech task was the test of auditory working memory (the letter-number sequencing [LNS]), which is known to share a strong association with scores on the forward and backward memory tests. The LNS is a particularly challenging test, as participants are required to perform a series of temporal sequencing tasks including manipulating a series of random numbers and letters into two separate sets and then repeating them back, the letters alphabetically and the numbers consecutively.

Pearl

Speech processing uses numerous cognitive resources including working memory, selective attention, and inhibition (Craik, 2007).

Hearing Loss and Alzheimer's Disease

Because of the high prevalence of hearing impairment among persons with a diagnosis of AD, coupled with the overlapping presentation between those with untreated hearing impairment and persons diagnosed with AD, there has been considerable interest in a possible connection between AD and hearing status. Gates et al (1996) speculated early on that low scores on the SSI-ICM may be predictive of dementia in older adults. Gates et al (2008a) recruited participants from the ACT sample discussed in an earlier section of this chapter. The two groups of ACT participants they recruited included the target group, categorized as memory impaired based on performance on a series of memory tests and on the Clinical Dementia Rating Test, and the non–memory-impaired group, categorized as participants who did not show memory impairment. The target group was further subdivided into AD and no-AD groups. All participants underwent pure-tone testing, electrophysio-

logical testing, including evoked potential testing, and a complete battery of central and cognitive tests including the SSI-ICM, the DSI, and the DDT plus such neuropsychological tests as the Trail Making test and the Stroop Color and Word test. The control group and the memory impaired with and without AD groups were comparable in terms of race, cardiovascular status, and word-recognition scores. With regard to pure-tone thresholds, the differences across groups were not clinically significant, and the vast majority of audiograms were consistent with a gradually sloping, high-frequency hearing loss. The control group was slightly younger and had a few more years of education.

The performance of the control group on each of the central auditory tests was significantly better than that of the memory impaired with and without AD groups. Within the memory-impaired groups, performance on the SSI-ICM was poorer in the AD group. The receiver operating curves (ROCs) for the CAPD tests) revealed the DSI test to be the most sensitive to memory loss in this sample. Further, mean differences in performance between the memory-impaired groups with and without AD occurred on the tests of CAPD; the target group with AD consistently performed more poorly on each of the three tests of CAPD as compared with the control group, yet the target group without AD also performed more poorly than the control group after adjusting for age and hearing level. Gates and colleagues concluded that because older adults with memory impairment do more poorly on tests of CAPD than do those without memory impairment, these tests should be part of the routine test battery for older adults.

Gates et al (2002) explored the possible role that central auditory processing ability may play in diagnosing AD. Participants were part of the dementia cohort established in 1976 of the Framingham Heart Study who first underwent a battery of neuropsychological tests between 1976 and 1978 and were identified as cognitively intact at that time. Participants undergoing central auditory testing, which included the SSI-ICM test, the Staggered Spondaic Word test, and a PI-PB function, had PTAs better than 35 dB HL to ensure that peripheral auditory sensitivity did not contaminate the test results. The authors defined CAPD as a low score (<50%) on the SSI-ICM test in either ear in the presence of normal bilateral (>80%) word-recognition scores (W-22) in each ear when the words were presented at 40 dB SPL for determining the PTA. Participants undergoing the central auditory tests were followed through 1998 or until the point of a probable diagnosis of dementia, death, or an abnormal score on the dementia screening test. Interestingly, of the 740 participants in the dementia cohort free of stroke and dementia at the time of the initial hearing test, 5% were assigned a probable diagnosis of AD; 2% were determined to be presenting with a CAPD, and of these 15 individuals 46.7% were labeled as having probable dementia, versus 4.6% of the participants who did not have a CAPD. The investigators noted that peripheral hearing loss did not explain the differences in prevalence of probable dementia of those with CAPD and those without CAPD; however, those with CAPD were older than those without CAPD. Although the sensitivity and specificity data were not strong enough to make a case for administering the SSI-ICM routinely, it was noteworthy that the time to diagnosis of probable dementia in those with CAPD was shorter than in those without CAPD, such that participants with the poorest SSI-ICM scores had the shortest time from testing to diagnosis of probable AD. Gates and colleagues theorized that frontal lobe executive control function may be a factor affecting performance on the SSI-ICM.

Pearl

Perception of speech is facilitated by listener expectations and linguistic context in large part due to the beneficial effects of top-down processing (Pichora-Fuller, 2008).

Implications of the Role of Cognition in Speech Understanding

The cognitive theory of aging posits that as people age, processing resources are overburdened when multiple levels of effortful processing is required (e.g., reduced acoustic information is available and the memory load is increased) (Gordon-Salant & Fitzgibbons, 2001). Aging is associated with reduction in the ability to process temporal aspects of speech (time-compressed speech) and nonspeech stimuli (e.g., gap detection tasks). Auditory temporal processing is mediated by several variables, including speed of information processing and syntactic complexity. It appears that older listeners may be able to compensate for age-related hearing loss by allowing their increased experience with language to enable them to take full advantage of semantic context (Wingfield, Poon, Lombardi, & Lowe, 1985). These findings are in keeping with the cognitive principle that there is an inverse relationship between amount of sensory information available and correct word recognition within a given context (Stewart & Wingfield, 2009). Global cognitive function, such as working memory, loss of cognitive control and ability to inhibit attention to irrelevant stimuli,

and increased listening effort and processing speed, contributes profoundly to the speech processing problems of older adults in isolation and in combination with central auditory processing deficits. The speech-specific cognitive declines (e.g., absence of linguistic redundancy) that contribute to the speech-understanding difficulties that emerge when testing older adults could perhaps be compensated for by rehabilitation programs (Pichora-Fuller, 2003a,b).

Pichora-Fuller (2003b) eloquently explained the variables that come into play for comprehension of discourse and subsequently for communication to take place. Simply put, the listener must be able to manipulate and integrate the "ongoing flow of information that is received" (p. S63) and store in memory portions of the message until the speaker completes the message. Not only is memory integral to comprehension, but selective attention and inhibitory control are critical as the message must be interpreted in the context of the social and physical (e.g., noise) environment. Pichora-Fuller (2010) suggested that although fluid intelligence, which includes working memory, processing speed, and attention, declines with age, interfering with speech understanding, crystallized intelligence or the ability to utilize context tends to be preserved, challenging audiologists to consider these factors in the diagnostic and rehabilitative process. In light of the complexity of the act of engaging in discourse, cognitive factors are critical even when audibility is restored and especially when the SNR is unfavorable, when the speech rate is altered (i.e., speeded), or when contextual support is limited (Pichora-Fuller, 2003b). The evidence presented in this section in a sense supports the information-degradation hypothesis as espoused by Baltes and Lindenberger (1997), namely that degraded input and slowing of the rate at which information is processed interact to hamper speech understanding. Although amplification theoretically can help to improve audibility, improve the SNR, and ease the effort necessary to listen, in fact cognitive and auditory training may be necessary to facilitate top-down processing and maximize any benefit to be realized.

Pearl

Establishing the underlying anatomical loci of an older adult's speech-understanding difficulties using reliable and valid approaches will lead to better and appropriately tailored intervention (Humes et al, 2011).

Speech Tests: Summarizing Remarks

Speech tests are essential in the evaluation of the elderly because they offer the clinician a means of assessing receptive communication function in a quasi-systematic manner using materials and procedures that potentially vary in complexity. They can be used to provide (1) objective quantifiable information about rehabilitative potential, (2) differential diagnostic information relating to the site of lesion, (3) data that can help to identify the etiology of the speech-understanding problems so typical of older adults, (4) information about probable diagnosis of AD, and (5) information about detrimental effects of central auditory deficits on functional performance with hearing aids. In fact, one could speculate that in large part the dissatisfaction with hearing aids may be due to distraction from and susceptibility to competing speech and background noise, slowed perceptual processing, temporal distortions, and cognitive challenges posed by a decline in working memory, inhibitory control, and the exploitation of resources used with effortful listening in the presence of syntactically complex stimuli, or when stimuli are presented at reduced presentation levels or in the presence of competing noise.

Audibility, especially of high-frequency sounds, figures prominently in the ability to understand speech especially when hearing levels exceed 30 dB HL in the higher frequencies (Humes, 2007). Measures of cognitive ability, including temporal order discrimination and central auditory processing ability, explain a considerable proportion of the variance in speech understanding in quiet and noise. According to Humes (2007), there is evidence that when audibility is restored via spectral shaping, nonauditory measures emerge and account for significant amounts of the variability in speech-recognition scores, replacing the role of hearing levels. Humes argues that when we spectrally shape speech through 4000 Hz, as is the case for well-fitted digital hearing aids, residual factors such as cognition and central processing underlie speech-recognition problems, underscoring the need for more favorable SNRs. **Table 6.11** summarizes the auditory and nonauditory issues that interact to affect speech understanding. This information serves as the basis for the protocol recommended for testing older adults being considered for some form of audiological intervention (Vaughan et al, 2008). **Table 6.12** summarizes the conclusions from the volume of studies on correlates of speech understanding among older adults. It is evident that performance on a wide variety of tests of speech understanding explains the extent to which the difficulties experienced by older adults are attributable to changes in the auditory periphery, changes in the central auditory nervous system, or generalized slowing across the cognitive domain.

Pearl

Speech testing in the presence of competing speech and dichotic speech testing are the most common test conditions used in speech testing over the past 25 years (Humes et al, 2011).

◆ Hearing Handicap/Participation Restrictions, Quality of Life, and Hearing Impairment

The discussion above isolates the peripheral, central, and cognitive variables that help to explain the individual variability in performance on speech tests among older adults. It is clear that individual variability is the rule rather than the exception. It is also evident that pure-tone and speech measures fall short in helping clinicians understand the behavioral consequences of a given hearing impairment or of speech understanding deficits. This has led to increasing interest in understanding the quality-of-life correlates of audiometric tests routinely administered. This functional information is important, because if consequences cannot be predicted from performance, this

Table 6.11 Summary of Functional Effects of Auditory and Nonauditory Changes Associated with Aging

Auditory or Nonauditory Age-Related Change	Functional Effect
Peripheral	Reduced hearing sensitivity due to distortions in cochlear mechanics and other peripheral changes
Central	Speech understanding deficits associated with changes in the brainstem pathways and nuclei
Cognitive	Speech understanding difficulties associated with age-related changes in the cortex that interfere with the ability to perform linguistic analyses of complex materials such as speech; hallmarks of cognitive aging include changes in working memory and processing speed

Source: Data from Vaughan, N., Storzbach, D., & Furukawa, I. (2008, Jul–Aug). Investigation of potential cognitive tests for use with older adults in audiology clinics. *Journal of the American Academy of Audiology, 19*, 533–541, quiz 579–580.

would underscore the important role such information plays in the routine test battery.

Chia et al (2007) assessed the association between hearing impairment and health-related quality of life as part of the BMHS in an attempt to quantify the burden of a chronic disease such as hearing impairment. Participants had a mean age of 67 years, with the majority presenting with mild bilateral hearing impairment; individuals with unilateral hearing impairment were also represented in the sample. Hearing levels of the participants were consistent with the cross-sectional data cited earlier in the chapter for individuals 80 years of age or older having a mild hearing loss in the low frequencies and a severe hearing loss in the higher frequencies. Approximately half of the participants reported perceiving some hearing problems. Health-related quality of life was measured using the Short-Form Health Survey (SF-36), which assesses eight dimensions of health status ranging from mental health to general health perceptions to social functioning. SF-36 scores were associated with bilateral rather than unilateral hearing loss, and the more severe the hearing loss, the poorer the scores on the dimensions of health measured by the SF-36, including physical functioning, social functioning, and general perceptions of health. Persons with hearing loss across all frequencies had poorer SF-36 scores than did those with a high-frequency hearing loss, and persons with a high-frequency hearing loss had comparable scores on the SF-36 to those without hearing loss. Finally, individuals perceiving a hearing loss also perceived their functional health and well-being to be problematic, based on the correlation between self-reported hearing problems and functional health status as measured by the SF-36. Dalton et al (2003), using participants from the Epidemiology of Hearing Loss Study (EHLS) and participants comparable in age to the above sample (mean age = 69 years), also noted a relation between hearing impairment and health-related quality of life. In their sample the severity of hearing impairment corresponded with health-related quality of life as measured on the SF-36, with those with more severe hearing loss perceiving their physical functional status to be poorer.

Table 6.12 The Matrix Underlying Speech Understanding in Older Adults

Peripheral hypothesis	Age has a greater effect on speech understanding in those with moderate to severe hearing loss	
	When pure-tone thresholds across age groups (e.g., 50 to 90 years) are held constant, speech recognition performance is comparable in quiet, and for low- and high-context sentence materials presented in babble	Dubno et al (1997)
	For speech presented in quiet and steady-state background noise at presentation levels ranging from 50 to 90 dB SPL, audibility is the primary factor underlying deficits in speech understanding; inaudibility of the higher frequencies is the main contributor to speech understanding problems in quiet and in the presence of steady-state noise in unamplified conditions	Humes and Dubno (2010)
	Audibility or peripheral hearing sensitivity accounts in part for deficits in understanding of time-compressed speech, reverberant speech, and when undistorted speech is presented in the presence of temporally interrupted noise; however, the nature of the background noise and of the distortion affects the amount of variance remaining unaccounted for	Gordon-Salant and Fitzgibbons (1993); Humes (2005); Humes and Dubno, (2010)
	Peripheral factors (e.g., elevated thresholds, broadened tuning curves, reduced compression) account for only a minimal amount of the variability in performance on tasks involving dichotic presentation of speech materials, and when background noise is temporally distorted	Humes and Dubno (2010)
	The relationship between speech understanding and high-frequency hearing is weaker for temporally distorted speech materials than when listening to speech in quiet or in the presence of steady-state noise, suggesting that other factors remain, such as central and cognitive, to account for the unexplained variance in scores	Humes and Dubno (2010)
	Mild hearing loss has little effect on performance on sentence in noise tests, provided the presentation levels are adequate to overcome loss of audibility	Neijenhuis, Tschur, and Snik (2004)
Central hypothesis	Age is a risk factors for moderate to severe central auditory processing dysfunction (CAPD)	Golding et al (2005)
	Subtle cognitive decline based on even a mild Mini-Mental Status Examination (MMSE) score is predictive of severity of CAPD	
	Older adults with central auditory deficits rate themselves as more handicapped than those without such disorders	Jerger, Oliver, and Pirozzolo (1990)
	Older adults have reduced ability to perceive stimuli presented to the left ear in a dichotic speech situation compared with younger adults, possibly because the signal from the left ear is conveyed through the corpus callosum	
	Dichotic tasks are good indicators of central auditory function	
	Noise and reverberation reduce the availability of temporal speech cues, compromising processing in these environments	
Cognitive hypothesis	Cognitive factors contribute to speech-understanding problems of older adults when speech is temporally degraded or background noise is temporally degraded; in fact, cognitive factors may come into play when speech is made audible through amplification	Humes and Dubno (2010)
Peripheral + central + cognitive	For aided performance to equal that of a younger sample, the entire speech area must be rendered audible and the signal-to-noise ratio must be restored and must be better than normal for older adults to function well	Humes and Dubno (2010)
	Age-related differences in speech processing exist even after accounting for hearing loss, especially on complex auditory processing tasks	

Table 6.12 Continued

Central + cognitive	Central auditory and cognitive declines are concomitant and, in some cases, CAPD precedes the onset of cognitive decline	Gates et al (2002)
	Performance on dichotic tests (selective versus divided attention) correlates with cognitive parameters and with age	Hällgren et al (2001)
	Scores on the left focusing condition of dichotic tests correlate more strongly with cognitive factors than do scores for the right focusing condition; a good working memory capacity is critical for the perception of materials to the left ear on a dichotic task	
	Speech processing in the temporal domain in the presence of fluctuating background noise is susceptible to age effects; when speech rate is increased, the ability to perform syntactic analysis and to process lexical cues is compromised	Pichora-Fuller and Souza (2003)

Wiley, Cruickshanks, Nondahl, and Tweed (2000) explored the prevalence of self-reported hearing handicap as measured using the HHIE-S and changes in perceived handicap as a function of age in a sample of 3471 adults participating in the EHLS. Several interesting trends emerged. The mean scores on the HHIE-S increased in women and men as a function of age, and in each age group the mean HHIE-S score for men was indicative of greater self-perceived hearing handicap/participation restrictions than for women. When participants were stratified by age, gender, and degree of hearing loss, it was clear that the prevalence of self-perceived handicap was greater for individuals with more severe hearing loss for both men and women. Interestingly, within degree of hearing loss categories, older men self-perceived their hearing loss to be less handicapping than did younger men. The authors conducted a logistic regression analysis to determine the probability of hearing handicap as a function of age, and found that the probability of self-reporting a hearing handicap decreased with increasing age, and gender did not have a significant role in this predictive model (Wiley et al, 2000).

Pugh and Crandell (2002) compared hearing handicap and functional health status in a sample of African-American and Caucasian older adults. The majority of participants in the study were between 60 and 80 years of age, with a very small proportion over 80 years. Approximately half of the participants were African Americans and half were Caucasians with essentially mild to moderate sensorineural hearing loss for the most part. Thresholds at 8000 Hz were poorer in the Caucasians than in the African Americans, and the latter group reported significantly lower educational levels. Mean HHIE scores were comparable, with both groups presenting with essentially mild self-perceived hearing handicaps. Similarly, scores on the SF-36 were comparable across groups as well. It was noteworthy that increasing levels of hearing loss produced lower functional health scores on the SF-36. The findings suggest that mild hearing loss contributes a comparable amount to the variability in self-perceived hearing handicap and functional health status in Caucasian and African-American older adults, with the more pronounced functional deficits arising when hearing levels approach 40 dB HL.

As part of the BMHS Sindhusake et al (2003), assessed the accuracy of a self-reported hearing handicap in predicting pure-tone thresholds. This is an important question, as lack of predictive accuracy confirms the need to measure handicap and impairment as part of the routine audiological evaluation to obtain a complete picture of the patient's hearing status. All participants underwent a complete audiological evaluation, completed the HHIE-S, and responded to a single question: "Do you feel you have a hearing loss?" The sample ranged in age from 55 to over 85, with the majority being between 55 and 75 years of age. With regard to hearing levels, the majority of participants presented with mild to moderate hearing impairments. Responses to the HHIE-S were highly predictive of moderate to marked hearing loss, whereas the response to the single question was more predictive of mild hearing loss than was the score on the HHIE-S. It was of interest that the HHIE-S was more predictive of hearing impairment in the younger sample, confirming the work of other researchers that individual differences in HHIE-S are accounted for by hearing impairment and cognitive and central factors, once again underscoring the importance of using a questionnaire to capture information not provided by the pure-tone assessment.

Chang, Ho, and Chou (2009) explored the association between hearing handicap as measured using the HHIE and a variety of audiological and nonaudiological variables in a sample of community-based older adults living in Taipei, Taiwan. Of the 1220 participants 65 years of age or older, 45.5% had a hearing impairment and 11.6% perceived a hearing handicap. The majority of participants presented with a moderate hearing loss. Mean HHIE-S scores increased with increasing hearing impairment, although the relation between hearing impairment and hearing handicap was weak, such that 78% of individuals with moderate hearing loss did not report a handicap. It is important to note that 45% of those with moderate to severe hearing impairments and 45% of those with self-perceived handicap used hearing aids, whereas only 5% of those without a hearing handicap used hearing aids. In this sample, those who rated their health as poor were more likely to self-report a hearing handicap. These findings once again highlight the import of assessing the self-perceived effects of hearing impairment as they cannot be predicted from the audiogram.

Absent a reliable and valid test of CAPD, whether an auditory processing disorder exists remains an important question because (1) difficulty understanding speech, especially in noise, a hallmark of CAPD, is one of the most frequent complaints of older adults presenting for audiological assessment and management; (2) the existence of a central auditory processing problem has a significant impact on an older adult's perception of the social and emotional handicap resulting from hearing loss; and (3) CAPD has a potential impact on the successful use of hearing aids. With regard to the second consideration, older adults with minimal, mild, or moderate sensorineural hearing loss and CAPD self-rate their psychosocial handicap to be significantly greater than do those individuals without CAPD. This is not the case for older adults with and without cognitive deficits (Jerger, Oliver, & Pirozzolo, 1990). It is noteworthy that hearing aids are less effective in reducing psychosocial handicap in older adults with CAPD than are frequency-modulated (FM) systems. An older adult with CAPD who receives a hearing aid must realize that hearing aids may be bothersome to the point that speech understanding in noise is poorer, often leading to hearing-aid rejection (Jerger, Chmiel, Wilson, & Luchi, 1995). Older adults with CAPD, with or without peripheral hearing loss, who consider themselves handicapped should be considered prime candidates for audiological intervention in the form of technology, counseling, and auditory or cognitive training. The recent report by Hartley, Rochtchina, Newall, Golding, and Mitchell (2010) confirms the role of responses to the Hearing Handicap Inventory as a measure of candidacy for targeted audiological interventions.

As part of the BMHS, Hartley et al (2010) administered a complete battery of tests including pure tones, speech and the HHIE-S to a sample of 2933 adults residing in Australia. Thirty-three percent of respondents had hearing levels in the better ear in excess of 25 dB HL. Eleven percent of those with hearing loss who owned hearing aids and of those, 24% of participants with hearing aids never used them. Unfortunately, 33% of those with hearing levels in excess of 60 dB HL did not own hearing aids, despite experiencing negative consequences of hearing loss. Only 4.4% of participants reported having used some form of hearing-assistive technology systems (HATS. Interestingly, non–hearing-aid owners were more likely to use an assistive technology for their television than were hearing-aid owners. The majority of users of HATS had hearing aids, but a minority of hearing-aid owners used assistive technology (Hartley et al, 2010). The logistic regression analysis found that age, increasing degree of hearing loss, and HHIE-S score were significantly correlated with hearing-aid and HATS usage. Interestingly, educational level, hearing-aid usage, and hearing level in excess of 40 dB HL were significantly associated with the use of HATS. Further, age, smoking, HHIE-S score, assistive listening devices (ALD) usage, and severity of hearing loss were most strongly associated with hearing-aid usage (e.g., smokers were less likely to use hearing aids), with the mean age of hearing-aid owners being 75 years. Given the predictive value of self-reported hearing handicap, audiologists should make every effort to use patient responses to target interventions and to guide decisions regarding hearing health care.

<table>
<tr><td>Pearl</td></tr>
<tr><td>Age-related changes and temporal aspects of cognitive processing play a critical role in the comprehension of everyday speech, as do individual differences in performance on tasks designed to measure speech comprehension (Pichora-Fuller, 2003b).</td></tr>
</table>

◆ A Test Battery Approach for Use with Older Adults

Most clinicians and researchers would agree that there is considerable variability among older adults in the pure-tone threshold data, in speech-recognition ability in demanding listening environments, in the reaction to a given hearing impairment, and in motivation for seeking out hearing health care services. Yet, age-related differences in speech-recognition ability in challenging listening environments are the rule rather than the exception, even after accounting for audibility. It is well accepted that the individual differences are attributable in part to age-related changes in central auditory and cognitive function (Harris, Dubno, Keren, Ahlstrom, & Eckert, 2009). In my view, given what we now know regarding the multi-faceted nature of presbycusis, we must approach the audiological evaluation as detectives seeking to find a solution to the dilemma with which we are confronted. We must gather enough data on each domain of function so that we can understand the needs and competencies of our patients, which will facilitate an individualized approach to intervention, be it technological, counseling, auditory-cognitive training, or some combination.

As a matter of philosophy, the diagnostic evaluation should be considered an integral part of or a first step in the treatment plan. Further, this era of health care reform demands the delivery of high-quality, evidence-based, cost-effective care. Only by exploring and understanding the patient's unique problems can we prescribe a treatment plan that will be effective for and responsive to the patient. To this end, I concur with Pichora-Fuller and Souza (2003) that communication is not a unimodal process. I urge the use of materials and test conditions that relate to real-life listening experiences and environments, and encourage assessment of the patient multimodally. Understanding the relative contribution of age changes in the brain versus age changes in the ear, their impact on function, the value added by assessing auditory-visual status, coupled with the patient's perceptions and expectations, should drive assessment and management (Gates et al, 2008b).

Assessment of the older adult should begin with a comprehensive functionally oriented case history, with a formal or informal caregiver or communication partner being present. The case history should be elicited in a systematic fashion, beginning with exploration of the patient's rationale for purchasing hearing health care services. Taking the case history is an opportunity to learn about the patient's attitudes toward hearing loss and hearing aids, and to gain insight into the communication-specific difficulties attributable to hearing loss. Further, given the link among hearing loss, hearing hand-

Table 6.13   Hearing Health Risk Appraisal Form

Health Condition	Yes	No
1. Do you smoke cigarettes?	+	–
2. Do you or a family member believe that you have difficulty hearing and understanding others?	+	–
3. Have you been told that you now have diabetes mellitus?	+	–
4. Have you been told that you now have cardiovascular disease?	+	–
5. Have you been told that you now have arthritis?	+	–
6. Are you taking aminoglycoside antibiotics, cisplatin, an antiinflammatory agent, or loop diuretics? If so, which ones?	+	–
7. Have you had a fall within the past year? If so, please describe. (If so, clinician should administer the Screening for Otological Functional Impairments [SOFI] shown in Table 6.15.)	+	–
8. Have you been told that you have low vision or blindness?	+	–
9. Have you been told that you are suffering from depression? (If so, clinician should administer the Patient Health Questionnaire [PHQ] Screener shown in **Table 6.14**.)	+	–

*Circle the "+" for yes and "–" for no

icap, and physical functional status, the perceived impact of the hearing loss on physical functional status should be explored. A thorough drug history should be taken along with a systems analysis to determine whether age-related changes in an organ system or a disease is responsible for or explains in part the etiology of the hearing impairment. The audiologist should record the names of all medications, including dosing, and the model number of hearing aids, if they are in use, and the ear settings. The Hearing Health Risk Appraisal Form shown in **Table 6.13** taps into the comorbid conditions that place older adults at risk for hearing impairment. This form can be completed quickly and it provides essential information for diagnosis, for counseling, and for referrals. The screening version of the Patient Health Questionnaire (PHQ-9) should be considered if the patient responds affirmatively to the question about depression **Table 6.14**). If patient appears at risk for depression but is not being treated, a referral back to the primary care physician is in order. As part of the case history, cognitive status should be screened using the MMSE or the digit symbol substitution test, which assesses executive func-

Table 6.14   Two-Question Patient Health Questionnaire (PHQ)

Name: _____   Date: _____
During the past month, have you often been bothered by:
(Administrator, please use a checkmark to indicate the answer)

	Yes	No
1. Little interest or pleasure in doing things	1	0
2. Feeling down, depressed, or hopeless	1	0

If the patient's response to *both* questions is no, the screen is negative.
If the patient responds yes to *either* question, consider asking more detailed questions or using the nine-item PHQ.

tion and is correlated with hearing loss (Lin, 2011). Using the MMSE, cognitive function can be classified as low (score of 18–21), intermediate (22–25), or high (26–30). Here, too, a referral is indicated if mild cognitive impairment (MCI) appears to be present.

At the time of the initial encounter, audiologists must have a great deal of patience during their interactions with older hearing-impaired individuals. Allow adequate time, as several conditions can interfere with the interview process, including cognitive dysfunction, speech deficits, and depression. A handheld amplifier, such as a PocketTalker, should be used if necessary to assist in taking a case history to ease the flow of the interview, if the patient is not a hearing-aid user or if the hearing aid is malfunctioning. If the patient is a hearing-aid user, it is helpful to watch him or her manipulate the hearing aid, as one can gain insight into the patient's motoric skills, fine motor skills, memory, and so on.

Following the case history, a communication profile should be taken to uncover the perceived communicative and psychosocial effects of a given hearing impairment on daily function. Self-assessment scales, which quantify the perceived effects of hearing loss on daily life, have emerged as instruments that reliably uncover the functional impact of unremediated and remediated hearing loss. For the most part, scores on questionnaires that assess communicative function, activity limitations, and participation restrictions bear an imperfect relation to hearing impairment, which explains why each domain should be explored independently. In fact, the findings of Jerger and Chmiel (1997) and Humes (2007), among others, have confirmed that perceived deficits associated with hearing impairment are factors independent of pure-tone and speech data. In selecting a self-assessment scale, the audiologist must consider its reliability, content validity, and the age of the patient. Further, the instrument selected by the clinician should fit the purposes and setting for which the instrument was intended. Most audiologists continue to dismiss the contribution of information contained in responses to self-report scales at baseline and throughout the relationship that evolves with the patient with hearing impairment. However, their value in screening, in assessing the functional impact of hearing loss, as a prognostic indicator, in monitoring patient status, and as an outcome measure is undeniable.

Because tinnitus and dizziness are prevalent among older adults, audiologists are encouraged to explore their significance for the patient. Several questionnaires quantify the individual's perception of the characteristics and physical, emotional, and social response to tinnitus and to dizziness (Newman, Sandridge, & Jacobson, 1998). For example, the Tinnitus Handicap Inventory (THI), which is similar to the HHIE in format and scoring, contains 25 items that explore the functional, emotional, and catastrophic reactions to tinnitus. The THI has high internal-consistency reliability and high test-retest reliability. Individuals can be classified according to the severity of their tinnitus using the THI. Scores ranging from 0 to 16 are indicative of no tinnitus, scores ranging from 18 to 36 suggest a mild tinnitus handicap, scores ranging from 38 to 56 suggest a moderate tinnitus handicap, and scores 58 and above suggest a severe tinnitus handicap. The THI should be administered to clients reporting tinnitus so that the necessary referral for otological evaluation or continued medical management can be made. Alternatively, the Screening for Otologic Functional Impairments (SOFI) is a reliable tool for screening for tinnitus, dizziness or hearing related problems (**Table 6.15**). I suggest that audiologists send the SOFI or any other self-report instrument and a health risk appraisal form to the patient prior to the first appointment with a notice confirming the date and time of the appointment; ask the patient to complete the forms and bring to the first appointment. If the patient answers yes to any of the dizziness items on the SOFI, which are taken from the Dizziness Handicap Inventory (DHI) developed by Newman, Jacobson & Spitzer (1996), the patient should be referred to the primary care physician, as dizziness places the patient at risk for falls. The primary care physician may decide to do a complete workup. Physical therapy and an assessment of the patient's environment, to reduce the probability of falls, may also be appropriate. Preliminary results based on a small sample size ($n = 19$) suggest that test-retest reliability of the SOFI is high (0.91) and scores bear a strong relationship to HHIE-S scores ($r > 0.80$).

Pearl

It is a good idea to begin the audiological examination with otoscopy to rule out the presence of collapsed canals or impacted cerumen as a source of error in the testing.

Once the many steps in the history have been completed, the audiologist should discuss the evaluation plan with the patient and move ahead quickly. If cerumen is present, it is within the audiologist's scope of practice to undertake cerumen management. If this course is chosen, the necessary precautions should be taken, including complete documentation of the procedure and successful outcome. If it appears that the external auditory canal walls will collapse under pressure from standard supra-aural earphone cushions, which is often the case in the elderly, especially those residing in nursing facilities, insert earphones should be used to reduce the threat to the validity of air-conduction thresholds posed by collapsed canals. Many audiologists routinely and justifiably use inserts.

Table 6.15 Screening for Otological Functional Impairments (SOFI)

Instructions: The purpose of this questionnaire is to identify any problems you are having that may relate to your ears, including hearing difficulties, dizziness, or tinnitus (ringing/buzzing/noises in your ears/head). Please circle either *Yes, Sometimes,* or *No* for each question. If you use hearing aids, please answer the way you hear while using the hearing aids. If you are not experiencing any difficulties, please indicate by circling *No*.

D-1	Because of feelings of dizziness, is it difficult for you to walk around the house in the dark?	Yes	Sometimes	No
D-2	Does dizziness interfere with your job or household responsibilities?	Yes	Sometimes	No
D-3	Does bending over increase your feeling of dizziness?	Yes	Sometimes	No
Dizziness score				
H-1	Does a hearing problem cause you difficulty when listening to the television or radio?	Yes	Sometimes	No
H-2	Does your hearing problem cause you to feel frustrated when talking to members of your family?	Yes	Sometimes	No
H-3	Does a hearing problem cause you difficulty when visiting with friends, relatives, or neighbors?	Yes	Sometimes	No
Hearing score				
T-1	Do you feel that you can no longer cope with your tinnitus?	Yes	Sometimes	No
T-2	Because of tinnitus, do you have trouble falling asleep or staying asleep at night?	Yes	Sometimes	No
T-3	Do you feel that you cannot escape your tinnitus?	Yes	Sometimes	No
Tinnitus score				
G-1	Do you feel that any difficulty with your hearing, dizziness, or tinnitus significantly restricts your participation in social activities such as going to restaurants, dancing, movies, or other events?	Yes	Sometimes	No
Global score				
Total score				

In the box below, please circle the number that corresponds with the severity of the given problem.

	Not at all severe									Extremely severe
Dizziness:	0	1	2	3	4	5	6	7	8	9	10
Hearing loss:	0	1	2	3	4	5	6	7	8	9	10
Tinnitus:	0	1	2	3	4	5	6	7	8	9	10

Source: From Weinstein, B., Newman, C., & Sandridge, S. (2009) Screening for Otologic Functional Impairments (SOFI). Personal communication.

Pure-tone air and bone-conduction thresholds and immittance testing are an essential part of the audiological test battery, providing baseline information about hearing and middle ear status. Routine test procedures should be used when the client's mental, cognitive, and physical health status allow. I recommend routine testing of the inter-octave frequencies through 8000 Hz to gain a comprehensive picture of the extent of high-frequency hearing loss and potential impact on speech understanding. It is a good practice to routinely ask about the presence of tinnitus in either ear before you begin instructing the patient, as the response may affect the decision to use a continuous or pulsed tone. It is well established that pulsed tones can help minimize the confounding effects of tinnitus on threshold levels. Instructions must be audible, straightforward, and redundant, using examples of sounds the patient will hear to minimize any confusion. It is a good idea to have one trial run before beginning the testing to ensure that the patient understands the response task. Further, the audiologist should emphasize that the patient should respond to the softest tone heard because the goal is to find the patient's best hearing levels. The latter should be reiterated for nursing home residents because clinical experience suggests that often they tend to respond when tones are most comfortable rather than minimally audible. Otoacoustic emissions are often routinely done for purposes of corroborating findings. This is critical in patients taking ototoxic medications and especially when older adults are undergoing a course of chemotherapy. **Table 6.16** lists the modifications that may be necessary with selected clients during pure-tone testing. I have found some of the adjustments invaluable with confused patients and the frail elderly.

Pearl

When testing nursing home residents, it is often preferable to begin the actual test session with speech testing rather than pure-tone threshold seeking, as speech materials have more face validity and enable the respondent to attend to the task more readily.

A battery of speech tests should follow pure tone and immittance testing. Spondee or speech recognition thresholds are important for intra-test reliability purposes. A speech-awareness threshold may be indicated, depending on the patient's cognitive status or expressive abilities. Next, speech recognition tests should be administered to gain full insight into the complexity of the deficits and to explore auditory visual speech recognition ability, which is important for counseling. In my view speech tests should be administered that explore some of the complaints expressed by the patient with hearing impairment and some of the potential cognitive deficits. For example, the information from the self-report completed at the outset may have revealed difficulty (1) in highly reverberant conditions, (2) with accented speech, (3) when multiple people are speaking simultaneously, (4) in the presence of noise or competing conversation, (5) when people speak quickly, or (6) when the SNR is unfavorable. Select the test or tests that are sensitive to these complaints, because, during counseling, clarifying and confirming the test results can be very important in terms of establishing rapport and respect. Also, it is important that you explore how well the person with

Table 6.16 Modifications to the Standard Test Battery

Behavior	Test Modification
Slowed response time	Slowed rate of tonal presentation, allowing the patient's pace to dictate the interstimulus interval
Working memory deficits	Repeat and simplify instructions
	Use gestures to supplement voice when instructing
	Allow an opportunity for practice
	Provide frequent conditioning/reconditioning trials
	Provide verbal reinforcement
Movement deficits	Evaluate different strategies for responding before initiating testing
	Select response strategy that is the most natural and reflexive
	Do not change response behavior too often
Failing attention	Take a break during the session if fatigue begins to set in
	Sessions should be short, no longer than 45 to 60 minutes
	Morning sessions are often preferable in terms of fatigue and attention

hearing impairment uses the semantic context as an aid to speech perception, especially in challenging situations. Thus, the use of sentence materials such as the SSI, the DSI, and the SPIN is essential. According to a recent report by Gates et al (2008a) the DSI in free-response mode is the most sensitive test for uncovering the presence of memory impairment. Keep in mind that vocabulary-related verbal measures tend to be resistant to age-related declines, so that if speech understanding is assessed with speech materials that are highly contextual, older adults may be able to compensate for peripheral or central-auditory deficits, thereby potentially masking "the true extent of auditory involvement, including any underlying central-auditory deficits" (Humes et al, 2011, p. 18).

Documenting whether the patient derives benefit from contextual information in the more demanding listening conditions is important in terms of counseling and rehabilitative recommendations (Gordon-Salant & Fitzgibbons, 1997; Pichora-Fuller, 2003b; Pichora-Fuller, Schneider, & Daneman, 1995). Similarly, how well the patient understands speech with and without visual cues is important during counseling and when developing a rehabilitation plan. All of the data gathered during speech testing will help to tap into the central and cognitive overlay that may influence the nature of the targeted intervention options you discuss with the patient with hearing impairment and the patient's communication partner.

The purpose of the speech testing will drive the audiologist's thinking regarding the choice of test material, the presentation level, and the nature of the noise competition. As the work of Humes (2007) and others suggests, the presentation level for word-recognition tests is critical, given the peripheral hearing loss with which most older adults present. The decision should be affected by the need to ensure audibility of the high-frequency speech spectrum by compensating for the high-frequency hearing loss. **Table 6.17** summarizes some of

Table 6.17 Factors to Consider When Evaluating Speech-Understanding Abilities of Older Adult

Peripheral status
   a. Magnitude of high-frequency hearing loss
   b. Temporal acuity: time compression or reverberation task
   c. Audibility of signal: suprathreshold, normal conversational level
   d. Use of visual cues
Cognitive status
   a. Performance on a screening test of cognitive status, such as the Mini-Mental Status Examination (MMSE)
   b. Test indicative of speed of mental processing, such as subtests of the Wechsler Adult Intelligence Scale (WAIS): forward or backward digit span subtest
Central auditory and cognitive status
   a. Performance on a speech in noise test (fluctuating noise)
   b. Dichotic task
   c. Sentence materials: importance of context
Environmental factors
   a. Distance between communicators
   b. Quiet, noise (e.g., multi-talker babble, competing noise)
   c. Reverberation
   d. Optical conditions (e.g., room illumination)
   e. Availability of visual cues
Self-perception of hearing handicap
   a. Reliable and valid measure of psychosocial and communicative handicap that bears a minimal relationship to pure-tone data (e.g., Hearing Handicap Inventory for the Elderly [HHIE], COSI, Abbreviated Profile of Hearing Aid Benefit [APHAB])

Source: From Erber, N., Lamb, N., & Lind, C. (1996). Factors that affect the use of hearing aids by older people: A new perspective. *American Journal of Audiology, 5,* 11–19. (Reprinted by permission.)

the variables the clinician should consider when measuring speech-understanding ability. If you wish to make a point about the role of visual cues in testing with and without cues in noise and in quiet, it can certainly provide the clinical with evidence to use during counseling sessions. Similarly, if the audiologist is attempting to understand why previously successful hearing-aid users are suddenly dissatisfied with their binaural hearing aids, the clinician may wish to assess peripheral and central auditory processing ability and compare findings to previous word-recognition scores. Having baseline central auditory tests against which to compare performance is very helpful. Evidence of a decline in scores relative to the baseline may implicate a central component. Absolute scores on central tests of binaural integration can help shed light on why a binaural fitting may be problematic. Finally, I would be remiss if I did not caution that because routine tests of central auditory function (e.g., SSI) tend to be unreliable and confounded by peripheral hearing, Humes et al (2011) recommend consideration of some of the nonspeech measures in the Test of Basic Auditory Capabilities (TBAC).

If, for example, you want to counsel the patient with hearing impairment regarding communication strategies and context, demonstrating the difference in performance use of monosyllabic words and sentence materials in quiet or noise can be helpful, especially when the communication partner is complaining of the patient's difficulty communicating in selected listening situations. The early findings of Gordon-Salant and Sherlock (1992), who explored the role of linguistic factors, including context, help to make the point about the importance of context, especially in the presence of noise competition. They explored the efficacy of adaptive frequency response (AFR) hearing aids in improving speech perception in

noise among a group of older hearing-impaired adults. Speech-recognition ability in the presence of noise was improved with AFR circuitry only when contextual cues were provided to aid in recognition.

Following the preliminary test battery, the patient and communication partner or caregiver should be counseled regarding the findings. The test results should be presented in a clear, concise manner, so that the purpose and outcome on each of the tests is understood. At this time it is important to discuss the patient's impressions of the findings and together make a decision regarding the next steps. If hearing aids are a consideration, it may be helpful to gather information regarding the patient's sense of self-efficacy and the stage of readiness. Clinical experience suggests that if the patient with hearing impairment and the communication partner are given well-defined targets, have reasonable expectations, and the intervention options are targeted to their communication needs, the patient's successful rehabilitation potential will be enhanced. We have an obligation to provide the patient with hearing impairment and the communication partner with enough information and options to make an informed decision. If the patient has no interest in pursuing hearing aids, he or she should be made aware of assistive technologies and communication strategies that can be effectively employed. If hearing aids are an option, experiencing firsthand how speech sounds through hearing aids can be very instructive.

Later chapters discuss counseling in more depth, but here is an outline of important steps to follow when counseling:

1. Assess the patient's perspective, sense of self-efficacy, and readiness before discussing rehabilitative interventions.

2. Advise the patient regarding diagnostic results, impressions, prognosis, potential for success, and risks and benefits of pursuing an intervention, be it medical or rehabilitative.
3. Agree on the next steps, the importance of compliance with the chosen treatment options, and the role and responsibilities of the communication partner or caregiver.
4. Assist in arranging for follow-up visits, and establish a possible rehabilitative time line if intervention is the option being pursued.

These four steps are used by many in primary care to improve the care of community-based older adults. Comprehensive patient-centered assessment, engagement of the family in treatment, evidence-based care planning, and counseling about targeted interventions will help increase the ranks of older adults with hearing loss who take the necessary steps to overcome their deficiencies in understanding speech in an effort to optimize their function so that their quality of life will improve (Boult & Wieland, 2010).

References

Aarts, N. L., Adams, E. M., & Duncan, K. R. (2003, Dec). Older adult performance on an altered version of the SSI test. *American Journal of Audiology, 12,* 137–145

Baloyannis, S. J., Mauroudis, I., Manolides, S. L., & Manolides, L. S. (2009, Apr). Synaptic alterations in the medial geniculate bodies and the inferior colliculi in Alzheimer's disease: A Golgi and electron microscope study. *Acta Oto-Laryngologica, 129,* 416–418

Baltes, P. B., & Lindenberger, U. (1997, Mar). Emergence of a powerful connection between sensory and cognitive functions across the adult life span: A new window to the study of cognitive aging? *Psychology and Aging, 12,* 12–21

Boult, C., & Wieland, G. D. (2010, Nov). Comprehensive primary care for older patients with multiple chronic conditions: "Nobody rushes you through". *Journal of the American Medical Association, 304,* 1936–1943

Chang, H. P., Ho, C. Y., & Chou, P. (2009, Oct). The factors associated with a self-perceived hearing handicap in elderly people with hearing impairment—Results from a community-based study. *Ear and Hearing, 30,* 576–583

Chia, E. M., Wang, J. J., Rochtchina, E., Cumming, R. R., Newall, P., & Mitchell, P. (2007, Apr). Hearing impairment and health-related quality of life: The Blue Mountains Hearing Study. *Ear and Hearing, 28,* 187–195

Committee on Hearing, Bioacoustics, and Biomechanics (CHABA); Working Group on Speech Understanding and Aging, Commission on Behavioral and Social Sciences and Education, National Research Council, Washington. (1988). Speech understanding and aging. *Journal of the Acoustical Society of America, 83,* 859–895

Cooper, J. C., Jr, & Gates, G. A. (1991, Oct). Hearing in the elderly—The Framingham cohort, 1983–1985: Part II. Prevalence of central auditory processing disorders. *Ear and Hearing, 12,* 304–311

Craik, F. I. (2007, Jul-Aug). The role of cognition in age-related hearing loss. *Journal of the American Academy of Audiology, 18,* 539–547

Crandell, C. C. (1991, Dec). Individual differences in speech recognition ability: implications for hearing aid selection. *Ear and Hearing, 12*(6, Suppl), 100S–108S

Crandell, C., Henoch, M., & Dunkerson, K. (1991). A review of speech perception and aging: Some implications for aural rehabilitation. *Journal of the Academy of Rehabilitative Audiology, 24,* 121–133

Cruickshanks, K. (2010). *Age related hearing loss: Demographics and risk factors.* Presented at the ARC meeting in San Diego, April 14. http://www.audiologynow.org/pdf/Aging/2010_ARC_Cruickshanks.pdf

Dalton, D. S., Cruickshanks, K. J., Klein, B. E., Klein, R., Wiley, T. L., & Nondahl, D. M. (2003, Oct). The impact of hearing loss on quality of life in older adults. *Gerontologist, 43,* 661–668

Divenyi, P. L., & Haupt, K. M. (1997a, Apr). Audiological correlates of speech understanding deficits in elderly listeners with mild-to-moderate hearing loss. II. Correlation analysis. *Ear and Hearing, 18,* 100–113

Divenyi, P. L., & Haupt, K. M. (1997b, Jun). Audiological correlates of speech understanding deficits in elderly listeners with mild-to-moderate hearing loss. III. Factor representation. *Ear and Hearing, 18,* 189–201

Divenyi, P. L., Stark, P. B., & Haupt, K. M. (2005, Aug). Decline of speech understanding and auditory thresholds in the elderly. *Journal of the Acoustical Society of America, 118,* 1089–1100

Dubno, J. R., Dirks, D. D., & Morgan, D. E. (1984, Jul). Effects of age and mild hearing loss on speech recognition in noise. *Journal of the Acoustical Society of America, 76,* 87–96

Dubno, J. R., Horwitz, A. R., & Ahlstrom, J. B. (2007, Feb). Estimates of basilar-membrane nonlinearity effects on masking of tones and speech. *Ear and Hearing, 28,* 2–17

Dubno, J. R., Lee, F. S., Matthews, L. J., Ahlstrom, J. B., Horwitz, A. R., & Mills, J. H. (2008, Jan). Longitudinal changes in speech recognition in older persons. *Journal of the Acoustical Society of America, 123,* 462–475

Dubno, J. R., Lee, F. S., Matthews, L. J., & Mills, J. H. (1997, Apr). Age-related and gender-related changes in monaural speech recognition. *Journal of Speech and Hearing Research, 40,* 444–452

Dubno, J. R., & Schaefer, A. B. (1992, Apr). Comparison of frequency selectivity and consonant recognition among hearing-impaired and masked normal-hearing listeners. *Journal of the Acoustical Society of America, 91*(4 Pt 1), 2110–2121

Erber, N., Lamb, N., & Lind, C. (1996). Factors that affect the use of hearing aids by older people: A new perspective. *American Journal of Audiology, 5,* 11–19

Frisina, D. R., & Frisina, R. D. (1997, Apr). Speech recognition in noise and presbycusis: Relations to possible neural mechanisms. *Hearing Research, 106,* 95–104

Gaeth, J. (1948). *A study of phonemic regression in relation to hearing loss.* Ph.D. dissertation, Northwestern University

Gatehouse, S., Naylor, G., & Elberling, C. (2003, Jul). Benefits from hearing aids in relation to the interaction between the user and the environment. *International Journal of Audiology, 42*(Suppl 1), S77–S85

Gates, G. A., Anderson, M. L., Feeney, M. P., McCurry, S. M., & Larson, E. B. (2008a, Jul). Central auditory dysfunction in older persons with memory impairment or Alzheimer dementia. *Archives of Otolaryngology–Head & Neck Surgery, 134,* 771–777

Gates, G. A., Beiser, A., Rees, T. S., D'Agostino, R. B., & Wolf, P. A. (2002, Mar). Central auditory dysfunction may precede the onset of clinical dementia in people with probable Alzheimer's disease. *Journal of the American Geriatrics Society, 50,* 482–488

Gates, G. A., Cobb, J. L., Linn, R. T., Rees, T., Wolf, P. A., & D'Agostino, R. B. (1996, Feb). Central auditory dysfunction, cognitive dysfunction, and dementia in older people. *Archives of Otolaryngology–Head & Neck Surgery, 122,* 161–167

Gates, G. A., Feeney, M. P., & Mills, D. (2008b, Dec). Cross-sectional age-changes of hearing in the elderly. *Ear and Hearing, 29,* 865–874

Gelfand, S. A., Piper, N., & Silman, S. (1986, Dec). Consonant recognition in quiet and in noise with aging among normal hearing listeners. *Journal of the Acoustical Society of America, 80,* 1589–1598

George, E. L., Zekveld, A. A., Kramer, S. E., Goverts, S. T., Festen, J. M., & Houtgast, T. (2007, Apr). Auditory and nonauditory factors affecting speech reception in noise by older listeners. *Journal of the Acoustical Society of America, 121,* 2362–2375

Golding, M., Carter, N., Mitchell, P., & Hood, L. J. (2004, Oct). Prevalence of central auditory processing (CAP) abnormality in an older Australian population: The Blue Mountains Hearing Study. *Journal of the American Academy of Audiology, 15,* 633–642

Golding, M., Mitchell, P., & Cupples, L. (2005, Jun). Risk markers for the graded severity of auditory processing abnormality in an older Australian population: the Blue Mountains Hearing Study. *Journal of the American Academy of Audiology, 16,* 348–356

Golding, M., Taylor, A., Cupples, L., & Mitchell, P. (2006, Apr). Odds of demonstrating auditory processing abnormality in the average older adult: The Blue Mountains Hearing Study. *Ear and Hearing, 27,* 129–138

Goldstein, E. (2002). *Sensation and perception.* Pacific Grove, CA: Wadsworth-Thomson

Gordon-Salant, S. (2006). Speech perception and auditory temporal processing performance by older listeners: Implications for real-world communication. *Seminars in Hearing, 27,* 264–268

Gordon-Salant, S. (1987a, Oct). Age-related differences in speech recognition performance as a function of test format and paradigm. *Ear and Hearing, 8,* 277–282

Gordon-Salant, S. (1987b, Oct). Consonant recognition and confusion patterns among elderly hearing-impaired subjects. *Ear and Hearing, 8,* 270–276

Gordon-Salant, S., & Fitzgibbons, P. J. (1993, Dec). Temporal factors and speech recognition performance in young and elderly listeners. *Journal of Speech and Hearing Research, 36,* 1276–1285

Gordon-Salant, S., & Fitzgibbons, P. J. (1995a, Jun). Comparing recognition of distorted speech using an equivalent signal-to-noise ratio index. *Journal of Speech and Hearing Research, 38,* 706–713

Gordon-Salant, S., & Fitzgibbons, P. J. (1995b, Oct). Recognition of multiply degraded speech by young and elderly listeners. *Journal of Speech and Hearing Research, 38,* 1150–1156

Gordon-Salant, S., & Fitzgibbons, P. J. (1997, Apr). Selected cognitive factors and speech recognition performance among young and elderly listeners. *Journal of Speech and Hearing Research, 40,* 423–431

Gordon-Salant, S., & Fitzgibbons, P. J. (2001, Aug). Sources of age-related recognition difficulty for time-compressed speech. *Journal of Speech, Language, and Hearing Research, 44,* 709–719

Gordon-Salant, S., & Sherlock, L. P. (1992, Aug). Performance with an adaptive frequency response hearing aid in a sample of elderly hearing-impaired listeners. *Ear and Hearing, 13,* 255–262

Grimes, A. M., Grady, C. L., Foster, N. L., Sunderland, T., & Patronas, N. J. (1985, Mar). Central auditory function in Alzheimer's disease. *Neurology, 35,* 352–358

Hällgren, M., Larsby, B., Lyxell, B., & Arlinger, S. (2001, Apr). Cognitive effects in dichotic speech testing in elderly persons. *Ear and Hearing, 22,* 120–129

Harris, L., Dubno, J., Keren, N., Ahlstrom, J., & Eckert, M. (2009). Speech recognition in younger and older listeners. *Journal of Neuroscience, 13,* 6078–6087

Hartley, D., Rochtchina, E., Newall, P., Golding, M., & Mitchell, P. (2010). Use of hearing aids and assistive listening devices in an older Australian population. *Journal of the American Academy of Audiology, 21,* 642–653

Helfer, K. (1991). Everyday speech understanding by older listeners. *Journal of the Academy of Rehabilitative Audiology, 24,* 17–34

Helfer, K. (2009). Older adults in complex listening environments. In *Conference proceedings: Hearing care for adults—The challenge of aging.* http://www.phonakpro.com/com/b2b/en/events/proceedings/archive/adult_conference_chicago2009.html.html

Helfer, K. S., & Wilber, L. A. (1990, Mar). Hearing loss, aging, and speech perception in reverberation and noise. *Journal of Speech and Hearing Research, 33,* 149–155

Humes, L. E. (1996, Jun). Speech understanding in the elderly. *Journal of the American Academy of Audiology, 7,* 161–167

Humes, L. E. (2002, Sep). Factors underlying the speech-recognition performance of elderly hearing-aid wearers. *Journal of the Acoustical Society of America, 112*(3 Pt 1), 1112–1132

Humes, L. E. (2005, Apr). Do "auditory processing" tests measure auditory processing in the elderly? *Ear and Hearing, 26,* 109–119

Humes, L. E. (2007, Jul-Aug). The contributions of audibility and cognitive factors to the benefit provided by amplified speech to older adults. *Journal of the American Academy of Audiology, 18,* 590–603

Humes, L. E., Burk, M. H., Strauser, L. E., & Kinney, D. L. (2009, Oct). Development and efficacy of a frequent-word auditory training protocol for older adults with impaired hearing. *Ear and Hearing, 30,* 613–627

Humes, L. E., & Christopherson, L. (1991, Jun). Speech identification difficulties of hearing-impaired elderly persons: The contributions of auditory processing deficits. *Journal of Speech and Hearing Research, 34,* 686–693

Humes, L., Christopherson, L., & Cokely, C.(1992). Central auditory processing disorders in the elderly: Fact or fiction? In J. Katz, N. Stecker, & D. Henderson (Eds.), *Central auditory processing: A transdisciplinary view.* St. Louis: Mosby Year Book

Humes, L. E., & Dubno, J. R. (2010). Factors affecting speech understanding in older adults. In S. Gordon-Salant, R. Frisina, A. Popper, & R. Fay (Eds.), *The aging auditory system.* New York: Springer

Humes, L., Dubno, J., Gordon-Salant, S., Lister, J., Cacace, A., Cruickshanks, K., et al. (2011). *Report from the American Academy of Audiology Task Force on Central Presbycusis.* http://www.audiology.org/resources/documentlibrary/Documents/20111208_AAA_TFCentPres_Report.pdf

Humes, L. E., Nelson, K. J., & Pisoni, D. B. (1991, Nov). Recognition of synthetic speech by hearing-impaired elderly listeners. *Journal of Speech and Hearing Research, 34,* 1180–1184

Humes, L. E., & Roberts, L. (1990, Dec). Speech-recognition difficulties of the hearing-impaired elderly: The contributions of audibility. *Journal of Speech and Hearing Research, 33,* 726–735

Humes, L. E., Watson, B. U., Christensen, L. A., Cokely, C. G., Halling, D. C., & Lee, L. (1994, Apr). Factors associated with individual differences in clinical measures of speech recognition among the elderly. *Journal of Speech and Hearing Research, 37,* 465–474

Jerger, J., Alford, B., Lew, H. L., Rivera, V., & Chmiel, R. (1995, Oct). Dichotic listening, event-related potentials, and interhemispheric transfer in the elderly. *Ear and Hearing, 16,* 482–498

Jerger, J., & Chmiel, R. (1997, Aug). Factor analytic structure of auditory impairment in elderly persons. *Ear and Hearing, 8,* 269–276

Jerger, J., Chmiel, R., Allen, J., & Wilson, A. (1994, Aug). Effects of age and gender on dichotic sentence identification. *Ear and Hearing, 15,* 274–286

Jerger, J., Chmiel, R., Wilson, N., & Luchi, R. (1995, Aug). Hearing impairment in older adults: new concepts. *Journal of the American Geriatrics Society, 43,* 928–935

Jerger, J., & Hayes, D. (1977, Apr). Diagnostic speech audiometry. *Archives of Otolaryngology, 103,* 216–222

Jerger, J., Jerger, S., Oliver, T., & Pirozzolo, F. (1989, Apr). Speech understanding in the elderly. *Ear and Hearing, 10,* 79–89

Jerger, J., Jerger, S., & Pirozzolo, F. (1991, Apr). Correlational analysis of speech audiometric scores, hearing loss, age, and cognitive abilities in the elderly. *Ear and Hearing, 12,* 103–109

Jerger, J., Oliver, T. A., & Pirozzolo, F. (1990, Apr). Impact of central auditory processing disorder and cognitive deficit on the self-assessment of hearing handicap in the elderly. *Journal of the American Academy of Audiology, 1,* 75–80

Lin, F. R. (2011, Oct). Hearing loss and cognition among older adults in the United States. *Journal of Gerontology: Medical Sciences, 66,* 1131–1136

Lin, F. R., Metter, E. J., O'Brien, R. J., Resnick, S. M., Zonderman, A. B., & Ferrucci, L. (2011, Feb). Hearing loss and incident dementia. *Archives of Neurology, 68,* 214–220

Lindenberger, U., & Baltes, P. B. (1997, Sep). Intellectual functioning in old and very old age: Cross-sectional results from the Berlin Aging Study. *Psychology and Aging, 12,* 410–432

Martin, J. S., & Jerger, J. F. (2005, Jul-Aug). Some effects of aging on central auditory processing. *Journal of Rehabilitation Research and Development-Supplement, 42*(4, Suppl 2), 25–44

Neijenhuis, K., Tschur, H., & Snik, A. (2004, Jan). The effect of mild hearing impairment on auditory processing tests. *Journal of the American Academy of Audiology, 15,* 6–16

Newman, C. W., Jacobson, G. P., & Spitzer, J. B. (1996, Feb). Development of the Tinnitus Handicap Inventory. *Archives of Otolaryngology–Head and Neck Surgery, 122,* 143–148

Newman, C. W., Sandridge, S. A., & Jacobson, G. P. (1998, Apr). Psychometric adequacy of the Tinnitus Handicap Inventory (THI) for evaluating treatment outcome. *Journal of the American Academy of Audiology, 9,* 153–160

Peelle, J. E., Troiani, V., Grossman, M., & Wingfield, A. J. (2011, Aug). Hearing loss in older adults affects neural systems supporting speech comprehension. *Journal of Neuroscience, 31,* 12638–12643

Pichora-Fuller K (2003a). Cognitive aging and auditory information processing. *International Journal of Audiology, 42,* 2S26–2S32

Pichora-Fuller, M. K. (2003b, Jul). Processing speed and timing in aging adults: Psychoacoustics, speech perception, and comprehension. *International Journal of Audiology, 42*(Suppl 1), S59–S67

Pichora-Fuller, M. (2008, Nov). Use of supportive context by younger and older adult listeners: Balancing bottom-up and top-down information processing. *International Journal of Audiology, 47*(Suppl 2), S72–S82

Pichora-Fuller, K. (2010). *Implications of cognitive factors for rehabilitation.* Paper presented at the ARC Audiology Now Conference. http://ebookbrowse.com/2010-arc-pichora-fuller-pdf-d66689644

Pichora-Fuller, M. K., Schneider, B. A., & Daneman, M. (1995, Jan). How young and old adults listen to and remember speech in noise. *Journal of the Acoustical Society of America, 97,* 593–608

Pichora-Fuller, M. K., & Singh, G. (2006, Mar). Effects of age on auditory and cognitive processing: Implications for hearing aid fitting and audiologic rehabilitation. *Trends in Amplification, 10,* 29–59

Pichora-Fuller, M. K. & Souza, P. (2003). Effects of aging on auditory processing of speech. *International Journal of Audiology, 42,* 2S11–2S16

Plomp, R., & Duquesny, A.(1982). A model for the speech-reception threshold in noise without and with a hearing aid. In O. Pedersen & T. Poulsen (Eds.), *Binaural effects in normal and impaired hearing. Scandinavian Audiology Supplement, 15,* 95–101

Pugh, K. C., & Crandell, C. C. (2002, Oct). Hearing loss, hearing handicap, and functional health status between African American and Caucasian American seniors. *Journal of the American Academy of Audiology, 13,* 493–502

Rossi-Katz, J., & Arehart, K. H. (2009, Apr). Message and talker identification in older adults: Effects of task, distinctiveness of the talkers' voices, and meaningfulness of the competing message. *Journal of Speech, Language, and Hearing Research, 52,* 435–453

Roup, C. M., Wiley, T. L., & Wilson, R. H. (2006, Apr). Dichotic word recognition in young and older adults. *Ear and Hearing, 17,* 230–240, quiz 297–298

Schneider, B. A., Daneman, M., & Murphy, D. R. (2005, Jun). Speech comprehension difficulties in older adults: cognitive slowing or age-related changes in hearing? *Psychology and Aging, 20,* 261–271

Schneider, B. A., Daneman, M., Murphy, D. R., & See, S. K. (2000, Mar). Listening to discourse in distracting settings: The effects of aging. *Psychology and Aging, 15,* 110–125

Sindhusake, D., Mitchell, P., Newall, P., Golding, M., Rochtchina, E., & Rubin, G. (2003, Jul). Prevalence and characteristics of tinnitus in older adults: The Blue Mountains Hearing Study. *International Journal of Audiology, 42,* 289–294

Souza, P., Boike, K., Witherell, K., & Tremblay, K. (2007). Prediction of speech recognition from audibility in older listeners with hearing loss: Effects of age, amplification and background noise. *Journal of the American Academy of Audiology, 18,* 54–65

Stach, B. A., Spretnjak, M. L., & Jerger, J. (1990, Apr). The prevalence of central presbyacusis in a clinical population. *Journal of the American Academy of Audiology, 1,* 109–115

Stewart, R., & Wingfield, A. (2009, Feb). Hearing loss and cognitive effort in older adults' report accuracy for verbal materials. *Journal of the American Academy of Audiology, 20,* 147–154

Strouse, A. L., Hall, J. W., III, & Burger, M. C. (1995, Apr). Central auditory processing in Alzheimer's disease. *Ear and Hearing, 16,* 230–238

Sweetow, R., & Sabes-Henderson, J. (2004). Components of communication. The case for LACE (listening and communication enhancement). *Hearing Journal, 57,* 32–38

Townsend, T. H., & Bess, F. H. (1980). Effects of age and sensorineural hearing loss on word recognition. *Scandinavian Audiology, 9,* 245–248

Tremblay, K. L., Piskosz, M., & Souza, P. (2003, Jul). Effects of age and age-related hearing loss on the neural representation of speech cues. *Clinical Neurophysiology, 114,* 1332–1343

Tremblay, K., & Ross, B. (2007, Jul-Aug). Effects of age and age-related hearing loss on the brain. *Journal of Communication Disorders, 40,* 305–312

van Rooij, J. C., & Plomp, R. (1990, Dec). Auditive and cognitive factors in speech perception by elderly listeners. II: Multivariate analyses. *Journal of the Acoustical Society of America, 88,* 2611–2624

van Rooij, J. C., & Plomp, R. (1992, Feb). Auditive and cognitive factors in speech perception by elderly listeners. III. Additional data and final discussion. *Journal of the Acoustical Society of America, 91,* 1028–1033

van Rooij, J. C., Plomp, R., & Orlebeke, J. F. (1989, Oct). Auditive and cognitive factors in speech perception by elderly listeners. I: Development of test battery. *Journal of the Acoustical Society of America, 86,* 1294–1309

Vaughan, N., Storzbach, D., & Furukawa, I. (2008, Jul-Aug). Investigation of potential cognitive tests for use with older adults in audiology clinics. *Journal of the American Academy of Audiology, 19,* 533–541, quiz 579–580

Weinstein, B., Newman, C., & Sandridge, S. (2009) *Screening for Otologic Functional Impairments (SOFI).* Personal communication

Wiley, T. L., Cruickshanks, K. J., Nondahl, D. M., & Tweed, T. S. (2000, Feb). Self-reported hearing handicap and audiometric measures in older adults. *Journal of the American Academy of Audiology, 11,* 67–75

Wiley, T. L., Cruickshanks, K. J., Nondahl, D. M., Tweed, T. S., Klein, R., & Klein, B. E. (1998, Jun). Aging and word recognition in competing message. *Journal of the American Academy of Audiology, 9,* 191–198

Wingfield, A. (1996, Jun). Cognitive factors in auditory performance: Context, speed of processing, and constraints of memory. *Journal of the American Academy of Audiology, 7,* 175–182

Wingfield, A., Poon, L. W., Lombardi, L., & Lowe, D. (1985, Sep). Speed of processing in normal aging: Effects of speech rate, linguistic structure, and processing time. *Journal of Gerontology, 40,* 579–585

III

Rehabilitation Considerations

Chapter 7

Audiological Rehabilitation/Communication Management: An Integrated Approach

I always tell people if I could choose between blindness or having a hearing loss, I would choose blindness. Hearing loss can be so terribly isolating.

—M.K., 76-year-old man with hearing loss for 30 years

I do not like these hearing aids; I am beginning to hear my wife.
—F.G., 80-year-old man

Hearing aids: the final indignity.
— L.G., 80-year-old woman with a series of age-related health issues

When asked if she notices a difference when she wears her hearing aids, she responded, "No, they are soooo annoying," and her husband responded, "Yes, she is so annoying when she does not have them on."

—66-year-old couple

Hearing aids have brought me back into the conversation. I no longer sit outside the circle but I am able to participate in the important social situations of everyday life.

—J.G., 77–year-old woman

People who work in the reception area of dispensing audiologists should learn how to talk to people who have hearing impairment. You would think that they would know how important it is to face the hearing impaired when they speak and to remove background noise that may interfere with communication.

—M.F., 60-year-old woman

If audiology is to survive as the dispenser of choice for quality hearing care, then the professional audiologist must take a hard look at the services that they offer that will substantiate the claim of "better care" and the "higher cost."

—T.Z., 60+-year-old hearing-aid user

To hear as well as my ears will allow in any given situation; that is my goal.

—R.H., 58 years old

◆ Learning Objectives

After reading this chapter, you should be able to

- understand that audiological rehabilitation is a holistic client-centered process that is a natural part of the hearing-aid delivery system;

- understand the theoretical underpinnings of counseling and the principles of counseling;
- understand that time constraints serve as an excuse for not providing the full range of services necessary to optimize audibility and communication and to reduce the functional deficits associated with hearing loss; and
- realize the value of outcomes assessment as a means of ensuring that treatment goals are realized.

◆ Overview

This chapter offers a contemporary view of audiological rehabilitation (AR), presents a framework in which audiologists can practice AR in tune with their understanding of the unique needs of older adults with handicapping hearing impairments, and discusses how clinicians can deal effectively with the special aspects of providing care to older patients with hearing loss by applying recent information about approaches that are of proven success. This chapter also emphasizes that AR is the responsibility of audiologists involved in the diagnosis and management of individuals with hearing impairments, activity limitations, and participation restrictions (Brummel-Smith, 1990). The organization of the chapter reflects my belief that AR is the vehicle for optimizing communication in hearing impaired persons with and without hearing aids. Further, the chapter takes into consideration the evolving health care system in which funding is minimal, time is money, and the need for accountability is great. These factors convince me more than ever of the importance of an AR program that is brief, efficient, and, above all, patient centered.

The work of Pichora-Fuller has been inspirational to me, and it is my hope that this chapter will lead some audiologists to explore how a patient's improved social interactions and active lifestyle facilitated in part by auditory and cognitive-based interventions may possibly slow cognitive decline in older hearing impaired adults. Further, the persons with hearing loss (PHLs) who I evaluate have inspired my thinking in this arena. I have learned that we must heed their advice and take into account their perspective. Summing up advice from persons with hearing loss (PHLs) who are members of Hearing Loss Association of America (formerly SHHH), Sorkin (1997) reported that PHLs:

"become frustrated, confused, even bitter when they realize that a hearing aid is not going to restore normal hearing in the same way that eyeglasses restore vision. When this happens, they become ineffective hearing-aid users or nonusers. Use of amplification is most successful when it is used by people with an understanding of the full range of modifications that a person needs to incorporate hearing loss into their life. People who enjoy such success understand that the effectiveness of a hearing aid increases with time and with experimentation, that hearing aids work better in certain situations than others, and that other assists—used in concert with a hearing aid—can often help someone function more effectively in a range of settings and situations (p. 54)."

Sorkin's suggestion to audiologists is an important one: "Listen to the patient and make sure that the intervention is adapted to the lifestyle and expresses the needs of the hard of hearing person."

Let's begin by underscoring one fact and ten myths, which we must address in our work with PHLs and health care professionals (Kochkin, 2010; Rejeski, Brawley, & Jung, 2009; Sweetow & Sabes, 2010):

Fact: Forty percent of Americans self-reported a moderate to severe hearing loss, yet only 9% of persons with mild hearing loss wear hearing aids, which is ironic as hearing aids and AR are the treatment of choice for more than 90% of persons with impaired hearing (Kochkin, 2010).

Myth 1: Hearing aids and cochlear implants restore hearing to normal.

Myth 2: Hearing aids eliminate all communication problems.

Myth 3: All hearing-aid users can achieve adequate speech recognition with hearing aids alone.

Myth 4: Most people with hearing aids do not like how they sound.

Myth 5: Advancements in digital technology have perfected hearing aids.

Myth 6: Stigma is no longer a deterrent to hearing-aid uptake.

Myth 7: Personal and device-related counseling are not effective tools for promoting acceptance of hearing aids.

Myth 8: Aural rehabilitation is an "added benefit" pursued at the conclusion of the hearing-aid fitting.

Myth 9: You cannot expect older adults to benefit from auditory training designed to assist in deriving meaning from auditory cues and the linguistic context.

Myth 10: Cognitive skills such as working memory, speed of processing, and executive control do not influence speech processing in older adults with or without hearing aids.

Hopefully after reading this chapter you will be convinced that debunking these myths is an integral part of AR.

◆ Principles of Geriatric Rehabilitation and Its Relation to Audiological Rehabilitation

Rehabilitation with older adults must be comprehensive in terms of the approach to assessment, and multidimensional in terms of the interventions. The purpose of rehabilitation with older adults, irrespective of the impairment, is to assist in recovering physical, psychological, and social skills that have been lost due to illness, disease, or injury; and to ensure that older adults can remain independent, maintain meaningful

social interactions, and live in environments that are personally satisfying (Lewis & Bottomley, 2008). Achievement of the highest possible level of function and quality of life is the priority (Brown, 2009). Given the important role of the family, the rehabilitation process demands participation of family members, caregivers, and communication partners. Although many of the techniques used to achieve rehabilitative goals are similar to those used with younger adults, the modalities, philosophy, and expected outcomes differ (Brown, 2009). Of utmost importance is engaging the older adult in a discussion regarding rehabilitative goals and expectations, and targeting interventions to achieve mutually agreed-upon goals and outcomes appropriate to the person with hearing impairment and the communication partner. Cognitive reserve, or the ability to compensate for cognitive changes as one ages, and executive function, or mental flexibility, will influence the design and course of treatment as well. Recognition of the variability across individuals in terms of cognitive changes and the ability to compensate for age-related cognitive changes is paramount and integral to the success of rehabilitation (Martin & Gorenstein, 2010).

Geriatric rehabilitation services are organized around a conceptual model of disability as adopted by the World Health Organization (WHO). In adopting a biopsychosocial view of health, the International Classification of Functioning, Disability, and Health (ICF) provides a framework for rehabilitation with older adults (WHO, 2001). Using the WHO model, interventions are designed to target a person's impairment and to modify limitations in activities and restrictions in participation deriving from the impairment. Characterizing decreases in function as a consequence of health conditions and environmental and personal factors, the ICF enables the audiologist to view the patient's hearing impairment in a context that helps the clinician generate a treatment plan. A problem at the organ level in older adults (e.g., peripheral damage, cognitive and central auditory processing decrements at the level of the brainstem and cortical regions) must be viewed in terms of its functional effects on the person, family, and society, and ultimately the nation at large within their physical or social environment (Lewis & Bottomley, 2008). When clinicians working in geriatric rehabilitation design an intervention, they must consider the effort the intervention requires and the impact it will have on an older adult's functional independence and quality of life. Rehabilitative interventions with older adults have high value when the treatment improves speech perception in the presence of various types of background noise, and improves the quality of life (Abrams, 2008). When using the ICF model to describe patients' function, as we will see later in the chapter, we must restore audibility resulting from organ-level deficits in individuals who vary considerably in their function, with the goal being to help them continue to effectively communicate with family and friends according to their level of expectation. The ICF model underscores the importance of focusing on how audiologists can help patients live a satisfying life with the existing hearing impairment (Brown, 2009). Using a biopsychosocial perspective acknowledges that aging is a complex phenomenon that involves the interrelationship among social, cultural, biological, and psychological processes, yet it is also a very personal experience (Morgan & Kunkel, 2011).

Functional capabilities must be assessed on an individual basis because of the individual variability characterizing older adults. Chronological age is not a reliable predictor of physical functional abilities, because of the heterogeneity of all of the variables that impact on physical, social, and mental well-being—three indices of functional outcomes (Lewis & Bottomley, 2008). Given this variability, older adults' subjective appraisal of their personal health status influences rehabilitative planning and outcomes. In fact, their appraisal is often at odds with that of the health care provider, but improvement resulting from intervention is correlated with the former. The patient's perspective is key because it "influences how he or she reacts to the symptoms, perceives his or her vulnerability, and perceives his or her abilities to perform a given activity" (Lewis & Bottomley, 2008, p. 163). One final fundamental principle of geriatric rehabilitation is that frequent and positive feedback regarding progress improves outcomes (Lewis & Bottomley, 2008).

Pearl

Knowing about an older adults' hearing status is important, but to plan meaningful interventions we must know how the condition affects their lives, especially their functional ability (Morgan & Kunkel, 2011).

◆ Audiological Management: A Holistic Approach

Audiological rehabilitation, auditory rehabilitation, and aural rehabilitation are terms used interchangeably to describe a patient management process designed for individuals who experience deficits in communication in a variety of listening environments and are seeking assistance to optimize communication efficiency. I prefer the term *audiological management* or *communication management*. The ability to maintain meaningful social interactions; reduce communication limitations; decrease participation restrictions; promote function, independence, quality of life, and well-being of older adults; and to slow down cognitive decline are important goals of audiological management (Boothroyd, 2010; Hickson, Worrall, & Scarinci, 2007; Pichora-Fuller, 2006; Sweetow & Sabes, 2010). Audiological management is a comprehensive program of hearing health care for persons with handicapping hearing impairments premised on the assumption that wearing a hearing aid is only a part of the solution to communication problems and their psychosocial manifestations (Hickson & Worrall, 2003; Trychin, 1995). Indeed, with communication and understanding spoken language as the ultimate goal, AR must be incorporated at the beginning of the management process rather than at the conclusion. Stated differently, a product orientation with the person with hearing impairment having a passive role should be replaced with a person-centered orientation with the person with hearing impairment assuming an active role in overcoming obstacles to communication success and achieving his or her goals (Hickson & Worrall, 2003; Sweetow & Sabes, 2010). Understanding the patient the audiologist

serves, providing appropriate support and counseling, maximizing communication success in everyday environments, and managing the consequences of hearing loss are integral to successful management programs (Tye-Murray, 2008).

At the heart of the management process is the concept of optimizing patient function and the patient's ability to extract auditory information from a degraded input (Kane, Ouslander, & Abrass, 2004; Pichora-Fuller, 2009). Management must (1) be interactive, aimed at restoring communication function and improving quality of life; (2) be person-centered, such that the preferences of the patient and family members are respected, and they are involved in decision making; (3) be practical and accessible; (4) involve a partnership between the audiologist and the patient; (5) be multifaceted, including provision of a hearing instrument in the context of psychological support, social supports, and environmental manipulation; (6) be adaptive, wherein there is a balance between the individual's attention span and performance or frustration threshold; (7) emphasize self-management; (8) entail frequent feedback; (9) include measurable outcomes that verify progress, as this is the foundation of evidence-based practice; and (10) reflect an understanding of the patient's cultural belief system (Besdine et al, 2005; Sweetow & Sabes, 2007).

Kane, Ouslander, and Abrass (2004) view optimal functioning as part of a fraction, with the numerator being the product of physical capabilities, medical management, and motivation, and the denominator being an estimate of the social, physical, and psychological environment. The resulting equation reads as follows: (physical capabilities × medical management × motivation)/(social, psychological, and physical environment). In their view, to optimize patient function, we must follow several steps: (1) remediate the chronic conditions that are responsive to treatment, and consider the patients physical capabilities when deciding on the appropriate intervention; (2) create a physical, social, and psychological environment that will be conducive to promoting independent function by reducing barriers to access; (3) ensure that caregivers and the patient believe that the patient can improve with the appropriate intervention; and (4) emphasize that a positive attitude matters, and provide frequent feedback regarding accomplishments, which helps to motivate and empower patients toward pursuing and sustaining the behavior in which they are engaged.

Pearl

Holistic management of the hearing impaired must reflect an understanding of the principles borrowed from social psychology and gerontology.

With its focus on human functioning rather than on disease, the ICF nomenclature (WHO, 2001) serves as the framework for a care plan necessary to optimize patient function. The International Classification of Impairments, Disabilities, and Handicaps (ICIDH-2) system is organized into two parts; one emphasizes functioning and disability, and the other acknowledges the role of contextual factors. In the context of the older adult, the term *impairment* carries a broader definition than

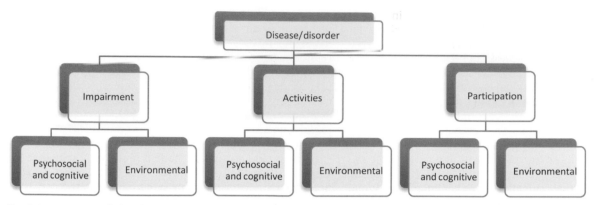

Fig. 7.1 International Classification of Impairments, Disabilities, and Handicaps (ICIDH-2) World Health Organization (WHO) classification system. [From World Health Organization (WHO). (2001) *International Classification of Functioning (ICF), Disability, and Health*. Geneva, Switzerland: World Health Organization.]

just hearing, and the terms *activity limitations* and *participation restrictions* replace the concepts of disability and handicap, which are more negative than the former terms. The domains of function to be assessed include lower level auditory function, auditory brainstem function, the level of the midbrain and the auditory cortex, activity limitations, and participation restrictions in the variety of situations in which persons with hearing impairment find themselves owing to the interaction between top-down and bottom-up processing deficits. Environments that are not conducive to successful communication and personal factors such as confidence, compensatory strategies, and adequacy of cognitive resources must enter into the equation when making management decisions. The WHO-ICF model allows for the fact that contextual factors will moderate or influence how the peripheral and central auditory systems interact during speech processing, and that degradation of the input will influence activity and participation levels (Gallun & Saunders, 2010). Extrapolating from a recent lecture by Tremblay and Pichora-Fuller (2011), using the ICF model we can consider the perceptual and cognitive processing difficulties as activity limitations and how these difficulties impact social roles and participation restrictions, with environmental and personal factors serving as either supports or barriers to communication. According to Gagne and Jennings (2011), we can conceive of our interventions as designed to restore or optimize participation in activities using expressed activity limitations and participation restrictions to formulate goals and to target particular problems.

The model of communication handicap in **Fig. 7.1** shows how contextual factors such as the listening environment might influence how a hearing impairment may contribute to activity limitations and participation restrictions. Similarly, the model shows how when we counsel the hearing impaired to use compensatory strategies to modify their environment, the direct result may be increased involvement in activities previously avoided, with perhaps less listening effort. The classification system emphasis is on the active role the person with hearing impairment plays in appraising the factors within themselves and in the environment to be manipulated to optimize function. It is an indispensable part of the process used to match a treatment plan to demands of the chronic

condition. At the heart of the model is the effect of the condition on function, and an understanding of the functions of audition can assist in understanding the consequences of hearing impairment.

◆ Functions of Audition

To best understand the impact of acquired hearing loss on older adults as conceptualized using the ICF model, familiarity with the functions of hearing and the resulting sense of loss as described by Ramsdell (1960) is important. Although proper communication entails several steps, including hearing, listening, comprehending, and responding, the ability to hear entails three important levels (Sweetow & Sabes, 2010): The fundamental level of hearing is the primitive level, which constitutes an unconscious link between the person with hearing loss and the environment. The primitive level of hearing might be conceived of as a basic physiological function. The ability to hear background sounds, such as birds singing and the hum of a car, contributes to our sense of being part of an alive world (Ramsdell, 1960). Prior to the advent of cochlear implants, persons with severe to profound hearing loss were often deprived of the ability to hear background noise and speech prosody, with potentially dramatic psychosocial consequences resulting from such deprivation. Loss at this level which goes untreated may trigger depressive reactions. Cochlear implantation has been shown to be an effective remedy for restoring the primitive level of hearing, and as such is considered a realistic intervention for older adults meeting the preestablished criteria (Orabi, Mawman, Al-Zoubi, Saeed, & Ramsden, 2006).

It is well accepted that hearing loss associated with the normal aging process does not tend to render the majority of older adults profoundly deaf, and thus rarely is there a need for restoration of the primitive level of hearing. However, we must keep in mind that we will be called on to serve adults who have been deaf all of their lives and are now aging. Of the 35 million people 65 years of age or older in the United States, 250,000 to 400,000 individuals have severe to profound hearing impairment, many of whom should be considered cochlear

Table 7.1 Level of Hearing and Impact on Function

Level of Hearing	Behavioral Consequence	Impact on Function When There is No Intervention
Inability to hear at the primitive level	Inability to hear environmental sounds and sounds of nature	Disorientation, isolation
Inability to hear at the signal warning level	Inability to hear warning and information sounds; inability to hear traffic noise	Insecurity in daily life
Inability to hear at the symbolic level	Inability to understand the spoken message	Unable to participate in conversation; difficult to maintain long-distance contacts using the telephone; unable to participate in social, religious, and cultural activities; impaired quality of life

implant candidates as restoration of the primitive level of hearing now can be a reality (Leung et al, 2005).

Moderately severe, severe, or profound hearing loss can compromise the signal/warning level or the second level of hearing. Ramsdell (1960) postulated that at this level, sound serves as an indicator of an outside stimulus or event and assists in locating the source of sound. In a sense, at this level, hearing serves to inform persons of dangers in the environment including the presence of smoke in the home, an oncoming vehicle, or a knock at the door. The ability to hear warning signals as well as background noise fosters a sense of security and independence. Thus, one's sense of safety and security in the home can be jeopardized when warning signals in the environment are inaudible. The ability to hear signals in the environment is an especially important goal for most hearing-impaired older adults, especially for those who live alone and for those suffering from cognitive problems, including dementia. According to Maslow's hierarchy of needs theory (Maslow, 1954), older adults are very motivated to pursue intervention when a chronic condition is a threat to their security or safety, either at home or in society at large. People first seek to satisfy their most basic needs, those necessary to survival (e.g., security and safety needs that may pose a threat or deprivation), after which they will seek to satisfy higher social, self-esteem, and self-actualization needs (Kotler & Clark, 1987). Use of hearing assistance technology, such as a smoke alarm that flashes, is an important step toward maintaining a sense of safety and security. Further, binaural hearing aids and directional technology enhances safety, as individuals report improved ability localizing sound and detecting danger signals from behind.

The function subserved by the third level of hearing, namely the symbolic level, is the ability to process complex symbols, which is at the heart of communication and a uniquely human ability. When hearing, the least complex of the elements leading to proper communication, does not function at this level, as is the case in individuals suffering from age-related declines in speech processing, older adults may be denied the pleasure of enjoying music; understanding family and friends when they speak; understanding at theater, lectures, or restaurants; and understanding colleagues at work. Hence, loss of the symbolic level of hearing is likely to diminish the quantity and quality of social interactions. Hearing-impaired individuals deprived of hearing at the third level may suffer from a loss of social independence. The resulting inability to communicate may interfere with life satisfaction and may have an impact on one's self-esteem and level of communicative confidence (Kemp, 1990). It is helpful to discuss these levels of hearing with persons with hearing impairment and their communication partner, as this helps them to better understand the impact of a hearing and communication deficit. **Table 7.1** summarizes the potential effects of loss of each of the levels of audition.

> **Pearl**
>
> Restoration, either in part or in full, of each of these levels of hearing via audiological management can help promote adjustment to deficits in communication and functional abilities associated with hearing loss.

◆ Consequences of Hearing Loss

Hearing loss negatively affects physical, cognitive, and behavioral functions, and the general quality of life, and is related to depression and dementia (Arlinger, 2003). Projections suggest that 10% of the population in Western countries experience a significant-enough hearing loss that it affects ordinary daily life (Arlinger, 2003). The deleterious effects of the hearing impairment can best be understood by combining an appreciation of the functions of audition and the important role played by communication with an appreciation of the profound effect cognitive and perceptual declines place on older adults. Recall that older adults often experience threshold elevations and difficulty understanding in quiet and demanding listening situations. Added to this, older adults often have to apply greater effort to understand, owing to decreased speed of processing, attentional deficits associated with reductions in inhibitory control, and reductions in working memory (Sweetow & Sabes, 2010). The latter cognitive deficits plus the additional cognitive effort necessary to understand in complex environments contributes to reductions in speech perception, creating a negative feedback loop. The interaction between top-down and bottom-up processing further complicates the challenges.

In general, the effects of sensorineural hearing loss are diverse, pervasive, and highly variable. The sensorineural hearing loss experienced by older adults has dramatic effects on communication and hence psychosocial and cognitive function. With regard to communication function, the primary deficit is difficulty in understanding speech or in identifying the target message from a background of noise (Anderson & Kraus, 2010). The most difficult situations include noisy backgrounds, environments with multiple speakers, and speaking with strangers, persons with accents, or people who speak quickly. Communication deficits attributable to the aging of the senso-rineural mechanism include difficulty communicating at home or at work, interpersonal difficulties, and difficulty under-standing speech from a distance, in the context of noise, and on the telephone. In addition, according to Arlinger (2003), communication deficits can also include a reduced ability to detect, identify, and localize sounds. Communication disabil-ity can place an individual at a disadvantage relative to others, leading to a handicap or a "disadvantage experienced through interaction with and adaptation to the environment" (Hyde & Riko, 1994, p. 348). It is often the case that the person with hearing impairment may not be aware of the extent of the speech understanding deficits and their effect on everyday function (Arlinger, 2003). Untreated hearing impairment has a profound effect on many aspects of the life experience rang-ing from physical health status, emotional well-being, mental health status, cognitive status, income level, family relation-ships, work performance, and ability to remain employed or to find employment (Kochkin, 2010). Although it has been well established that persons with hearing impairment suffer from depression, social isolation, poor social interactions, cognitive dysfunction, reduced emotional and social well-being, the ef-fects of family members, in particular on communication part-ners is not as well studied.

I reviewed the literature on the impact of hearing loss, on hearing-aid uptake, and on functional hearing-aid benefit, and found that the effects of hearing loss are first felt in the emo-tional domain. As the hearing impairment becomes more se-vere and more obvious, it impacts social situational function. Findings from an early study that I conducted support this theory. I investigated the relation between audiological mea-sures and objective and subjective social isolation in a sample of older male veterans with adult-onset mild to moderately severe sensorineural hearing loss (Weinstein, 1980). Objec-tive isolation was quantified using the Objective Present Isola-tion Scale, which quantifies contacts with significant others, participation in leisure and recreational activities, and living arrangements. Subjective isolation was quantified using the Subjective Social Isolation Scale, which quantifies interest in engaging in activities, feelings of loneliness, feelings of inferi-ority, and satisfaction with the quality and quantity of social interactions. Both these scales are homogeneous subscales of the Comprehensive Assessment and Referral Evaluation (CARE), a semistructured interview that was developed by Gurland et al (1977–1978). The extent of subjective social isolation (e.g., loneliness, withdrawal) was more highly related to severity of hearing impairment and self-perceived hearing handicap than was the extent of objective isolation (e.g., engagement in so-cial activities, visiting friends/family).

Correlations between audiometric measures and feelings of subjective social isolation ranged from 0.40 to 0.52, whereas the correlation between audiometric measures and feelings of objective isolation was 0.25. It was noteworthy that not until the hearing loss became moderately severe did it have an im-pact on involvement in social activities, such that the majority of persons with moderately severe sensorineural hearing loss

lived alone, rarely socialized, kept problems to themselves, rarely visited friends and relatives, rarely engaged in leisure activities, rarely spoke on the telephone, and rarely engaged in volunteer activities. In contrast, although a mild hearing loss left a large proportion of participants feeling upset, nervous, and handicapped, the extent of their involvement in daily ac-tivities was not diminished in response to the hearing impair-ment. It was of interest that individuals who were considered to be isolated both objectively and subjectively had poorer hearing and were more handicapped than those who were not isolated. I concluded that early on, hearing loss is felt in terms of its psychological impact, and as it progresses, it curtails social life (Weinstein, 1980), which is in keeping with the data on hearing-aid uptake that suggests that the majority of older adults who own hearing aids buy them when the hearing loss approaches a moderate to moderately severe level, and that they wait close to 10 years after first noting a hearing loss be-fore they seek intervention. Counseling the hearing impaired is therefore a critical part of the diagnostic and management process, if we are to encourage them to seek an intervention for their communication difficulties.

Several recent studies have demonstrated that hearing loss has an adverse effect on functional status, cognitive function, and emotional, behavioral, and social well-being. Arlinger (2003) contends that hearing loss can result in a poorer quality of life, isolation, reduced social activity, and increased symptoms of depression. Increasing difficulties communicating combined with the aforementioned changes account for the finding that hearing impairment may inhibit a person's ability to function independently and hence compromise quality of life (Bess, Lichtenstein, Logan, Burger, & Nelson, 1989b; Garstecki & Erler, 1996; Mulrow et al, 1990b; Uhlmann, Larson, Rees, Koepsell, & Duckert, 1989).

The reactions to hearing loss can be categorized into several domains as shown in **Table 7.2** (Tremblay & Pichora-Fuller, 2011; Trychin, 2002). The audiologist working with older adults must be familiar with each of the reactions as part of the man-agement process and should focus on addressing and possibly ameliorating some of these deleterious consequences. Keep in mind that personality, lifestyle, support system, attitude, and physical health status all contribute to the extent and complexity of the psychosocial reaction to a given hearing impairment, which in large part explains the incomplete rela-tion between measured impairment and the psychological response. Van Vliet (2005) summarized the relevance of psy-chosocial correlates of hearing loss, stating that "psychosocial factors and their effects on behavior related to hearing aid use are very complex and require a more prominent place in as-sessment and fitting protocols than exist within the current standard of care" (p. 415). Further, hearing loss has a deleteri-ous effect on income and is a factor associated with unemploy-ment among the hearing impaired (Kochkin, 2010).

Although hearing aids are technologically very advanced and mitigate the effects of hearing loss, the proportion of hearing-aid users has not changed in more than 50 years, with less than one fourth of the hearing impaired using hearing aids; four million people who could benefit from hearing aids have not purchased them (Kochkin, 2010; Kochkin et al, 2010). Fur-ther, close to 12% of hearing-aid owners are not using their hearing aids. The reasons for nonuse are listed in **Table 7.3**, and

Table 7.2 Possible Responses to and Consequences of Hearing Loss

Emotional reaction	May include shame, anger, frustration, embarrassment, depressive symptoms
Interpersonal reaction	May include social withdrawal, social isolation, confusion, loss of intimacy in relationships
Cognitive reaction	Increased effort necessary to comprehend especially in suboptimal situations; difficulty processing speech; cognitive capacity affects speech understanding in complex and fluctuating listening situations, and attentional deficits; deficits in working memory; changes in mental status; hearing loss is associated with incident dementia; hearing loss negatively effects cognitive reserve; dementia (Lin, Metter, O'Brien, Resnick, Zonderman & Ferrucci, 2011; Lunner & Sundewall-Thorén, 2007).
Participation restrictions	Withdrawal from previous involvement in community activities; avoidance of interpersonal interactions because of the strain associated with communicating; experiences social rejection
Physical reaction	Sleep problems, fatigue, muscle tension, feeling unsafe
Safety	As hearing loss increases, so to do concerns about safety
Health status	Self-rating of health worse as hearing levels increase in severity; patient is perceived by others to have compromised cognitive function
Activity limitations	Difficulty to detect environmental sounds such as telephone ringing, difficulty localizing the sound source, difficulty understanding accented speech, speech in noise, and speeded speech

Sources: Data from Trychin, S. (2002). *Guidelines for providing mental health services to people who are hard of hearing.* San Diego: University of California, San Diego; Laplante-Lévesque, A., Hickson, L., & Worrall, L. (2010, Mar). Rehabilitation of older adults with hearing impairment: A critical review. *Journal of Aging and Health, 22,* 143–153; and Tremblay, K., & Pichora-Fuller, K. (2011). Rehabilitating older ears and older brains. Paper presented at Audiology Now, Chicago, April.

it is probable that the lack of use accounts for the persistent psychosocial problems experienced by persons with hearing loss. This table can be helpful in informing the audiological management process.

Several investigators have explored the reaction of older adults to hearing impairment, and there is agreement that there is a high degree of individual variability in the reactions of older adults to hearing loss, ranging from complete acceptance and positive personal adjustment to feelings of displacement, anger, and withdrawal. Hence, it is important to qualitatively and quantitatively assess each patient. Many investigators sampled non–hearing-aid users to determine the psychosocial and functional impacts of hearing impairment, and others evaluated hearing-aid users to determine the beneficial effects of hearing aids, indirectly demonstrating the impact of hearing impairment on well-being.

Strawbridge, Wallhagen, Shema, and Kaplan (2000) conducted a longitudinal study of the negative effects of self-reported hearing loss on physical health, physical functioning, mental health, and social functioning outcomes in a sample of older adults. Participants were involved in the Alameda County Longitudinal Study of Health and Mortality, which began in 1965 and included a sample of close to 7000 older adults ranging in age from 50 to 102 years, with a mean age of 65 years. Although objective measures of hearing status were not administered, the findings of self-reported difficulty hearing were noteworthy and were compared primarily to self-reports of

Table 7.3 The Reasons Why the Hearing Impaired Do Not Use Hearing Aids

Poor benefit
Poor fit
Lack of comfort
Unsatisfactory performance in noise
Little positive word-of-mouth endorsement

Source: Data from Kochkin, S., Beck, D., Christensen, L., Compton-Conley, C., Fligor, B., Kricos, P., McSpaden, J., Gustav Mueller, H., Nilsson, M., Northern, J., Powers, T., Sweetow, R., Taylor, B., & Turner, R. (2010). Marke Trak VIII: The impact of the hearing healthcare professional on hearing aid user success. *Hearing Review, 17,* 12, 14, 16, 18, 23, 26, 27, 28, 30, 32, and 34.

physical health status, physical functional status, mental health status, and social functioning. Although self-reported hearing loss tends to yield a lower prevalence of hearing loss than do objective data, the trends here were similar to hearing loss prevalence using objective measures of hearing status. Men had a higher prevalence of self-reported hearing loss than did women, and self-reported hearing loss became more prevalent with increasing age. Interestingly, the authors found that those reporting moderate to severe difficulty hearing and understanding had an increased likelihood of self-reported mental health problems, were more likely to be depressed, had more difficulty performing activities of daily living, and were more likely to rate their health as poor. Moderate self-reported hearing loss appeared to detract dramatically from interpersonal relationships and had a negative effect on morale. Finally, Strawbridge and colleagues found that self-reported hearing loss is longitudinally associated with common measures of disability and independence level, namely activities of daily living (ADLs), instrumental activities of daily living (IADLs), and physical performance. ADLs address such activities as walking, grooming, dressing, and eating with or without assistance, whereas IADLs address use of the telephone, ability to shop for and prepare meals, ability to manage money, and ability to do light housework, for example. The fact that self-reported hearing loss is associated with functional outcomes is important, given the role that decrements in ADL and IADL play in decisions to institutionalize older adults and in determining eligibility for home care services.

Dalton et al (2003) conducted a population-based longitudinal study of the effects of hearing loss on quality of life and functioning of older adults. Participants were enrolled in the Epidemiology of Hearing Loss Study (ELHS-2) conducted in Beaver Dam, Wisconsin. Information on global functioning was obtained from interviews that asked about ADLs and IADLs during the month prior to the interview. Health-related quality of life was assessed using the Short-Form Health Survey (SF-36), which measures eight domains of health status, including physical functioning, pain, general health perception, social functioning and emotional and mental health. Mean age of the participants was 69 years; 51% of participants had some degree of hearing loss (27% had a mild loss and 24% had a moderate to severe loss). The majority of persons with impaired hearing were non–hearing-aid users (85%). Self-reported hearing handicap, defined based on scores on the screening version of the Hearing Handicap Inventory for the Elderly (HHIE-S), increased with increasing hearing impairment, such that 22% of persons with mild hearing loss had a self-perceived handicap, as did 56% of persons with a moderate to severe hearing loss (i.e., HHIE-S score >8) (Ventry & Weinstein, 1983). Interestingly, younger participants with mild, moderate, or severe hearing impairment (52–69 years) were more handicapped than older participants (70–97 years). After controlling for age, sex, and education participants with moderate to severe hearing loss were 34 times more likely to have a self-reported handicap than were participants without hearing loss. Overall, 52% of participants admitted to having communication difficulties, such as difficulty understanding their physician, difficulty understanding on the telephone, and difficulty understanding conversation when several people are talking. The odds of experiencing communication difficulties increased with hearing loss severity with even a small proportion of participants with normal hearing reporting communication difficulties. Similarly, severity of hearing loss was associated with impairments in ADL and IADL, after controlling for chronic conditions such as arthritis and impaired visual acuity. HHIE-S score >8 and self-report of communication difficulties were significantly associated with reduced SF-36 scores in all domains of function including the physical health and bodily pain sections. Similarly, severity of hearing impairment was associated with lower Physical Health Component (e.g., physical and general health) and Mental Health Component (social, mental health) scores.

Cox, Alexander, and Gray (2007) conducted a cross-sectional survey of the contribution of nonaudiometric variables including personality to self-reported hearing handicap and hearing impairment. The mean age of the participating women was 75 years, and the mean age of the men was 73 years. The 205 participants had bilateral symmetrical mild to moderately severe sensorineural hearing loss. The study sheds light on the role personality characteristics may play in terms of noise tolerance or aversiveness to noise and in terms of activity limitations as measured using the Abbreviated Profile of Hearing-Aid Benefit (APHAB) and participation restrictions based on scores on the HHIE. For example, participants who scored higher on the Extraversion, Openness, and Agreeableness scales were less likely to report that environmental sounds were unpleasant, whereas those who scored higher on the Neuroticism scales were more likely to have a negative reaction to environmental sounds. Interestingly, higher scores on the Neuroticism scale were associated with more activity limitations and participation restrictions, whereas lower Extraversion scores were associated with higher APHAB and HHIE scores. Personality traits had a stronger relationship to self-report scores than to the audiogram. The score on the Neuroticism scale accounted for 21% of the variance in scores on the HHIE, with higher neuroticism associated with more participation restrictions. Neuroticism accounted for 11% of the variance in APHAB scores such that higher neuroticism was associated with more activity limitations. Hearing impairment did not bear a strong relationship to the trait of neuroticism, whereas it was strongly associated with self-reports of listening and communication difficulties. The study findings demonstrate that individuals with the same audiometric results can report different types of difficulty in the real world that are related to personality traits, which in turn are tapped in self-report tests such as the HHIE and the APHAB. This conclusion underscores the role of self-report in routine assessment of older adults.

The National Council on the Aging (NCOA) commissioned the Seniors Research Group to conduct a national survey of older Americans, with the goal being to quantify the social, psychological, and functional effects of hearing loss, and to compare effects on quality of life between seniors who use hearing aids and those who do not (NCOA, 1999). A total of 2304 persons with hearing impairment responded, and an additional 2090 communication partners responded to a parallel questionnaire asking about their partners' communication difficulties. The findings from the NCOA study confirmed that adults over 50 years of age with untreated hearing loss are more likely than adults over 50 years of age with comparable hearing loss but who use hearing aids to experience depression, anger, and frustration, and to be less engaged socially. Further, compared with adults who use hearing aids, those who do not are more likely to report feeling sad and anxious, to be less social active, and to report experiencing emotional turmoil and insecurity. Finally, the hearing-impaired respondents who owned hearing aids were more likely than nonusers to be involved in organized social activities and attend activities at a local senior center. Similarly, the hearing-aid users reported that the hearing aids improved their family relationships, mental health, and quality of life. Interestingly, the communication partners observed more benefits from the partner's use of hearing aids than did the hearing-aid users. Again, this survey demonstrated directly and indirectly the negative effect of hearing impairment on quality of life.

Mulrow et al (1990b) conducted comprehensive cross-sectional studies of the relationship between hearing impairment and quality of life in a sample of 204 elderly male veterans selected from a primary care clinic. Quality of life was defined according to two disease-specific and three generic measures that have been standardized on older adults. The disease-specific measures were the HHIE, which assesses the self-perceived emotional and social effects of hearing loss, and the Quantified Denver Scale of Communication Function (QDS). The QDS quantifies the perceived communication difficulties secondary to hearing impairment. The generic measures were the Short Portable Mental Status Questionnaire (SPMSQ), which yields information about cognitive function; the Geriatric Depression Scale (GDS), which assesses affect; and the Self-Evaluation of Life Function (SELF), which assesses function in several domains, including physical disability, social satisfaction, aging, depression, self-esteem, and personal control.

Hearing loss in this sample of older hearing-impaired adults was associated with significant social, emotional, and communication handicaps, as mean scores on the HHIE and QDS were significantly higher for the hearing-impaired group than for the non–hearing-impaired group. In contrast, mean scores on the GDS and the SELF did not differ for the groups with and without a hearing impairment. Similarly, mental status was intact for both groups of subjects. As the extent of the perceived social and emotional dysfunction was considerable for this sample (i.e., 66% had HHIE scores >42, indicative of severe handicap, and 16% had HHIE scores between 18 and 40, indicative of mild to moderate handicaps), the authors concluded that hearing loss has an adverse effect on quality of life. A follow-up randomized trial of hearing-aid rehabilitation indicated that hearing-aid intervention was effective at reducing the communication difficulties, psychosocial handicaps, and depressive and cognitive symptoms experienced by the majority of hearing-impaired older men in this sample. In light of the reduction in depressive symptoms and psychosocial handicap, it is tempting to infer a causal relation between hearing loss and these symptoms.

Bess, Lichtenstein, and Logan (1990) reported on the association between hearing loss in older adults and scores on tests of hearing disability and global dysfunction. The Sickness Impact Profile (SIP), a 136-item scale that assesses psychosocial function in a behavioral context, was the index of functional health status, and the HHIE-S was the hearing-specific measure for disability. The authors noted a graded association between measurable hearing impairment and functional health status, such that persons with increasing levels of hearing impairment (speech frequency pure-tone average) demonstrated increased levels of psychosocial and physical dysfunction as measured on the SIP. For example, on the physical scale that assesses ambulation, mobility, and body care/movement, mean SIP scores increased from 3.3 for those with no impairment to 18.9 for those with a loss of 41 dB HL or greater. Thus, on the physical subscale, a SIP score change of 2.8 will occur with each 10-dB increase in hearing loss (Bess, Lichtenstein, Logan, & Burger, 1989a). Further, higher HHIE-S scores were associated with higher SIP scores, suggesting a relation between hearing disability and global dysfunction (Bess et al, 1990). Once again, these findings link hearing loss to functional disability and handicap and demonstrate the importance of including this information in the rehabilitative assessment. Efforts to improve hearing with hearing aids can result in meaningful improvements in quality of life in general and functional status in particular.

More data are accumulating documenting a link between hearing loss and cognitive status in persons diagnosed with senile dementia. The major findings of studies on hearing loss in persons with dementia are as follows:

1. Hearing loss is independently associated with incident all-cause dementia (Lin et al, 2011).
2. Central auditory processing difficulties may be an early marker for dementia; individuals with low scores on the Synthetic Sentence Identification with Ipsilateral Competing Message (SSI-ICM) were more likely to develop clinical dementia several years after the initial testing (i.e., 3 to 12 years later); auditory speech-processing problems appear predictive of future manifestations of senile dementia (Gates, Beiser, Rees, D'Agostino, & Wolf, 2002).
3. Hearing loss is more prevalent in older adults with dementia (Weinstein & Amsel, 1986).
4. Older adults with dementia are likely to have more severe hearing loss than those without dementia (Uhlmann et al, 1989; Weinstein & Amsel, 1986).
5. The risk of dementia increases as a function of increasing hearing loss, after adjusting for potentially confounding variables such as depression, number of primary prescriptions, and age (Uhlmann et al, 1989).

6. Unremediated hearing loss lowers performance on aurally administered diagnostic tests used to quantify the severity of senile dementia (Weinstein & Amsel, 1986).
7. Hearing aids lower scores on tests of cognitive function, suggesting improved mental status with hearing-aid use.
8. Hearing impairment bears a significant relationship to scores on the Mini-Mental Status Examination (MMSE) based on a case–controlled study (Uhlmann et al, 1989)

Given the high prevalence of senile dementia among older adults, especially those residing in institutions, and the high prevalence of hearing loss, it is likely that the two disorders will co-occur in a large proportion of older adults. According to Arlinger (2003), uncorrected hearing loss has been significantly correlated with reduced cognitive abilities. Detection and treatment of hearing loss is therefore critical if we are to optimize cognitive processing, especially for those with compromised abilities. Further unremediated hearing loss can confound the diagnosis of dementia, and often exacerbates the behavioral manifestations of senile dementia. Similarly, lack of familiarity with the behavioral characteristics of persons with dementia can jeopardize the validity of the audiological assessment and interfere with the benefits to be derived from audiological interventions, such as hearing aids and hearing assistance technologies. Approximately one third of the "oldest old" population, or those age 85 or over, report moderate or severe memory problems according to a U.S. Census Bureau report (Bergman, 2006). Accordingly, audiologists should informally assess mental status in persons being considered for intervention by asking simple questions that yield information regarding memory and orientation, or by administering a validated instrument such as the SPMSQ (Pfeiffer, 1975). Any in-service training of physicians or nurses should always include information on the relation between cognitive status and hearing status in older adults.

Several investigators have indirectly documented the effects of hearing impairment on quality of life by demonstrating how hearing-aid use alleviates the social and emotional handicaps experienced prior to using hearing aids. Chisolm et al (2007) conducted a systematic review of health-related quality of life and hearing aids. Their review of 16 studies focusing almost exclusively on adults revealed that hearing-aid use yields an improvement in health-related quality of life by reducing the psychological, social, and emotional effects of sensorineural hearing loss. The study by Vuorialho, Karinen, and Sorri (2006) was not part of Chisolm et al's review, but these authors also found that improvements in scores on the HHIE-S were associated with hearing-aid use, leading them to conclude as well that hearing aids help to alleviate the social and emotional consequences of hearing loss. As is evident from **Table 7.4**, hearing loss is associated with many negative emotional and social behaviors that are reversed in part by the use of hearing aids.

Evidence is beginning to mount documenting that hearing loss affects communication with one's family, friends, and co-workers. Communication partners have to put more effort into communication with PHLs; they need to speak more slowly and be more articulate, they must face the PHL, and they must adjust their distance. As a consequence of these increased demands, friends and family members may have fewer contacts with the hearing-impaired person, leading to the person's iso-

Table 7.4 Multidimensional Benefit of Hearing Aids (N = 4000)

Greater earning power (especially the top 60% of hearing losses)

Improved interpersonal relationships, greater intimacy, reduction in discrimination toward the person with the hearing loss

Reduction in difficulty associated with communication, especially among those with severe to profound hearing loss

Reduction in anger and frustration

Reduction in the incidence of depression and depressive symptoms

Enhanced emotional stability

Reduced anxiety symptoms

Improved self-efficacy

Improved cognitive functioning

Improved health status

Enhanced group social activity

Improved mental, emotional, and physical health

Improved quality of conversation

Less effort required to communicate

Improved ease of listening

Source: Data from Kochkin, S. (2005). *The impact of treated hearing loss on quality of life.* http://www.betterhearing.org/aural_education_and_counseling/ articles_tip_sheets_and_guides/hearing_loss_treatment/quality_of_life _detail.cfm.

lation (Arlinger, 2003). The qualitative evidence demonstrating that hearing impairment affects the psychosocial function of the communication partner is noteworthy (Brooks, Hallam, & Mellor, 2001). Given the centrality of communication in intimate relationships, and the listening effort required to communicate with a spouse, the stress associated with having to serve "as the ears" of PHLs affects the spouse's engagement in and enjoyment of previously enjoyed social activities.

Hearing loss has an effect on intimate relationships and places unexpected tensions on marital relationships (Scarinci, Worrall, & Hickson 2008). The stress and frustration often associated with the need to repeat what has been said, to speak louder, and to speak in close proximity with one's face visible has been well documented (Preminger & Meeks, 2010). Scarinci et al (2008) conducted a qualitative study of 10 couples who were married for well over 25 years, and at the time of the study one of the partners had a hearing loss whereas the other had normal hearing. The majority of participants had moderate hearing loss for over 5 years. Participants ranged in age from 60 to 83 years (mean, 70 years). Although six out of the ten participants with hearing loss owned hearing aids, only two reported using them. The goal of the study was to identify the effects of hearing impairment on the relationships and the impact of hearing loss on retirement, and to explore the communication strategies employed as well as the effect on the communication partner of the person with hearing loss accepting or denying hearing loss. It was noteworthy that the spouses reported that hearing impairment had an effect on nearly all tasks and everyday activities, on their relationship, on their emotional status, and on participation in activities. The spouses expressed concerns about the safety of the PHL, and notably they reported feeling embarrassed especially because of the need to use repair strategies to facilitate communication. The communication partners noted that retirement tended to exacerbate the effect of the hearing impairment on their relationship, as they were spending much more time together and were communicating more frequently. One final

theme was that most of the spouses commented that the PHLs for the most part denied having a hearing impairment, attributing their difficulties to external factors rather than to a hearing impairment.

One of the sources of conflict is that communication partners and PHLs often do not agree on the nature or the extent of the effect of the hearing impairment on quality of life, especially prior to pursuing amplification. Newman and Weinstein (1986) demonstrated that although prior to amplification PHLs tend to view their hearing impairment as being more significant than did their communication partners, following hearing-aid use the congruence in perceived hearing-related quality of life is remarkable. Similarly, Stark and Hickson (2004) also reported improvements in understanding for both the PHLs and communication partners in selected listening situations following hearing-aid use, including in the presence of background noise, when the television is turned to a high volume, and during small group conversations. Hence, when working with the PHLs and communication partners, the perspective of the different parties should inform the rehabilitative agenda.

◆ The Effects of Hearing Loss: Discussion

Untreated hearing impairment in older adults restricts one or more dimensions of quality of life, including physical functional status and cognitive, emotional, and social function. Hence, the consequences are far reaching, global, and cumulative. Because pure-tone and speech-recognition ability bear an imperfect relationship to self-perceived activity limitations and participation restrictions, the effects must be measured directly by questioning both PHLs and their communication partner. It is incumbent on the audiologist to ensure that management decisions are based on both the audiometric data and on expressed functional ability in the communicative and psychosocial domains. As expressed by Howard "Rocky" Stone (1990), the audiologist must be aware of the psychosocial needs of the whole person and not just focus on the technology, and this information will set the stage for intervention. Consistent with the biopsychosocial philosophy espoused above, Gagne, Jennings, and Southall (2009a) make an interesting point regarding our view of PHLs. People with hearing loss do not have a hearing handicap; rather, in selected situations they may experience a handicap because of their hearing impairment. By extension, the goal of audiological management is to improve audibility and speech understanding so that older adults can communicate effectively in noisy situations, in restaurants, or in other problematic situations. Finally, it is important to note that the length of time that PHLs have been dealing with the consequences of their hearing loss will have direct impact on the quality of their lives and their functional abilities (Abrams & Chisolm, 2009).

◆ Principles Underlying Audiological Management of Older Adults with Hearing Impairment

Prior to discussing the components of a comprehensive management program, a discussion of the assumptions and principles underlying audiological management is essential. This discussion uses concepts from social psychology and geriatric medicine and rehabilitation. At the heart of each of the philosophies discussed below is that the person with hearing loss may need to change or unlock certain behaviors and learn complex new skills to achieve successful outcomes. This is the challenge audiologists must accept. The integral principles, strategies, and philosophies discussed here are motivational interviewing, collaborative self-management, self-efficacy beliefs, the transtheoretical stages of change model, expectations confirmation theory, motivational dynamics, and learning theory (Margolis, 2004; Sweetow & Sabes, 2010).

Motivational Interviewing

Both an assessment strategy and an intervention, motivational interviewing (MI) is a patient-centered approach to counseling designed to promote intrinsic motivation and to reduce motivational barriers to behavior change, with the end result being the achievement of positive outcomes during the rehabilitative encounter (Miller and Rollnick, 2002; Wagner & McMahon, 2004). MI is designed to promote strong, collaborative relationships between clinician and client so as to reduce resistance to behavior change and increase motivation toward realizing target behaviors. The art of MI is that the clinician encourages the patient to talk freely about the problem as he or she sees it without fear of being judged. This first step of eliciting information is imperative, as it sets the stage for the clinician's learning from the PHL about his or her beliefs, attitudes, and readiness. It is the responsibility of the clinician to elicit and understand the patient's perspective in terms of concerns, expectations, intrinsic motivation, needs, feelings, and level of functioning. It is imperative that the PHL be understood within his or her psychosocial context and in accordance with his or her value system, as one's cultural orientation will inform the course and content of intervention. The clinician must create a favorable environment for open discussion, facilitating personal exploration of the problem, as this will empower the PHL. The clinician typically asks the PHL for permission to provide information in the form of filling any knowledge gaps to assist in forming a collaborative relationship. Shared decision making is essential, with the clinician having an appreciation for the degree to which the patient wants to be involved. A key principle of MI is that the audiologist must be directive and must adhere to the principle of unconditional positive regard, empathy, and genuineness while steering the patient to initiate and maintain a behavior. Finally, if the patient is provided with new information, the clinician should elicit feedback to make sure the patient understands the new information and to explore further the patient's feelings about the new information. The key elements of MI are listed in **Table 7.5**. MI is considered successful when two conditions are met: (1) The clinician must be directive, relying on the viewpoint of the patient, while helping to resolve ambivalence about behavior change. (2) The motivation to change behavior must be unlocked, as intrinsic motivation is key to positive outcomes. **Table 7.6** lists strategies for unleashing the intrinsic motivation of the PHL. During MI, patients with hearing loss must come to appreciate the value of intervention for which behavior change is necessary, in terms of benefits relative to costs (e.g., psychological, monetary), that a successful outcome is probable, and that there are few barriers in their social or psychological environment that will preclude behavior change consistent with a successful rehabilitation outcome (Wagner & McMahon, 2004).

Motivation is increased when clients perceive their rehabilitative goals to be valuable, achievable, sustainable, and supported by the environment. The strategies the clinician employs successfully in MI to benefit the PHL are open-ended questions, affirmations, reflections, and summaries, which can be remembered by the acronym OARS (Wagner & McMahon, 2004).

Table 7.5 Five Principles to Which the Clinician Must Adhere for Motivational Interviewing to Be a Success

Principle	Definition	Advantage
Roll with resistance	Persons with hearing impairment have the opportunity to explore their viewpoints with a clinician who has unconditional positive regard, allowing patients to come up with the solution through an open exchange	Allows persons with hearing impairment to explore new perspectives and to find answers on their own
Express empathy	Allowing patients to see that you understand and accept their feelings, that they are viewed as the expert on their condition, that you have confidence in their ability to perform the skills necessary to succeed at a particular task	Helps to develop rapport, minimizes resistance to change, enhances self-esteem
Avoid arguments	Arguments or dissonance between the patient and clinician should be avoided as this promotes resistance to change	Helps person toward self-recognition of the problem
Develop and explore discrepancy	Persons with hearing impairment see the dissonance between their present situation and their personal goals and values	A discrepancy between present and future values or conditions can motivate change
Support self-efficacy	Persons with hearing impairment must come to see that they are capable of changing behavior and succeeding; that you have confidence in their ability to perform the skills necessary to succeed at a particular task; they must believe that performing a particular behavior will result in the desired health outcome	Belief in possibility of change is an important intrinsic motivator; likelihood of behavior change is increased if participants believe in their ability to change and execute the actions required

Sources: Data from Wagner, C. C., & McMahon, B. T. (2004). Motivational interviewing and rehabilitation counseling practice. *Rehabilitation Counseling Bulletin, 47,* 142–161; and Miller, W., & Rollnick, S. (Eds.). (2002). *Motivational interviewing: Preparing people for change* (2nd ed.). New York: Guilford Press.

Table 7.6 Key Approaches to Be Used by Clinicians to Unlock Intrinsic Motivation and Behavior Change

Encourage small steps toward change
Reinforce efforts toward change
Be positive
Explore feelings when patients reject recommendations
Examine advantages and disadvantages of behavior change
Promote autonomy
Ask open-ended questions
Empower patients
Take a relationship-centered approach
Help patients gain confidence by considering ways to achieve goals and gain additional skill by de-emphasizing limitations and focusing on assets—affirmation
Involve patients in all aspects of decision making related to the rehabilitation process—reflections
Do not focus on threatening topics
Be interactive and facilitative
Be patient focused
Understand patients' perception of the value of behavior change
Accept that patients are the expert on their condition
Provide environmental supports to promote change
Provide unconditional positive regard

Sources: Data from Miller, W., & Rollnick, S. (Eds.) (2002). *Motivational interviewing: Preparing people for change* (2nd ed.). New York: Guilford Press.

Collaborative Self-Management

Collaborative self-management is closely aligned with many of the principles underlying MI. Self-management involves a partnership among the patient, the health care professional, and family members/caregivers (Rejeski et al, 2009). More specifically, Rejeski and colleagues define self-management as a process that "involves self-regulatory strategies taken by patients, who use their personal skills as well as those of health care professionals and supportive others to detect and manage their symptomatology and improve function" (p. 326). Self-management of health behavior is closely allied with adherence, and thus it is imperative that audiologists understand the factors that promote self-management, as they are responsible for helping patients to take charge of their condition and for making informed decisions about their management. At the heart of self-management is collaboration between all parties. The audiologist should do the following to promote adherence: (1) determine the patient's preference for each aspect of the treatment regimen; (2) ensure that the patient has the skills necessary to implement your recommendations; (3) introduce new concepts gradually over time rather than at the first session; (4) break down complex tasks into actions that can be handled sequentially; (5) begin the intervention with a step that the patient can easily accomplish, to foster a sense of control and success; (6) enlist family support; (7) gradually reduce the role of the audiologist so that the patient assumes responsibility for all behaviors relating to the intervention process; (8) be patient oriented; (9) customize treatment; (10) repeat everything you say and everything you ask the patient to practice; and (11) enlist support from family members, and include them in the partnership. Incorporating these principles into each encounter with the patient helps ensure self-management and a successful outcome. **Table 7.7** summarizes the key elements of collaborative self-management.

Table 7.7 Key Elements of Collaborative Self-Management

1. Clinician, person with hearing impairment, and communication partner must work together to help manage the client
2. Focus should always remain on the client's needs, abilities, values, preferences, and areas of possible behavior change
3. Family members, caregivers, and all others in the support network should be welcomed as partners in care
4. All partners in the "caring network" should share information and create a step-by-step action plan together to guide management
5. The roles of the clinician are to provide information, provide resources, provide supportive care, engage the patient, and engage in collaborative action planning

In focusing on these elements, the audiologist should always remember the role of reciprocal determinism, or the interdependence among personal factors, client behavior, and the environment, as change in one element affects the others.

Self-Efficacy

The concept of self-efficacy is at the heart of audiological management as well (Rollnick, Mason, & Butler, 2001; Smith & West, 2006). Self-efficacy refers to an individual's confidence or expectations about the ability to change or master a behavior or belief in the ability to carry out or succeed with a task. Patients with hearing impairment must come to see that they are capable of changing behavior and succeeding at the task before them (Miller & Rollnick, 2002; Rollnick et al, 2001). Confidence in the ability to make a change is related to the way in which an individual approaches a specific threat such as a chronic condition like hearing loss (Smith and West, 2006). Self-efficacy beliefs are relevant to rehabilitation with older adults, as they influence motivational level and contribute to one's ability to grasp new skills and to learn new activities (Miller & Rollnick, 2002; Smith & West 2006). **Table 7.8** lists the factors that influence self-efficacy beliefs.

Individuals who believe they will be able to succeed and who believe that their behavior will likely lead to a favorable outcome are considered to be strongly motivated and to have high self-efficacy (Bandura, 1997). The feeling of high self-efficacy is conducive to behavior change and ultimate success. Treatment outcomes are directly dependent on patients' beliefs about what they are capable of learning or activities they are capable of performing. Additionally, people with high self-efficacy are likely to set challenging goals and to develop strategies to realize their goals For example, a PHL believing that he or she can overcome the negative effects of hearing loss by learning new skills and gaining mastery over a technology is important for goal setting and achieving success. Health care providers must understand the motivation to seek professional assistance to overcome the activity limitations and participation restrictions associated with hearing loss. This enables them to work effectively and collaboratively on strategy setting and documenting that in fact the hearing aid is having the desired effect (Zimmerman and Kitsantas, 2007). Self-efficacy is nurtured when the hearing health care professional provides encouragement about the patient's actions or new behaviors, reinforces the patient by discussing the tangible evi-

Table 7.8 Factors Influencing How Individuals Achieve Self-Efficacy Beliefs

Sources of Self-Efficacy Beliefs	Direction of Influence	How to Achieve Self-Efficacy
Mastery experience	Successful performance or outcomes raise self-efficacy	Practice
Vicarious experience	Similarity to others or the belief that others are slightly better heightens self-efficacy	Model or "the other" should be similar in terms of age, gender, hearing status, etc.
Verbal persuasion	When others express belief in the person's ability and capability to accomplish a task	Positive feedback that is associated with success
Physiological and affective states	When the person with hearing impairment experiences a positive emotional state and positive thoughts	Experiencing positive thoughts and feelings rather than feeling anxious and stressed

Sources: Data from Bandura, A. (1997). Self-efficacy: The exercise of control. New York: W.H. Freeman; Smith, S. L., & West, R. L. (2006, Jun). The application of self-efficacy principles to audiologic rehabilitation: A tutorial. *American Journal of Audiology, 15,* 46–56; and Schunk, D., & Usher, E. (2011). Assessing self-efficacy for self-regulated learning. In B. Zimmerman & D. Schunk (Eds.), *Handbook of self-regulation of learning and performance.* New York: Routledge.

dence of the value of interventions (e.g., verbal persuasion), provides reassurance that many people experience similar challenges and successes when they proceed with audiological intervention (e.g., vicarious experience), and affirms that success requires time and patience. It is important to build into the intervention sessions opportunities to experience positive emotions, as this will promote self-efficacy (e.g., affective states). Hence, the clinician should begin with an easier skill so that the person with hearing impairment can experience success before proceeding to a more challenging task, and should make sure the physical environment is free of distractions so as to reduce stress and tension. Supplying written material or e-material following the session to reinforce what went on during the session can reduce stress and anxiety during subsequent training sessions (Smith & West, 2006).

Self-efficacy appears to mediate the extent of distress associated with visual impairment and by extension possibly hearing loss too (Lewis & Barrett, 2011). Lewis and Barrett (2011) explored the relation among functional or self-reported visual status, life satisfaction, magnitude of depressive symptoms, and social and psychological resources. The psychological resource measure was self-efficacy, or the extent to which respondents felt they had control over their own life circumstances. The authors found that the level of self-efficacy had the greatest effect on the relation between functional visual status and quality of life. The level of self-efficacy accounted for 35% of the effect of functional visual impairment on magnitude of depressive symptoms, and 60% of the effect on life satisfaction. This finding suggests that perhaps improving self-efficacy could reduce the negative effects of hearing loss, and it seems reasonable to believe that audiologists might consider targeting interventions at promoting self-efficacy, as this could be a variable mediating the relation between hearing impairment and many negative consequences. Hence, promoting self-efficacy should be built into counseling sessions with the PHL, be it during the hearing-aid fitting or during discussions about intervention options.

> **Pearls**
>
> Self-efficacy is an important influence on behavior and is an integral component of the transtheoretical stages of change model. An individual's belief in the possibility of change is a key motivator.

Transtheoretical Stages of Change Model

The transtheoretical stages of change model (TTM) espoused by Prochaska and DiClemente (1983) offers a model for understanding the process of behavior change and the series of stages through which people pass during intentional behavior change. A theoretical model of behavior change, the TTM has been the basis for developing effective interventions to promote health behavior change in numerous areas including smoking cessation and cancer prevention. It is an integrative model, as shown in **Fig. 7.2**, as it incorporates principles from other theories, including self-efficacy beliefs. The stages of change model relies heavily on emotional and cognitive factors as instruments of behavior change, and focuses on decisional balance or decision making in which the patient is engaged. The model holds that individuals must be ready for change if they are to embrace the recommendations of hearing health care professionals. Familiarity with the stages of readiness for change helps guide the clinician in matching the treatment to patient readiness to accept intervention, and familiarity with barriers to change can help the clinician anticipate and avoid factors that can pose obstacles to change.

Several assumptions underlie the TTM. The TTM includes a temporal domain, as it implies that change occurs over time,

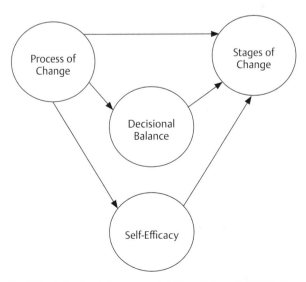

Fig. 7.2 Behavioral change model. [From Kricos, P. (2006). Personal communication.]

Table 7.9 Stages of Change and Decisional Balance

Stage	Mental Set	Decisional Balance	Recommended Intervention
Precontemplation	Unaware that an impairment exists; unwilling to or uninterested in changing the status quo; uninformed, unmotivated	Reluctant, resigned, rationalization; not aware of advantages of intervening; disadvantages outweigh advantages	Provide a menu of options including educational materials; show empathy and optimism
Contemplation	Acknowledge that a problem exists and willing to consider solving the problem	Struggle to understand the condition, the causes, and possible solutions; gather information about intervention options; open to information about hearing impairment; advantages of taking action tend to equal disadvantages of taking action; more aware of the advantages of intervening but still cognizant of the disadvantages	Audiological assessment, provide positive listening experiences with HATs in selected listening situations (e.g., television, theater); have patient meet with new and satisfied hearing-aid users; educational materials about success of interventions for hearing impairment, completion of self-report questionnaires about effects of hearing impairment
Preparation	Deciding and preparing to make a change; individual is ready and committed to take action; ready to take action within about 1 month	Advantages equal disadvantages, but scale is tipping toward the advantages	Administer self-report such as the HHIE, counseling session regarding the value of hearing aids and the fitting process; provide a menu of intervention options
Action	Individual has decided to consult with a professional and has scheduled an appointment	Individual has adequate self-efficacy, which helps to increase likelihood of taking action and experiencing success; needs encouragement and positive feedback to ensure action is taking place and that patient is following protocols	Hearing-aid fitting and/or HATS, orientation, counseling, follow-up; Listening and Communication Enhancement (LACE) program
Maintenance	The acclimatization and adjustment phase	Requires continued orientation, counseling, and rehabilitation to ensure outcome is positive and intervention outcomes meet and exceed expectations; advantages and cost benefit of intervening must exceed disadvantages and cost of not intervening	Short-, medium-, and long-term follow-up; send periodic email communication with tips on hearing aids and hearing loss; completion of checklists or self-report scales demonstrating progress

Sources: Data from Prochaska, J. O., & DiClemente, C. C. (1983, Jun). Stages and processes of self-change of smoking: Toward an integrative model of change. *Journal of Consulting and Clinical Psychology, 51,* 390–395; and DiClemente, C. C., & Velasquez, M. (2002) Motivational interviewing and the stages of change. In W. R. Miller & S. Rollnick (Eds.). (2002). *Motivational interviewing:* Preparing *people for change* (2nd ed.). New York: Guilford.

moving from behavioral intention (before target behavior change takes place) to maintenance of behavior for a specific period of time. The decisional balance construct reflects the individual's relative weighing of the importance of the pros relative to the importance of the cons (Janis & Mann, 1985). The decisional balance chosen by the patient mediates the decision to move from one stage to the next. Patients may weigh the perceived advantages and disadvantages, the pros and cons, the importance of moving forward, and their confidence in their ability to move forward as they proceed through the different stages. According to the TTM, people are most likely to change their behavior if they are doing so for personal reasons without the prodding of outsiders and if the pros tend to outweigh the cons. The self-efficacy construct represents the confidence that the patient has regarding embarking on the target behavior. Self-efficacy tends to increase as one goes through the stages. The assumptions that underlie the stages of change model include the fact that change in behavior, especially in older adults, occurs gradually, change is incremental, and pa-

tients moving through the series of stage changes can be assisted in this process by a skilled clinician.

As depicted in **Table 7.9** and **Fig. 7.3**, there are five stages that people tend to go through as part of the process of behavior change. Individuals move from being uninterested, unaware, or unwilling to make a change (precontemplation), to considering the possibility of making a change (contemplation), to being prepared to make a change (preparation), to taking action (action), and finally maintaining the new behavior (maintenance). It is our responsibility, possibly through screening programs (which include information about hearing loss) and counseling during diagnostic and rehabilitation sessions, to help persons with hearing impairment move from the precontemplation to the action phase or move them along the readiness-to-change continuum as depicted in **Fig. 7.4**. When it is clear, based on the patient's own decisional balance sheet, that the pros and benefits of seeking intervention are equal to or exceed the cons and the cost, PHLs will be prepared to take action. We might assume that they perform their own

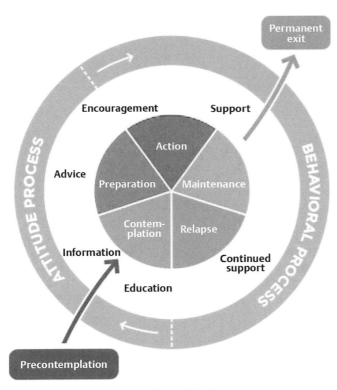

Fig. 7.3 The stages of change. [From the Ida Institute, www.idainstitute.com]

1 BENEFITS OF STATUS QUO	2 COSTS OF STATUS QUO
No need to hear anymore than I do now!	**I can't really think of any.**
Are there any situations you avoid because of your hearing difficulties?	*You never feel exhausted when you are in group contexts?*
Have you considered that your communication partners may be unhappy or dissatisfied because you miss out on things?	*Would your communication partners agree to that?*
	I will feel excluded from social contexts.
I do not have a hearing problem!	*In which situations do you feel excluded?*
You never find that people mumble?	**I might lose my job!**
Have you experienced any situations in which it is difficult to hear?	*Is it only in job situations that you have hearing problems?*
3 THE POTENTIAL COSTS OF CHANGE	4 THE POTENTIAL BENEFITS OF CHANGE
Hearing aids whistle!	**I can participate more.**
Have you experienced that?	**It will be less tiring for me if I don't have to pretend that I know what people are talking about.**
Other people might not like me because hearing aids are unattractive!	
What do you think when you see other hearing-aid users?	**It will help me keep my job.**
Have you considered that the relationship to other people might suffer if you can't hear them or you misunderstand them?	**There will be less conflicts in the family.**
	Acknowledge the response and ask if there are any other benefits—get as many benefits as possible.

Fig. 7.5 The cost-benefit box. [From the Ida Institute, www.idainstitute.com]

cost-benefit analysis, and it is our responsibility to make them aware of the benefits to facilitate their analysis, as is shown in **Fig. 7.5.**

Table 7.9 shows that people in different stages have different patterns of thinking and require different types of intervention. Matching the stage to the intervention can help patients progress toward acceptance of what the clinician and patient agree is most appropriate. In our role as clinician counselor, we should offer a menu of options or strategies that will be helpful as the patient works through the various stages. **Table 7.9** also summarizes some of the issues patients confront as they make a decision and some approaches that may be helpful during their decisional balancing act. Each stage presents a particular challenge to the audiologist, but the contemplation stage of readiness is the most complex. Individuals are often stuck in the contemplation stage, as they have acknowledged that a problem exists but they are reluctant to commit to taking action (DiClemente & Velasquez, 2002). Feedback about the impact of the impairment, the efficacy of interventions,

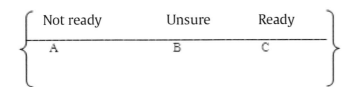

Fig. 7.4 Readiness-to-change continuum. [From Rollnick, S., Mason, P., & Butler, C. (2001). *Health behavior change a guide for practitioners.* New York: Churchill-Livingstone.]

and encouragement regarding their potential to succeed with intervention are strategies for helping to move these individuals toward the preparation stage. Shifting the decisional balance for these individuals and helping them to overcome their ambivalence requires patience and time (DiClemente & Velasquez, 2002). Once the decisional balance tips and the individual is prepared to take action, the challenge for the audiologist is to work collaboratively with the patient to develop intervention options from which the patient can choose and which are informed by responses to various questionnaires regarding activity limitation, participation restrictions, and expectations.

When individuals enter the action phase, they schedule the appointment for an evaluation and follow up with the recommended intervention, but they will continue to need positive feedback and counseling and require realistic assurances regarding what outcomes they can come to expect. It is critical that you continue to emphasize the value of better hearing, better speech understanding, and improved cognitive function, including less effort involved in listening and the slowing of cognitive aging. It is helpful to think of readiness as a con-

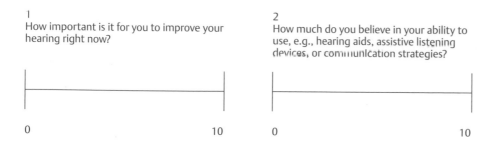

1
How important is it for you to improve your
hearing right now?

2
How much do you believe in your ability to
use, e.g., hearing aids, assistive listening
devices, or communication strategies?

0   10   0   10

The lines go from '*0 = not at all*' to '*10 = very much.*'

Fig. 7.6   The Ida Institute assessment continuum line. (From the Ida Institute, www.idainstitute.com.)

tinuum from not ready, to unsure, to ready, and individuals gradually approach the "ready" end of the continuum when they think it is important enough to intervene and they feel that they have the confidence to proceed. This conceptualization of readiness should help inform the approach to working with the hearing impaired and moving them toward action. Clinicians should consider asking each patient to rank themselves along a continuum representing their readiness to make a specific change and let this guide the evaluation and management process (**Figs. 7.4 and 7.6**) (Rollnick et al, 2001).

The Ida Institute tools can be helpful in determining patients' stage of readiness to pursue treatments, where patients are in the change process, and their level of self-efficacy. As shown in **Fig. 7.6**, a high score (e.g., 9 or 10) on the line suggests that it is important for patients to improve their ability to hear. This would suggest that motivation is high to attempt the target behavior. Similarly, a score of 9 on the second line suggests that the patient's sense of self-efficacy is high and consistent with a likelihood of a successful outcome, should intervention be pursued. Another approach to assessing readiness and self-efficacy is to use a modified version of the HHIE that includes a global self-efficacy question and questions about motivation (**Table 7.10**). If scores on the line or the HHIE suggest that the patient is motivated but the patient does not feel he or she has the ability to use hearing aids or communication strategies to improve understanding, then counseling to promote the patient's self-efficacy and strategies training to promote a sense or responsibility for health outcomes along with positive feedback or experiences will be important. The use of the cost-benefit analysis Ida Institute tool shown in **Fig. 7.5** as part of counseling to help patients see the value added or advantages of being able to communicate better with others can be helpful. A recent study by Milstein and Gershteyn (2011) found that the stage of change relates directly to the self-perceived hearing handicap and hearing-aid uptake.

Building on a study by Milstein and Weinstein (2002), Milstein and Gershteyn (2011) explored the relationship between self-reported stage of change and hearing-aid uptake in a sample of 30 adults with hearing impairment. Participants were asked to label the stage that best represented where they consider themselves by choosing one of the following four statements:

Stage 1: I do not think I have a hearing problem, and therefore nothing should be done about it.
Stage 2: I think I have a hearing problem. However, I am not yet ready to take any action to solve the problem, but I might do so in the future.
Stage 3: I know I have a hearing problem, and I intend to take action to solve it soon.
Stage 4: I know I have a hearing problem, and I am here to take action to solve it now.

Of the 30 participants who sought an initial audiological evaluation, 27 chose one of the two high stages of readiness—nine chose stage 3 and 18 chose stage 4. Participants who were in these stages of readiness were more likely to comply with the recommendation for amplification than were participants

Table 7.10   Modification of the Hearing Handicap Inventory for the Elderly (HHIE)

E Do you feel handicapped by a hearing loss?	Yes	Sometimes	No
MI Is it important for you to feel less handicapped by your hearing problem?	Yes	Sometimes	No
S Does a hearing problem cause you to have arguments with family members?	Yes	Sometimes	No
MI Is it important for you to have fewer arguments with family members because of your hearing loss?	Yes	Sometimes	No
S Does a hearing problem cause you difficulty when listening to the TV or radio?	Yes	Sometimes	No
MI Is it important for you to have less difficulty understanding when listening to the TV or radio?	Yes	Sometimes	No
S Does a hearing problem cause you difficulty when in a restaurant with relatives or friends?	Yes	Sometimes	No
MI Is it important for you to have less difficulty understanding when in a restaurant with relatives or friends?	Yes	Sometimes	No
SE If you decided that you wanted to hear/understand others better, do you feel that you could take the necessary actions to attempt to overcome any difficulties attributable to your hearing loss?	Yes	Sometimes	No

Abbreviations: E, emotional; MI, motivational interviewing; S, social/situational; SE, self-efficacy.
Source: From author's personal communication with Montano and Chisolm. (Reprinted by permission.)

in the two lower stages of readiness; 76% of participants who pursued amplification considered themselves to be in stage 4. Hence, using the categorizations above seems to have predictive validity as indicators of hearing-aid use. The majority of individuals in the more advanced stages also considered themselves to have a handicap based on HHIE-S scores. Specifically, the majority of participants (17 of 18) who scored 14 or higher on the HHIE-S were in stage 4.

Kochkin (2007) developed a hearing solution adoption model that dovetails nicely with the concept of a decisional balance sheet and with the stages of change model. PHLs must first accept that they actually have a physical challenge. It is likely that PHLs who do not yet accept that a hearing loss exists rarely come to our clinics, so we must come up with ways of reaching them. We must develop approaches, possibly through screening or counseling, to reach and change the attitudes of those who deny the existence of a physical impairment (those in the precontemplation stage). These individuals present a tremendous challenge, requiring educational efforts, including public service announcements about the challenges posed by unidentified hearing impairment. Kochkin's (2007) conceptualization may provide the key to helping move the 23 million adults who admit to hearing loss toward acceptance of the need for an intervention be it surgical or medical, or products such as hearing aids, hearing-assistance technologies (HATs), or cochlear implants. Some solutions to dealing with people in the four stages are shown in **Table 7.11**.

Expectations-Confirmation Theory

Another principle that underlies the management process is development of clinical expectations or benchmarks. Kane et al (2004) suggest that the use of benchmarks is an approach that is applicable when working with older adults with chronic conditions. In part this is at the heart of expectations-confirmation theory, whereby satisfaction is a function of the match between expectations and perceived performance (**Fig. 7.7**). Patients should be apprised of how they are progressing, and should receive regular feedback either in writing or in graphic form regarding their performance. As long as performance is as expected or is better than predicted, there is no need to make adjustments to the intervention. If the course changes or the patient is not deriving the benefit expected, there should be a reassessment and the intervention modified. The use of benchmarks during ongoing management is bound to expectations-confirmation theory (aka "disconfirmation of expectations" model). Expectations-confirmation theory posits that expectations, coupled with perceived performance, affect patient satisfaction, which is mediated through positive disconfirmation or negative disconfirmation (Spreng, Mackenzie, & Olshavsky, 1996). If performance exceeds expectations (positive confirmation), satisfaction with intervention will result. If a performance falls short of expectations (negative disconfirmation), it is likely that the patient will be dissatisfied with the intervention (Spreng et al, 1996). Expectations are the benchmark against which patients judge performance. Hence, when communication participation (e.g., performance) matches communication performance expectations, hearing-impaired patients will be satisfied, whereas if communication participation performance falls short of the benchmark, they will be

dissatisfied. In the case of older adult hearing-aid users, personal experience from patients and health care professionals who work with older adults suggests that communication performance especially in suboptimal listening situations often falls short of expectations, hence dissatisfaction, frustration, and disillusionment with the intervention or with the hearing health care professionals tend to ensue. To ensure that expectations are realized, hearing-aid users must accept their hearing loss rather than consider it a disgrace or a stigma. They should not hide their hearing aids, thereby hiding the hearing loss. If performance is to match expectations, acceptance of hearing loss is key. If hearing-aid users accept hearing loss and hearing aids, so will the people to whom they are speaking. Acceptance of hearing loss and motivation to overcome its consequences are conditions for hearing-aid satisfaction and success (Ross, 1996).

Principles of *learning theory* and how the theory impacts recall of new information must be incorporated when working with persons with hearing loss and their communication partners. Margolis (2004) and Sweetow and Sabes (2010) recommend incorporating some of the following strategies to maximize retention of new information. I will begin with some general principles and then proceed to more specific recommendations. In general, best practice dictates active participation of the learner, using multiple modalities when presenting new information, providing immediate and positive feedback regarding performance, avoiding information overload, and making sure to be repetitive regarding important information. With regard to active participation, interactivity and feedback regarding progress is important. The term *multiple modalities* refers to supplementation of auditory information with written or pictorial materials. To promote retention, it is important that there is a direct correlation between the amount of information being presented and retention; hence, every effort should be made to avoid presenting too much information at one session. In addition to the above principles, the primacy effect is of the utmost importance; thus, during counseling or audiological management sessions it is productive to present the most important information first, as it will be remembered more often. **Table 7.12** includes more specific strategies that derive from learning theory.

There is considerable overlap across the principles discussed above. It is imperative that audiologists develop their own approach to synthesizing the information and to use of the materials based on what is most beneficial to the patient. Keeping in mind the patient-centered nature of audiological management will make it easier to incorporate some of the principles discussed above.

◆ Components of the Process of Audiological Management

Boothroyd (2010) advocates a progressive and holistic approach to audiological management, which includes, but is not limited to, optimizing audibility via the provision of devices such as hearing aids, cochlear implants, HATs, or bone-anchored hearing aids (BAHAs). Even when audibility is restored via sensory management, communication problems often persist, and especially compromised is speech understanding in complex

Table 7.11 A Decisional Balance Sheet or a Hearing-Solution Adoption Sheet

Possible Explanations	Possible Solutions
Denial–Precontemplation	
Patients do not realize they have a hearing problem	Screening + informational counseling; encourage reevaluation of current behavior; encourage self-exploration; explain and personalize the risk
Patients know at some level, but will not admit to having a hearing loss	Screening + educational counseling; encourage reevaluation of current behavior; encourage self-exploration; explain and personalize the risk
Patients know they have a hearing loss but do not realize it is a problem for others	Screening + self-help groups + administer questionnaire to a family member or caregiver that assesses their perception of the individual's activity limitations, participation restrictions; explain results and personalize their susceptibility
Contemplation–Preparation	
Patients are aware that they have a hearing loss, but there are many obstacles and barriers to overcome before they adopt concept of a hearing intervention	Screening + informational counseling + administer questionnaire that assesses the perception of the individual's activity limitations, participation restrictions, and quality of life; explain results on the latter and personalize their susceptibility; referral to an audiologist; explain responses and discuss possible solutions
Obstacles to Adoption	
Socioeconomic factors	
Cost	Marketing regarding added value of hearing aids
Lack of transportation	Mobile vans for the homebound; home visits for the homebound; help patient identify social support
Psychological/personality variables	
Anxiety	Screening + informational counseling + handicap assessment; encourage self-exploration; explain and personalize the risk; reinforce long-term benefits and internal rewards
External stigma	
Lack of motivation	
Family resistance	Informational counseling
Fear of being considered incompetent or failing	Informational counseling
Unwilling to relinquish the benefits of having a hearing loss!	Screening + informational counseling; identify and assist in problem solving regarding obstacles
Afraid of doctors	Screening + informational counseling
Bad experience with hearing aids	Informational counseling re: efficacy and value
Emotional status	Screening + informational counseling
Vanity	Screening + informational counseling
Communication difficulties not significant enough to warrant intervention	Screening + informational counseling; encourage self-exploration, not action; explain and personalize the risk
Physiological factors	
Motor coordination problems	Hearing-assistance technologies (HATs)
Visual acuity	
Cognitive status	
Health status	
Incentives	
Reduce stress associated with hearing loss	
Alleviate embarrassment of not following conversation	
Enhanced life satisfaction and quality of life	
Will hear and understand grandchildren	
Easier to communicate	

Sources: Data from Kricos, P. (2006). Personal communication; Trychin, S. (2001). Why don't people who need hearing aids get them? *Hearing Loss, 22,* 15–19; and Kochkin, S. (2007). Marke Trak VII: Obstacles to adult non-user adoption of hearing aids. *Hearing Journal, 60,* 24–50.

listening environments. Focusing solely on sensory management ignores the important link to cognitive processing, which helps the brain reconnect listeners with their impaired ears and it does not address listening and comprehension, all important components of communication (Pichora-Fuller, 2006; Sweetow & Palmer, 2005). A more holistic and progressive approach to management that goes beyond the restoration of audibility is especially important for those who have been fit with hearing aids but rarely use them because of persisting communication problems (unsuccessful users) and those who wear their hear-

ing aids but experience communication and psychosocial challenges that they find frustrating and limiting. Individuals who have bottom-up problems and difficulty analyzing acoustic information may have persistent problems because they have not learned how to maximize top-down processing, including the use of working memory, repair strategies, context, and knowledge of the language to help disambiguate the message (Hickson et al, 2007; Tremblay & Pichora-Fuller, 2011).

Central to a progressive and holistic approach to management are four essential steps integral to effective communication,

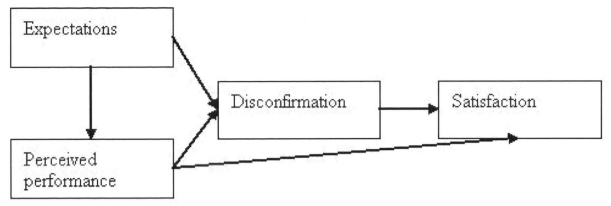

Fig. 7.7 Expectations confirmation theory (disconfirmation of expectations model) [From Oliver, R. (1977). Effect of expectation and disconfirmation on postexposure product evaluations—An alternative interpretation. *Journal of Applied Psychology, 62,* 480.]

namely hearing, listening, comprehension, and communication (**Fig. 7.8**) (Sweetow & Sabes, 2006). Hearing is a passive function, whereas listening is an active function. Sweetow and Sabes (2006) also contend that although comprehension is a unidirectional function, it entails a bidirectional transfer of information such that improved listening will follow from improved comprehension and communication, and enhanced listening skills will lead to better comprehension and communication. Impediments to successful communication include bottom-up processing problems arising from a distorted auditory signal associated with peripheral hearing loss, less efficient top-down processing abilities arising from cognitive declines or cognitive constraints, lack of adequate compensatory strategies, and loss of communicative confidence or self-efficacy (Sweetow & Sabes, 2010). **Table 7.13** shows how one might assess the outcome of each of the steps involved in communication.

A progressive and holistic program of management should include the following: a communication needs assessment; sensory management and orientation, including counseling about HATs; auditory/visual/cognitive/perceptual training in-cluding training in speech perception and conversational skills; communication strategies counseling; personal adjustment counseling; and short-term, medium-term, and long-term cognitive, perceptual, and functional outcome assessment (i.e., verification). Communication management could be done individually, in a group, or in hybrid ways combining face-to-face sessions with Web-based training. It should target both the person with hearing impairment and the communication partner, be evidence based, and include booster sessions that provide additional opportunity for feedback regarding progress and for monitoring of progress or lack of progress. **Table 7.14** shows components of a progressive approach to management of effective communication, along with intervention strategies and potential outcomes. The remainder of the chapter addresses these different components.

Step 1: Needs Assessment

At the heart of rehabilitation with older adults is a multifaceted needs assessment that will set the stage for individualizing

Table 7.12 Strategies to Promote Optimal Retention During Counseling and Audiological Rehabilitation Sessions

Provide concrete instructions

Use short words and sentences, as these are easy to understand

Maintain records that allow you to plot progress over time, as this can be used to show the effects of training

Keep environmental distractions to a minimum when counseling or during treatment sessions

Be explicit when giving instructions

Make sure to consider the patient's beliefs, wants, and needs during counseling and rehabilitation sessions

Use materials for auditory or cognitive training that are challenging, interesting, and graded in terms of difficulty, but match level of difficulty to ability as you want to avoid frustration

Pace sessions based on patient's reaction time, psychomotor, and cognitive abilities

Sources: Data from Margolis, R. (2004). Boosting memory with informational counseling. *Asha Leader, 9,* 10–11, 28; and Sweetow, R. W., & Sabes, J. H. (2010, Oct). Auditory training and challenges associated with participation and compliance. *Journal of the American Academy of Audiology, 21,* 586–593.

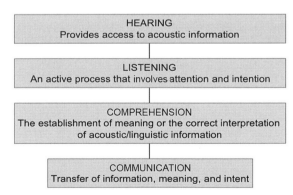

Fig. 7.8 Effective communication. [From Sweetow, R. W., & Sabes, J. H. (2006, Sep). The need for and development of an adaptive Listening and Communication Enhancement (LACE) program. *Journal of the American Academy of Audiology, 17,* 538–558; and Sweetow, R. W., & Sabes, J. H. (2010, Oct). Auditory training and challenges associated with participation and compliance. *Journal of the American Academy of Audiology, 21,* 586–593.]

Table 7.13 Components of Effective Communication

Component	Function	Intervention	Outcome
Hearing	Access to acoustic information	Hearing-aid fitting, hearing-assistance technology	Real ear, functional gain
Listening	Hearing with both intention and attention	Hearing aid or hearing-assistance technology + communication management	Speech testing: QuickSIN™, HINT
Comprehension	Correct interpretation of acoustic/linguistic information	Speech perception training: speech in babble, time-compressed speech, competing speech, working memory, and missing word exercises	Speech testing: QuickSIN™, HINT, competing speaker task
Communication	Effective use and transmission of information	Speech perception training: speech in babble, time-compressed speech, competing speech, cognitive training; working memory and missing word exercises; strategies training	HHIE, speech testing, CSOA, tests of working memory and speed of processing, and functional communication

Abbreviations: CSOA, Communication Scale for Older Adults; HHIE, Hearing Handicap Inventory for the Elderly; HINT, Hearing in Noise Test.
Source: Data from Sweetow, R., & Henderson-Sabes, J. (2004). The case for LACE: Listening and auditory communication enhancement training. *Hearing Journal. 57,* 32–40.

treatment goals and will serve as a foundation for the treatment plan to be effected. A starting point for individualized goal setting, the functional communication needs assessment (FCA), helps the audiologist to identify the appropriate interventions options. It includes a battery of objective and subjective measures that will help assess related functions beyond the information provided by the routine pure-tone and speech testing, including cognitive, social, emotional, and physical health status (Sweetow, 2007). Given the large individual differences and the fact the speech understanding in noise is a complex process representing the continuous interplay between top-down and bottom-up processing, the objective measures conducted as part of the needs assessment must go beyond the traditional tests used to assess audibility and word recognition ability in quiet. The baseline assessment must tap

into the cochlear distortions, impaired frequency, and temporal resolution that attend hearing loss and the difficulty understanding speech in complex listening environments typical of older adults. Further, we must gain insight into cognitive status in such areas as speed of processing, working memory, attention, use of context information, semantic knowledge, and listening strategies, given their role in speech understanding and auditory visual integration (Boothroyd, 2007; Cox et al, 2007; Kiessling et al, 2003; Pichora-Fuller & Singh, 2006; Sweetow, 2007; Yueh et al, 2005). Objective measures are selected that provide insight into speech-processing ability, specifically listening, comprehending, and communicating (Pichora-Fuller, 2006). According to Pichora-Fuller (2006), listening is a process that involves mental effort and hearing with intention and attention for purposeful activities; comprehend-

Table 7.14 Progressive Management to Promote Effective Communication

Communication Needs Assessment	Sensory Management and Orientation	Auditory/Auditory Visual/Cognitive/Perceptual and Listening and Conversational Skills Training	Counseling: Personal Adjustment and Communication Strategies	Outcome Assessment/Verification
Includes objective auditory objective measures of speech perceptual abilities,[1] subjective functional measures, measures of cognitive status (working memory, which includes storage and processing aspects of the incoming message),[2] screening of visual status	Consideration of sensory aids, implants; hearing-assistive technologies; wireless technologies as potential realistic options	Hearing and listening must be integrated; training in use of acoustic, linguistic, and visual cues; training in use of lexical, sentence, and narrative context; memory and speed of processing training; training in extracting speech signal from noise; training in use of visual cues	Counseling regarding hearing tactics, repair strategies, positioning for both the person with hearing impairment and the communication partner; personal adjustment counseling pertaining to speech understanding deficits	Beyond validation of the adequacy of the fit in electroacoustic terms is verification that the intervention is effective in promoting speech understanding, in reducing the psychosocial impact of the hearing impairment on function, and possibly in promoting cognitive function

[1]QuickSIN™, Hearing in Noise Test (HINT), acceptable noise levels (ANLs), dichotic tests, rapid compressed speech.
[2]Measures of verbal memory ability include Hopkins Verbal Learning Test, Rey Auditory-Verbal Learning Test, the Rivermead Behavioral Paragraph Recall Test, the Visual Letter Monitoring Test, and working memory such as a test of reading span (Foo, Rudner, Rönnberg, & Lunner, 2007; Willis et al, 2006).
Sources: Data from Boothroyd, A. (2010). *You have a new hearing aid: So what?* Now what? Paper Presented at Starkey Innovation in Action Symposium. Minneapolis, Minnesota; Sweetow, R. W., & Sabes, J. H. (2006, Sep). The need for and development of an adaptive Listening and Communication Enhancement (LACE) program. *Journal of the American Academy of Audiology, 17,* 538–558; and Sweetow, R. (2009). *Five ideas to better meet the hearing needs of older people.* Paper presented at the Adult Conference: The Challenge of Aging, Chicago.

ing entails reception of information, meaning, and intent; and communicating is a bidirectional transfer of information between two people. Further, cognitive resources and auditory-processing ability impact the ability to listen, comprehend, and communicate, and interact to influence activity and participation levels. Further, the degree and configuration of the peripheral hearing loss impacts communication performance, as does cognitive status (Cox, McCoy, Tun, & Wingfield, 2008).

Because vision adds redundancy and makes cues available that can help a person to identify sounds when auditory cues are reduced, auditory visual integration of the spoken message in complex listening situations, especially under informational masking conditions, for example, should be assessed (Kiessling et al, 2003). Information on the ability to integrate visual input with auditory input is also critical, as it will inform counseling, the nature of the auditory-visual integration training, and communication strategies training. As part of the baseline assessment of speech processing ability, I would include speech comprehension in noise measures including the QuickSIN,™ the Hearing in Noise Test (HINT), which is considered to be a clinically relevant and an ecologically valid speech in noise tests, and possibly a measure of auditory temporal processing or sequencing such as the time-compressed (60%) sentence and word tests (Cox et al, 2008; Foo, Rudner, Rönnberg, & Lunner, 2007). Ideally, at least two tests of speech understanding in complex situations should be completed, varying the nature of the noise competition, the speed of the speech, the signal-to-noise ratio (SNR), and the presence or absence of visual cues. This menu of tests will uncover deficits in auditory processing that will serve as the basis for perceptual or auditory training to address listening difficulties, especially in adverse listening environments (Pichora-Fuller, 2006). Cognitive tests might include the Visual Letter Monitoring Test as described by Gatehouse, Naylor, and Elberling (2003), which contains elements of both memory and processing speed, the Visual Rhyme Test described by Hällgren, Larsby, Lyxell, and Arlinger (2001), which measures speed of phonological processing, or the Stroop (1935) test, which is widely used in studies on cognitive plasticity and is a general measure of cognitive flexibility and control of the effects of cognitive interference. In addition to being important for auditory visual integration, performance on the cognitive tests will influence the time constants recommended at the time of the hearing-aid fitting. Hence, all of the above areas should be assessed if audiologists are committed to a holistic approach to management. Unfortunately, health care economics is likely to influence the time allotted for the assessment but the more we learn at the front end, the greater the likelihood that the needs of the PHL will be met.

The subjective needs assessment as described by Sweetow (2007) includes gathering data that will shed light on the individual's practical abilities and needs. Specifically, the subjective assessment will yield information about functional communication goals, expectations, and well-being. Hearing-related function, namely activity limitations and communication participation restrictions, should be assessed against the backdrop of environmental, personal, physical, and cognitive factors. These metrics are more sensitive to hearing effects, and are often referred to as hearing-specific quality-of-life measures as compared with health-related quality-of-life measures, which is an umbrella concept that incorporates all dimensions of the WHO International Classification of Functioning and Disability, including body, activity, and participation (Abrams, 2008; Stark & Hickson, 2004; WHO, 2001). Each category of quality-of-life measure serves as a benchmark against which the value of treatment can be measured and in some way provides information on well-being. Asking the patient to self-assess their circumstance places a greater focus on the patient's individual needs when designing a management plan and that of the communication partner (Benjamin-McKie, 2006). It provides the clinician with information about the patient's attitude, listening needs, and the range of listening circumstances that are most problematic. They also shed light on the behavioral and psychosocial consequences (e.g., activity limitations and participation restrictions) of the numerous speech-understanding difficulties for the individual, family members, and potentially for society at large. These difficulties cannot be predicted from the audiogram because of the individual variability in response to a given impairment, but should be targeted as part of the management process. Cox (2003, p. S91) eloquently listed reasons why patient self-report about communication function has gained traction:

> Second, we need to recognize that there are many domains of real-life outcome that cannot be accessed in the laboratory. After all, why do people seek hearing aids? It is not because they have a hearing impairment. It is because they cannot carry out their daily activities as they want to, or because they cannot participate in their family, social, and cultural lives in the way that they want to. In other words, people seek hearing aids because they are experiencing activity limitations or participation restrictions, or both (WHO, 2001). The traditional hearing aid outcome measures cannot readily grasp activity limitations or participation restrictions, because these problems are very individualized—they depend on personal circumstances, family situation, lifestyle, etc. To quantify them, we need self-report data. Third, even when we are able to simulate real-world conditions in the laboratory, we usually find that laboratory outcome measures do not closely resemble the client's impression of real-life outcome in the simulated situation. Cox concludes by stating that the variance in laboratory data describes less than 40% of the variance in real-life data. Self-report measures are increasing in use, because they give us a scientifically defensible way to validly measure the real-life success of the hearing aid fitting. (p. S90–91)

According to Abrams (2008) health-related quality of life (HRQOL) can be conceptualized as the value assigned to one's life as modified by one's impairments, functional states, perceptions, and social opportunities. HRQOL instruments can be classified as health status measures or preference-based measures. Health status measures include questionnaires that assess disease-specific or generic consequences of hearing impairment. Self-report findings from standardized questionnaires are important for helping the clinician decide what approaches to include in the management process and are key for assessing outcomes.

Information about expectations should be gathered, as this too will help with setting management priorities (Gatehouse, 2003). It is important to emphasize that expectations should be based on accurate information, as unrealistic expectations can interfere with management outcomes, and it is well established that hearing-impaired people have expectations that are unreasonable. In accordance with expectations-confirmation theory, patients' expectations must be in alignment with what the management promises to deliver for a good outcome (Gatehouse, 2003). A variety of self-report questionnaires are available to the clinician for assessing disablement, attitudes, perceived listening needs, and expectations—all factors that will affect management decisions. I refer to these as income measures, borrowing from terminology introduced by Johnson and Danhauer (2002).

We are attempting to manage the patient, and given the array of interventions we can maximize clinical effectiveness by gaining as much insight into the patient as possible (Gatehouse, 2003). Structured interview, using self-report instruments that are reliable, sensitive, and valid for the purposes of the assessment, is the ideal approach. The setting in which the history is taken should be free of distractions. It is often helpful to obtain information from a variety of sources, as often there are discrepancies between expectations and perceptions. Open-ended questions can serve as an excellent supplement to standardized questionnaires (Kane et al, 2004).

Patient preferences and expectations are of paramount importance when planning the management protocol (Kane et al, 2004). Patient preference measures assess the extent to which individuals would prefer to be in perfect health or, at the other extreme, terminally ill (Abrams, 2008); most people prefer to be healthy. Older adults' self appraisal of their health is intertwined with their psychological well-being and is predictive of rehabilitation outcomes (Lewis & Bottomley, 2008). Older adults often underreport potentially important symptoms due to cultural differences, educational backgrounds, fears, or because of the assumption that what they are experiencing is part of the normal aging process. In fact, the majority of older adults rate their health positively, although whites have higher self-rated health than do blacks or Hispanics (Morgan & Kunkel, 2011). Further, perceived potential for overcoming a chronic or medical condition correlates with improvement and achievement of functional goals. Self-report measures should be quick, easy to administer, scorable, and reliable. Assessment of the patient's communication environment is important as well, as alterations in the physical environment may be necessary to promote understanding and patient safety.

Given the memory problems that are prevalent as people age, Benjamin-McKie (2006) suggests that at times using pictures to help elicit responses to the self-report questionnaires can be productive. The impact of the hearing impairment on the communication partner must be considered at the outset, as this too will inform the treatment plan and outcomes. Gatehouse (2003) suggests that the clinician should question the patient and family members regarding the priority they attach to selected listening needs, activity limitations, and psychosocial sequelae, as this can influence the management options offered. At the Ida Institute, this is referred to as the communication partnership. Each partner must acknowledge how the hearing loss is limiting and restricting participation in the enjoyment of shared activities. Further, each partner must accept responsibility to work together to attempt to improve communication, and must be willing to commit to the steps necessary to improve the partnership. This is something that can be assessed by observing the person with hearing impair-

ment and the communication partner communicate (Lind 2009), and by asking the communication partner questions about his or her perceptions of the difficulty. (The communication partner could be a spouse or an adult child.) Asking the partner to rate his or her perception of the importance of being able to communicate in selected situations can be helpful. For example, Montano (2010) suggests asking one of the following questions to initiate the dialogue and to begin sharing emotions and feelings: (1) How important is it for you that your husband improve his hearing right now? (2) How important is it to you that your mother be able to participate in family conversations? Some already existing measures such as the International Outcomes Inventory for Significant Others (IOI-SO) or the HHIE-SP (Noble, 2002 can be helpful in understanding the perceptions of a communication partner, notably the spouse. Alternatively, shared goals can be developed by using a template such as the one that can be found on the Ida Institute web page (http://idainstitute.com/tool_room/topics/communication_partners/).

In selecting a scale, it is imperative that the questionnaire be psychometrically robust, appropriate to the population for which it will be used, and appropriate for the desired purpose. For example, the Hearing Handicap Inventory for Adults was standardized on young adults and would not be appropriate for an elderly person. Similarly, the HHIE was standardized on noninstitutionalized older adults and is not valid for nursing home residents. The Significant Other Assessment of Communication (SOAC) is a companion scale to the Self-Assessment of Communication (SAC) and is not appropriate for a person with a hearing impairment. The audiologist must also consider the reason for utilizing a self-assessment questionnaire. If the audiologist merely wants to quickly screen an older adult to determine the need for an audiometric referral, short questionnaires such as the SAC or the HHIE-S would be appropriate. If, however, the clinician wants to design an individualized intervention program, then a more comprehensive questionnaire such as the HHIE, the Client-Oriented Scale of Improvement (COSI), or the APHAB might prove more effective. A comprehensive questionnaire would give the clinician a more complete picture of the areas of communication or psychosocial function warranting change, so that a client-centered rehabilitation plan can be implemented. If the audiologist needs to identify family counseling needs, then scales with companion versions such as the HHIE, the IOI, and the SAC might be appropriate because of the availability of spousal versions.

As older adults with hearing impairment and their family members often have difficulty communicating with one another, information from a significant other gathered at the start of intervention can be helpful. Typically, a discrepancy exists between ratings of handicap by the significant other and that of the person with hearing impairment. In contrast to the findings of Newman and Weinstein (1986), who found that the PHL rates the consequences to be more significant than does the communication partner, Jerger, Chmiel, Florin, Pirozzolo, and Wilson (1996) found that at baseline (prior to intervention) significant others tend to judge the handicap as being slightly greater than does the patient. Interestingly, following intervention with hearing aids or ALDs, the perceived residual handicap is judged about the same by both the PHL and the communication partner. Responses of family members or a caregiver to a self-report questionnaire can be used during counseling sessions to develop empathy for the person with hearing loss and to set realistic expectations for communicating in difficult listening situations.

Finally, if the audiologist wants to focus on hearing-aid benefit, then perhaps a questionnaire such as the Hearing Aid Performance Inventory (HAPI), developed by Walden, Demorest, and Hepler (1984), or the Shortened Hearing Aid Performance Inventory (SHAPI), described by Schum (1994), may be appropriate. The latter scale provides the hearing-aid user with an opportunity to rate hearing-aid benefit in a variety of situations. The SHAPI was designed to be used with older adults purchasing hearing aids. Subjects in the normative study were older hearing-aid users residing in New Zealand (Schum, 1994).

Special Consideration

Questionnaires that assess activity limitations, communication participation restrictions, and quality of life should be administered at several intervals during the management process to document outcomes.

Table 7.15 lists the questionnaires and scales that are integral to the assessment process. Each of the scales listed in column one can be helpful in identifying listening needs, attitudes, expectations, and the difficulties the patient has in performing everyday hearing-related tasks, and in unraveling the barriers to carrying out routine ADLs. In short, questionnaires

such as the Speech, Spatial, and Qualities of Hearing Scale (SSQ) help evaluate speech understanding difficulties in challenging listening situations not available on an audiogram. The choice of measures to use depends in large part on the dimension(s) of real-world outcome the clinician wishes to measure and on the unique life circumstances of a given patient.

Available research supports a multidimensional needs assessment, as scores on income measures often do not bear a strong correlation to one another and are differentially predictive of outcomes. The results of the large-scale cross-sectional survey conducted by Cox et al, (2007), who claim that "self-report data from standardized questionnaires occupy a key position in hearing health care" (p. 142), support this claim. They found that unaided problems reported on the HHIE and APHAB reflect auditory lifestyle demands and personality, so they do capture differences among individuals with similar audiograms, which are designed to gauge problems arising from audibility (Singh & Pichora-Fuller, 2010). They also noted that expectations data from the Expected Consequences of Hearing-Aid Ownership (ECHO) are predictive of long-term fitting outcomes, so it is important to quantify expectations as part of the needs assessment.

The needs assessment is integral to holistic management, and yields information distinct from that which is gleaned from the audiogram and from real ear measures (Cox et al, 2007). Information from self-report questionnaires serves as the basis for designing an individualized management plan. Responses to self-report questionnaires are pertinent when counseling both the hearing impaired and family members, and when doing communication strategies auditory-visual training,

Table 7.15 Income Measures: Assessment of Listening Difficulties, Activity Limitations, and Participation Restrictions

Hearing-Related Function, Activity Limitations, or Participation Restrictions
Hearing Handicap Inventory for the Elderly (HHIE) (Ventry & Weinstein, 1982)
Client Oriented Scale of Improvement (COSI) (Dillon, James, & Ginis (1997)
Abbreviated Profile of Hearing Aid Benefit (APHAB) (Cox & Alexander, 1995)
Communication Profile for the Hearing Impaired (CPHI) (Erdman & Demorest, 1990)
The Self-Assessment of Communication (SAC) (Schow & Nerbonne, 1982)
IOI-HA-SO (International Outcome Inventory for Hearing Aids–Significant Others) (Noble, 2002)
Speech, Spatial, and Qualities of Hearing Scale (SSQ)[1] (Gatehouse & Noble, 2004)
International Outcomes Inventory–Hearing Aids (IOI-HA)[2] (Cox & Alexander, 2002; International Outcomes Inventory-Alternative Interventions (IOI-AI) (Noble, 2002)
Glasgow Hearing Aid Benefit Profile (GHABP) (Gatehouse, 1999)
Speech, Spatial, and Qualities of Hearing Scale (SSQ) (Gatehouse & Noble, 2004)[3]
Expectations and Goals
Expected Consequences of Hearing Aid Ownership (ECHO) (Cox & Alexander, 2000)
Attitude
Hearing Attitudes to Rehabilitation Questionnaire (HARQ) (Brooks & Hallam, 1998)
Attitudes Toward Loss of Hearing Questionnaire (ALHQ) (Saunders & Cienkowski, 1996)
Health-Related Quality-of-Life Measures
Sickness Impact Profile (SIP) (Bergner, Bobbitt, Carter, & Gilson,1981)
Medical Outcome Survey Short-Form-36 (MOS SF-36) (Ware & Sherbourne, 1992)
World Health Organization Disability Assessment Schedule (WHO-DAS II) (McArdle, Chisolm, Abrams, Wilson, & Doyle, 2005)

[1]Assesses subjective experience of hearing disability and quantifies spatial hearing abilities in realistic listening situations with a focus on binaural hearing (Singh & Pichora-Fuller, 2010).
[2]Assesses function in seven areas: use, benefit, activity limitations, satisfaction, participation restrictions, impact on others, and quality of life.
[3]A 43- item questionnaire that assesses speech hearing and spatial and sound quality.
Sources: Data from American Academy of Audiology. (2006). Guidelines for the audiologic management of adult hearing impairment. *Audiology Today, 18,* 1–44; and Meister, H., Walger, M., Brehmer, D., von Wedel, U., & von Wedel, H. (2008). The relationship between pre-fitting expectations and willingness to use hearing aids. *International Journal of Audiology, 47,* 153–159.

and they serve as the basis for measuring benefit from intervention. It is important to raise the issue of the mode of administration of questionnaires, which is typically a self-administration method or a face-to-face interview. Reliability of responses varies with presentation mode, with a cost to reliability when patients are asked to complete questionnaires on their own without an interviewer present (Singh & Pichora-Fuller, 2010; Weinstein, Spitzer, & Ventry, 1986). For example, Singh and Pichora-Fuller (2010) suggest that the interview may be preferable to the self-administration mode, as responses are less variable, and self-administration calls into play additional cognitive resources. If these resources are overtaxed, then the quality of the data may be poorer than would be the case if a face-to-face interview were used. In contrast, the self-administration mode has other advantages, including the fact that respondents are more likely to report socially undesirable behaviors when completing the questionnaire on their own, and that individuals are less prone to the social pressure of an interviewer if they complete the questionnaire on their own (Singh & Pichora-Fuller, 2010).

Pearl

Multidimensional needs assessment using self-report questionnaires yields a more fully realized understanding of the patient's situation (Cox et al, 2007).

Step 2: Sensory Management and Orientation

Boothroyd (2007) suggests that the provision of devices to address auditory function and communication should be comprehensive and dependent on the patient's auditory ability, cognitive ability, communicative function, and motivational level, among other factors. Options range from hearing aids to implantable devices to HATs. The explicit goal is to optimize audibility and speech comprehension in commonly encountered simple and complex listening situations. It is important to verify that the recommended device is performing according to a given standard and is providing ample audibility, comfortable listening, and adequate speech understanding. Verification techniques can be employed for this purpose, and to determine the magnitude of benefit in selected domains and the satisfaction the person with hearing impairment is achieving. Integral to sensory management is the hearing-aid orientation for those who have received hearing aids.

Step 3: Counseling

Counseling is a key part of communication management, as it enhances participation, addresses emotional and practical limitations, and improves participation and quality of life (Boothroyd, 2007). As audiologists and rehabilitation professionals, we must form effective therapeutic relationships with PHLs and their communication partners. An understanding of counseling principles is critical if we are to achieve optimal outcomes with our older patients. In short, our work with PHLs is designed to facilitate adjustment to hearing impairment so that they can adapt to the challenges imposed by hearing

impairment, with the ultimate goal being to ensure enhanced quality of life, optimal care, improved communication skills. A recent field survey conducted by Kochkin and colleagues (2010) found that new and experienced hearing-aid users reported receiving 1.2 hours of counseling over the first 2 months of their hearing-aid fitting. Those surveyed indicated the fitting process required on average 2.5 visits. Interestingly, the authors defined counseling as "explaining care and maintenance of the hearing aids" (p. 16). The survey included a separate question about hours spent in auditory rehabilitation (not defined), and new users were more likely to attend a group aural rehabilitation session than were experienced users (18% vs. 9%). Only 5% of those surveyed received a self-help video or auditory retraining therapy or were referred to a self-help group such as the Hearing Loss Association of America. The authors did not attempt to relate counseling and audiological rehabilitation to the success of the fittings, but it is noteworthy that 25% of new users used their hearing aids less than 2 hours per day, and 68% of new users reported that they were satisfied with their hearing aids as compared with 75% of experienced users. The authors also noted that respondents rated as below-average in terms of success as a hearing-aid user were less likely to receive personal counseling from the hearing health professional than were those considered above-average in terms of success, and were less likely to receive advice regarding ancillary counseling tools, such as auditory retraining software, self-help material, or referral to a self-help group than those individuals rated above-average in terms of success.

These findings, although from a mail survey, shed light on the status of counseling services delivered by hearing health professionals and underscore the importance of paying greater attention to counseling principles and practice among audiologists. It is hoped that the predominantly technological focus will soon give way to a more patient-centered focus, which may help in terms of word-of-mouth advertising, increased hours of hearing-aid use, improved patient satisfaction and hearing-aid utility, and increased numbers of PHLs who embrace hearing aids.

Counseling is an ongoing, facilitative process that entails a working alliance, a collaboration, and a partnership. According to Erdman (2009), counseling is the "means by which we facilitate patients' realization of the confidence and skills they need to manage their hearing problems effectively" (p. 171). More specifically, the overall objectives of counseling are to (1) support PHLs as they works through any hearing-related issues, (2) help PHLs make important decisions regarding their condition, (3) clarify questions and issues surrounding the problems that derive from the hearing impairment, (4) help PHLs make important decisions pertaining to their hearing, and (5) facilitate adjustment to both the consequences of hearing impairment and the intervention recommended to overcome any associated difficulties (McDonald & Haney, 1997).

With the experience of hearing impairment as the centerpiece, the patient's needs, motivations, and perceptions provide the context and the focus of counseling. A biopsychosocial model that is patient or client centered should prevail rather than a biomedical top-down model or professional-centered approach with the disorder or disease as the focal point. Several conditions are unique to the client-centered approach if therapeutic goals are to be achieved (Raskin & Rogers, 1989): empathic listening, focusing on patients' needs and perceptions, determining goals and strategies, reciprocal positive unconditional regard and acceptance of patients and their narrative, counselor congruence, warmth and genuineness on the part of the clinicians, and patient engagement in the process (Erdman, 2009). A clinical interview at the outset punctuated by open-ended questions and affirmations will set the stage for the personal narrative to unfold and form the centerpiece of the therapeutic process. Open-ended questions such as "What brings you to my office today?" or "Tell me about your hearing problem" or "What made you decide to make an appointment to see an audiologist today?" are effective in encouraging PHLs to begin to tell their story. It is hoped that the fears, concerns, and desires of the person with hearing impairment will be communicated to the audiologist who must listen attentively, focusing on verbal and nonverbal cues. Excellent attending and listening skills on the part of the audiologist will help to foster a productive patient–practitioner alliance. Allowing the narrative to unfold by offering supportive silence, and by posturing oneself by leaning forward and maintaining eye contact, communicates involvement and investment in the patient. According to Erdman, ample evidence exists in the literature supporting semi-structured interviews driven by open-ended questions, as they help put the patient at ease, deepen the working alliance, and foster positive outcomes. It is important to note that if the clinician feels a need to probe for additional information, it should be done sparingly so as not to distract patients from what is on their mind.

Although patient-centered counseling as advocated by Rogers (1951) has as a goal empowering the person with hearing impairment and the communication partner to emerge as partners in an alliance designed to help manage and overcome the ramifications of the patient's condition as they see it, motivational interviewing, as discussed in an earlier section of this chapter, is more directive, with the focus being to remove barriers or obstacles to behavior change. Stated differently, although client-centered counseling and motivational interviewing have as their focus self-determination and patient empowerment, the former is nondirective whereas the latter is directive, promoting the self-efficacy that is integral to the process (Erdman, 2009). Further, motivational interviewing is designed specifically to promote motivation and barriers to change, so it sets the stage for client-centered counseling once patients are ready for behavior change and have confidence in their ability to succeed at an intervention (Wagner & McMahon, 2004). It is critical to emphasize that motivation plays a critical role in the success of counseling endeavors, because if the person with hearing loss is not invested in the counseling venture, the likelihood of success is diminished (Wagner & McMahon, 2004).

Table 7.16 Key Elements of Patient-Centered Counseling (PCC)

Element	Goal/Purpose
Patient	Eliciting and understanding the patient's perspective or narrative—concerns, ideas, expectations, illness experience, needs, feelings, and functioning
Biopsychosocial	Understanding the patient within his or her unique psychosocial context and the health system context
Clinician	Reaching a shared understanding of the problem and its treatment with the patient that is concordant with the patient's values and motivations
Relationship	Helping patient to share power and responsibility by involving the patient as well as family members in the choices associated with intervention

Source: Data from Epstein, R. M., Franks, P., Fiscella, K., Shields, C. G., Meldrum, S. C., Kravitz, R. L., et al. (2005, Oct). Measuring patient-centered communication in patient-physician consultations: Theoretical and practical issues. *Social Science and Medicine, 61,* 1516–1528.

The key elements of a patient-centered approach are listed in **Table 7.16**. The fourth element entails involving the PHLs in all aspects of decision making that relate to the intervention, focusing on assets and de-emphasizing negative aspects of their situation, and being uncritical when acknowledging and exploring, which are key ingredients of successful counseling (Wagner & McMahon, 2004). The setting of goals should be dictated by the difficulties or problems described by the PHL, and solutions for obtaining specific goals must be acceptable.

English (2008) argues that "the effectiveness of audiological rehabilitation is contingent on the audiologist's counseling skills" (p. 93). She acknowledges that counseling requires many skill sets, not often acquired until one is engaged in active clinical practice (Atkins, 2007). The counseling model used with older adults proposed by McDonald and Haney (1997), which is displayed in **Fig. 7.9,** dovetails with the key elements of PCC. For example, items 2 and 7 in **Fig. 7.9** would be considered relationship factors, whereas item 1 might be considered a patient factor.

The first step in the process is to understand clients as social and psychological beings with their own understanding of their experience with hearing loss. This step is followed by establishment of a rapport, which includes being an empathic listener and a respectful professional (McDonald & Haney, 1997). We must understand how PHLs feel about their hearing impairment: do they own it, or in their view is it someone else's problem (English, 2008)? How do they feel about hearing aids, cochlear implants, or assistive technologies? Do they have biased assumptions about their value, their cost, and the public impression about hearing aids in particular? Where do they fit in terms of their readiness and in terms of their willingness to change the status quo? Once we understand PHL in the context of the latter issues, we are ready to work with them to set goals and priorities. Counseling goals should be established based on comprehensive assessment of patient needs, with their motivational level informing the course of counseling. In the document on preferred practice patterns,

---

Pearl

Self-determination, which is central to rehabilitative counseling and motivational interviewing, implies that persons with the hearing impairment should make their own decisions, set their goals, and decide on how to achieve their goals (Wagner & McMahon, 2004).

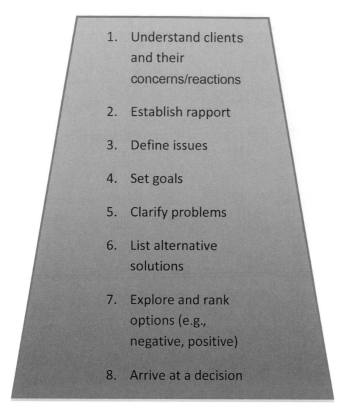

1. Understand clients and their concerns/reactions

2. Establish rapport

3. Define issues

4. Set goals

5. Clarify problems

6. List alternative solutions

7. Explore and rank options (e.g., negative, positive)

8. Arrive at a decision

Fig. 7.9 Counseling model for use with older adults. [Modified from McDonald, P., & Haney, M. (1997). *Counseling the older adult: A training manual in clinical gerontology* (2nd ed.). San Francisco: Jossey-Bass.]

the American Speech-Language-Hearing Association (ASHA, 2006) emphasizes the importance of being sensitive to cultural factors that influence the perspective of persons with hearing impairment. Cultural factors and racial differences are major considerations in terms of self-rated health (SRH), wherein individuals are asked to rate their health on a 5-point Likert-type scale. Results of the 2006 National Health Interview Survey revealed that 69% of white adults reported excellent or good health as compared with 56% of black adults (U.S. Department of Health and Human Services, 2007). This disparity exists even when controlling for sociodemographic variables and correlates of self-reported health. Interestingly, when whites and blacks were compared at the same level of health functioning, whites continued to rate their health more favorable than did blacks (Spencer et al, 2009). The differences have been interpreted in many ways, but one conclusion is that black adults may have different views about health that might lead to negative health assessments. As health pessimism could influence outcomes with interventions, counseling with black adults may have to focus on self-efficacy principles. Further the five A's model of behavior change discussed below will be helpful.

Regarding cultural factors, Chang, Ho, and Chou (2009) explored perceptions of hearing handicap in a sample of 1220 adults aged 65 years or older in Taiwan, China. They found that only 21.4% of subjects with moderate to profound hearing loss

had an HHIE-S score greater than 10, which differs dramatically from samples of veterans and older adults in the United States. Similarly, Maratchi (2011) compared differences in the way ethnicity influences choices with regard to hearing aid use in a sample of Caucasian and Chinese-American men and women with comparable hearing levels and perceptions of hearing handicap. Interestingly, Caucasian women's hearing-aid acceptance rate was 57%, Chinese-American women's hearing-aid acceptance rate was 14%, Caucasian men's hearing-aid acceptance rate was 57%, and Chinese-American men's hearing-aid acceptance rate was 43%. **Figure 7.10** captures the differences. These two studies serve to demonstrate how cultural differences may inform counseling.

Similarly, cultural differences in health literacy inform the content of counseling. In their seminal article on cultural considerations in counseling, Sue, Arredondo, and McDavis (1992) expound on the beliefs, attitude, and knowledge necessary for counselors to be culturally competent. Two important beliefs and attitudes culturally skilled counselors possess is the ability to value and respect differences and to recognize that the counselor's cultural background and experiences may "color" or bias the patient-centered process. Regarding knowledge, the authors contend that culturally skilled counselors are knowledgeable about communication style differences and know how to anticipate the impact these differences may have on the counseling process. They suggest that culturally skilled counselors seek out training experiences that will enrich their understanding of how to be most effective when working with people from different cultures. They also acknowledge that culturally skilled counselors are familiar with how mental health and health issues are impacted by ethnic and racial differences. Finally, culturally skilled counselors are aware of when the mismatch between their linguistic skills and that of their patients necessitate referral to outside resources, use of interpreters to facilitate the counseling process, or a hybrid approach to counseling wherein traditional healers or spiritual leaders may play a role in the therapeutic process. These cultural considerations should increasingly be emphasized and deployed during counseling regarding hearing aids and hearing loss.

Glasgow, Emont, and Miller (2006) developed the five A's model of behavior change to be used as part of health behavior change counseling. This approach is instructive for clinicians working with persons with hearing impairment as it provides a template for the "script" audiologists should use when counseling. The five A's are shown in **Table 7.17** and are reduced to user-friendly fragments. As shown, the first step in counseling is to assess the needs, values, expectations, and motivations of the person with hearing impairment and ideally those of the communication partner. Options for eliciting this information have already been presented and include use of a formal questionnaire coupled with nondirective, open-ended questions. The client's perspective and priorities are central to establishing collaborative goals at this stage. The perspective of the communication partner is critical as well. Consistent with the health belief model espoused by Becker et al (1979), barriers to and perceived benefits of a behavior must become apparent at this stage as they will influence the recommended actions. Here is where cultural sensitivity on the part of the audiolo-

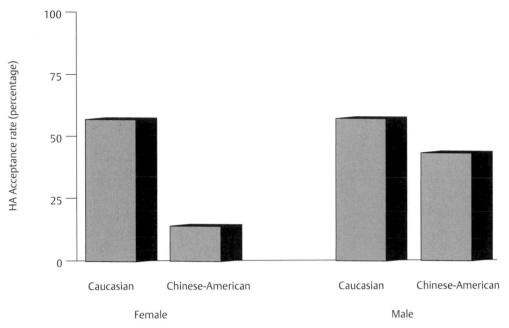

Fig. 7.10 Summary of reported choices with regard to wearing a hearing aid (HA) for Chinese-American and Caucasian older adults.

gist is crucial. Consistent with the philosophy of Gagne and Jennings (2011), the first step is to identify and assess the problems (e.g., participation restrictions, activity limitations, psychosocial consequences), to be sure they are understood.

Next, we must advise the patient of the available options, be they medical interventions or rehabilitative interventions depending on data from the assessment, including the patient's motivational level, transtheoretical stage of change, hearing status, and self-perception. Specifically, possible solutions should be identified and possible implications associated with choosing a particular solution discussed (Gagne & Jennings, 2011). Next, the clinician and patient must agree on the solution, goals, and realistic intervention options, be they hearing aids, cochlear implants, or hearing-assistance technologies, or just counseling. Once there is agreement, the audiologist should collaborate with the patient on developing a comprehensive action plan that should be discussed and written down. Stated

differently, this is the point at which the acceptable solutions are implemented. The final stage entails arranging for the professional who will work closely with the patient to execute the intervention plan and to address compliance issues. As part of this aspect of counseling, it is the responsibility of the clinician implementing the plan to evaluate the impact and consequences of the intervention program and to include compliance-improving strategies to optimize outcomes. Further, directing patients to self-help groups or to group audiological rehabilitation is critical for educating patients and for providing opportunities for social interaction (e.g., Hearing Loss Association of America). **Table 7.18** lists some compliance-improving strategies that Sweetow (2009) suggests can help optimize outcomes. Finally, conditions for terminating rehabilitation based on outcomes data should be established and agreed upon by the patient and audiologist. **Table 7.19** presents a simple checklist that I have modified from the article by Glasgow and colleagues (2006) for use during counseling to record the activities or have prompts available during the session.

Kuntze, Van Der Molen, and Born (2009) discuss the basic skills necessary for effective counseling. As audiologists have little background in counseling, and as counseling plays such an important role in audiological practice, it is worth isolating the skill set they discuss. They confirm that the three stages of counseling as discussed above include problem clarification, wherein patients' difficulties associated with their condition are clarified; helping them gain new insight into their problems; and formulating strategies to address the issues identified in the first two stages. The first stage requires seven basic counseling skills, and the second stage requires four or five basic skills. These counseling communication skills are shown in **Table 7.20**. For the most part, these skills are relevant to the audiologist when counseling about adjustment to and coping

Table 7.17 The Five A's Model of Health Behavior Change Counseling

	Areas in Which to Implement
Assess	Patient level of behavior, beliefs, and motivations
Advise	Patient based on personal health considerations
Agree	Person with hearing impairment and clinician must agree on a realistic set of goals
Assist	To anticipate psychosocial or environmental barriers and develop an action plan
Arrange	Follow-up support in the community, with affiliated health professionals or with an audiologist

Source: Data from Glasgow, R. E., Emont, S., & Miller, D. S. (2006). Assessing the delivery of the 5 "A's" for patient-centered counseling: Alternatives and future directions. *Health Promotion International, 21*, 2245–2255.

Table 7.18 Checklist to Promote Compliance with Recommendations

Strategy	Addressed	
Provide clear instructions orally and in writing regarding technology, communication strategies	Yes	No
Provide feedback about progress	Yes	No
Simplify instructions (e.g., return visits; hearing-aid use schedule) and present them using multiple modalities	Yes	No
Have systems in place to generate reminders regarding appointments	Yes	No
Listen to patients and respect their input and that of their communication partner	Yes	No

Source: Data from Sweetow, R. (2009). *Five ideas to better meet the hearing needs of older people.* Paper presented at the Adult Conference: The Challenge of Aging, Chicago.

with the hearing loss. Mastery of these skills can take some time, but based on limited evidence, patients have rated clinicians as being effective when they used the counseling skills with them. Further, they claim that they were satisfied with the therapeutic encounter when the skills were used.

Pearl

A holistic approach emphasizing counseling and communication strategies is critical to successful audiological management (Hawkins, 2005).

Counseling Content

Informational counseling about the hearing aid and assistive technologies is important, as is personal-adjustment counseling. Personal-adjustment counseling is a facilitative process that assists persons with hearing impairment in coping effectively with their communicative difficulties and helps patients resolve adjustment problems (Erdman, 1993). Personal-adjustment counseling can enable patients to see that a hearing aid is effective in helping them overcome the consequences of hearing

impairment, thereby enhancing the chance of achieving maximal functioning, life satisfaction, and self-esteem (Kemp, 1990). Throughout the counseling process, patients come to understand how hearing loss can have an impact on important aspects of their daily life and that hearing aids can restore some of the functions lost because of hearing impairment. One goal of personal-adjustment counseling is to help the hearing impaired adapt to a life that has been permanently changed by a chronic condition. A chronic condition such as sensorineural hearing loss cannot be cured, yet we should make every attempt through counseling to help the patient resolve the life changes associated with hearing impairment. Some of the changes on which to focus are decreased social independence, compromised life satisfaction, and diminished self-esteem. To the extent that rehabilitation programs help people deal with these changes, they are successful. It is thus beneficial to focus the hearing impaired on the potential outcomes of AR, targeting improvements in these latter domains of function.

Maintenance of independence (i.e., autonomy) is a desired goal of individuals suffering from a chronic condition such as hearing impairment. Two psychological processes interact to enable a person suffering from a handicapping chronic condition to live independently (Kemp, 1990). First, the individual must learn the skills necessary to compensate for the effects of hearing loss, and to enable performance of the tasks necessary for daily life and for familial relationships. PHLs must learn to use a hearing aid in social and communicative situations as a first step toward restoring independence. Family members, communication partners, and caregivers must be integrated into each phase of the counseling process to facilitate adaptation to the many settings in which the older adult is expected to function, be it at home, in a nursing facility, or in an assisted living setting (Kane et al, 2004). To this end, we must work with PHLs and their family members to structure an environment that is safe and conducive to functional independence, and if necessary safety devices should be installed in the home. If hearing loss threatens the security of a PHL, it will produce alienation and jeopardize a sense of independence.

The second psychological process that promotes independence is assertiveness, and development of an open, positive, and realistic attitude regarding hearing loss and hearing-aid

Table 7.19 Checklist to Document Counseling Activities

Check If Completed	Activity	Description
	Assess	Client completed needs assessment and received feedback on hearing health behaviors and objective test results; provide written list to client
	Advise	Client received advice about recommendations for behavior change specifically targeted to his or her condition; make sure to include client ideas and beliefs when discuss treatment plan
	Agree	Achievable goals were collaboratively set with the client and approaches to addressing hearing health issues were communicated clearly; make sure to empower client
	Assist	Action plan established, including strategies for problem solving, and necessary referrals made; helped client resolve issues so that he/she could meet goals and improve hearing health; discussed communication strategies with communication partner and how to best communicate in difficult situations
	Arrange and address	Followed up with client to see if client followed through on goals and to receive feedback on progress made and needs relating to the intervention or condition; address factors that will promote compliance with recommended interventions

Source: Data from Glasgow, R. E., Emont, S., & Miller, D. S. (2006). Assessing the delivery of the 5 "A's" for patient-centered counseling: Alternatives and future directions. *Health Promotion International, 21,* 2245–2255.

Table 7.20 Communication Skills Basic to Each Stage of Counseling

Stage of Counseling	Counseling Skill	Purpose
Problem clarification	Minimal encouragements	Brief verbal responses intended to encourage client and to show that the client is receiving attention
	Asking questions	Help clients to clarify their problem using their own words
	Paraphrasing	Clinicians restate in their own words the gist of what the client has described
	Reflection of feeling	Clinician attends to and shows an understanding of the emotional aspects of the client's narrative
	Concreteness	Help clients be as precise as possible in describing their problem by paraphrasing, asking questions, and reflecting
	Summarizing	Clinician structures what has been said by stating in order the points raised by the client
	Situation clarification	Clinician discusses ambiguities or misunderstandings that may arise in the relationship between clinician and client
Gaining new insights	Advanced accurate empathy	Clinician provides an interpretation of the client's narrative, providing a sharper and possibly more constructive view of the issues at hand
	Confrontation	Clinician provides a perspective about clients' viewpoint that differs markedly from their perspective
	Positive relabeling	Clinician applies a positive spin to the parts of the problem described by the client that may have been negative, thereby altering the client's negative self-image
	Directness	Clinician provides clients with a perspective on the consequences of their behavior

Source: Data from Kuntze, J., Van Der Molen, H., & Born, M. (2009). Increase in counseling communication skills after basic and advanced microskills training. *British Journal of Educational Psychology, 79*, 175–189.

use (Kemp, 1990). During counseling sessions, especially with the old-old, efforts must be made to facilitate development of these attitudes. Older adults should be encouraged to admit to hearing loss, to offer cues to facilitate communication, and to offer visible reminders to everyone about behaviors that interfere with or facilitate communication (Glass, 1990). These steps will avoid the tendency for hearing-impaired individuals to be stigmatized or to be mistakenly labeled as "confused" or "forgetful" because of failure to remember what they in fact never heard. As will be discussed later in the chapter, assertiveness training and participation in self-help groups with other hearing-impaired persons and hearing-aid users can promote the attitudes necessary for independence despite a significant hearing impairment.

Audiologists often pay lip service to the concept of life satisfaction and its importance to older adults. The "topic of life satisfaction after disability is crucial in rehabilitation" (Kemp, 1990, p. 45). Some older adults, especially late-deafened adults, may question the purpose or value of life when confronted with a devastating chronic condition such as a handicapping hearing impairment. Rather than confront it and attempt to alleviate it, the older adult will retreat and succumb to depression, declines in physical functional status, and possibly cognitive deficits (Bess et al, 1990; Herbst & Humphrey, 1980). Maintenance of intimate relationships and feelings of belonging are integral to life satisfaction.

Pleasurable experiences such as those that derive from our senses (e.g., hearing music) and the experience of success with daily activities are important sources of life satisfaction. According to Kemp (1990), disabling chronic conditions are a great source of psychological pain for older adults, and the goal of rehabilitative interventions should be to increase the pleasure-to-pain ratio, to make life satisfying. Audiologists should begin to emphasize life satisfaction as a key outcome of hearing-aid use as a means of promoting this form of inter-vention. The work of Mulrow et al (1990a) demonstrates the contribution of hearing-aid use to life satisfaction.

Special Consideration

Older adults are often unaware of the contribution of hearing loss to life satisfaction, and thus it is incumbent on audiologists to link the benefit of hearing aids to life satisfaction when counseling the elderly.

Experiencing success also contributes to life satisfaction among older adults, which is why positive feedback is so important (Kemp, 1990). Examples of conditions conducive to feelings of success among the hearing impaired include restoration of the ability to communicate with family members or caregivers and of the feeling of belonging and of intimacy, renewed enjoyment of television and radio, or, at the most basic level, hearing a baby cry or the water run. The ability to successfully engage in communicative behaviors once lost contributes to feelings of life satisfaction. Another psychological variable contributing to life satisfaction among older adults is "having a sense of meaning or purpose in life" (Kemp, 1990, p. 44). Similarly, feelings of apathy, loss of self-esteem, and feelings of worthlessness, which are typical signs of depression, also compromise life satisfaction in older adults. A reduction in sensory input deriving from hearing loss is linked to depression, and hearing aids have proven successful in reversing depression in selected older adults. Thus, it is incumbent on audiologists to emphasize to the hearing impaired and their families the potential role hearing aids may play in the management of this prevalent affective disorder.

Whereas life satisfaction relates to people's appraisal of their life, self-esteem follows from people's appraisal of themselves

(Kemp, 1990). The onset of a chronic condition, such as impaired hearing, may diminish people's self-esteem because of the stigma often associated with hearing impairment, which affects how PHLs are viewed by others (e.g., as handicapped, stupid, or dumb), and because it may interfere with what a person can do such as engaging successfully in leisure or group activities. These variables are the ingredients from which self-esteem arises, and the greater the extent to which each is diminished, the greater the probability that the individual will suffer from poor self-esteem. Once the counseling sessions are complete, it should be clear that the interference with communication, the loss of self-esteem, depression, the loss of independence, and the decrease in functional ability associated with hearing loss are temporary, thanks to the hearing aid and assistive technologies delivered in the context of AR.

Step 4: Auditory Training, Speech Perception Training, and Communication Management

It is well accepted that perceptual training to improve communication and speech recognition in noise is an important part of any management program with older adults (Boothroyd, 2007). However, there is considerable inconsistency among audiologists in the language used to describe communication programs for hearing-impaired adults. To some the term *auditory training* is too narrow and the term *speech perception training* is too restrictive. We need to distinguish between the terms *speech perception training* and *communication management* and then further fine tune these terms. According to Laplante-Lévesque, Hickson, and Worrall (2010), speech perception training encompasses auditory training, speech-reading training, and auditory visual training, whereas communication management refers to programs that target communication strategies/hearing tactics, conversational fluency, assertiveness training, stress management, and personal adjustment (i.e., counseling). I think of synthetic auditory training programs as a form of communication management, as they emphasize top-down processing with a focus on teaching skills necessary to communicate, including communication strategies and the use of repair strategies (Sweetow & Sabes, 2009).

Given the cognitive skills integral to speech understanding in adverse listening situations, and considering the literature on cognition and cognitive plasticity, I believe a better term for auditory training is *auditory/cognitive perceptual training,* because hearing aids merely restore audibility and are not effective at restoring the frequency resolution caused by damage to the outer hair cells, nor can they correct the declines in central auditory and cognitive function concurrent with aging. I urge audiologists to use a more global definition of auditory training in light of emerging data that declines in cognitive function (e.g., memory reasoning, speed of processing) can be restored via cognitive training, and there is a positive transfer effect such that cognitive training improves functional outcomes (Willis, Tennstedt, Marsiske, Ball, Elias, Koepke, et al, 2006). By combining hearing-aid use with auditory/cognitive perceptual training, which Sweetow and Sabes (2006) do with the Listening and Communication Enhancement (LACE) program, the added value associated with hearing aids would be tremendous.

Essential for helping persons with hearing impairment to integrate linguistic, acoustic, and environmental information, auditory/cognitive perceptual training entails the application of formal listening procedures and cognitive exercises to optimize the activity of speech perception (Boothroyd, 2010; Sweetow & Sabes, 2009). Sweetow and Sabes (2009) define auditory training as a process, be it analytic, synthetic, or a combination, which is designed to enhance the ability of persons with hearing impairment to interpret auditory experiences by maximally using their residual hearing. According to Tye-Murray (2008), auditory training has as its goals assisting persons with hearing impairment to develop their ability to recognize speech and to interpret auditory experiences using the auditory signal. Auditory training is premised on the principle that training can help promote auditory capacity, and can help individuals maximize their use of residual hearing. The goal is to help enhance the ability to use whatever sound is available in both ideal and adverse listening situations, and because understanding in adverse listening situation is the goal, cognitive skills and training must come into play. That is to say, part of the perceptual training includes manipulation of cognitive variables that influence comprehension and speech understanding, especially in noise.

There are several options for providing auditory/cognitive training and training in communication strategies and conversational repair strategies. Individual training coupled with either group or home-based training is the best option. Sweetow and Sabes (2006) outlined essential design criteria for comprehensive yet practical communication programs, and although they primarily pertain to home-based training, some of the recommendations are appropriate for individual and group training as well. According to Sweetow and Sabes, any communication management program must be cost-effective, practical, easily accessible, interactive, and sufficiently difficult so as to maintain interest while minimizing fatigue. In addition, there should be ample opportunity to provide reinforcement, the content should match the patient's skill level, and exercises should proceed at the appropriate pace and include both analytic and synthetic listening training. Finally, feedback should be provided to both the patient and the clinician to appropriately monitor progress, and the patient should bear some level of responsibility with respect to the final outcome.

As shown in **Table 7.21,** available communication management programs differ on several variables including delivery mode (e.g., clinician led and individual or group training, or self-directed computer-assisted self-instruction); content (e.g., communication strategies, cognitive training); session duration and number of sessions; and target audience (e.g., hearing-aid user, people with hearing impairment regardless of hearing-aid use, communication partner and person with hearing impairment (Boothroyd, 2010; Laplante-Lévesque et al, 2010). Some of the advantages of individual, group, or self-directed computer-assisted training are listed in **Table 7.21.**

The LACE program is a hybrid approach as it includes communication management, speech perception, and cognitive training. Designed to enhance the ability to communicate by training the brain to utilize a combination of auditory and cognitive skills, LACE is one of the most widely used of the computer, DVD or internet based training programs. The primary

Table 7.21 Options for Delivery of Auditory Training, Speech Perception Training, or Communication Management to the Hearing Impaired

Option and Examples	Advantage
Individual Analytic auditory training	Individualized and tailored, can provide immediate feedback and reinforcement, can monitor balance between success and learning opportunity based on individual performance, pacing matched to individual needs
Group Active Communication Education (ACE) program	All members of the group share the stigma of hearing loss, supportive milieu, and conducive to all members sharing feelings; hearing loss is typical rather than deviant, not too costly, ideal environment for teaching communication strategies via role playing, reinstates feeling of belonging
Computer assisted or computer aided Listening and Communication Enhancement (LACE),[1] Computer-Assisted Speech Perception Evaluation and Training (CASPER),[2] Computer-Assisted Speech Training (CAST),[3] CasperSent[4]	Inexpensive, self-pacing, person with hearing impairment assumes responsibility for success, individualized attention, pacing is individualized, private, nonthreatening, interactive

[1]http://www.neurotone.com/index.html.
[2]http://www.hearingresearch.org/.
[3]http://www.cochlearamericas.com/Support/2427.asp.
[4]Software available on DVD, which is an expansion of the original CASPER program (Boothroyd, 1987).
Sources: Data from Preminger, J. E. (2007). Issues associated with the measurement of psychosocial benefits of group audiologic rehabilitation programs. *Trends in Amplification, 11*, 113–123; Boothroyd, A. (2010). *You have a new hearing aid: So what?* Now what? Paper Presented at Starkey Innovation in Action Symposium. Minneapolis, Minnesota; and Sweetow, R. W., & Sabes, J. H. (2010, Oct). Auditory training and challenges associated with participation and compliance. *Journal of the American Academy of Audiology, 21*, 586–593.

goals of LACE are enhancement of listening and communication skills and confidence levels, and training of the brain to use skills to compensate for gaps created by hearing impairment. Interactive and sentence based, LACE can be completed using the standalone DVD version in 10 sessions, which typically translates into a half-hour commitment per day totaling 5 hours of training over a period of 2 weeks. Training is conducted at the hearing-aid user's most comfortable listening level. Key features include self-pacing and adaptivity, meaning that training progresses at the listener's own speed and is adaptive in that the training activities are not too hard or too easy (Olson, 2011). It includes three types of interactive and adaptive tasks: (1) training exercises to promote cognitive skills (e.g., auditory working memory and speed of processing); (2) interactive communication tasks to improve the use of communication strategies, context, and linguistics to derive meaning from the spoken message; and (3) exercises using time-compressed competing speech, and speech in a background of noise. The degraded speech training exercises includes sentence-based tasks in situations typically problematic for persons with hearing impairment. The cognitive training exercises are designed to improve the cognitive skills that are important for speech understanding in noisy situations. **Figure 7.11** displays the listening situations included in LACE. A typical exercise for many of the simulations may take the form of an omitted word, thereby challenging the listener to take advantage of context and linguistic knowledge especially when acoustic components are missing (Sweetow & Sabes, 2007). Communication strategy activities includes discussion of suggested "hearing tactics" and strategies to promote effective communication, such as facing the speaker when sitting in a noisy environment. **Table 7.22** describes the training exercises.

The LACE program has some unique features (**Table 7.23**): (1) the difficulty level of tasks is adaptive, based on the accuracy of the response; (2) it provides stimulating training exercises in a variety of areas; and (3) it provides exercises to discourage the use of maladaptive compensatory tactics (Sweetow & Sabes, 2006). The PHL sets the volume of the speakers, calibrates the system, and selects the topic that will be the basis for the sentences used in the training for the day's activities. A few studies have verified the outcomes with LACE and have identified the variables predictive of outcomes following LACE training. Sweetow and Sabes (2006) conducted a multi-site study of the effectiveness of LACE with 65 participants ranging in age from 28 to 85 years. The majority of participants were experienced hearing-aid users, 85% of whom wore binaural hearing aids. The impact of the training on off-task outcome measures such as speech understanding, use of communication strategies, self-reported handicap, working memory, and speed of processing was assessed after the 4-week trial with LACE. Further, on-task training outcomes were assessed to determine the adequacy of training materials and of the time frame allotted for the training. Training effects were noted on many of the off-task outcome measures, including the measure of speed of processing and working memory. Further, the majority of participants showed improved performance on the QuickSIN™ at two presentation levels, on the Hearing Handicap Inventory for the Elderly (HHIE) or the Hearing Handicap Inventory for Adults (HHIA), and on the Communication Scale for Older Adults (CSOA-s). Interestingly, gains made during training were maintained over an 8-week time frame. Although 20% of participants dropped out of the study, evidence is mounting in the cognitive psychology literature regarding patient acceptance of Web-based training in the cognitive domain among older adults. Hence, audiologists should encourage hearing-aid users to use LACE as a means of promoting improvements in speech understanding, working memory, and speed of processing, and reductions in communication handicaps. Ideal candidates for LACE training are those with difficulty understanding speech in noise and those who have and perceive themselves to have

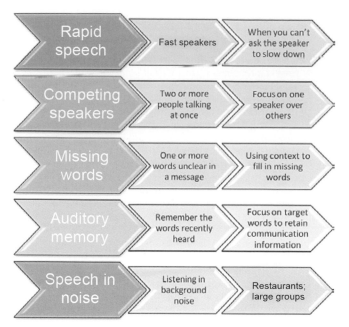

Fig. 7.11 Simulated situations exercises included in Listening and Communication Enhancement (LACE) program. (From Rachel Marcus, Au.D., student class assignment. Reprinted by permission.)

a significant hearing impairment and handicap. What remains to be worked out is whether the cost of LACE is bundled into the hearing-aid fitting or if LACE is considered an add-on. Of course using LACE on the internet is cost-effective. To some extent the answer will depend on the view of the audiologist in terms of the integral role of AR in the hearing-aid fitting process.

Sweetow and Sabes (2006) extended the above investigation to determine candidacy for LACE training. They found that older subjects and those with more severe hearing loss took less time than their counterparts to complete the training.

Table 7.22 Listening and Communication Enhancement (LACE™) Training Exercises

Area of Skill Trained	Training Activities and Conditions
Degraded speech	Multi-talker speech babble (SB), time-compressed or rapid speech (TC), competing speech (CS)
Cognitive skill training	Exercises designed to improve auditory working memory and speed of processing
Communication strategies	Helpful hints regarding management of the acoustic environment, assertive listening skills, realistic expectations

Source: Data from Sweetow, R. W., & Sabes, J. H. (2006, Sep). The need for and development of an adaptive Listening and Communication Enhancement (LACE) program. *Journal of the American Academy of Audiology, 17,* 538–558.

Further, the more severe the hearing loss, the greater the improvement on the QuickSIN™ and on the HHIE. Similarly, those who perceived greater initial handicap on the HHI showed the greatest improvement on the HHI and on the QuickSIN™. Similarly, those participants who did not have effective communication strategies at the start of the training showed the greatest improvement on the CSOA-S scale. Further, the poorer the baseline performance on the QuickSIN™, the better the post-training performance. Although computerized training may not be ideal for all persons with hearing impairment, the findings of Sweetow and Sabes (2007) confirm data from social psychology, suggesting that those individuals most motivated to improve listening skills tend to complete the training program and to benefit from it. The latter individuals are those who are older, with poorer HHIE scores at the outset, and with more difficulty understanding speech in noise. I concur with the conclusions of Sweetow and Sabes that counseling and motivational interviewing would be the approach with the best yield in terms of identifying candidates likely to succeed with LACE training. It would be interesting if patients with reduced cognitive function who do poorly on speech-understanding

Table 7.23 Features of LACE

Delivery Mode	Outcomes	Training Time Required	Features Across Training Activities
Home computer version	Improved listening	Daily, 30 minutes	Feedback following each stimulus presentation in form of a graph at the end of the training session displaying progress since the beginning of the session
DVD player attached to a television or computer monitor	Improved cognitive skills	Five days per week	Tracking allows the audiologist to track patient progress, assuming the patient consents
	Improvement in use of communication strategies	Total of 10 hours	
	Improved speech perception	Four weeks	
	Improved ability to fill in the "gaps" in situations wherein audibility is compromised		
	Reductions in magnitude of self-reported handicap		

Sources: Data from Sweetow, R. W., & Sabes, J. H. (2007, Jun). Technologic advances in aural rehabilitation: Applications and innovative methods of service delivery. *Trends in Amplification, 11,* 101–111; and Sweetow, R. W., & Sabes, J. H. (2006, Sep). The need for and development of an adaptive Listening and Communication Enhancement (LACE) program. *Journal of the American Academy of Audiology, 17,* 538–558.

tasks in the presence of varying amounts of background noise when fitted with hearing aids having fast-activating compression would improve if LACE were part of the fitting protocol (Lunner & Sundewall-Thorén, 2007).

Hickson et al (2007) evaluated the effectiveness of the Active Communication Education (ACE) program, a community-based group program designed for older people with hearing impairment irrespective of hearing-aid use. The ACE program is facilitated by an audiologist or speech pathologist. In contrast to LACE, the ACE program runs for 5 weeks, 2 hours per week. The ideal number of persons in the group is 6 to 10 including both persons with hearing impairment and their communication partner. The ACE program consists of a series of modules about everyday communication activities typically problematic for older adults. The modules chosen derive from an initial analysis of problematic communication settings for group participants. The group sessions are interactive, with a focus on problem solving using practical communication strategies. Using a double-blind randomized-controlled trial, the authors found that participation restrictions, activity limitations, and well-being improved in participants undergoing the ACE training, and improvements in these domains of function were sustained 6 months after the intervention. Participant feedback on the ACE program showed that the participants benefited from learning about communication strategies. The authors also noted that participants' initial awareness of and positive attitude toward their hearing impairment were predictive of success. Similarly, a pilot study conducted by Hickson and Worrall (2003) found that participants in the ACE intervention group experienced a greater reduction in HHIE scores than did those in the control group, again underscoring the value of the ACE in terms helping to resolve communication challenges. In a sense, their findings confirm that the self-perception that a problem exists indicates candidacy for intervention, given its relationship to successful outcomes. Some of the modules in the ACE program are communication activities that have proven difficult for the hearing impaired, including using the telephone in noisy situations, discussions in a restaurant or at the dinner table, and watching television.

The ACE program is not prescriptive; rather, the group defines and prioritizes the communication situations that are most problematic, especially those associated with activity limitations and participation restrictions (Hickson & Worrall, 2003). Further, emphasis is placed on the role of the communication partner and on how he/she may assist in helping the person with hearing impairment to overcome communication difficulties. In contrast to more traditional rehabilitation programs, Hickson and Worrall (2003) suggest that ACE uses a social model approach relying on expressed situational difficulties in the listeners' environments and shared decision making among the clinician and group members on how to optimize communication. As an example, if the communication activity the group members identify as problematic is conversing in noise, the session proceeds as described in **Table 7.24**. ACE focuses on communication and repair strategies (**Table 7.25**), so it has more of a communication management approach than does LACE, which is more comprehensive in scope.

The role of cognitive factors in speech processing under varying conditions of noise is becoming increasingly apparent. Audiologists planning on doing individual or group rehabilitation

Table 7.24 Sample Active Communication Education (ACE) Program Module for Difficulty Conversing in Noisy Situations

Objectives of the Session	Sample Session Flow
Work through the problem-solving process using a setting in which participants admit having difficulty	Introduction to session Participants identify one of the noisy situations listed in the handout they receive at the outset
Identify skills necessary for improved communication in noise	Suggestions for how to improve the listening environment and optimize communication are listed on a white board in the room
Practice skills necessary for requesting that speakers clarify what they are saying	Discuss further repair strategies after discussions reveal that the modifications to the environment are not sufficient for resolving communication difficulties Divide into groups and practice repair strategies for given situations
Work through the problem-solving approach for a situation unique to each participant	Participants discuss a particular situation that is problematic for them and the group helps to work through the problem-solving process

sessions should embed cognitive training exercises in each stage of the management process to boost signal processing and to improve outcomes (Craik, 2007). The exercises should promote motor learning, memory retrieval (e.g., teaching mnemonic strategies for remembering verbal material), working memory (e.g., Categorization Working Memory Span [CWMS] tasks), and speed of processing (e.g., visual search and divided attention tasks) (Borella, Carretti, & De Beni, 2008; Willis et al, 2006). Also, during group or individual sessions, every effort should be made to avoid interference from outside distractions (Craik, 2007).

The value of cognitive-based training has been demonstrated on numerous occasions, and of interest are studies using auditory-based training. A recent randomized-controlled trial that included an experimental treatment consisting of exercises designed to improve speed and accuracy of auditory information processing demonstrated the effectiveness of auditory-based computerized cognitive training intervention that included manipulation of temporal variables (Smith et al, 2009). Specifically, six computerized exercises that were designed to improve the speed and accuracy of auditory information processing were completed by those in the experimental group. The computer-based exercises continuously adjusted the task difficulty to the user performance in an effort to maintain an 85% correct response rate. Reinforcement for correct trials was in the form of accumulation of points coupled with animations. The authors found that cognitively-based training improved the speed and accuracy of central auditory system function. The duration of the training was 5 days per week, 1 hour per day, for 8 weeks, which amounted to a total of 40 hours. This is just one of several studies document the value of cognitive-based training, and it is incumbent on audiologists

Table 7.25   Main Objectives of LACE and Strategies Used to Achieve Them

Objective	Strategy and Task
Enhance listening and communication skills	Listening to degraded speech and speech in single talker and multi-talker babble; auditory memory exercises vary in level of difficulty
Get the person with hearing loss more involved	Listening to speech in babble; interactive communication strategies
Improve the level of confidence of the person with hearing loss	Listening to speech in babble; auditory memory exercises vary in level of difficulty; interactive communication strategies
Provide person with hearing loss with a set of communication strategies	Missing-word exercise to promote speed of processing and use of linguistic and contextual cues; interactive communication strategies
Help patient to recognize that hearing aids address audibility, and it is the responsibility of persons with hearing loss to understand that they have to work to improve listening and communication skills	Listening to speech in babble; missing-word exercise to promote speed of processing, auditory closure, and use of linguistic and contextual cues

to couple this with hearing-aid fittings and traditional auditory training.

Communication strategies training (including conversational repair strategies) is an all-inclusive approach that entails the collective use of communication strategies, auditory training, and auditory–visual integration (AVI) training to maximize the communication potential of persons with hearing impairment (Tye-Murray, 2008). Assuming a conversational fluency perspective, Lind (2009) adds to the discussion by introducing a conversationally oriented intervention model that focuses on bringing patterns of conversational repair under the control of the communication partner to help promote the flow of communication or to prevent communication breakdown, which often occurs when the communication partner does not understand the speaker's message. Marrying his perspective with that of Tye Murray, communication strategies training entails teaching of strategies to enhance the listener's performance when he or she cannot be understood or is unable to understand and when communication partners do not understand each other, resulting in a communication breakdown.

The goal of strategies training is to instruct PHLs and their communication partners in the use of selected strategies to minimize potential communication breakdowns associated with reduced sensory input (Tye-Murray & Witt, 1997). Integral to strategies training is assertiveness training, which in this context implies that the person with hearing loss is taking control and affecting the outcomes (Kemp, 1990). To explain, assertiveness training encourages persons with hearing impairment to stick up for their rights, seek answers to questions, and take responsibility for improving communication and avoiding communication breakdowns. It gives people a sense of control and a sense of self-efficacy when confronted with difficult listening situations (Abrahamson, 1995). Consistent with self-efficacy principles, imbuing individuals with the ability and power to intervene and make a difference goes a long way toward setting the stage for success.

Two classes of communication strategies can be used by the hearing impaired to resolve communication breakdowns: facilitative and receptive repair strategies. There are several types of facilitative and receptive repair strategies, including anticipatory, receptive repair, instructional, or constructive strategies (Abrahamson, 1997; Sweetow & Sabes, 2006; Tye-Murray, 2008; Tye-Murray & Witt, 1997). **Table 7.26** defines the classes of communication strategies used to resolve a communication

breakdown, which I am defining as a situation that takes place when the communication partners do not understand one another, requiring that one of the partners recognize that a breakdown has taken place and choose a course of action in terms of a repair strategy (Tye-Murray, 2008). Facilitative strategies are used to affect speech-recognition performance, the communication environment, the communication partner's presentation of a message, and the message itself. Facilitative strategies are most effectively employed when they are informative and specific, and they may be used to improve the client's speech recognition skills; the communication environment, so as to structure it to be most favorable for the listener; and the communication partner.

One facilitative communication strategy is message tailoring, in which persons with hearing impairment try to structure their phrasing to control the answer given by the communication partner. For example, rather than using open-ended questions, persons with hearing impairment might ask a question that includes response choices. Instructional strategies are facilitative in that they can be used to influence the speaking behaviors of the communication partner (e.g., "slow down," "face me, please") and to influence the way in which the message is delivered or can be tailored (e.g., use short sentences) (Tye-Murray, 2008). In contrast, constructive strategies, another form of facilitative strategy, are used to effect a change in the communication environment, thereby promoting speech reception. Anticipatory strategies used by the person with hearing impairment are facilitative, as they affect the reception of the spoken message. It entails advanced planning before a communication encounter takes place. For example, keeping abreast of current events prior to going out with people interested in world events can help one better fill in the blanks when words are missed, thereby minimizing the number of communication breakdowns that take place.

Adaptive strategies are also facilitative, as they are used to minimize communication difficulties by influencing reception of the spoken message. Examples of anticipatory strategies include anticipating the content of the conversation based on the context (e.g., job interview versus going to a lecture on current events) and anticipating flow of conversation based on conversational style and sequences (**Fig. 7.12**). The strategy depends on linguistic variables, the linguistic environment, or the linguistic context. Specifically, linguistic redundancy can enable the individual to fill in the information when a com-

Table 7.26 Classes of Communication Strategies

Classes of Communication Strategies	Definition	Factors or Persons Being Influenced to Promote Reception of the Spoken Message	Examples of Strategy
Facilitative strategies	Counseling the speaker on how to best structure the message and the listening environment to enhance understanding	Listening environment, the speaker, structure of the message	Instructional, message, tailoring, and constructive strategies to optimize the environment; examples include the following: make sure room is well lit and free of distractions; use short sentences rather than long ones
Receptive repair strategies	A strategy used by the person with hearing impairment when he or she does not understand the message, resulting in communication breakdown; used to influence reception of the spoken message	Person with hearing impairment	Ask the speaker to slow down; make sure speaker is facing the person with hearing impairment when speaking
Communication breakdown	A situation that takes place when the communication partners do not understand one another	Communication partners	One of the communication partners must recognize that a breakdown has taken place and choose a course of action in terms of a repair strategy

Source: Data from Tye-Murray, N. (2008). *Foundations of aural rehabilitation: Children, adults, and their family members.* Clifton Park, NY: Thomson/Delmar Learning.

munication breakdown takes place. That is, knowledge of language (e.g., how sounds and words are strung together) and anticipating the content of the conversation, can supplement auditory input. Similarly, the context may define the topic of conversation (e.g., world events may define a discussion), and this is a critical aspect of discourse (Houston & Montgomery, 1997). The "context and general knowledge can disambiguate the sensory stream" (Houston & Montgomery, 1997, p. 148).

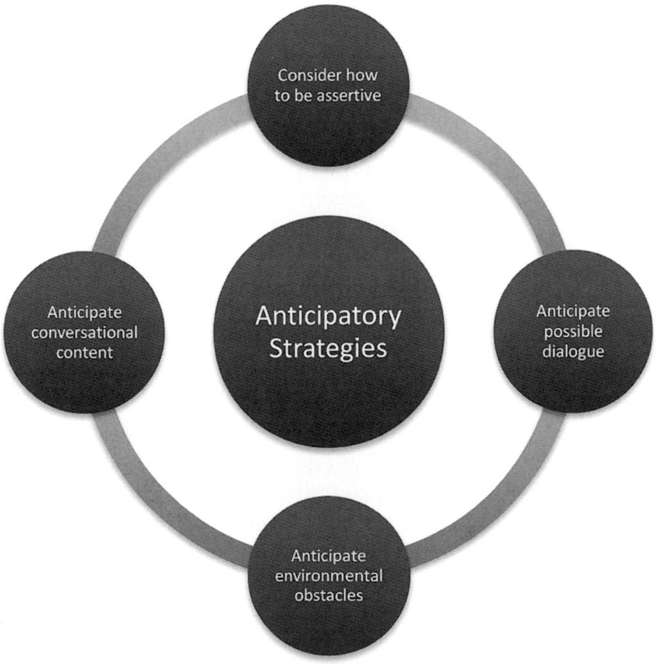

Fig. 7.12 Suggested anticipatory strategies.

As part of strategies training in this area, the audiologist should encourage the patient to keep abreast of current events because remaining current can aid in the comprehension of compromised auditory and visual input. Persons with hearing impairment feel more comfortable participating in conversation when they have contextual knowledge as a backup. Linguistic knowledge can be a valuable resource to help overcome communication breakdowns associated with very rapid speech or speech amidst distracting background noise.

A final type of facilitative strategy is one that affects the communication environment, such as lighting, distance from the speaker, and the presence of noise and visual distractions. Thus, facilitative strategies are used to modify the environment to improve communication. Environmental manipulation training helps to improve conversational fluency (Laplante-Lévesque et al, 2010)). The focus of environmental manipulations strategies training is to ensure that the patient and communication partner understand that the environment is an information field. It assists individuals in understanding events, making decisions, and taking appropriate actions (Steinfeld, 1997). Steinfeld (1997) suggests that it is important to emphasize that the ability to detect a signal such as speech depends in large part on the strength of the input relative to the information field in the background, namely noise or visual distractions (**Fig. 7.13**). One way of increasing signal strength or of improving the SNR is through hearing aids, but they have to be supplemented by reduction or avoidance of noises within the environment such as reverberation from air-conditioning machinery or background music. Additional suggestions include closing the door of a meeting room to eliminate noise from the hallway, turning off the computer in the home or office to eliminate electromagnetic interference, and turning off the television, radio, or computer printer to eliminate background noise when speaking.

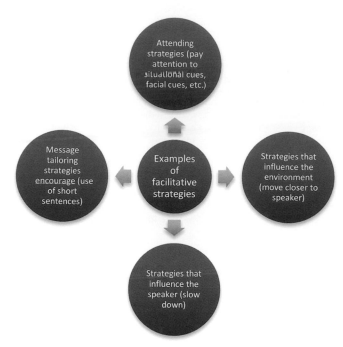

Fig. 7.13 Examples of facilitative strategies that affect the reception of the message and the environment.

Lighting is an important environmental variable to be manipulated during discourse. The patient should be reminded of the importance of adequate room lighting at all times and of minimizing glare from the light. Older adults require more light because their pupils are smaller, allowing less light in. Use of natural light should be encouraged, but blinds should be adjusted to prevent streams of bright, glaring light. Older adults should avoid talking in an area where there is glare from windows or mirrors. The light should always be focused on the speaker's face for optimal viewing.

Receptive repair strategies are important tactics used when the communication partner cannot be understood. Examples of repair strategies include asking the communication partner to rephrase the message, to elaborate it, to repeat it, to simplify it, or to summarize it. In my view, such specific repair strategies are preferable to nonspecific repair strategies such as saying "What?" or "Huh?" (Tye-Murray, 2008). Finally, as part of counseling regarding communication strategies, the clinician should make sure to review the three steps involved in repairing communication breakdowns. Role playing each of the stages involved in the repair process can be very helpful. The three stages are detecting a communication breakdown, choosing a course of action to repair it, and implementing the selected repair strategy. Persons with hearing impairment should be encouraged to use constructive repair strategies, rather than to pretend that they understand by either disregarding what is said or using a facial expression or language that suggests that the message was understood (e.g., bluffing). Assertiveness training is integral to strategies training, as it helps persons with hearing impairment resolve communication problems when they occur or reduce their occurrence in the first place. Repair strategies and assertive listening skills provide directions to

the communication partner about how to rectify a breakdown in communication.

Pearl

The environment is an information field that can facilitate receptive communication.

Special Consideration

The environment can be viewed as a type of assistive technology that can be manipulated to compensate for age-related sensory losses (Steinfeld, 1997). Knowledge of realistic strategies for preventing or reducing communication breakdowns and changing communication behaviors should be considered a vehicle that can empower people with hearing impairments, introducing an element of equity into previously threatening situations (Trychin, 1995).

Although it is perhaps a bit outdated, the WATCH program described by Montgomery (1994) is a simple but effective approach to teaching communication strategies. WATCH is an acronym for the strategies discussed above:

W = Watch the speaker's mouth, not his or her eyes.
A = Ask specific questions.
T = Talk/tell about your hearing loss.
C = Change or modify the environment so it is free of distractions.
H = Acquire hearing health care knowledge.

The W component covers some of the facilitative strategies used by the patient with hearing impairment to improve speech recognition. Also, the importance of attending to the speaker's facial expressions, gestures, and intonation to facilitate speech recognition can be stressed here. The A component includes facilitative communication strategies to be used with the communication partner, including instructional strategies. For example, the communication partner should be urged to repeat or rephrase a message when it is unclear, to provide additional information that might help convey the message, or to use gestures. The T component entails encouraging persons with hearing impairment to inform communication partners that they have a hearing loss and to provide constructive strategies to optimize speech reception. The person with hearing impairment, for example, may be encouraged to say, "I have a hearing loss; can you please face me when you are talking?" or "The lighting in this restaurant is not adequate as I need to see your face to help improve my ability to understand what is being said." The C component entails the client, communication partner, and audiologist discussing the situations that are difficult and how to modify them to one's advantage. Constructive strategies can be used to affect the listening environment, or instructional strategies can affect how the message is delivered. For example, speaking on the telephone is often difficult for persons with hearing impairment. Repair strategies such as verification or confirmation about what has been said by providing feedback about whether the message was recognized are helpful in this situation; if the listener has difficulty hear-

Table 7.27 Communication Strategies for the Person with Hearing Impairment and the Caregiver

Hearing-Aid User	Communication Partner
Ensure that you can see the speaker's face	Ensure the listener can see your face when you are speaking
Make sure that you are in a well-lit area	Make sure that you are communicating in a well-lit area
Do not be afraid to ask the speaker to repeat or further clarify what was said	Verify that your message was communicated and rephrase when necessary
Look for facial and body cues for content	Use facial expressions and body language to enhance the message
Communicate in situations with minimal noise	Communicate in situations with minimal noise
Do not be afraid to ask the speaker to slow down their rate of speech	Speak clearly and not too quickly
Do not look away from the speakers/try to communicate from another room	Do not walk away while talking/communicate from another room
Look for clues of topic changes to maximize context	Clearly distinguish topic changes
Do no be embarrassed about not being able to hear the complete message	It is not the listeners' fault if they cannot understand, do not make them feel embarrassed
Ask for the message to be written down if oral communication proves difficult	Write down part of the message if oral communication isn't working
Do not pretend you understood if you did not	Do not assume the message was correctly received
Be patient	Be patient

Source: From Rachel Marcus, Au.D. student. (Reprinted by permission)

ing numbers, the speaker can be asked to count from zero to the correct number and then stopping (Abrahamson, 1995). The H component entails informing the patient and communication partner about resources available for hearing loss, hearing health care, assistive technology, and consumer organizations. **Table 7.27,** developed by Rachel Marcus, one of my doctoral students, is an example of a handout for persons with hearing impairment and their communication partner that delineates and depicts some of the strategies listed above that are incorporated in the WATCH program.

Auditory–visual integration training is typically done in concert with training in the use of hearing tactics or communication strategies (Laplante-Lévesque et al, 2010). It is premised on the fact that speech understanding is a multisensory phenomenon that requires the integration of audition, vision, and cognitive processing. AVI training improves speech-recognition ability by helping the individual utilize input from several modalities, most notably auditory and visual (Garstecki, 1988;

Montgomery, 1991). Stated differently, AVI training optimizes receptive communication skills during interactive verbal communication by incorporating auditory input, visual sensual information, and nonverbal associational cues into the communication exchange (Gagne, 1994). An important principle of AVI training is to ensure that communication partners understand the variables that affect speech understanding and can be manipulated to optimize communication interplay. **Table 7.28** outlines the principles on which AVI training are based.

An important feature of AVI training is that the audiologist includes a communication partner and role playing in the conversation; the challenge is to elicit the cooperation of both speaking partners. The communication partner must make every effort to apply what he or she has been taught to ensure that the appropriate message has been delivered and received. From the outset, the fact that proficiency in visual speech understanding requires instruction and practice should be emphasized. The fact that access to auditory cues as provided by

Table 7.28 Principles Underlying Auditory–Visual Integration (AVI) and Listening in Complex Listening Situations

1. Visual speech cues play a highly significant role in speech perception, acquiring increased significance after hearing becomes impaired (Walden & Grant, 1993).
2. Normal-hearing and hearing-impaired persons tend to look at the talker, consciously or unconsciously, to maximize input from visual cues.
3. The person with hearing impairment can learn to supplement auditory input with secondary cues (e.g., visual input) to promote speech understanding.
4. The auditory-visual communication process requires skills that can be naturally acquired, some that can be slowly acquired, and neurological and cognitive abilities that we now know are amenable to change and training.
5. Nonverbal association cues or relevant talker characteristics include facial expressions, situational cues, contextual cues, and message-related extrafacial gestures, and visual sensual information is available from the speaker's articulatory movements (e.g., lip, tongue, and jaw movements) (Gagne, 1994).
6. Similarity between the target message and competing message increases both energetic (overlap in spectral energy) and informational masking (confusion between target and competing speaker) (Helfer, 2009).
7. As the signal-to-noise ratio decreases (or increases) the amount of energetic masking, so the need for visual cues to supplement the message similarly decreases (or increases).
8. Visual cues help when informational masking is maximum (e.g., 2–3 competing voices) because they help to fill in masked phonetic information.
9. Availability of visual cues is more beneficial when competition is speech rather than noise.
10. Familiar voices are easier to understand than unfamiliar voices in complex listening environments.

Source: Data from Helfer, K. (2009). *Older adults in complex listening environments.* Paper presented at the Adult Conference: The Challenge of Aging, Chicago.

hearing aids or assistive technology is a key part of AVI training must be emphasized as well. It is helpful to provide a brief overview of the distinctions among selected phonetic units, as this can help make a case for the importance of a multisensory approach to speech perception. The person with hearing impairment carries the biggest load in AVI training (Trychin, 1997). As discussed above in the communication strategies section he/she must (1) inform others about the existence of hearing loss and speech-understanding difficulties; (2) inform speakers about what to do to be understood; (3) politely remind the speaker how to communicate effectively; and (4) model the desired communication behavior. Modeling the desired behavior or teaching effective communication behaviors serves as encouragement and inducement for others (e.g., people with hearing loss should speak at the rate and loudness level they desire in others).

Individualization of the multisensory process involved in multisensory speech perception is of the utmost importance as the linguistic knowledge, cultural perspective, and cognitive processing skills one brings to the situation affect how older listeners must relearn to balance bottom-up (signal–driven) and top-down (knowledge-driven) processing (Pichora-Fuller, 2009). That is, when the auditory mechanism is deficient, the person with hearing loss must rely on linguistic knowledge and cognitive skills to facilitate understanding of the spoken message.

Integral to AVI training is discussion of the variables affecting receptive communication ability, which are summarized in **Table 7.29**. Each should be discussed, with the audiologist demonstrating the appropriate behavior to the patient and the communication partner and with each role playing the correct behavior, many of which are shown in **Table 7.27** above. For example, mouth movements should be natural, not exaggerated; hands should not cover or obscure the face; and the speaker should always face the listener so that the face is in full view. As regards the rate of speech, the speaker should not talk too rapidly but rather at a moderate rate. The speaker should try to speak at a slightly louder than normal level, but not so loud that facial movements are exaggerated. The speaker should avoid dropping his or her voice at the end of sentences. Pitch should be normal, not too high and not too low. The speaker should not speak with food in the mouth nor while chewing gum. The speaker should be encouraged to use facial expressions to complement what is being said. For example, a joke might be accompanied by slight laughter, a happy story by a smile. The findings of Helfer (1998) underline the importance of instructing the communication partners that speaking clearly when conversing face to face with older adults aids communication. She found that the older the listeners, the more poorly they recognized conversational speech with auditory and visual speech cues, and the greater the benefit derived from the talker's speaking clearly. Helfer reported that "the difference between [auditory]-only perception of conversational speech and [auditory-visual] perception of clear speech was approximately 30%, far greater than the benefit obtained from either speaking clearly or using visual speech cues in isolation" (p. 240).

The personal variables listed in **Table 7.29** pertain more to the person with hearing loss. The listener must be instructed to set the stage by admitting to the existence of hearing loss.

Table 7.29 Factors that Affect Receptive Communication

Speaker Variables
  Mouth movements
  Speech prosody including intonation, stress, and rhythm
  Loudness of voice
  Pitch of voice
  Accent
  Dialect
  Visibility of articulators
  Objects in the mouth
  Facial expressions
  Diction
  Familiarity to the person with hearing impairment
Physical or Personal Variables Pertaining to the Person with Hearing Impairment
  Severity of hearing impairment; residual hearing
  Cognitive status
  Hearing-aid use
  Visual acuity (wear glasses if necessary to view speaker's face)
  Physical functional status
  Listening skills
  Attention span
  Age
  Motivational level
  Linguistic skills
Environmental Variables
  Acoustic factors (room acoustics)
  Lighting
  Distractions
  Viewing angle
  Distance
  Understandability of the masker[1]
Linguistic Variables
  Topic awareness
  Context awareness
  Semantic variables
  Syntactic considerations
Variables Pertaining to the Message
  Length of the message
  Context
  Linguistic complexity
  Providing the listener with information about the message helps reduce the effects of informational masking
  Meaningfulness of the message[2]
Cognitive Variables (Helfer, 2009)
  Efficiency of inhibitory mechanisms[3]
  Processing speed affects the ability to switch attention from speaker or from topic of conversation
  Efficiency of working memory, especially explicit storage and processing functions[4]
  Presence of attentional difficulties[5]
  Executive control
  Verbal inference making

---

[1]When the competing message is not understandable to the listener, it produces less informational masking.
[2]Older adults are affected more than younger adults by the meaningfulness of the masker (Helfer, 2009).
[3]If inhibitory mechanism is less efficient, the listener will have a reduced ability to either attend to the target message or ignore the competing message.
[4]Reductions in working memory will produce problems processing simultaneous or multiple speakers and will detract from speech-reading ability (Foo, Rudner, Rönnberg & Lunner (2007).
[5]Contributes to difficulty in noise and difficulty when distractions are present.

Consistent with the transtheoretical stages of change model, acceptance of hearing loss and its impact on communication is the first step to successful communication with or without hearing aids. Trychin (1997) suggested that people often postpone informing others about their hearing loss because they themselves are embarrassed and have not fully accepted responsibility for it. They prefer to wait until there is an obvious communication breakdown rather than using anticipatory strategies as discussed above. Failure to be forthcoming about hearing loss often leads to unnecessary misunderstandings and erroneous assumptions about the listener, and there often is a stigma effect (Trychin, 1995). When persons with hearing impairment are stigmatized (e.g., as being old or mentally slow), their social identity can be devalued in various social contexts (Gagne, Southall, & Jennings, 2009b).

The person with hearing loss may not have good listening habits, and time should be spent during AVI in developing this aptitude. Good listening habits increase confidence and can help the person with hearing loss concentrate on the spoken message (Kricos & Holmes, 1996). The following are some tips for promoting listening skills: (1) listen intently yet remain relaxed, (2) show interest and understanding when others are talking by maintaining eye contact and attentive body language, (3) use guessing skills to fill in the blanks for words not heard clearly, (4) disregard background noise, (5) maintain good eye-lip contact, (6) sit within 3 to 6 feet of the speaker, and (7) do not give up prematurely. Kricos and Holmes (1996) reported that active listening training is an effective treatment for helping individuals with hearing impairment improve their auditory-visual recognition of speech especially in a background of noise. Today, three-dimensional avatars/electronic speaking faces that generate speech-related acoustic and optical information (such as facial gestures) are being used to help promote spoken language understanding (Lansing, 2009). As the use of synthetic talkers shows promise for enhancing the understanding of spoken content, audiologists should continue to explore these applications in rehabilitation settings.

Some of the sessions promoting visual speech perception should focus on the communication partners, who also must be taught compensatory communication strategies to facilitate understanding. Caissie et al (2005) argue that communication breakdowns often occur because the speech of the communication partner may be rapid, unclear (words are blurred), or inaudible. Accordingly, communication partners should be taught how to break a complex idea into short phrases, to produce clearer speech, to produce more easily understandable messages, or perhaps to work with a frequency-modulation (FM) system using proper microphone placement and techniques (Pichora-Fuller, 1997). They should know why it is important to speak slowly and to make mouth movements visible, to use nonverbal cues, to respond to requests for clarification, and to repeat/clarify during communication breakdowns (Erber & Heine, 1996). When communicating with persons with hearing impairment, the communication partner should always make sure that the message has been understood. It is often helpful to repeat what has been agreed upon to keep misunderstandings to a minimum. Message-related gestures are very helpful as well as writing the message down to supplement what is available through audition and speech reading. Of utmost importance, communication partners must try to avoid showing their feelings of frustration and annoyance with the difficulty associated with getting a message across. Often, it is the communication partner rather than the person with hearing impairment who needs advice about coping and overcoming the consequences of hearing impairment. Communication partners must also be counseled regarding the influence of the environment on speech reception. Hence, they need to know how to recognize poor communication environments and create optimal conditions for communicating, including rearranging furniture and reducing distractions such as glare and noise.

Caissie et al (2005) explored the benefit of clear speech for improving speech recognition by the person with hearing impairment. Clear speech has several distinct features including a decreased speaking rate, lengthening of consonants and vowels, expansion of acoustic vowel spaces, and increase in the decibel level of the long-term spectra of clear speech. A commercially available clear speech program was used as part of their study, and the talkers were trained to use clear speech strategies. The goals of the study were (1) to determine the effect of clear speech training on speech understanding, and (2) to determine if the speech of individuals undergoing clear speech intervention is more easily perceived than the speech of those who were merely instructed to speak more slowly and more clearly. The authors found that the intelligibility of the speech of communication partners was improved by basic instructions to speak clearly; however, the speech of the communication partner who underwent clear speech intervention was more intelligible, resulting in better speech-recognition scores. The authors concluded, therefore, that training communication partners to use clear speech may promote speech understanding of persons with hearing impairment. Hence, an intervention session with the communication partner focusing on clear speech techniques in addition to handouts describing various communication strategies can be beneficial.

Kramer, Allessie, Dondorp, Zekveld, and Kapteyn (2005) also found that involvement of the communication partner is of value in the audiological rehabilitation process. They designed a home-based education program for older adults with hearing impairment and their communication partner. The program included training in communication strategies, speech reading, hearing-aid use, and information regarding additional technical devices. Persons with hearing impairment and their communication partners were randomly assigned to either the experimental or the control group. The mean hearing level of participants in each group ranged from 53 to 56 dB HL. Those assigned to the experimental group underwent a home-based program along with their hearing-aid fitting, whereas those in the control group merely were fit with hearing aids. The home education program was self-administered and presented via videotape or DVD. The content ranged from demonstration of how communication strategies can resolve communication breakdowns to discussion of coping strategies and demonstration of how speech is perceived. The goal of the program is to raise problem awareness, to enhance communication, and to provide information about consequences of hearing loss. The home-based course was completed over 5 to 12 weeks. Self-report instruments were completed to determine the efficacy of the intervention. The results showed increased awareness of the benefits of speech reading, improved interaction, as well as improved quality of life and satisfaction on long-term measures in the training group only. Interestingly, 90% of the participants in the experimental group reported using the strategies reviewed in the home-based program. The communication partners and participants with hearing impairment in the experimental group also reported an increased awareness of the benefits of speech reading and improved interactions with their communication partners. Their study confirmed the value of an active listening program in combination with hearing aids for both communication partners and persons with hearing impairment.

The role of higher order cognitive capacity cannot be underestimated when discussing speech-reading or auditory-visual integration. Specifically, when the speech signal is degraded, as is the case in persons with hearing impairment when portions of the auditory component are lost, the visual components of speech assume greater importance (Foo et al, 2007). For optimal reception of an audiovisual signal, working memory, especially higher order complex storage and processing functions (e.g., visual strategy), assume considerable importance. The reason working memory is so important is that when a degraded message is received, long-term memory is recruited to help match semantic and phonological representations established over time. If the listener is unable to find a stored representation for the perceived signal, speech understanding will be compromised. Working memory plays an even greater role when speech reading in the presence of noise. It is notable that reading span, which bears a strong relation to age (0.65) and a minimal relation to pure-tone average (–0.37), is a cognitive test that assesses simultaneous storage and semantic processing capacity. As cognitive training including memory training and speed of processing training has beneficial short- and long-term effects, audiologists should consider including cognitive training in any auditory-visual integration intervention. The LACE program has considerable potential in that it includes some cognitive training exercises, but generally it needs to be supplemented with memory training exercises such as reasoning training, wherein we teach strategies

for finding the patterns in a letter or word series and teaching mnemonic strategies such as visualization or association for remembering verbal materials (Willis et al, 2006). Strategies training, auditory-visual integration training, and auditory/cognitive training are important components of communication management. Providing advice to persons with hearing impairment and their communication partners on how to modify their behavior to accommodate hearing loss can empower older adults and relieve them from some of the worries and anxieties associated with communication breakdowns. It is imperative that audiologists provide with hearing-aid fittings some form of instruction, be it home-based, individual, or group, about all facets of communication management. Including communication partners in the exchange is beneficial as well, and should be pursued.

Communication Management: A Group or Individual Process?

An issue worthy of consideration is whether any or all aspects of communication management should be a group or an individual process. The typical group rehabilitation session includes communication strategies training, speech perception/auditory training exercises, informational lectures, hearing-aid orientation lectures, and some form of personal adjustment counseling to assist group members to cope with their hearing loss. **Table 7.30** lists the topic areas typically included in group sessions or in audiological rehabilitation sessions based in the home (Preminger, 2011). Preminger emphasizes the value of a mix of content and exercises, particularly lectures and role playing exercises, that afford the opportunity to manage/solve specific communication breakdowns and to help to resolve some of the emotional challenges posed by hearing impairment.

Hawkins (2005) cited the opinion of Chisolm, Abrams, and McArdle (2004), who postulated that one of the most important benefits derived from short-term group rehabilitation potentially may be the pivotal role it plays in the decision to keep using hearing aids, which remains the focus of counseling

Table 7.30 Sample Topic Areas for Group Audiological Rehabilitation (AR) Sessions

Strategy	Sample Topic Area
Communication strategy training	Discussion of and practicing the varieties of facilitative and reception repair strategies; assertiveness training; value of facial cues, gestures to supplement auditory cues; discussion of importance of speech reading
Speech perception training	Auditory training exercises: hybrid that combines analytic and synthetic speech perception training; discuss importance of finding and looking at the target speaker, as this will help to maximize availability of visual speech cues
Informational lectures	Orientation to hearing aids; expectations regarding valued of hearing aids; hearing-assistive technologies; hearing loss and speech perception—what is the audiogram telling us?
Psychosocial exercises	Discussion of how it feels to have a hearing loss; discussion of impact on family; discussion of coping strategies
Group problem identification and problem-solving exercises	Identification of problem situations (e.g., inability to hear communication partner in separate room); discussion of solutions and role playing of solutions and instructional strategies (e.g., ability to see speaker's face is more beneficial when competition is speech and not competing noise (Helfter & Freyman, 2005)

Source: Data from Preminger, J. E. (2011). Group audiologic rehabilitation for adults and their communication partners. *ASHA Leader* http://www.asha.org/publications/leader/2011/110705/group-audiologic-rehabilitation-for-adults-and-their-communication-partners/

sessions in which audiologists are engaged. Preminger (2011) contends that the greatest benefit is in the quality-of-life improvements associated with multifaceted group programs, and points out that although there is little objective evidence of improved speech perception, anecdotal reports of participants in group AR include improvements in auditory and visual speech perception. The systematic review by Hawkins (2005), which included eight randomized-controlled trials, three cohort studies, and one case study, also underscored the value of group AR with adults. Although most of the studies were weak in terms of design and in the variety of outcome measures used, it was evident that group AR is associated with psychosocial benefits, higher level of assertiveness, and improved use of communication strategies, which was greater than in individuals who obtained hearing aids but did not partake in group AR. The beneficial effects of group sessions on hearing-aid retention was affirmed by the findings of Northern and Beyer (1999), who found that hearing-aid return rates were lower in individuals participating in group AR than in those not participating. They reported that the percentage of PHLs who returned their hearing aids because they were dissatisfied was 3% among the 3080 individuals who attended at least one post-fitting AR group session. In contrast, the hearing-aid return rate among the 7187 persons with hearing loss who did not attend a post-fitting sessions was 9%. The systematic review of the value of individual AR conducted by Sweetow and Palmer (2005) found that there is little evidence supporting the effectiveness of individual auditory training.

Consistent with my commitment to educating audiologists to use an evidence base, the following discussion begins with the theoretical and moves to an evidence base. Several systematic reviews have addressed this issue, but our esteemed colleague, Dr. Mark Ross believes that the group process he experienced during World War II had the most enduring impact on his adjustment to his hearing loss. Sharing experiences with others who have hearing impairment, with others who are first learning to use hearing aids, and with others who are struggling to accept hearing impairment can be a very powerful part of the remediation process. Based on an extensive review of the literature, it appears that the cost utility of post–hearing-aid fitting group audiological rehabilitation is clear; the value of individualized auditory/perceptual training and active communication training is questionable; and the participation of significant others in the group process helps foster improvements in the self-reported hearing handicap (Abrams, 2008; Preminger, 2003).

Abrams, Chisolm, and McArdle (2002) conducted a cost-utility analysis comparing short-term group post–hearing-aid fitting with audiological rehabilitation (HA+AR group) with hearing-aid use alone in a sample of male and female veterans, with a mean age in the various groups ranging from 73 to 74.5 years and mean four-frequency pure-tone averages ranging from 34.5 to 35.7 dB HL. All participants had binaural hearing aids that were fitted at no cost to the patient. The group AR sessions for those assigned to the HA+AR group were 2 hours log and met once a week for 4 weeks. The first session provided an overview of the hearing process and communication strategies training, the second session provided auditory training and discussed strategies for improving communication in adverse listening conditions; the third session provided a dis-

cussion of environmental management and communication repair strategies; and the final session focused on hearing-assistive technologies and community resources for the hearing impaired.

Abrams et al (2002) calculated the change in quality of life as a function of each treatment approach, and found that the improvement in mental component score (which assessed mental health, role limitations due to physical health problems, and social functioning) was greater in the HA+AR group; the difference did not reach statistical significance, but according to the clinical utility analysis this difference was clinically significant. Specifically, the cost-utility analysis showed that the combined treatment modality was more cost-effective in terms of quality-adjusted life years (QALYs) than hearing aids alone. Preminger (2003, 2011) has added considerably to the literature base on group intervention with adults by discussing the psychosocial value of group AR programs, and she has outlined the important issues to consider when mounting group programs. Among the most important factors that impact group dynamics are the heterogeneity of the group (experienced versus inexperienced hearing-aid users), the content of the session, and the training of the facilitator or group leader.

Chisolm et al (2004) conducted a very interesting study using a veteran population to determine the cost-effectiveness of hearing aids alone as an intervention as compared with hearing aids delivered in the context of group AR. The experimental group was fit with hearing aids and participated in four 2-hour group rehabilitation sessions focusing on communication strategies and counseling regarding coping with the hearing loss. The control group did not undergo any AR. The outcome measure used in the cost-effectiveness analysis was quality of life, using the Medical Outcomes Study (MOS) Short-Form Health Survey modified for veterans (SF-36V), which measures health-related well-being, social functioning, and mental health. Participants experienced short-term improvement in their use of communication strategies and in their adjustment to the hearing loss, whereas those just receiving hearing aids did not. Unfortunately, the improvement experienced by participants in the experimental group was not sustained, and after 1 year the groups were comparable in terms of adjustment to hearing loss and the use of strategies. It was noteworthy that the authors found no difference between the control and experimental groups in scores on various scales of the SF-36V. However, when they looked at changes due to the intervention in terms of cost, they found that the cost of treatment per QALY gained with hearing aids alone differed from the cost of treatment per QALY gained when hearing aids were delivered in the context of group AR. In the control group the cost of hearing aids alone was $60.00 per QALY gained, whereas the addition of group AR reduced the cost of the intervention to $31.91 per QALY gained. These data are very powerful, especially in today's health care environment. Their work underscores the importance of follow-up as part of any AR program.

The systematic review conducted by Hawkins (2005) focused on the effectiveness of counseling-based adult group AR programs. He concluded that these programs provide short-term reduction in self-perception of hearing handicap with potentially better use of communication strategies and hearing aids, and lead to improvements in self-perceived quality of life. He reported the group AR approach offers individuals with hearing loss the opportunity to share their feelings and to discuss problems and solutions with others. Psychosocial outcomes associated with group AR are better than outcomes achieved by those not participating in group sessions. In addition, group AR serves as a time- and cost-effective treatment measure if home-based training is not realistic. Hawkins was unable to draw conclusions about the long-term benefits of group AR due to the paucity of longitudinal studies in this area.

Abrams, Chisolm, Guerreiro, and Ritterman (1992) demonstrated that benefit from hearing aids, namely improvements in emotional and social function, can be enhanced when a hearing aid is dispensed in the context of a counseling-based AR program. They divided their sample of older adults with mild to moderate sensorineural hearing loss into three treatment groups. Each group completing the HHIE at baseline and at the 2-month follow-up. In addition, treatment group I received a hearing aid and participated in 3 weeks of counseling-based AR, which included an overview of the anatomy of the ear, an overview of hearing and communication, discussions about speech reading, and an overview of ALDs. Treatment group II received a hearing aid accompanied by a brief counseling session. Group III served as the control group and only completed the HHIE.

Mean HHIE scores for each group were comparable at baseline. Two months after the hearing-aid fitting, there was a clinically and statistically significant reduction in HHIE scores for treatment groups I and II, but not for the control group. Interestingly, subjects obtaining the hearing aid and counseling-based AR experienced more significant reductions in psychosocial handicap than did those who obtained the hearing aid without rehabilitation. Further, self-perceived psychosocial handicap was reduced in 45% of subjects in treatment group I versus 18% of subjects in treatment group II. This study demonstrates that the self-perception of hearing handicap can be significantly reduced in persons who have used hearing aids and have participated in a counseling-based AR program. Hence, it underlines the value of counseling-based AR in the hearing-aid delivery process.

Primeau (1997) found that AR and/or hearing-aid modifications can promote hearing-aid benefit among older adults who initially did not appear to be benefiting from their hearing aids. In his study, 139 older adults were fitted with hearing aids. Benefit was assessed in the handicap domain using the HHIE-S. The 95% confidence interval for significant benefit was an improvement of 10 or more points in the score on HHIE-S from the unaided to the aided condition. Primeau's data were impressive in that 81% of subjects fitted with hearing aids appeared to be benefiting in the psychosocial domain. However, some subjects were not, in that unaided HHIE-S scores were comparable to aided HHIE-S scores at the 6-week follow-up. The group not benefiting obtained some form of intervention consisting of counseling and/or hearing-aid modifications. Following the additional intervention, benefit in the psychosocial domain was recomputed by combining the hearing aid plus rehabilitation group with the original group, and the percentage benefiting improved to 90%. His data confirm the conclusions of Abrams et al (1992) regarding the contribution of rehabilitation to end-user satisfaction and benefit. Taylor and

Jurma (1999) assessed the relative efficacy of group audiological rehabilitation programs with adults as well. They concluded that group audiological rehabilitation as a supplement to initial post-fitting counseling can help reduce the handicap associated with hearing loss and help maintain it at a stable level.

As communication partners often experience stress and anxiety associated with the effort of communicating with persons with hearing impairment, it is logical to assume that including them in an AR program can be beneficial. Stark and Hickson (2004) assessed hearing-specific and health-related quality of life of a sample of older adults with hearing impairment and their communication partners, primarily their significant others, prior to and 3 months following hearing- aid fitting, and they confirmed the beneficial effects on both parties. They found that hearing-specific quality of life for significant others improved after the hearing-aid fitting.

Preminger (2003) examined the effect on hearing-related quality of life of the PHL when spouses were included in group AR sessions, and found that not only did PHLs experience improvements in hearing-related quality of life, but those who attended with a communication partner experienced the most benefit. Preminger and Meeks (2010) built on this study to determine the effects of group AR, specifically training in communication strategies and exercises to promote psychosocial adjustment, on the PHL and their communication partner. The PHLs were hearing-aid (n = 34) or cochlear-implant users (n = 2) for at least 3 months, and they all passed a cognitive screen. Thus, 36 couples participated in the study; the majority of the PHLs were men. Communication partners were required to have hearing levels (pure-tone averages) better than 30 dB HL in the better ear. All the PHLs had experienced participation restrictions and activity limitations attributable to their hearing impairment, based on responses to the Hearing Handicap Inventory (HHI) (all had scores poorer than 20). The participants with hearing loss also had QuickSIN™ scores of 25 or less. The mean pure-tone average of participants in the control (traditional) and experimental AR groups was 53 to 54 dB HL, and mean HHI scores were 56% for those in the control group and 61% for those in the experimental group. The spouses or communication partners also perceived that the PHL was experiencing difficulty, as the mean score on the HHI for spouses ranged from 46 to 48%. As was the case in the study by Newman and Weinstein (1986), the PHL did report greater hearing-related quality of life issues than did the communication partner. Participants also completed the Perceived Stress Scale (PSS) to determine degree of stress associated with the communication breakdowns and their sequelae, along with the Philadelphia Geriatric Center Positive and Negative Affect Rating Scale (ARS), which measures mood or affect. Finally, to quantify communication in the marriage, the Primary Communication Inventory (PCI) was completed, providing as estimate of the perceptions of each couple participating in the study.

Then, AR classes were held separately for the PHLs and the communication partners. The class content for the PHLs in the experimental group included lectures about hearing loss and hearing-assistive technologies, exercises in communication strategies, and psychosocial exercises. The class content for the communication partners in the experimental group

Table 7.31   AR for Communication Partners of Persons with Hearing Loss (PHLs)

Topic Area	Focus of Exercises	Sample Exercises
Psychosocial	1. Problems encountered when living with a person with hearing loss 2. Role of the communication partner in minimizing the activity limitations and participation restrictions occasioned by hearing loss 3. Overview of expected communication problems typically associated with hearing loss	Participants given predetermined questions and prompts regarding scenarios as a way to begin discussions among group members
Communication strategies	1. Discussion of how to resolve communication breakdowns using repair strategies, instructional strategies, etc. 2. Discussion of the role and import of visual cues	Exercises to demonstrate the importance of speech reading in difficult listening situations
Clear speech	1. Participants were shown visual and auditory examples of clear speech and of conversational speech	Communication partners were asked to repeat what they heard when lips were not visible and utterances were presented in a background of noise

included lectures with a focus on psychosocial considerations, clear speech training (e.g., slow down when you speak), and communication strategies training. The specifics of the classes for the communication partners are shown in **Table 7.31**. Classes consisted of four to six participants, and were conducted for 90 minutes once a week for 4 weeks.

The major findings of the study are as follows:

1. Communication partners who participated in an AR program developed a better understanding of their PHLs' hearing-related quality of life than did the communication partners who did not participate in AR programs.
2. PHLs participating in the AR program showed significant improvements in hearing-related quality of life. When PHL participated in an AR program, their communication partners experienced small hearing-related quality of life benefits.
3. As a result of the intervention, the assessment by communication partners of the extent of the hearing-related quality of life sequelae was more congruent with that of the PHLs.
4. PHLs reported experiencing better communication with their communication partner following the intervention, which may be why the communication partners adjusted their rating of the extent of the hearing-related quality of life challenges.

Group programs should include communication partners, should be short term (3 to 6 weeks in duration), and should provide sufficient time for an instructional component and for group discussion. Topics for group AR classes could include (1) hearing loss and the audiogram, (2) troubleshooting hearing aids, (3) hearing-assistive technologies to supplement hearing aids, (4) the importance of clear speech, (5) conversational repair strategies to facilitate communication, (6) environmental manipulation, and (7) assertiveness and advocacy. The communication partners who also have a hearing loss should have assistive technologies available to make sure that their hearing loss does not interfere with their effectiveness, and the PHL should wear hearing aids during the sessions. Preminger and Meeks (2010) suggest that the homogeneity of group

membership in terms of retirement status and work history may be important to the group dynamic.

Bally (2009) considers homogeneous groups to be more effective than heterogeneous groups. Homogeneity should apply to the hearing loss severity, type of technology (e.g., hearing aids versus cochlear implants), communication ability, and age. The gender mix may be a factor as well. The timing of classes is an important consideration to capture the largest audience. A morning and possibly an early evening session may be advantageous. It is worth noting that the group leader has a very important charge in terms of the dynamic of the group and setting the stage for a positive outcome.

The characteristics of the group leader/facilitator and the way in which he/she executes responsibilities affect the efficacy of the group intervention. According to Bally (2009), it is incumbent on the group leader to foster a supportive and safe environment, especially as regards confidentiality. The group leader should model excellent communication strategies and should encourage participants as they to learn to communicate. The group leader should encourage spontaneous conversation regarding experiences related to the topic at hand. Members of the group should be encouraged to offer positive feedback to one another in their efforts to achieve their goals. The group leader also should provide positive feedback, and end each session by reinforcing the "take-away" message and by underscoring the collective and individual contributions of the group.

A group environment is a wonderful opportunity for individuals with hearing loss to share experiences and provide each other with support and a sense of belonging. Further, a group environment enables members to learn from each other, and to serve as role models and sources of social and moral support. According to Preminger (2011), Bally (2009), and Abrahamson (1997), group rehabilitative sessions are an important supplement to individual sessions for the following reasons:

- They provide a support network for the hearing impaired and their family members and foster sympathetic and empathic relationships.
- They empower the individual to assume responsibility for the hearing loss.
- They confirm some of the negative effects of hearing loss.

◆ They help to set realistic expectations regarding the consequences of hearing loss and the benefits of hearing aids.

◆ They help participants to recognize their own experiences and feelings based on the difficulties expressed by others in the group, and serve as a vehicle for identification with others.

◆ They help to alleviate the stigma often associated with hearing impairment.

◆ They provide opportunities for social interaction.

◆ They provide a supportive network outside of the family structure.

◆ They help to validate feelings about hearing loss and the use of technologies and communication strategies to optimize communication function.

◆ They promote compliance with recommendations regarding hearing-aid use and use of communication strategies.

◆ They promote self-confidence and self-esteem and develop optimism about living with hearing loss.

◆ They enable collaborative problem solving.

◆ They enhance self-efficacy.

◆ They reduce the self-perceived activity limitations and participation restrictions associated with hearing loss.

The evidence regarding the outcomes achieved with AR, be it individual, group, or home-based, supports the value of group or home-based intervention to facilitate adjustment to hearing aids. However, the quality of the evidence regarding efficacy of AR is limited, and opportunities abound for additional research in the area. When conducting or reviewing the research in the area, as Gatehouse (2003) points out, the clinician should look at outcomes from two perspectives, namely the extent to which the intervention has improved patients' quality of life and addressed their communication needs, and the extent to which residual problems remain demanding supplemental intervention. Hence, the short- and long-term benefits of AR are areas requiring investigation. Similarly, cost utility or cost-effectiveness should be calculated as part of any study, as this is of interest to third-party payers, especially given the current health care climate. It is our responsibility as audiologists to provide each patient with the best possible care based on the execution of evidence-based practice principles. This will foster greater acceptance of rehabilitation recommendations and better treatment outcomes. As with all treatment protocols, audiologists should apply an evidence-based approach to the provision of audiological management. This approach involves a careful evaluation of high-quality research as the basis for management decisions (Boothroyd, 2007). A greater evidence base will also elevate the quality of the treatments available to the elderly. Finally, the value of support groups for persons with hearing impairment and their communication partners has been documented anecdotally, and audiologists should make every effort to educate their patients about the many advocacy and support groups focused on hearing impairment.

Pearl

Group AR positively impacts on the emotional consequences of hearing impairment.

Self-Help Groups

Several consumer organizations serve as a resource for older adults with hearing impairments and their families. The largest self-help/consumer group that focuses on hearing loss and deafness is the Hearing Loss Association of America (HLAA; http://www.hearingloss.org), which has local chapters in communities across the country (http://www.hearingloss.org/chapters/index.asp). The latter Web address provides maps showing the location of over 200 chapters. HLAA prides itself on providing support and understanding, information about community resources, information about hearing aids and cochlear implants, tips for coping with hearing loss, and communication strategies. HLAA members benefit from information-sharing and advocacy; HLAA activities are directed and driven by the membership. The premise underlying the formation of self-help organizations is that participation can facilitate the coping and acceptance process. It is a relief to be with others who know how it feels and who routinely experience the frustration and embarrassment of trying to manage when not being able to hear what is being said (Glass, 1990). The Association of Late Deafened Adults (http://www.alda.org) is an advocacy group for persons who have lost some or all of their hearing. It provides a community to help PHLs live happy and satisfying lives.

The Better Hearing Institute (BHI) is a not-for-profit corporation that has as its mission education of the public about the neglected problem of hearing loss and what can be done about it. The BHI works to erase the stigma that prevents millions of people from seeking help for hearing loss, writes extensively about the negative consequences of untreated hearing loss, and educates the public about treatment options. BHI has a wonderful Web site with resources for persons with hearing impairment (http://www.betterhearing.org). Organizations for older adults, including the American Association of Retired Persons (AARP) and consumer organizations such as the Consumers' Union, develop and disseminate educational materials about hearing aids and associated technology, which can be invaluable. Audiologists should make available information about organizations and resources that can be helpful to persons with hearing impairment. Working collectively, we can help improve the quality of life of persons with hearing loss and their family members.

Pearl

Learning from others with similar conditions can provide the patient with information beyond what professionals are taught in graduate school.

Step 5: Outcomes Assessment

The final step of any program of communication management is outcomes assessment. This stage is one of the greatest challenges facing audiologists and one of the most important steps in the process. Most health care professionals acknowledge the importance of outcome measurement to verify that the needs of the person with hearing impairment have been met and that the goals have been realized, and to determine the residual needs that remain and continue to be addressed. Yet how to measure effectiveness remains elusive and an issue upon which audiologists have difficulty agreeing. In my view it is quite simple: we decide on what outcome to measure and on how to measure it. It is incumbent on the audiologist to match the treatment goal to the outcome domain and to the patient's expectations. **Table 7.32** presents a taxonomy that might help the audiologist decide on the measure based on the domain that is problematic. There are a multiplicity of outcome domains that have emerged, in part because of empirical data demonstrating the weak correlation across the various domains and because of the differences in the strength of the correlations between audiological data and various outcome measures. Applying the ICIDH language to outcomes taxonomy, one can interpret the statement that the PHL is experiencing improved communication function at the activity level as meaning that the PHL was able to hear more sounds and better understand speech in a variety of contexts as a result of intervention. Similarly, if one says that there is evidence that the level of participation in selected activities has increased, then we can interpret this as meaning that the PHL is a more active participant in important activities. By extension, if we measure quality of life, we can determine if it has been positively impacted.

As is evident from **Table 7.32**, subjective self-report measures assess benefit and communication effectiveness across many contexts, situations, and environments. In selecting outcome measures, the income measures and the initial interview should determine the domain, the goals of treatment, and the measure to be used. For example, from the outset responses to the ECHO may show that the person with hearing impairment has unrealistic expectations regarding the efficacy of hearing aids in selected situations, so if counseling addresses the expectations, it would be important to determine if the patient's expectations have become more realistic as a result of the counseling intervention. Similarly, if responses to the COSI suggest that patients want to enjoy life again and to be able to watch television without raising the volume to a level that is annoying to family members, then the audiologist would re-administer the COSI to see if in fact intervention improved quality of life and if television viewing is less of a problem. If the PHL still has difficulty with television viewing, even with a new set of hearing aids, the audiologists might consider recommending television ears or an infrared system. Alternatively, if the PHL owns hearing aids that can connect wirelessly to the television and other media devices and communication devices, such as cellular phone, then this option should be explored.

If we learn from baseline responses to a self-report measure such as the HHIE that particular situations are problematic and have led to both activity limitation and participation restrictions (e.g., the patient has difficulty understanding family and friends, and thus visits them less often), then we want to make sure when the intervention is completed little residual disability remains. It is not enough to pay lip service to merely administering outcome measures; rather, it is important to review responses with patients to ensure that the difficulties have been appropriately addressed and that the problem has been resolved. Similarly, if the communication partners provided parallel information on the self-report instrument they completed, it is important to see if they perceive that the problem was addressed by the intervention. If the feedback from the PHL and from the communication partner are aligned following intervention, then this is an additional and important outcome.

As shown in the examples and evidence reviewed above, benefit from hearing aids and communication management can be measured directly in terms of degree or amount of change by comparing the initial responses and test score to the final responses and test score following the intervention. Clinically significant endpoints are used as a referent for defining effectiveness of an intervention. A confirmation of subjective benefit on a hearing-specific questionnaire typically emerges if the difference score achieves significance based on the 90% or the 95% confidence interval established for the particular measure, which is suggestive of clinically significant improvement attributable to the intervention. The confidence intervals often differ based on the mode of administration and the type of technology, and are questionnaire dependent. For example, on the APHAB, clinically significant benefit is defined for a 90% confidence interval, as an improvement score of five or more points on all three communication subscales (ease of communication [EC], reverberation [RV], and background noise [BN]) (Cox, 1997). An alternate way to determine benefit using the APHAB is to compare the response of the PHL against the normative sample described by Cox (1997). In contrast, the critical difference values associated with the HHIE are 18.7 using a face-to-face administration, 19.2 using face-to-face/paper-and-pencil administration, rising to 36 using a paper-and-pencil administration on each occasion. Hence, using a paper-and-pencil administration, the standard error of measurement is large and it is more difficult to detect change with a high level of confidence.

The audiologist must be familiar with the psychometrics of the outcome measure, which could determine the mode of administration to be used. If a person with a moderate sensorineural hearing impairment went to the audiologist for a hearing aid and communication management and had an initial score on the HHIE of 60%, and following the fitting and a 3-week period of intervention the score improved to 30%, then the difference exceeds the 95% critical difference for a face-to-face administration and the patient is considered to have made dramatic improvement. However, the audiologist must look at the residual activity limitations and examine each item to see if there is any additional intervention, such as a trial with LACE, that could improve the situation even further. If there is further intervention, it would be important to reassess patient function possibly 6 months later and also after 1 year to ensure that the beneficial outcomes are sustainable. Residual activity limitations are the difficulties the PHL continues to have in hearing-related activities such as understanding speech (Cox, 2003). The magnitude of the residual activity limitations will depend on the demands of that person's lifestyle. In contrast, residual participation restrictions are the unresolved problems or barriers that the PHL continues to encounter that curtail his or her involvement in routine activities such as attending religious services. Another such restriction is that the patient feels frustrated because of difficulty understanding family members.

Table 7.32 Outcomes Taxonomy for Communication Management

Domain	Function	Purpose	Sample Items or Methodology
Impairment	Improved audibility	Verify electroacoustic characteristics of the hearing aid, verify REAR, speech mapping	Probe Tube Measures; Articulation Index (AI),
Activity limitations at time the intervention begins and residually; self-reports	Communication function, subjective experience of psychosocial function or difficulty in performance of an activity at the individual level	Verify that activity limitations have been reduced due to intervention; determine magnitude of residual activity limitations	APHAB: sample item (Cox & Alexander, 1995) Instructions: Circle the answer that comes closest to your everyday experience: With my hearing aids. . . I miss a lot of information when I am listening to a lecture. The answer continuum ranges from Always to Never; COSI: Sample item: Instructions: Indicate specific needs in order of significance; rate degree of change and final ability; IOI sample item: Think about the situation where you most wanted to hear better, before you got your present hearing aid(s). Over the past 2 weeks, how much has the hearing aid helped in that situation? SSQ (Gatehouse & Noble, 2004): Sample item. You are talking with one other person and there is a TV on in the same room. Without turning the TV down, can you follow what the person you are talking to says? The answer continuum ranges from Not at all to Perfectly
Participation restrictions at time the intervention begins and residually; self-reports	The disadvantage or difficulties an individual may have in terms of manner or extent of involvement in social relationships, participation in community activities, or engagement at work	Verify that the PHL is disadvantaged in fewer situations due to intervention; determine magnitude of residual participation restrictions	HHIE: Sample item (Ventry & Weinstein, 1982): Instructions: Answer Yes, Sometimes, or No for each question. Now that you have hearing aids. . . Does a hearing problem cause you to use the phone less often than you would like? Yes, Sometimes, No; APHAB, IOI: residual participation restrictions: Think again about the situation where you most wanted to hear better. When you use your present hearing aid(s), how much difficulty do you STILL have in that situation?
Impact on others; patient-centered self-report	How hearing impairment is perceived by a spouse or communication partner to interfere with activities or to circumscribe participation in preciously enjoyed activities	Determine if, from the perspective of the communication partner or significant other, the intervention has had a positive impact on activities and engagement; how has hearing impairment impacted family constellation (Cox, 2003)?	IOI-HA-SO (Noble, 2002): Sample item: Over the past 2 weeks, with his or her present hearing aid(s), how much have your partner's hearing difficulties affected the things you can do? The answer continuum ranges from Very much to Not at all; HHIE-SP
Health-related quality of life; patient-centered self-report	How has hearing impairment affected functional health status, self-perceptions, emotional status	Verify that hearing intervention has had a positive impact on quality of life	IOI-HA: Sample item: Considering everything, how much has your present hearing aid(s) changed your enjoyment of life? The answer continuum ranges from Worse to Very much better; MOS SF-36; SIP; SF-36V
Expectations; patient-centered self-report	What the PHL expects in terms of how he/she will function with hearing aids and how he/she may be perceived by others	Determine the extent to which expectations are realistic in terms of performance with the hearing aid	ECHO

Table 7.32 Continued

		Data logging will provide objective data on how often and what proportion of the day is spent with	
Device usage; self-report	Are hearing aids being worn by the PHL?	hearing aids on	Provides an objective measurement of daily use
Cognitive function	Slow down cognitive aging; improve speech understanding in complex listening situations as listening effort is reduced	Measures of working memory, processing speed, resource allocation, or listening effort	Provides an index of change in cognitive function associated with intervention

Abbreviations: APHAB, Abbreviated Profile of Hearing-Aid Benefit; COSI, Client-Oriented Scale of Improvement; ECHO, Expected Consequences of Hearing-Aid Ownership; HHIE, Hearing Handicap Inventory for the Elderly; HHIE-SP, Hearing Handicap Inventory for the Elderly-Spouse; IOI-HA-SO, International Outcome Inventory for Hearing Aids–Significant Others; MOS SF-36, Medical Outcomes Study Short-Form Health Survey; REAR, real ear aided responseSF-36V, a multi-item scale that measures eight general health concepts in two major domains, namely mental and physical functioning, as modified for veterans (Abrams et al, 2002); SIP, Sickness Impact Profile; SSQ, Speech, Spatial, and Qualities of Hearing Scale.
Sources: From Abrams, H. (2008). What's the value of better hearing? Here are some ways to calculate it. *Hearing Journal, 61,* 10–15; and Cox, R. M. (2003, Jul). Assessment of subjective outcome of hearing aid fitting: Getting the client's point of view. *International Journal of Audiology, 42*(Suppl 1), S90–S96.

In addition to measuring outcomes experienced by the PHL or the communication partner, it is beneficial to quantify the overall outcomes in one's practice setting using a cost-utility analysis, a cost-effectiveness analysis, or a cost-benefit analysis. Program evaluation data objectively reports the proportion of persons in one's practice who demonstrated clinically significant benefit attributable to intervention. Cost-effectiveness can be determined by calculating the cost of treatment for the hearing-related QALYs gained. When audiologists calculate a QALY, they examine the cost of an intervention protocol relative to a universal standard of a given domain such as quality of life (Abrams et al, 2002). In contrast, a cost-benefit analysis entails measuring outcome by comparing the money spent with the money gained or saved; therefore, costs and benefits are assigned monetary units. When conducting a cost-utility analysis, the costs of an intervention are measured in monetary units, and this is then standardized against life-expectancy as measured using a valid measure of quality of life. Mulrow et al (1990a) were among the first to project the quality of life years based on scores on the HHIE attributable to a hearing-related intervention. They found that the above techniques are helpful when large organizations are looking to reallocate resources. If an audiologist can demonstrate the QALYs gained from hearing aids and communication management, perhaps this would lend support to the expansion and sustainability of the audiology program. Using data from their cost-utility analysis comparing two different interventions, Abrams et al (2002) demonstrated that hearing aids plus AR cost $32 per QALY gained as compared with $60 for hearing aids alone, so from the point of view of resource allocation it appears that hearing aids in combination with AR is cost-effective.

The majority of audiologists do not verify or validate the efficacy of their intervention using objective measurements. However, given health care economics and the evidence pointing to the value of audiological interventions, I strongly advocate that audiologists consider measuring short-, medium-, and long-term outcomes. If the PHL and the communication partner are asked to complete a questionnaire to determine communication efficiency, activity limitations, and participation restrictions at the outset, then this information can help

define treatment goals and a treatment plan. Following the intervention (e.g., 6 weeks to 3 months following the start of intervention) it should be a matter of routine that the audiologist has the PHL and the communication partner complete the same scales, and the scores should be compared and discussed. If residual activity limitations and participation restrictions remain, then perhaps the hearing aid could be adjusted and a home-based intervention could be recommended, and the audiologist might also consider supplementing hearing aids with assistive technology if indicated based on the responses. If each quarter audiologists analyze their outcome data, and can demonstrate that a large percentage of their patients benefited from the intervention, then this information can be used to market one's services and practice. In my view the cost-effectiveness data could highlight the value of audiological interventions for persons with hearing impairment. How powerful it would be to use cognitive function as an outcome measure and to demonstrate that hearing aids and communication management slow the cognitive decline and that the beneficial effects are transferable to everyday function! Audiologists should begin to realize that by gathering evidence that our interventions add value, we are promoting our profession and the quality of the life of those we serve.

◆ An Integrated Approach to Communication Management: Final Considerations

In preparing to write this book, I have observed audiologists as they work with older adults, I have studied the dispensing practices of audiologists, I have worked with supervisors in university clinics and in hospitals and rehabilitation centers who are supervising doctoral students, and I have accompanied many of my elderly aunts to get their first, second, or third set of hearing aids. Sadly, the management approach seems to remain focused on the technology rather than on the PHL or the outcomes, despite what the ICIDH framework suggests. The literature addresses the individual differences that characterize people as they age, and emphasizes the importance of a patient-centered approach to older adults. It seems that the proportion of people with hearing loss who use hearing aids has not changed in 50 years, despite tremendous technological advances. Audiologists are convinced that all they have to do is sell the hearing aids, see the customer for an average of 1.2 hours of counseling during the first 2 months of the hearing-aid fitting process, and fit the typical patient with hearing aids in 2.5 visits (Kochkin et al, 2010). As verified by Kochkin and colleagues (2010), few patients enrolled in audiologic rehabilitation, receive a self-help book, view a self-help video, are referred to a self-help group, or receive auditory retraining therapy, and nearly 13% of new users wind up not using their hearing aids.

This content of this chapter was informed by a question that has inspired me throughout my career: How can we do right by the patient with hearing impairment and do right by ourselves? In my view, the challenge for the audiologist is to empower each patient to become a satisfied and successful hearing-aid user who experiences fewer communication breakdowns and a more satisfying quality of life. We must accomplish this even with the cloud of tremendous changes in health care hanging over our heads and with our autonomy constantly being threatened. Seeing communication management as the core of what we do, with hearing aids possibly serving as a fulcrum, may give us the best chance of distinguishing ourselves from other professionals who merely sell hearing aids. Health care economics demands that, however sophisticated and expensive the technology, the bottom line, for our survival as a profession, is that we must prove that the patient can hear better, can understand better, and can function better in daily life. Further, if we can demonstrably show other professionals, including physicians, attorneys, nurses, how much less effort is required of them to communicate when the PHL has the tools necessary to overcome communication breakdowns, then we will be a sustainable profession. Dispensing hearing aids within the context of an integrated rehabilitation program can move us close to our goals.

I think we can be most successful as professionals if we keep our goal in mind: that we want to make sure we have succeeded in helping persons with hearing loss and their communication partners to realize their goals and aspirations regarding overcoming the functional consequences of the communication breakdowns they experience. An outcome dimension that is most familiar to practitioners is benefit in the hearing-related domain or how much the hearing aid changes activity limitations; another outcome dimension is the social and psychological changes associated with being able to communicate more effectively; another dimension is the reduction in the amount of residual activity limitations and participation restrictions associated with improved communication (Cox, 2003). An improved sense of safety and security in the home and a reduction in the burden on family, friends, and care-givers is an important outcome for home-bound older adults, which we rarely think about because we rarely make home visits. Another outcome dimension is improved quality of life and care for older adults with multiple chronic conditions who want to remain vibrant and who want to continue to contribute to society despite the constraints posed by difficulty understanding.

Individual differences are a hallmark of the aging process. Bergman (2006) reports that more differences exist among older adults than in any other age group. Due to the changing demographics, we can expect that the elderly population, a large group that now spans a broad age range, will continue to present with diverse and multifaceted issues. Many older adults will continue to lead very active lives professionally and personally, and will have a host of communication needs. Conversely, some older adults may have very limited communication demands. As such, older adults will have varying needs in terms of audiological rehabilitation services with regard to the level of sophistication and technology required. In addition, the elderly population in the coming years will also represent a diverse group in terms of race and ethnicity, so it is imperative that we provide culturally sensitive treatment for this growing population.

The elderly of tomorrow will be a heterogeneous group with a range of AR needs that audiologists will need to be able to address. I see audiological rehabilitation or communication management as inextricably intertwined with the hearing-aid fitting. In fact, you cannot do one without the other. I do not believe hearing aids can cure the hearing impairment. Hearing aids in conjunction with rehabilitation can reduce activity limitations and participation restrictions, can improve function, and reduce any residual deficits associated with hearing impairment. It is important to always keep in mind that a person with hearing impairment does not cause his or her functional communication deficit. People with hearing impairment experience communication problems to the extent that they have difficulty interacting with people in their environment (Kemp, 1990). Communication breakdowns can be reduced by helping the person to become more comfortable with the condition and with other's reactions to it, and by communication partners becoming more accepting of and accommodating of the person with a disabling hearing impairment. Thus, family members, the patient, and the hearing health care professional are the agents of change who will determine the outcomes of the rehabilitation process. Family education and support, improvement of functional abilities, psychological support, social integration and acceptance, and empowerment should be our goals, as through communication management we help older adults with hearing impairments overcome the activity limitations and participation restrictions associated with communication breakdowns.

References

Abrahamson, J. (1995). Effective and relevant programming. In P. Kricos & S. Lesner (Eds.), *Hearing care for the older adult*. Boston: Butterworth-Heinemann

Abrahamson, J. (1997). Patient education and peer interaction facilitate hearing aid adjustment. *Supplement to Hearing Review, 1*, 19–23

Abrams, H. (2008). What's the value of better hearing? Here are some ways to calculate it. *Hearing Journal, 61*, 10–15

Abrams, H., & Chisolm, T. H. (2009). Measuring health-related quality of life in audiologic rehabilitation. In J. Montano & J. Spitzer (Eds.), *Adult audiologic rehabilitation*. San Diego: Plural Publishing

Abrams, H. B., Chisolm, T. H., Guerreiro, S. M., & Ritterman, S. I. (1992, Oct). The effects of intervention strategy on self-perception of hearing handicap. *Ear and Hearing, 13*, 371–377

Abrams, H., Chisolm, T. H., & McArdle, R. (2002, Sep-Oct). A cost-utility analysis of adult group audiologic rehabilitation: Are the benefits worth the cost? *Journal of Rehabilitation Research and Development, 39*, 549–558

American Academy of Audiology. (2006). Guidelines for the audiologic management of adult hearing impairment. *Audiology Today, 18*, 1–44

American Speech-Language-Hearing Association (ASHA). (2006). *Preferred practice patterns for the profession of audiology.* www.asha.org/policy1

Anderson, S., & Kraus, N. (2010, Oct). Sensory-cognitive interaction in the neural encoding of speech in noise: A review. *Journal of the American Academy of Audiology, 21*, 575–585

Arlinger, S. (2003, Jul). Negative consequences of uncorrected hearing loss—A review. *International Journal of Audiology, 42*(2, Suppl 2), S17–S20

Atkins, C. (2007). Graduate Slp/Aud clinicians on counseling: Self perceptions and awareness of boundaries. *Contemporary Issues in Communication Science and Disorders, 34*, 4–11

Bally, S. (2009). Group therapy and group dynamics in audiologic rehabilitation. In J. Montano & J. Spitzer (Eds.), *Adult audiologic rehabilitation* (pp. 283–304). San Diego: Plural Publishing

Bandura, A. (1997). *Self-efficacy: The exercise of control.* New York: W.H. Freeman

Becker, M. H., Maiman, L. A., Kirscht, J. P., Haefner, D. P., Drachman, R. H., & Taylor, D. W. (1979). Patient perceptions and compliance: Recent studies of the health belief model. In R. B. Haynes & D. L. Sackett (Eds.), *Compliance in health care.* Baltimore: Johns Hopkins University Press

Benjamin-McKie, A. (2006). The use of illustrations as an adjunct to administration of the cosi with aging patients. In *Seminars in hearing—The aging auditory system: considerations for rehabilitation. Proceedings from the National Center for Rehabilitative Auditory Research (NCRAR), 2005* (pp. 27, 330–336). New York: Thieme

Bergman, M. (2006). The oldest old—New challenges and responsibilities for audiologists. *Seminars in Hearing, 27*, 215–227

Bergner, M., Bobbitt, R. A., Carter, W. B., & Gilson, B. S. (1981, Aug). The Sickness Impact Profile: Development and final revision of a health status measure. *Medical Care, 19*, 787–805

Besdine, R., Boult, C., Brangman, S., Coleman, E. A., Fried, L. P., Gerety, M., et al; American Geriatrics Society Task Force on the Future of Geriatric Medicine (2005, Jun). Caring for older Americans: The future of geriatric medicine. *Journal of the American Geriatrics Society, 53*(6, Suppl), S245–S256

Bess, F. H., Lichtenstein, M. J., & Logan, S. A. (1990). Making hearing impairment functionally relevant: Linkages with hearing disability and handicap. *Acta Otolaryngolica Supplement (Stockholm), 476*, 226–231

Bess, F. H., Lichtenstein, M. J., Logan, S. A., & Burger, M. C. (1989a, Dec). Comparing criteria of hearing impairment in the elderly: A functional approach. *Journal of Speech and Hearing Research, 32*, 795–802

Bess, F. H., Lichtenstein, M. J., Logan, S. A., Burger, M. C., & Nelson, E. (1989b, Feb). Hearing impairment as a determinant of function in the elderly. *Journal of the American Geriatrics Society, 37*, 123–128

Boothroyd, A. (1987). Casper, computer-assisted speech-perception evaluation and training. In *Proceedings of the 10th Annual Conference of the Rehabilitation Society of North America* (pp. 734–736). Washington, DC: Association for Advancement of Rehabilitation Technology

Boothroyd, A. (2007, Jun). Adult aural rehabilitation: What is it and does it work? *Trends in Amplification, 11*, 63–71

Boothroyd, A. (2010). *You have a new hearing aid: So what? Now what?* Paper Presented at Starkey Innovation in Action Symposium. Minneapolis, Minnesota

Borella, E., Carretti, B., & De Beni, R. (2008, May). Working memory and inhibition across the adult life-span. *Acta Psychologica, 128*, 33–44 10.1016/j.actpsy.2007.09.008

Brooks, D. N., & Hallam, R. S. (1998, Aug). Attitudes to hearing difficulty and hearing aids and the outcome of audiological rehabilitation. *British Journal of Audiology, 32*, 217–226

Brooks, D. N., Hallam, R. S., & Mellor, P. A. (2001, Jun). The effects on significant others of providing a hearing aid to the hearing-impaired partner. *British Journal of Audiology, 35*, 165–171

Brown, C. (2009). Rehabilitation. In J. Hazzard, J. Ouslander, M. Tinetti, S. Studenski, K. High, & S. Asthana (Eds.), *Hazzard's geriatric medicine and gerontology.* New York: McGraw-Hill

Brummel-Smith, K. (1990). Introduction. In B. Kemp, K. Smith, & J. Ramsdell (Eds.), *Geriatric rehabilitation.* Boston: College Hill

Caissie, R., Campbell, M. M., Frenette, W. L., Scott, L., Howell, I., & Roy, A. (2005, Mar). Clear speech for adults with a hearing loss: Does intervention with communication partners make a difference? *Journal of the American Academy of Audiology, 16*, 157–171

Chang, H. P., Ho, C. Y., & Chou, P. (2009, Oct). The factors associated with a self-perceived hearing handicap in elderly people with hearing impairment—Results from a community-based study. *Ear and Hearing, 30*, 576–583

Chisolm, T. H., Abrams, H. B., & McArdle, R. (2004, Oct). Short- and long-term outcomes of adult audiological rehabilitation. *Ear and Hearing, 25*, 464–477

Chisolm, T. H., Johnson, C. E., Danhauer, J. L., Portz, L. J., Abrams, H. B., Lesner, S., et al. (2007, Feb). A systematic review of health-related quality of life and hearing aids: Final report of the American Academy of Audiology Task Force on the Health-Related Quality of Life Benefits of Amplification in Adults. *Journal of the American Academy of Audiology, 18*, 151–183

Cox, L. C., McCoy, S. L., Tun, P. A., & Wingfield, A. (2008, Apr). Monotic auditory processing disorder tests in the older adult population. *Journal of the American Academy of Audiology, 19*, 293–308

Cox, R. M. (1997). Administration and application of the APHAB. *Hearing Journal, 50*, 32–48

Cox, R. M. (2003, Jul). Assessment of subjective outcome of hearing aid fitting: Getting the client's point of view. *International Journal of Audiology, 42* (Suppl 1), S90–S96

Cox, R. M., & Alexander, G. C. (1995, Apr). The abbreviated profile of hearing aid benefit. *Ear and Hearing, 16*, 176–186

Cox, R. M., & Alexander, G. C. (2000, Jul-Aug). Expectations about hearing aids and their relationship to fitting outcome. *Journal of the American Academy of Audiology, 11*, 368–382, quiz 407

Cox, R. M., & Alexander, G. C. (2002, Jan). The International Outcome Inventory for Hearing Aids (IOI-HA): Psychometric properties of the English version. *International Journal of Audiology, 41*, 30–35

Cox, R. M., Alexander, G. C., & Gray, G. A. (2007, Apr). Personality, hearing problems, and amplification characteristics: Contributions to self-report hearing aid outcomes. *Ear and Hearing, 28*, 141–162

Craik, F. I. (2007, Jul-Aug). The role of cognition in age-related hearing loss. *Journal of the American Academy of Audiology, 18*, 539–547

Dalton, D. S., Cruickshanks, K. J., Klein, B. E., Klein, R., Wiley, T. L., & Nondahl, D. M. (2003, Oct). The impact of hearing loss on quality of life in older adults. *Gerontologist, 43*, 661–668

DiClemente, C. C., & Velasquez, M. (2002). Motivational interviewing and the stages of change. In W. R. Miller & S. Rollnick (Eds.), *Motivational interviewing: Preparing people for change* (2nd ed.). New York: Guilford

Dillon, H., James, A., & Ginis, J. (1997, Feb). Client Oriented Scale of Improvement (COSI) and its relationship to several other measures of benefit and satisfaction provided by hearing aids. *Journal of the American Academy of Audiology, 8*, 27–43

English, K. (2008). Counseling issues in audiologic rehabilitation. *Contemporary Issues In Communication Science and Disorders, 35*, 93–101

Epstein, R. M., Franks, P., Fiscella, K., Shields, C. G., Meldrum, S. C., Kravitz, R. L., et al. (2005, Oct). Measuring patient-centered communication in patient-physician consultations: Theoretical and practical issues. *Social Science and Medicine, 61*, 1516–1528

Erber, N., & Heine, C. (1996). Screening receptive communication of older adults in residential care. *American Journal of Audiology, 5*, 38–46

Erdman, S. (1993). Counseling hearing impaired adults. In J. Alpiner & P. McCarthy (Eds.), *Rehabilitative audiology: Children and adults* (2nd ed.). Baltimore: Williams & Wilkins

Erdman, S. (2009). Audiologic counseling: A biopsychosocial approach. In J. Montano & J. Spitzer (Eds.), *Adult audiologic rehabilitation.* San Diego: Plural Publishing

Erdman, S., & Demorest, M. (1990). CPHI manual: A guide to clinical use. Simpsonville, MD: CPHI Services

Foo, C., Rudner, M., Rönnberg, J., & Lunner, T. (2007, Jul-Aug). Recognition of speech in noise with new hearing instrument compression release settings requires explicit cognitive storage and processing capacity. *Journal of the American Academy of Audiology, 18*, 618–631

Gagne, J. P. (1994). Visual and audiovisual speech perception training: Basic and applied research needs. In J. P. Gagne & N. Tye-Murray (Eds.), *Research in audiological rehabilitation: Current trends and future directions. Journal of the Academy of Rehabilitative Audiology, Monograph Supplement, 27*, 133–159

Gagne, J. P. & Jennings, M. (2011, July). Incorporating a client-centered approach to audiologic rehabilitation. *Asha Leader*

Gagne, J., Jennings, M., & Southall, K. (2009a). The International Classification of Functioning: Implications and applications to audiologic rehabilitation. In J. Montano & J. Spitzer (Eds.), *Adult audiologic rehabilitation.* San Diego: Plural Publishing

Gagne, J. P., Southall, K., & Jennings, M. (2009b). The psychological effects of social stigma. In J. Montano & J. Spitzer (Eds.), *Adult audiologic rehabilitation* (pp. 63–92). San Diego: Plural Publishing

Gallun, F. J., & Saunders, G. H. (2010, Oct). The ear-brain system: Approaches to the study and treatment of hearing loss. *Journal of the American Academy of Audiology, 21*, 564–566

Garstecki, D. (1988). Speechreading with auditory cues. *Volta Review, 90*, 161–177

Garstecki, D., & Erler, S. (1996). Use of the communication profile for the hearing impaired with mildly hearing impaired adults. *Journal of Speech and Hearing Research, 39*, 28–42

Gatehouse, G. (1999). The Glasgow Hearing Aid Benefit Profile: Derivation and validation of a patient-centered outcome measure for hearing aid services. *Journal of the American Academy of Audiology, 10*, 80–103

Gatehouse, S. (2003). Rehabilitation: Identification of needs, priorities and expectations, and the evaluation of benefit. *International Journal of Audiology, 42,* 2s77–2s83

Gatehouse, S., Naylor, G., & Elberling, C. (2003, Jul). Benefits from hearing aids in relation to the interaction between the user and the environment. *International Journal of Audiology, 42*(Suppl 1), S77–S85

Gatehouse, S., & Noble, W. (2004, Feb). The Speech, Spatial, and Qualities of Hearing Scale (SSQ). *International Journal of Audiology, 43,* 85–99

Gates, G. A., Beiser, A., Rees, T. S., D'Agostino, R. B., & Wolf, P. A. (2002, Mar). Central auditory dysfunction may precede the onset of clinical dementia in people with probable Alzheimer's disease. *Journal of the American Geriatrics Society, 50,* 482–488

Glasgow, R. E., Emont, S., & Miller, D. S. (2006). Assessing the delivery of the 5 "A's" for patient-centered counseling: Alternatives and future directions. *Health Promotion International, 21,* 2245–2255

Glass, L. (1990). Hearing impairment in geriatrics. In B. Kemp, K. Brummel-Smith, & J. Ramsdell (Eds.), *Geriatric rehabilitation.* Boston: College Hill

Gurland, B., Kuriansky, J., Sharpe, L., Simon, R., Stiller, P., & Birkett, P. (1977–1978). The Comprehensive assessment and Referral Evaluation (CARE)—Rationale, development and reliability. *International Journal of Aging and Human Development, 8,* 9–42

Hällgren, M., Larsby, B., Lyxell, B., & Arlinger, S. (2001, Apr). Cognitive effects in dichotic speech testing in elderly persons. *Ear and Hearing, 22,* 120–129

Hawkins, D. B. (2005, Jul-Aug). Effectiveness of counseling-based adult group aural rehabilitation programs: A systematic review of the evidence. *Journal of the American Academy of Audiology, 16,* 485–493

Helfer, K. (2009). *Older adults in complex listening environments.* Paper presented at the Adult Conference: The Challenge of Aging, Chicago

Helfer, K. S. (1998, Jun). Auditory and auditory-visual recognition of clear and conversational speech by older adults. *Journal of the American Academy of Audiology, 9,* 234–242

Helfter, K., & Freyman, R. (2005). The role of visual speech cues in reducing energetic and informational masking. *Journal of the Acoustical Society of America, 117,* 842–849

Herbst, K. G., & Humphrey, C. (1980, Oct). Hearing impairment and mental state in the elderly living at home. *British Medical Journal, 281,* 903–905

Hickson, L., & Worrall, L. (2003, Jul). Beyond hearing aid fitting: Improving communication for older adults. *International Journal of Audiology, 42* (Suppl 2), S84–S91

Hickson, L., Worrall, L., & Scarinci, N. (2007, Apr). A randomized controlled trial evaluating the active communication education program for older people with hearing impairment. *Ear and Hearing, 28,* 212–23

Houston, K., & Montgomery, A. (1997). Auditory-visual integration: A practical approach. *Seminars in Hearing, 18,* 141–151

Hyde, M., & Riko, K. (1994). A decision-analytic approach to audiological rehabilitation. In J. P. Gagne & N. Tye-Murray (Eds.), *Research in audiological rehabilitation: Current trends and future directions. Journal of the Academy of Rehabilitative Audiology, Monograph Supplement, 27,* 337–374

Janis, I., & Mann, L. (1985). *Decision making.* New York: Free Press

Jerger, J., Chmiel, R., Florin, E., Pirozzolo, F., & Wilson, N. (1996, Dec). Comparison of conventional amplification and an assistive listening device in elderly persons. *Ear and Hearing, 17,* 490–504

Johnson, C., & Danhauer, J. (2002). *Handbook of outcomes measurement in audiology.* New York: Delmar Learning

Kane, R., Ouslander, J., & Abrass, I. (2004). *Essentials of clinical geriatrics* (2nd ed.). New York: McGraw-Hill

Kemp, B. (1990). The psychosocial context of geriatric rehabilitation. In B. Kemp, K. Smith, & J. Ramsdell (Eds.), *Geriatric rehabilitation.* Boston: College Hill

Kiessling, J., Pichora-Fuller, K., Gatehouse, S., Stephens, D., Arlinger, S., Chisolm, T., et al. (2003). Candidature for and delivery of audiological services: Special needs of older people. *International Journal of Audiology, 42,* S92–S101

Kochkin, S. (2005). *The impact of treated hearing loss on quality of life.* http://www.betterhearing.org/aural_education_and_counseling/articles_tip_sheets_and_guides/hearing_loss_treatment/quality_of_life_detail.cfm

Kochkin, S. (2007). Marke Trak VII: Obstacles to adult non-user adoption of hearing aids. *Hearing Journal, 60,* 24–50

Kochkin, S. (2010). Marke Trak VIII: The efficacy of hearing aids in achieving compensation equity in the workplace. *Hearing Journal, 63,* 19–26

Kochkin, S., Beck, D., Christensen, L., Compton-Conley, C., Fligor, B., Kricos, P., McSpaden, J., Gustav Mueller, H., Nilsson, M., Northern, J., Powers, T., Sweetow, R., Taylor, B., & Turner, R. (2010). Marke Trak VIII: The impact of the hearing healthcare professional on hearing aid user success. *Hearing Review, 17,* 12, 14, 16, 18, 23, 26, 27, 28, 30, 32, and 34

Kotler, P., & Clark, R. (1987). *Marketing for health care organizations.* Englewood Cliffs, NJ: Prentice Hall

Kramer, S. E., Allessie, G. H., Dondorp, A. W., Zekveld, A. A., & Kapteyn, T. S. (2005, May). A home education program for older adults with hearing impairment and their significant others: A randomized trial evaluating short- and long-term effects. *International Journal of Audiology, 44,* 255–264

Kricos, P. (2006). Personal communication

Kricos, P. B., & Holmes, A. E. (1996, Aug). Efficacy of audiologic rehabilitation for older adults. *Journal of the American Academy of Audiology, 7,* 219–229

Kuntze, J., Van Der Molen, H., & Born, M. (2009). Increase in counseling communication skills after basic and advanced microskills training. *British Journal of Educational Psychology, 79,* 175–189

Lansing, C. (2009). Visual speech perception in spoken language understanding. In J. Montano & J. Spitzer (Eds.), *Adult audiologic rehabilitation* (pp. 244–265). San Diego: Plural Publishing

Laplante-Lévesque, A., Hickson, L., & Worrall, L. (2010, Mar). Rehabilitation of older adults with hearing impairment: A critical review. *Journal of Aging and Health, 22,* 143–153

Leung, J., Wang, N. Y., Yeagle, J. D., Chinnici, J., Bowditch, S., Francis, H. W., et al. (2005, Dec). Predictive models for cochlear implantation in elderly candidates. *Archives of Otolaryngology–Head and Neck Surgery, 131,* 1049–1054

Lewis, C., & Bottomley, J. (2008). Geriatric rehabilitation: A clinical approach (3rd ed.). Englewood Cliffs, NJ: Pearson-Prentice Hall

Lewis, R. K., & Barrett, A. E. (2011). Visual impairment and quality of life among older adults: An examination of explanations for the relationship. *Journal of Gerontology: Social Science, 66B,* 364–373

Lin, F. R., Metter, E. J., O'Brien, R. J., Resnick, S. M., Zonderman, A. B., & Ferrucci, L. (2011, Feb). Hearing loss and incident dementia. *Archives of Neurology, 68,* 214–220

Lind, C. (2009). Conversation repair strategies in audiologic rehabilitation. In J. Montano & J. Spitzer (Eds.), *Adult audiologic rehabilitation* (pp. 217–243). San Diego: Plural Publishing

Lunner, T., & Sundewall-Thorén, E. (2007, Jul-Aug). Interactions between cognition, compression, and listening conditions: Effects on speech-in-noise performance in a two-channel hearing aid. *Journal of the American Academy of Audiology, 18,* 604–617

Maratchi, T. (2011). The perceived effects of hearing loss in Chinese-Americans and caucasians. Doctoral dissertation, The Graduate Center, City University of New York

Margolis, R. (2004). Boosting memory with informational counseling. *Asha Leader, 9,* 10–11, 28

Martin, J., & Gorenstein, M. (2010). Normal cognitive aging. H. Fillit, K. Rockwood, & K. Woodhouse (Eds.), *Brockelhurst's textbook of geriatric medicine and gerontology* (7th ed.). Philadelphia: Saunders Elsevier

Maslow, A. (1954). *Motivation and personality.* New York: Harper & Row

McArdle, R., Chisolm, T. H., Abrams, H. B., Wilson, R. H., & Doyle, P. J. (2005). The WHO-DAS II: Measuring outcomes of hearing aid intervention for adults. *Trends in Amplification, 9,* 127–143

McDonald, P., & Haney, M. (1997). *Counseling the older adult: A training manual in clinical gerontology* (2nd ed.). San Francisco: Jossey-Bass

Meister, H., Walger, M., Brehmer, D., von Wedel, U., & von Wedel, H. (2008). The relationship between pre-fitting expectations and willingness to use hearing aids. *International Journal of Audiology, 47,* 153–159

Miller, W., & Rollnick, S. (Eds.). (2002). *Motivational interviewing* (2nd ed.). New York: Guilford Press

Milstein, D., & Gershteyn, A. (2011). *Elderly, questionnaires, and compliance with rehabilitation poster.* Presented at Audiology Now, Chicago

Milstein, D. & Weinstein, B. (2002). Effect of information sharing on follow-up after hearing screening for older adults. *Journal of the Academy of Rehabilitation Audiology, 20,* 43–58

Montano, J. (2010). *Engaging Communication Partnerships.* http://idainstitute.com/tool_room/topics/communication_partners

Montgomery, A. (1991). Aural rehabilitation—Review and preview. In G. Studebaker, F. Bess, & L. Beck (Eds.), The Vanderbilt Hearing Aid Report II. Parkton, MD: York Press

Montgomery, A. (1994). Treatment efficacy in adult audiological rehabilitation. In J. P. Gagne & N. Tye-Murray (Eds.), *Research in audiological rehabilitation: Current trends and future directions. Journal of the Academy of Rehabilitative Audiology, Monograph Supplement, 27,* 317–336

Morgan, L., & Kunkel, S. (2011). *Aging, society and the life course.* New York: Springer

Mulrow, C. D., Aguilar, C., Endicott, J. E., Tuley, M. R., Velez, R., Charlip, W. S., et al. (1990a, Aug). Quality-of-life changes and hearing impairment. A randomized trial. *Annals of Internal Medicine, 113,* 188–194

Mulrow, C. D., Aguilar, C., Endicott, J. E., Velez, R., Tuley, M. R., Charlip, W. S., et al. (1990b, Jan). Association between hearing impairment and the quality of life of elderly individuals. *Journal of the American Geriatrics Society, 38,* 45–50

National Council on the Aging (NCOA). (1999). *The consequences of untreated hearing loss in older persons.* Washington, DC: NCOA

Newman, C. W., & Weinstein, B. E. (1986). Judgments of perceived hearing handicap by hearing-impaired elderly men and their spouses. *Journal of the Academy of Rehabilitative Audiology, 19,* 109–115

Noble, W. (2002, Jan). Extending the IOI to significant others and to non-hearing-aid-based interventions. *International Journal of Audiology, 41,* 27–29

Northern, J., & Beyer, C. (1999). Reducing hearing aid returns through patient education. *Audiology Today, 20,* 315–326

Oliver, R. (1977). Effect of expectation and disconfirmation on postexposure product evaluations—An alternative interpretation. *Journal of Applied Psychology, 62,* 480

Olson, A. (2011). Listening and communication enhancement training (LACE[tm]) DVD version. *Ear and Hearing, 32,* 266–268

Orabi, A. A., Mawman, D., Al-Zoubi, F., Saeed, S. R., & Ramsden, R. T. (2006, Apr). Cochlear implant outcomes and quality of life in the elderly: Manchester experience over 13 years. *Clinical Otolaryngology, 31,* 116–122

Pfeiffer, E. (1975, Oct). A short portable mental status questionnaire for the assessment of organic brain deficit in elderly patients. *Journal of the American Geriatrics Society, 23,* 433–441

Pichora-Fuller, M. (1997). Assistive devices for the elderly. In R. Lubinski & D. Higginbotham (Eds.), *Communication technologies for the elderly: Vision, hearing and speech.* San Diego: Singular

Pichora-Fuller, K. (2006). Perceptual effort and apparent cognitive decline: Implications for audiologic rehabilitation. In C. Palmer (Ed.), *The aging auditory system: Considerations for rehabilitation. Seminars in Hearing.* New York: Thieme

Pichora-Fuller, K. (2009). Using the brain when the ears are challenged helps healthy older listeners compensate and preserve communication function. In *Hearing care for adults* From the journal Trends in Amplification, March 2006 vol. 10 no. 1 29-59. http://tia.sagepub.com/content/10/1/29.abstract

Pichora-Fuller, K. M., & Singh, G. (2006, Mar). Effects of age on auditory and cognitive processing: Implications for hearing aid fitting and audiologic rehabilitation. *Trends in Amplification, 10,* 29–59

Preminger, J. E. (2003, Dec). Should significant others be encouraged to join adult group audiologic rehabilitation classes? *Journal of the American Academy of Audiology, 14,* 545–555

Preminger, J. E. (2007). Issues associated with the measurement of psychosocial benefits of group audiologic rehabilitation programs. *Trends in Amplification, 11,* 113–123

Preminger, J. E. (2011). Group audiologic rehabilitation for adults and their communication partners. *ASHA Leader* http://www.asha.org/publications/leader/2011/110705/group-audiologic-rehabilitation-for-adults-and-their-communication-partners/

Preminger, J. E., & Meeks, S. (2010, May). Evaluation of an audiological rehabilitation program for spouses of people with hearing loss. *Journal of the American Academy of Audiology, 21,* 315–328

Primeau, R. (1997). Hearing aid benefit in adults and older adults. *Seminars in Hearing, 18,* 29–37

Prochaska, J. O., & DiClemente, C. C. (1983, Jun). Stages and processes of self-change of smoking: Toward an integrative model of change. *Journal of Consulting and Clinical Psychology, 51,* 390–395

Ramsdell, D. (1960). The psychology of the hard of hearing and deafened adult. In H. Davis & S. Silverman (Eds.), *Hearing and deafness.* New York: Holt, Rinehart, and Silverman

Raskin, N., & Rogers, C. (1989). Person-centered therapy. In R. J. Corsini & D. Wedding (Eds.), *Current psychotherapies* (4th ed., pp. 155–194). Itasca, IL: Peacock

Rejeski, W., Brawley, L., & Jung, M. (2009). Self-management of health behavior in geriatric medicine. In J. Hazzard, J. Ouslander, M. Tinetti, S. Studenski, K. High, & S. Asthana (Eds.), *Hazzard's geriatric medicine and gerontology.* New York: McGraw-Hill

Rogers, C. (1951). *Client-centered therapy.* Boston: Houghton Mifflin

Rollnick, S., Mason, P., & Butler, C. (2001). *Health behavior change a guide for practitioners.* New York: Churchill-Livingstone

Ross, M. (1996). You've done something about it! Helpful hints to the new hearing aid user. *HLAA Journal, 17,* 7–11

Saunders, G. H., & Cienkowski, K. M. (1996). Refinement and psychometric evaluation of the Attitudes to Loss of Hearing Questionnaire (ALHQ). *Ear and Hearing, 17,* 505–519

Scarinci, N., Worrall, L., & Hickson, L. (2008, Mar). The effect of hearing impairment in older people on the spouse. *International Journal of Audiology, 47,* 141–151

Schow, R., & Nerbonne, M. (1982). Communication screening profile uses with elderly clients. *Ear and Hearing, 3,* 133–147

Schum, D. (1994). Personal adjustment counseling. In J. P. Gagne & N. Tye-Murray (Eds.), *Research in audiological rehabilitation: Current trends and future directions. Journal of the Academy of Rehabilitative Audiology, Monograph Supplement, 27,* 223–236

Schunk, D., & Usher, E. (2011). Assessing self-efficacy for self-regulated learning. In B. Zimmerman & D. Schunk (Eds.), *Handbook of self-regulation of learning and performance.* New York: Routledge

Singh, G., & Pichora-Fuller, K. M. (2010, Oct). Older adults' performance on the speech, spatial, and qualities of hearing scale (SSQ): Test-retest reliability and a comparison of interview and self-administration methods. *International Journal of Audiology, 49,* 733–740

Smith, G. E., Housen, P., Yaffe, K., Ruff, R., Kennison, R. F., Mahncke, H. W., et al. (2009, Apr). A cognitive training program based on principles of brain plasticity: Results from the Improvement in Memory with Plasticity-Based Adaptive Cognitive Training (IMPACT) study. *Journal of the American Geriatrics Society, 57,* 594–603

Smith, S. L., & West, R. L. (2006, Jun). The application of self-efficacy principles to audiologic rehabilitation: A tutorial. *American Journal of Audiology, 15,* 46–56

Sorkin, D. (1997). Consumer and hearing aids: The SHHH perspective. *Seminars in Hearing, 18,* 49–56

Spencer, S., Schulz, R., Rooks, R., Albert, S., Thorpe, R., Brenes, G., et al. (2009). Racial differences in self-rated health at similar levels of physical functioning: An examination of health pessimism in the health, aging, and body composition study. *Journal of Gerontology, B, Psychological Sciences and Social Sciences, 64b,* 87–94

Spreng, R. A., Mackenzie, S. B., & Olshavsky, R. W. (1996). A reexamination of the determinants of consumer satisfaction. *Journal of Marketing, 60,* 15

Stark, P., & Hickson, L. (2004, Jul-Aug). Outcomes of hearing aid fitting for older people with hearing impairment and their significant others. *International Journal of Audiology, 43,* 390–398

Steinfeld, E. (1997). Architecture as a communication medium. In R. Lubinski & D. Higginbotham (Eds.), *Communication technologies for the elderly: vision, hearing, and speech.* San Diego: Singular

Stone, H. (1990, July-Aug). Hearing health care in the 1990s. *Audiology Today,* 14–17

Strawbridge, W. J., Wallhagen, M. I., Shema, S. J., & Kaplan, G. A. (2000, Jun). Negative consequences of hearing impairment in old age: A longitudinal analysis. *Gerontologist, 40,* 320–326

Stroop, J. R. (1935). Studies of interference in serial verbal reaction. *Journal of Experimental Psychology, 18,* 643–662

Sue, D., Arredondo, P., & McDavis, R. (1992). Multicultural counseling competencies and standards: A call to the profession. *Journal of Counseling and Development, 70,* 477–486

Sweetow, R. (2007). Instead of hearing aid evaluation, let's assess functional communication ability. *Hearing Journal, 60,* 26–31

Sweetow, R. (2009). *Five ideas to better meet the hearing needs of older people.* Paper presented at the Adult Conference: The Challenge of Aging, Chicago

Sweetow, R., & Henderson-Sabes, J. (2004). The case for LACE: Listening and auditory communication enhancement training. *Hearing Journal. 57,* 32–40

Sweetow, R., & Palmer, C. V. (2005, Jul-Aug). Efficacy of individual auditory training in adults: A systematic review of the evidence. *Journal of the American Academy of Audiology, 16,* 494–504

Sweetow, R. W., & Sabes, J. H. (2006, Sep). The need for and development of an adaptive Listening and Communication Enhancement (LACE) program. *Journal of the American Academy of Audiology, 17,* 538–558

Sweetow, R. W., & Sabes, J. H. (2007, Jun). Technologic advances in aural rehabilitation: Applications and innovative methods of service delivery. *Trends in Amplification, 11,* 101–111

Sweetow, R. & Sabes, J. H. (2009). Auditory training. In J. Montano & J. Spitzer (Eds.), *Adult audiologic rehabilitation.* San Diego: Plural Publishing

Sweetow, R. W., & Sabes, J. H. (2010, Oct). Auditory training and challenges associated with participation and compliance. *Journal of the American Academy of Audiology, 21,* 586–593

Taylor, K., & Jurma, W. (1999). Study suggests that group rehabilitation increases benefit of hearing aid fittings. *Hearing Journal, 52,* 48–54

Tremblay, K., & Pichora-Fuller, K. (2011). *Rehabilitating older ears and older brains.* Paper presented at Audiology Now, Chicago, April

Trychin, S. (1995). Counseling older adults with hearing impairments. In P. Kricos & S. Lesner (Eds.), *Hearing care for the older adult.* Boston: Butterworth-Heinemann

Trychin, S. (1997). Coping with hearing loss. *Seminars in Hearing, 18,* 77–86

Trychin, S. (2001). Why don't people who need hearing aids get them? *Hearing Loss, 22,* 15–19

Trychin, S. (2002). Guidelines for providing mental health services to people who are hard of hearing. San Diego: University of California, San Diego

Tye-Murray, N. (2008). *Foundations of aural rehabilitation: Children, adults, and their family members.* Clifton Park, NY: Thomson/Delmar Learning

Tye-Murray, N., & Witt, S. (1997). Communication strategies training. *Seminars in Hearing, 18,* 153–165

Uhlmann, R. F., Larson, E. B., Rees, T. S., Koepsell, T. D., & Duckert, L. G. (1989, Apr). Relationship of hearing impairment to dementia and cognitive dysfunction in older adults. *Journal of the American Medical Association, 261,* 1916–1919

U.S. Department of Health and Human Services. (2007). Early release of selected estimates based on data from the 2006 National Health Interview Survey. http://www.cdc.gov/nchs/about/major/nhis/released 200706.htm#11

Van Vliet, D. (2005, Jul-Aug). The current status of hearing care: Can we change the status quo? *Journal of the American Academy of Audiology, 16,* 410–418

Ventry, I. M., & Weinstein, B. E. (1982, May-Jun). The hearing handicap inventory for the elderly: A new tool. *Ear and Hearing, 3,* 128–134

Ventry, I. M., & Weinstein, B. E. (1983, Jul). Identification of elderly people with hearing problems. *American Speech-Language-Hearing Association, 25,* 37–42

Vuorialho, A., Karinen, P., & Sorri, M. (2006, Nov). Counselling of hearing aid users is highly cost-effective. *European Archives of Oto-Rhino-Laryngology, 263*, 988–995

Wagner, C. C., & McMahon, B. T. (2004). Motivational interviewing and rehabilitation counseling practice. *Rehabilitation Counseling Bulletin, 47*, 142–161

Walden, D. E., Demorest, M. E., & Hepler, E. L. (1984, Mar). Self-report approach to assessing benefit derived from amplification. *Journal of Speech and Hearing Research, 27*, 49–56

Walden, B., & Grant, K. (1993). Research needs in rehabilitative audiology. In J. Alpiner & P. McCarthy (Eds.), *Rehabilitative audiology: Children and adults.* Baltimore: Williams & Wilkins

Ware, J. E., Jr, & Sherbourne, C. D. (1992, Jun). The MOS 36-item Short-Form Health Survey (SF-36). I. Conceptual framework and item selection. *Medical Care, 30*, 473–483

Weinstein, B. (1980). *Hearing impairment and social isolation in the elderly.* Ph.D. dissertation, Columbia University

Weinstein, B., & Amsel, L. (1986). Hearing loss and senile dementia in the institutionalized elderly. *Clinical Gerontologist, 4*, 3–15

Weinstein, B. E., Spitzer, J. B., & Ventry, I. M. (1986, Oct). Test-retest reliability of the Hearing Handicap Inventory for the Elderly. *Ear and Hearing, 7*, 295–299

Willis, S. L., Tennstedt, S. L., Marsiske, M., Ball, K., Elias, J., Koepke, K. M., et al; ACTIVE Study Group (2006, Dec). Long-term effects of cognitive training on everyday functional outcomes in older adults. *Journal of the American Medical Association, 296*, 2805–2814

World Health Organization (WHO). (2001). *International Classification of Functioning (ICF), Disability, and Health.* Geneva, Switzerland: World Health Organization

Yueh, B., McDowell, J. A., Collins, M., Souza, P. E., Loovis, C. F., & Deyo, R. A. (2005, Oct). Development and validation of the effectiveness of [corrected] auditory rehabilitation scale. *Archives of Otolaryngology–Head and Neck Surgery, 131*, 851–856

Zimmerman, B., & Kitsantas, A. (2007). Reliability and validity of Self-Efficacy for Learning Form (SELF) scores of college students. *Journal of Psychology, 215*, 157–163

Chapter 8

Sensory Management

Now that my listening problems have finally been solved with my binaural programmable hearing aids, can you help me out with my laptop computer? Then my troubles will be over.

—M.F., 74-year-old musician and retired teacher

I wish hearing aids were more convenient to use and more beneficial when wearing them.

—A.K., 83-year-old man

I wish I could sleep with my hearing aids; they help me feel so much safer.

—M.B., 78-year-old woman

An untreated hearing loss is more noticeable than hearing aids

-Dr. Sergei Kochkin

It seems to me that what my audiologist does the best is the knowledge of hearing aids available to her, but I have the feeling she knows just how to make her services as financially lucrative to herself as possible, with the customer playing second fiddle.

C.W., 79-year-old woman

◆ Learning Objectives

After reading this chapter, you should be able to

- discuss the demographics of hearing-aid use;
- discuss the audiological and nonaudiological variables essential to a successful hearing-aid fitting;
- articulate the generic and disease-specific outcomes associated with hearing-aid use;
- discuss the importance of hearing assistance technologies as a supplement to hearing aids or as a targeted intervention;
- discuss implantable hearing devices as an option for older adults with hearing impairment;
- discuss the stages of readiness and personality variables affecting hearing-aid candidacy; and
- discuss the value and components of a comprehensive approach to hearing-aid orientation.

◆ Part 1: Hearing Aids

Hearing aids, hearing assistance technologies (HATs), implantable devices, and associated audiological rehabilitation are the intervention of choice for older adults with hearing impairments that are associated with communication breakdowns, activity limitations, participation restrictions, and compromised quality of life. Hearing aids drive the rehabilitation process, and manufacturers are committed to reducing the size of high-performing hearing aids by loading them with advanced features so that they will be increasingly acceptable to those with hearing impairment. Some of the high-tech features include digital noise reduction technology, digital feedback reduction, and directional microphone technology, but they have not proven to be advantageous in a laboratory setting. Until recently, these features were reserved for high-end products, but increasingly they are included in hearing aids spanning a wide range of price points (Johnson, 2008). In fact, more than 80% of all hearing-aid fittings in 2007 included feedback reduction, noise reduction, and directional technologies (Johnson, 2007). More hearing aids are water resistant, a feature of considerable importance to older adults. There is evidence that telecoil use and wireless technology is on the rise, which bodes well for their usefulness with various forms of HATs and the more widespread acceptance of hearing-loop systems.

According to a recent survey of consumers, good times lie ahead for the hearing-aid industry, with satisfaction rates high and the average age of first-time users trending lower. Interestingly, for hearing aids manufactured within the past 4 years, customer satisfaction is now at 78%, and the proportion of people reporting that they do not use their hearing aids has declined dramatically to 7.5% from 10% in 2004 (Kochkin, 2010). However, hearing-aid market penetration has remained stable over the past half century, barely breaking 25% of all persons with hearing impairment. But Boothroyd (2007) projects that hearing aids of the future have great promise, thanks to technological advances. He contends that "to the extent that the marriage of hearing aid and wireless technology can remove some of the barriers to adoption, we may finally see inroads into the problem of low penetration" (p. 10).

Long-term satisfaction with hearing aids and quality-of-life improvements are critical if audiologists are going to successfully close the gap between prevalence of hearing loss and hearing-aid use and acceptance (Kochkin, 2011a). Positive outcomes are associated with best-practice patterns, which include a person-centered approach to the therapeutic process. Management of the person with hearing impairment must begin with a comprehensive and systematic intake and a targeted treatment plan, and conclude with documentation of outcomes (Valente et al, 2006a). The intervention of choice, be it hearing aids, HATs, or counseling, must be tailored to patients' residual auditory area and based on an understanding of their activity limitations, participation restrictions, and motivations, and on quality-of-life considerations. For example, an infrared system to boost television understanding may be a starting point for those who reject hearing aids because their primary difficulty is television viewing. Positive experiences with this targeted intervention may lead to the subsequent adoption of hearing aids. Alternatively, for a teacher who is hearing impaired and misunderstands questions posed by students in the classroom, perhaps a behind-the-hearing aid with an integrated frequency-modulated (FM) receiver or a hand-held, beam-forming microphone array is indicated because the more traditional features have not helped to overcome the teacher's unique communication difficulties. It is critical that we use the pre-fitting appointment to gain insight into the communication needs of persons with hearing impairment and of their communication partners, as this input will be a determinant of their ultimate satisfaction and benefit.

This chapter discusses a person-centered approach to auditory management that can increase hearing-aid market penetration, maximize benefit, and narrow the gap between expectations and user satisfaction. The focus is on best practices related to auditory technologies, with the centerpiece being collaboration among the patient, the audiologist, and the family or caregiver. The technology is part of the arsenal but is not the driver of the process, and given the dynamic nature of auditory technologies the focus of the chapter is on considerations unique to older adults rather than on the hearing instrument per se. Textbooks on hearing aids and courses in the typical Au.D. program generally provide an in-depth understanding of the technological aspects of hearing instruments. This chapter will enable the reader to apply information specific to older adults to their working knowledge of hearing aids, HATs, and implantable hearing devices. Our challenge as audiologists serving the hearing impaired is to inspire trust and foster relief. Our clients must trust that we have the professional training and knowledge to help them overcome their communication difficulties, and may be inspired by the relief they feel when we help them overcome the burden of their communication difficulties.

◆ Demography of Hearing-Aid Use

Of the 34 million persons who have hearing difficulty in the United States, fewer than 25% use hearing instruments, repre-

senting a gap of over 25 million people (Kochkin, 2009). The average age of these nonusers is 59.9 years, and the average age of hearing-aid users is 71.1 years (Kochkin, 2012). Institutional barriers continue to plague the industry, such that despite the great number of technological advances, the proportion of the hearing impaired who use hearing aids has remained stable since 1950. Individuals continue to wait between 7 to 12 years before buying a hearing aid (English, 2008; Kochkin, 2010). A recent study conducted by Consumer Reports (2009) found that, from the perspective of those purchasing hearing aids, our industry continues to be plagued by high-priced hearing aids, mediocre fittings, lack of information, lack of verification and validation, and lack of third-party payer support for hearing aids; the U.S. Department of Veterans Affairs (DVA) pays for hearing aids for veterans. Consumers see the high price of hearing aids as a barrier to hearing-aid ownership, but see third-party payment or installment plans as a possible relief valve (Johnson, 2008). Further, we now know that including clinical verification and validation techniques in our audiology practice has a positive impact on consumer satisfaction, especially when these findings are conveyed to the patient (Kochkin, 2011a).

Reflecting on the historical correlation between the state of the economy and the fate of the hearing-aid industry, Kirkwood (2009) reported that despite the global economic turmoil, dispensers have been relatively sanguine regarding hearing-aid sales; 43% of survey respondents anticipated selling more hearing aids in 2009 than in 2008, with a 3.4% increase in unit sales by manufacturer during the first quarter; 34% expected sales to remain the same; and only 19% projected a downturn in sales. In fact, overall hearing-aid unit sales in 2009 rebounded dramatically in both the private sector and in the DVA (Strom, 2010). Although net unit sales were up in 2009, net revenue was not as bright, with patients seeking less costly devices.

As compared with 2009, there remains cause for cautious optimism as of this writing. Hearing-aid sales increased by 4.9% overall in the first quarter of 2011 as compared with 2010 (Hj Report, 2011). Although hearing-aid sales were relatively flat in 2010 and 2011, 2.9% more hearing aids were sold in 2010 than in the second quarter of 2009 with a slight increase in sales from 2011 over 2010 (Hj Report, 2010, 2011). In 2010, nearly 2.7 million hearing aids were sold in the U.S. hearing-aid market, representing 1.5 million patients. Behind-the-ear (BTE) hearing aids maintained their position as the most popular device, representing 69% of the total market share in the first quarter of 2011, which represents an increase from the first half of 2010, when the market share was 66%, and from 1998, when the market share was only 19% (Hearing Industries Association, 2010; Kochkin, 2011b). Similarly, at the midpoint of 2010, manufacturers had sold 1,341,122 hearing aids, which is 4.2% ahead of the 1,287,390 sold in the first half of 2009, not insubstantial considering the global economy (Hj Report, 2010). **Figure 8.1** captures the trend in net hearing-aid sales from 2000 to 2010. In 2010, 40% of BTE units sold were receiver-in-the-canal (RIC) units. **Figure 8.2** captures the change in market penetration over nearly two decades, with the crossover point occurring in 2006 with the advent of innovations in the industry including open fittings, RIC fittings, and receiver-in-the-ear (RITE) fittings (Strom, 2010).

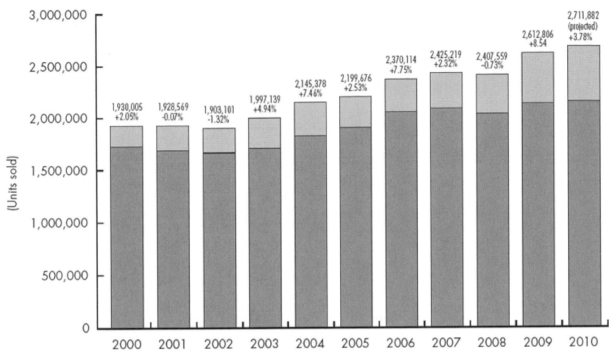

Fig. 8.1   Unit sales of hearing aids and percentage change from 2000 through 2010. [From Kirkwood, D. (2010). In troubled economic times, the hearing aid industry remains an island of stability. *Hearing Journal, 63*, 11–12, 14, 16.]

The hearing health-care industry is undergoing interesting changes among professionals engaged in dispensing as well as those in practice settings, and this translates into some novel trends in overall sales patterns. In 2008, 63% of persons dispensing hearing aids were audiologists, as contrasted to 1989 when only 48% were audiologists. In contrast, in 2008, 31% of dispensers were hearing-instrument specialists as contrasted to 57% in 1989! **Figure 8.3** captures the trends in terms of the percentage of hearing-aid fittings performed by audiologists, hearing-aid specialists, and physicians. It is not surprising that the average number of hearing aids sold in 2008 varied by practice setting and by professional. Audiologists in private

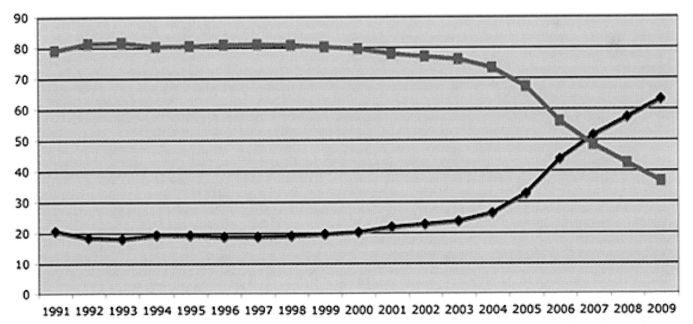

Fig. 8.2   Market penetration of behind-the-ear (BTE) hearing aids *(black)* and in-the-ear (ITE) hearing aids *(gray)* from 1991 through 2009. [From Strom, K. (2010). A market update and the top-so trends in hearing care, Part 1. *Hearing Review.* http://www.hearingreview.com/issues/articles/2010-05_01.asp.]

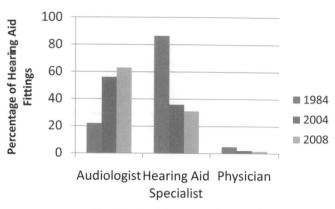

Fig. 8.3 Hearing-aid fitting by hearing health care professional as perceived by the consumer. [From Kochkin, S. (2009). MarkeTrak VIII: 25 year trends in the hearing health market. *Hearing Review. 16*, 12–31.]

practice reported the highest mean number of units sold per month (18), as contrasted with the mean number sold by audiologists in hospitals/clinics (10). Hearing-instrument specialists sold a mean of 17 units per month, whereas audiologists working in a physician's office sold a mean of 14 per month (Kirkwood, 2009). Interestingly, a recent survey by Kochkin et al (2010) found that the occupation of the professional fitting hearing aids explained less than 0.5% of the variability in whether the fitting protocol was successful, which is rather sobering especially since physicians are the gatekeepers of health care from the perspective of older adults. The DVA fit more hearing aids in 2009 than ever before, with purchases representing 17% of the total domestic market. According to Strom (2010), the DVA is responsible for almost 20% of all hearing aids sold in the U.S. The DVA has more than doubled (2.4 times) the number of units sold between 2000 and 2009, whereas non-DVA dispensing activity increased by only 1.23 times during the same period. The latter increase is due in large part to an aging population of close to 24 million veterans.

Geographic trends in hearing-aid sales are noteworthy. California, Texas, Florida, and New York remain the states selling the largest number of hearing aids, but in several areas there were dramatic increases in the number of hearing aids purchased from manufacturers. Specifically, Montana, North Dakota, and Washington, DC, recorded a rise in the number of units purchased, whereas sales of hearing aids in South Dakota and North Carolina slid (Kirkwood, 2010). Across the country, hearing-aid sales in 2007 were marked by continued growth in high-tech features, such that 77% of hearing aids sold had directional microphone technology, 89% included noise-reduction technology, 90% incorporated feedback-reduction technology, and 59% included a data-logging feature (Johnson, 2008). A higher percentage of hearing aids sold by audiologists in 2007 included directional technology, noise-reduction technology, feedback-reduction technology, and data-logging technology. It is cause for optimism that between 2004 and 2007, 53% of current hearing-aid users had never owned hearing aids. This in part may be due to the availability of mini-

BTEs, which have a greater appeal among persons with less severe hearing loss, among new users, and among persons still in the work force (Kochkin, 2011b). The advantages of the mini-BTEs for the elderly include reduction of the occlusion effect; better sound quality; less visibility due to the use of thin tubes; minimization, which provides the ability to camouflage by matching the color to the client's hair or skin color; and the possibility of being fit immediately and walking out with hearing aids (Johnson, 2008).

> ### Pearl
> Hearing-instrument ownership is highly related to age, even when the degree of hearing loss is considered.

According to Kochkin (2012), the average age of new hearing-aid users in the U.S. is 71.1 years, which, as is evident from **Fig. 8.4**, represents a slight increase since 1991. The majority of persons (40%) who own hearing aids report having moderate to severe hearing loss as compared to 9% with mild hearing loss. Audiologists, family physicians, and ear, nose, and throat (ENT) physicians are more likely to recommend against hearing aids for those with mild hearing loss than for those with moderate to severe hearing loss, and family physicians are more likely than ENT physicians to refer persons with hearing impairment for additional testing. The primary reason for purchasing hearing aids is the perception that hearing loss has worsened, or the influence of family members, primarily a spouse (Kochkin, 2009). According to Kochkin's (2009) report on 25-year trends in the hearing-aid industry, as compared with 1989, fewer family physicians and ear physicians are referring people for hearing aids. People with hearing loss are more likely to be retired or employed part-time than are those without hearing impairment. The majority of hearing-aid owners perceive themselves as having a moderate to severe hearing loss. Despite the apparent age-related dependence of

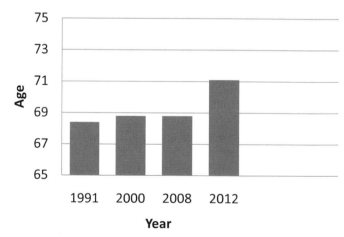

Fig. 8.4 Average age of new hearing-aid users. [From Kochkin, S. (2009). MarkeTrak VIII: 25 year trends in the hearing health market. *Hearing Review. 16*, 12–31; and Kochkin, S. (2012). MarkeTrak VIII: The key influencing factors in hearing aid purchase intent. *Hearing Review, 19*, 12–25.]

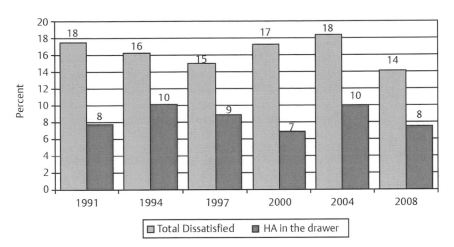

Fig. 8.5 Hearing-aid (HA) dissatisfaction rates. [From Kochkin, S. (2010). Marke-Trak VIII: Customer satisfaction with hearing aids is slowly increasing. *Hearing Journal, 63,* 19–20, 22, 24, 26, 28, 30–32.]

hearing-aid use, the majority of older adults with hearing loss do not use hearing instruments. According to a variety of surveys, it appears that only 18 to 20% of older adults with hearing loss use hearing aids. As is shown in **Fig. 8.5,** hearing-aid dissatisfaction appears to be on the decline, but the change over the past few years does not appear to be dramatic. **Table 8.1** shows a more complete picture of hearing-aid owners, many of whom have owned hearing aids for 4 years or less.

> ### Pearl
>
> The majority of hearing instrument users are older adults. The majority of older adults do not use hearing instruments.

The major barriers to hearing-aid adoption among those with admitted hearing loss fall into 11 key areas (Kochkin, 2007): 1) experience with hearing aids, (2) financial considerations, (3) attitudes toward hearing aids, (4) degree of hearing loss, (5) lack of need, (6) visual/manual dexterity issues, (7) recommendations from professionals, (8) recommendations of family/friends, (9) stigma, (10) trust, and (11) lack

Table 8.1 Characteristics of Hearing-Aid Owners

- 55% are first-time users
- 60% male
- 69% purchase behind-the-ear (BTE) hearing aids
- 91% have difficulty conversing in noise
- 53% perceived themselves to have a moderate loss
- 78% are binaural users
- 97 to 99% of hearing-aid owners use digital hearing aids
- 69 years is the average age of new users
- 71 years is the average age of hearing-aid owners
- 8% of hearing-aid owners report not using their hearing instrument at all
- 76% of hearing-aid users are satisfied (an increase from versus 60% in 1989)

Sources: Adapted from Kochkin, S. (2009). MarkeTrak VIII: 25 year trends in the hearing health market. *Hearing Review, 16,* 12–31; and Kochkin, S. (2010). Marke-Trak VIII: Customer satisfaction with hearing aids is slowly increasing. *Hearing Journal, 63,* 19–20, 22, 24, 26, 28, 30–32.

of knowledge. These reasons echo the earlier findings of Fino, Bess, Lichtenstein, and Logan (1991), who confirmed that hearing-impaired elderly who elected not to pursue amplification believed that hearing aids are too conspicuous, too expensive, too noisy, and called attention to one's hearing handicap. What is most surprising is that despite the technological advances and the miniaturization of hearing aids, negative attitudes continue to persist. Accordingly, the next section discusses these reasons, as they lend support to adoption of a more systematic and analytic approach to the pre-fitting process, in which the audiologist seeks to dispel the many myths about hearing aids. The section begins with an in-depth discussion of why hearing-impaired individuals decide against purchasing hearing aids and ends with a checklist that is an amalgam of other checklists, such as those developed by members of the Hearing Loss Association of America and by Consumer Reports (2009). These may be helpful to consumers when purchasing hearing aids.

◆ Factors Affecting Decisions Regarding Hearing-Aid Use

Let's begin with a discussion of nonadoption rates and how consumer perceptions and problem recognition contribute to this phenomenon. Among individuals with admitted hearing loss surveyed by Kochkin (2007), the majority were of the opinion that their hearing loss (1) was not severe enough; (2) was not of the variety that could be alleviated with hearing aids; (3) did not warrant intervention, given the frequency-specific nature of the loss; or (4) was in one ear only, thereby negating the need for a hearing aid. Many respondents did not see the need for a hearing aid because of their current life circumstance, because they have more pressing priorities, or because the hearing loss has not yet disrupted their life. Perceptions regarding financial issues also proved constraining, such as that hearing aids were not worth the expense, that the benefits did not justify the expense, that hearing aids were too costly to maintain and therefore unaffordable, and that a less costly device could serve their needs. Interestingly, respondents to the survey also expressed concerns with specific

Table 8.2 Obstacles to Hearing-Aid Uptake and Solutions

Obstacle	Solution
Problem recognition	Improved professional and consumer education; screening
Financial constraints	Sharing of information regarding cost-benefit; clarity regarding maintenance costs
Attitude toward hearing aids	Improved information about hearing-aid features
Health professional's advice	Marketing efforts aimed at education regarding hearing-aid value and candidacy

features or shortcomings of hearing aids. Specific deterrents included the perception that hearing aids do not fit well, do not work in noisy or in crowded situations, produce an annoying whistle/feedback, are a hassle and difficult to use, cannot be used with the telephone, and are of limited utility. Other major deterrents were the belief that hearing aids did not meet expectations and that they were a poor value. The stigma associated with hearing-aid use was also a reason for nonadoption. Respondents felt that hearing aids were too noticeable and made people look too old, disabled, or mentally challenged.

Interestingly, advice from health professionals, opinions of one's spouse, and negative experiences of friends who have used hearing aids also influenced the decision of many respondents to shy away from a hearing-aid purchase. According to Kochkin's (2007) projections, negative word of mouth or the negative experiences of other hearing-aid owners were factors in the decision of 4.4 million hearing-impaired individuals to refrain from purchasing hearing aids. Kochkin concluded that "the key driver to positive attitudes toward hearing aids is a substantial customer base deriving benefit at a perceived high value" (p. 50). Hence, since the "consumer's journey" is so important, how can audiologists realistically influence the journey in a positive way? **Table 8.2** summarizes some of the obstacles identified by Kochkin and includes some simple solutions. Solutions begin with a perspective on what it is we are trying to accomplish when working with older adults with a hearing impairment that is perceived to be impacting communication and daily life.

> **Pearl**
>
> Once older adults commit to purchasing a hearing instrument, they are no longer stigmatized by the hearing loss or hearing aid.

◆ Process-Based Approach to Interventions with Hearing Aids, Hearing Assistance Technologies, or Implantable Devices

The hearing-instrument fitting process should be seen in the context of a comprehensive audiological rehabilitation program, in which the responsibility of the audiologist is to facilitate the reduction in communication disability and psycho-

social handicap associated with a hearing impairment via an acceptable intervention, such as hearing aids. The hearing-aid fitting and the use of HATs are an integral part of the management process. In accordance with the World Health Organization's International Classification of Function, Disability, and Health (WHO-ICF) framework, the purpose of technology-based interventions is to reduce the auditory impairment, optimize the individual's auditory activities of daily living, and minimize participation restrictions (Chisolm et al, 2007). Optimally, amplified speech levels should be placed within the individuals' residual dynamic range (DR) such that amplified speech is audible and the DR is maximized (i.e., as wide as possible) without causing uncomfortable loudness (Hawkins, 2011). Of necessity, the process must begin with the assessment of auditory function. The goals of the initial assessment are multifaceted: (1) diagnosis of the extent of the hearing impairment and speech understanding difficulties, (2) determination of the activity limitations and participation restrictions concomitant with the hearing impairment (i.e., self-perceived difficulties), (3) assessment of clients' readiness for intervention, and (4) documentation of clients' baseline goals and expectations regarding the intervention.

As self-reported hearing disability and stage of change have repeatedly been identified as factors which are predictive of intervention uptake and success, it is incumbent on audiologists to take the time to quantify these two variables (Laplante-LeVesque, Hickson, & Worrall, 2012). Additional nonauditory variables which must be considered when making decisions about the appropriate intervention include working memory, mental status, visual status, and health-related quality of life. If after the initial assessment a decision is made to proceed with a hearing-aid fitting, then selecting the device and its features, and the acoustic verification of the match to the target are a critical part of the process, as acoustic accuracy of the fit sets the stage for the validation, which is a more subjective, patient-driven process (Schum, 2009). Following the fitting, the person with hearing impairment returns for the post-fitting session, the purpose of which is to determine if the prescribed target meets the individual's needs from the perspective of speech understanding and subjective preferences. At this session the audiologist adjusts the prescribed gain and output across frequencies, assesses acoustic accuracy and appropriateness, conducts further counseling, and schedules another verification visit.

> **Pearl**
>
> If the maximum output exceeds the hearing-aid user's loudness discomfort level, then the hearing aid is likely to be rejected or used in a limited number of situations (Hawkins, 2011).

The Pre-Fitting Session

As is shown in **Fig. 8.6**, the first step in the selection/fitting process is the pre-fitting, which entails administering tests that the audiologist uses to identify a hearing-aid candidate along with delineation of the client's expressed needs and the concerns of the communication partner. The nature of the au-

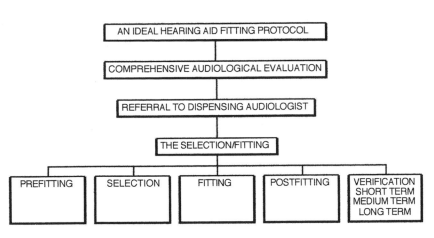

Fig. 8.6 The steps in the selection/fitting process.

ditory impairment should be described, along with its consequences, and the client's readiness, expectations, and motivational level should be assessed. The hearing impairment should be viewed in the context of the individual's physical, social, psychological, and environmental context as shown in **Table 8.3**. The assessment must be approached from a functional and holistic perspective that will serve as the basis for identifying individuals who are likely to both use and benefit from hearing-aid technology. It will also help to establish a pretreatment performance baseline against which the outcome of the intervention can be judged. The outcome(s) of a treatment relative to an established baseline will ultimately serve as the barometer for the person with hearing impairment and the communication partner in terms of the benefit justifying the investment of time and money.

Auditory Factors

Impairment, or the measurable loss of hearing function, is described in terms of the extent of hearing loss for pure-tone and speech signals in quiet and in noise and in terms of loudness discomfort. Impairment measures in the hearing-aid selection and fitting process help to (1) establish he appropriateness of hearing aids, HATs, a cochlear implant or a bone-anchored hearing aid (BAHA); (2) set realistic expectations regarding auditory and nonauditory benefits of hearing aids or implantable devices; (3) establish and verify selected electroacoustic characteristics and features of the prescribed hearing aid(s); (4) decide on hearing-aid and receiver/earmold style; (5) select the appropriate ear(s) to fit, hearing-aid arrangement (binaural, contralateral routing of signal [CROS]), and features; and

(6) establish the dynamic range of hearing necessary to optimize the fitting. Loudness discomfort levels (LDLs) in each ear using headphones and across frequencies are important impairment measures to determine at the pre-fitting, to assist in decisions regarding the output sound pressure level target with a 90-dB input (OSPL90) and maximization of the dynamic range. LDL is critical for setting acceptable output levels, as dissatisfaction with loud sounds is a major reason for hearing-aid rejection. It is commonly accepted that low LDLs are associated with unsuccessful hearing-aid use. According to Shi, Doherty, Kordas, and Pellegrino (2007), speech-in-noise tests and LDL conducted at the pre-fitting tend to reduce the number of hearing-aid adjustments at the follow-up fitting and promote satisfaction over time.

Impairment measures, primarily threshold measures, can help to determine whether a medical therapy is indicated; that is, is there a condition or pathology that can be remediated via medical or surgical intervention? The presence of impacted cerumen is a condition requiring immediate attention. Cerumen management falls within the purview of audiologists and it is a continuing maintenance issue when the Lyric hearing aid is prescribed. Regarding cerumen management, I would refer older adults vulnerable to infection, especially those suffering from diabetes and cancer to a physician. If there is a medical contraindication to hearing-aid use, referral to a physician and medical clearance are necessary steps prior to the hearing-aid selection and fitting. In the absence of a medically treatable condition, the audiologist next considers the severity of hearing impairment, symmetry, auditory response area, the hearing configuration, type of hearing loss, speech perception as measured possibly using a speech-in-noise test,

Table 8.3 Domains of Function to Consider When Selecting Hearing-Aid Candidates

Communication Status	Physical	Psychological	Sociological	Environmental
Impairment	Manual dexterity	Motivation	Lifestyle	Safety needs
Activity limitations	Physical health status (e.g., diabetes)	Cognitive	Familial-support (communication partner)	
Participation restrictions	Technological savvy	Readiness	Financial factors	
	Visual status	Personality	Life events	
		Expectations		
		Self-efficacy		

presence of a central auditory processing dysfunction (CAPD), cognitive problems, or binaural interference. Although the latter variables are not necessarily the primary determinants of candidacy for hearing aids, they do influence decisions regarding the hearing-aid style (e.g., Lyric versus mini-BTE), hearing-aid features, desireability of a binaural fitting, hearing-aid arrangement, electroacoustic response, as well as outcomes (Cox, Schwartz, Noe, & Alexander, 2011b). Communication strategies necessary to optimize performance can be used to set realistic expectations, and can be decisive in the decision to recommend one rather than two hearing aids. Further, configuration of hearing loss may affect decisions regarding electroacoustic characteristics of the hearing aid, features, type of fitting (e.g., open canal), and maximum high-frequency gain setting before feedback, whereas symmetry of hearing loss may figure into the decision regarding the arrangement (e.g., monaural or a binaural fitting; CROS/biCROS) rather than the candidacy. The level of impairment will drive the gain, output settings, and optimal frequency characteristics, yet most audiologists acknowledge that comparisons between general fitting methods for nonlinear hearing aids reveal large differences in prescribed gain–frequency response shape and in overall gain (Smeds, 2004).

To restore normal loudness perception to the impaired ear, threshold and suprathreshold data will affect optimal compression threshold settings, attack and release times, and maximum output or OSPL90 settings. Pure-tone findings are likely to inform decisions regarding the fitting method, be it those that advocate a loudness equalization approach (e.g., National Acoustic Laboratory-Revised, Profound [NAL-RP], National Acoustics Laboratory-Noninear [NAL-NL1], or the Cambridge formula), or those that advocate a loudness normalization approach (e.g., desired sensation level [input/output] [DSL (i/o)], loudness growth in 1/2-octave bands [LGOB]) (Kuk, 2008). Regarding appropriateness of tube fittings with the advent of feedback suppression circuitry, the upper range of the hearing loss that can be fit with open-fit digital hearing aids will be defined by the severity (e.g., 70 to 80 dBHL in higher frequencies) and configuration (Valente & Valente, 2008). Auditory response area and level of impairment may affect the auditory benefits to be derived from hearing aids and can help the audiologist to explain what patients can and cannot expect from hearing aids. Prevalence of dead regions, or regions along the cochlea where inner hair cells may be extensively damaged or where neurons are functioning poorly, may be a consideration for the features (e.g., noise-reduction circuitry, directional microphones, frequency-modulated [FM] systems) to be recommended when fitting hearing aids and in determining candidacy for cochlear implants (Preminger, Carpenter, & Ziegler, 2005). Testing for cochlear "dead regions" also can help set realistic expectations, select frequencies to be amplified, and select the most appropriate features (e.g., digital noise reduction when low-frequency dead regions are present). This is a major consideration given that dead regions may be present in 25% of the adult clinical population with moderate to severe hearing loss, although the data are variable. Recently, Cox, Alexander, Johnson, and Rivera (2011a) found prevalence to be 31% among hearing-aid users in their sample who tested positive for dead regions of at least one frequency

(Preminger, et al, 2005). Vinay and Moore (2007), who reported a prevalence as high as 57%, recommend measuring dead regions in older adults in whom the hearing loss exceeds 60 dB HL at a frequency at or below 2000 Hz, as the findings may affect the frequencies to be amplified. While not standard procedure to measure dead regions, and despite the variability in the data on prevalence of dead regioins, when individuals perform poorer than expected in adverse listening situations when aided,clinicians may wish to consider a clinical measure such as the threshold equalizing noise (TEN) test for determining dead regions (Moore, Huss, Vickers, Glasberg, & Alcántara, 2000). The rational for performing the test is that some audiologists have speculated that high-frequency amplification may be contraindicated when dead regions are noted in individuals with high frequency thresholds poorer than 60dBHL (Cox et al, 2011a).

The speech-understanding problems experienced by older adults often have a central auditory or cognitive basis, and these deficits can compromise the benefit from hearing aids. Hence, part of the candidate selection process should include a speech test capable of identifying individuals with potential CAPD, and possibly a cognitive test of working memory, given the impact of working memory on decisions regarding selected hearing-aid features. In my view, all hearing-aid candidates should be screened for the presence of CAPD, especially experienced hearing-aid users who are finding their hearing aids ineffective. The ideal central auditory test for screening hearing-aid candidates remains elusive (e.g., dichotic sentence identification [DSI], synthetic sentence identification [SSI]), but most would agree it should be quick and easy to administer, it should tap into temporal deficits and dichotic listening, and it should be free of the confounding effects of mild to moderate peripheral hearing loss. Candidates' mental status should be screened using the Mini-Mental State Examination (MMSE), as the scores may have impact on the decision to recommend hearing aids, and function on the MMSE may be an important baseline against which to assess outcome.

Although the magnitude of benefit cannot be predicted from the severity of the hearing loss, the severity may contribute to our understanding of the nature or quality of benefit and may influence the choice of interventions to supplement hearing-aid use such as communication strategies and cognitive-based auditory training. Further, restoration of the ability to hear warning signals and environmental sounds is an important outcome for older adults with profound hearing loss. In contrast, enhanced speech understanding in quiet and noise might be the primary outcome for persons with mild to moderately severe hearing loss. Similarly, in the case of a high-frequency hearing loss, hearing aids using an open-fit and feedback suppression technology can effectively restore the audibility cues inherent in high-frequency consonant sounds contributing to improved understanding. For persons with a bilaterally symmetric hearing loss, binaural hearing aids will provide for more balanced hearing, improved localization ability, and ease of listening than will a monaural hearing aid (hearing aid worn in just one ear). Persons with cognitive deficits and CAPD may be expected to experience extreme difficulty understanding in less than optimal conditions as well as on the telephone.

Evidence is beginning to emerge that acceptance of background noise or acceptable noise level (ANL) is predictive of hearing-aid success (Cunningham & Friesen, 2005). ANL, defined as the difference between the most comfortable listening level for running speech and the maximum background noise level that the hearing-impaired listener is willing to accept, can be assessed in a sound field as part of the pre-fitting evaluation using a paradigm described by Nabelek, Frey-aldenhoven, Tampas, Burchfiel, & Muenchen (2006) and Cunningham & Friesen (2005). The ANL can be completed in 2 to 3 minutes using test materials (running speech, multi-talker babble) available at standard audiology clinics. These authors recommend that loudspeakers should be located at a 0- and 180-degree azimuth for presentation of the stimuli. The patient is asked to listen to recorded speech in a sound field and adjust it to a most comfortable listening level (MCL). Multi-talker babble is next introduced as background noise and the listener is asked to adjust the level to the highest level acceptable while still following the recorded speech (background noise level [BNL]). The ANL is calculated by subtracting the BNL from the MCL (MCL – BNL), so that the lower the ANL and the more noise the hearing-impaired client is willing to accept, the better the hearing-aid outcome in terms of hearing-aid use and satisfaction (Cunningham & Friesen, 2005). According to Cunningham and Friesen (2005) ANL does not vary with age or hearing-aid acclimatization, and high ANLs should not deter an audiologist from recommending hearing aids. With the advent of directional microphones and noise-reduction technology, audiologists are urged to measure ANLs to decide on hearing-aid features and possible recommendations for remote microphone HATs. Ahlstrom, Horwitz, and Dubno (2009) also found that hearing-aid users had more hearing-aid benefit based on ANL scores, in that they tolerated more babble aided than unaided, confirming the value of ANL measures in the hearing-aid fitting. Nabelek et al (2006) claim that they can predict hearing-aid use with 85% accuracy using the ANL, so audiologists are encouraged to include this simple test as part of the pre-fitting assessment. Nabelek et al suggest that patients with low ANLs (<7 dB) are likely to emerge as successful hearing-aid users, whereas patients with ANLs >13 dB are likely to become unsuccessful users wearing hearing aids only occasionally. Of course, persons having difficulty with background noise should be considered candidates for directional-microphone, noise-reduction technology, and auditory and communication strategies training.

While only 25% of audiologists routinely measure speech in noise measures prior to the hearing aid fitting, in my view it should be a routine part of the audiological evaluation/pre-fitting. I find the data essential for selection of features, to inform the counseling process, for determining client expectations, and for highlighting some of the speech-understanding difficulties attributable to hearing impairment. The clinician must determine which speech measures to use as part of the pre-fitting based on the goal of the test, and then proceed to identify the material and test protocol. Widely used tests of speech recognition in noise include the Connected Speech Test (CST), the Hearing-in-Noise Test (HINT), and the Quick Speech-in-Noise Test (QuickSIN). Using signal-to-noise ratio (SNR) as the metric, the QuickSIN provides an estimate of the patient's unaided intelligibility in noisy situations relative to quiet at various predetermined audible presentation levels. If the QuickSIN reveals a large SNR, this information will provide a basis for counseling regarding realistic hearing-aid expectations, communication strategies, and the necessary technology and features to recommend (Shi et al, 2007). The QuickSIN can be used to help provide objective evidence regarding candidacy for directional microphones and or an FM system.

The test metric for the HINT is the SNR as well. A bracketing procedure is used to determine the SNR that allows for 50% correct recognition of sentences. Taylor and Bernstein (2011) suggested using pre-fitting test results from the QuickSIN and the ANL to better understand the difficulties the patient is experiencing in noise and to use a matrix they developed to communicate the challenges. They described a four-quadrant matrix wherein they plot results from the QuickSIN and ANL tests, which can be used to help establish realistic expectations for hearing-aid use prior to the initial trial period with hearing aids. They developed the Red Flag Matrix to identify patients at risk for annoyance from noise or speech-understanding difficulties in noise so as to both counsel and select features to help ameliorate the difficulty. The four quadrants that emerged when plotting results of the ANL on the ordinate and QuickSIN results on the abscissa are as follows: (1) Q1, the lower left-hand corner, is the clear zone because unaided QuickSIN and ANL scores are in the near-normal or mild SNR loss range; (2) Q2, the upper left-hand corner is the at risk zone as patients in this quadrant have near normal or mild SNR loss QuickSIN scores and elevated ANL scores; (3 Q3, the upper right hand corner, is also an at risk zone for difficulty understanding in noise and with annoyance as they have significant SNR loss on the QuickSIN and significant ANL scores; and (4) Q4 in the lower right hand corner with patients in this quadrant having no measurable annoyance problems, but a significant SNR loss and would be considered at-risk for having difficulties with speech intelligibility in noise but evidence of sound annoyance problems (Taylor & Bernstein, 2011).

Evidence for my emphasis on more nontraditional speech testing (i.e., in noise, using sentence materials) lies in the cognitive psychology literature discussed in Chapter 3 and in the discussion in a later section on cognitive status to consider during the hearing-aid fitting. Auditory systems susceptible to the effects of aging are slower and more asynchronous than an intact auditory system, making listening in adverse conditions more cognitively demanding (Schneider & Pichora-Fuller, 2000). Accordingly, cochlear damage and possibly other age-related differences in auditory processing affect speech understanding both by reducing the amount of information coming through the perceptual channel and because effortful listening consumes cognitive resources that could otherwise be allocated to the storage of information in working memory (Pichora-Fuller, 2006; Pichora-Fuller, Schneider & Daneman, 1995; Wingfield & Stine-Morrow, 2000; Wingfield & Tun, 2001). In essence, the cognitive decrements that can be uncovered using speech tests simulating adverse listening conditions can tap into the reduced ability to remember what has been said, by providing a "noisier" signal for the brain to interpret.

Pearl

When counseling potential hearing-aid users, impairment data and results of speech tests should be used to help set realistic expectations. Hearing and speech measures are critical in decisions regarding hearing-aid candidacy for older adults with postlingual profound hearing loss who are not eligible for conventional amplification because of a limited auditory response area. These individuals should be made aware of findings suggesting that the prognosis for use of cochlear implants in the older adult population with bilateral severe to profound sensorineural hearing loss is impressive.

The problems that result from a hearing impairment are conceived of in terms of the extent of auditory difficulties experienced by the listener and are affected in part by the auditory demands of a given situation, environmental factors, and context (Hyde & Riko, 1994). The activity limitations and participation restrictions are best measured by a self-report approach in which the perception of communication abilities in a variety of daily listening situations and the consequences of the breakdowns are enumerated. The Abbreviated Profile of Hearing-Aid Benefit (APHAB) is widely used for assessing activity limitations. The Client-Oriented Scale of Improvement (COSI), a personalized inventory of unmet needs relative to the hearing loss and "met needs" relative to the hearing-aid intervention, is widely used for uncovering situational difficulties (Dillon, James, & Ginis, 1997; Gatehouse, 1999). The COSI is not a questionnaire; rather, the clinician acts as a facilitator while the patient identifies up to five situations perceived to be the most impacted by the hearing impairment. Persons with hearing loss are encouraged to cite emotional consequences of the hearing impairment as well (Abrams, 2009). In contrast, the Hearing Handicap Questionnaire (HHQ) (Gatehouse & Noble, 2004) is a 12-item questionnaire that measures hearing disability as defined by the International Classification of Impairments, Disabilities, and Handicaps (ICIDH-2) system (WHO, 2001). Total scores range from 12 to 60, with higher scores signifying greater disability. Finally, the Speech, Spatial, and Qualities of Hearing Scale (SSQ) developed by Gatehouse and Noble is a questionnaire designed to evaluate

the consequences of hearing impairment across three hearing domains: speech (e.g., "You are in a group of about five people in a busy restaurant. You can see everyone in the group. Can you follow the conversation?"); spatial (e.g., "Do you have the impression of sounds being exactly where you expect them to be?"); and qualities (e.g., "Do other people's voices sound clear and natural?"). There are a total of 43 questions, each requiring a response along a 10-point Likert scale. The anchors differ depending on the specific question. Although the SSQ evaluates domains not addressed by other hearing-specific questionnaires (i.e., spatial and quality attributes), the length of the SSQ and response task may present significant challenges to elderly patients (Abrams, 2009).

Similarly to activity limitations assessment, participation restrictions assessment, construed as the nonauditory problems resulting from diminished auditory capacity and the auditory demands of real-life situations, is also critical (Hyde & Riko, 1994). According to the ICIDH system, hearing impairment affects the patient, the family/caregiver, and often society. The Hearing Handicap Inventory for the Elderly (HHIE) and its companion version for spouses (HHIE-SP) can be of assistance in uncovering perceived emotional and social consequences (Ventry & Weinstein, 1982. Information on participation restrictions and activity limitations can be helpful in deciding on candidacy for a hearing aid and in counseling the candidate and family members regarding realistic expectations from hearing-aid use, and the score serves as a baseline against which to judge outcomes with hearing aids.

Many of the auditory pre-fitting considerations discussed in this section are incorporated in the Characteristics of Amplification Tool (COAT), a self-report pre-fitting tool developed by Sandridge and Newman (2006), who were concerned that the Hearing-Aid Selection Profile (HASP) was too lengthy to be used by clinicians in a busy clinical setting. The most recent version of the COAT (**Table 8.4**) includes 11 items that enable the audiologist to engage with the hearing impaired client to consider the listening needs, motivation, and aspects of hearing aids (e.g., style, level of technology, cost) that the client considers important. According to the instructions accompanying the COAT, persons with hearing impairment are asked to list three situations in which they feel they need hearing aids

Table 8.4 Items or Areas Included on the Characteristics of Amplification Tool (COAT)

1. Top three situations in which patient needs hearing aids
2. Rating of the importance the patient assigns to improved hearing
3. Rating of how motivated the patient is to wear and use hearing aids
4. Rating of expectations: how well patient thinks hearing aids will work
5. Rating in order of importance the factors the patient considers most important in the decision to buy hearing aids (e.g., cosmetic factors including visibility and size of hearing aid, audibility or improved ability to hear and understand, improved ability to understand in noise, and financial considerations regarding the cost of the hearing aid)
6. Preference as to how automatic the hearing aid should be (e.g., manual adjustment of volume control and programs or automatic adjustment)
7. Needs regarding cellular phone (e.g., Bluetooth compatible, T-coil)
8. Needs regarding use of iPod or personal music player with hearing aids
9. Preferences as to style of hearing aid, based on visual images provided by audiologist
10. Degree of self-efficacy ranging from low self-efficacy with little confidence in ability to succeed with hearing aids, to high self-efficacy and confidence in ability to succeed with hearing aids
11. Preferences as to price range for hearing aids ranging from a basic level hearing aid to a premium hearing aid

Source: Adapted from Sandridge, S., & Newman, C. (2006). *Improving the efficiency and accountability of the hearing aid selection process using the COAT.* Article archives www.audiologyonline.com.

the most; they are then asked to rate how important it is for them to hear better, and how motivated they are to use hearing aids. Expectations are assessed by asking how well they think modern hearing aids will work. Finally, they are asked to rank order the most important factors in their decision to buy hearing aids, such as the size of the unit, ability to hear and understand, understanding in noise, and the cost of hearing aid. The person with hearing loss is shown pictures of hearing aids ranging from entry-level, basic digital aids to premium digital aids with costs ranging from $1500 to $6000. Although not extensively validated, the items on the COAT can also serve as a checklist to ensure that the important auditory and non-auditory factors that figure into the fitting are addressed. **Figure 8.7** displays the images and template for the COAT.

Laplante-LeVesque et al (2012) conducted a comprehensive study of factors associated with hearing-aid uptake and hearing-aid outcomes in a sample of older adults with a median age of 69. Specifically, they explored the predictive value of a large variety of audiological and nonaudiological variables, including age, gender, living situation, education, application for subsidized hearing services, severity of hearing impairment, time since onset of hearing impairment, stage of change, self-reported hearing disability, locus of control, concerns about hearing-aid cost, and uptake of intervention services. Interestingly, those less likely to pursue an intervention had high communication self-efficacy and low socioeconomic status. Those more likely to pursue interventions were those eligible for subsidized hearing services and those who had higher contemplation scores in terms of the stages of change. Participants completing a communication program had higher socioeconomic status, which was associated with greater reduction in self-perceived disability on the HHQ. Further, higher initial self-reported hearing disability on the HHQ was associated with greater reduction in self-reported hearing disability for participants who obtained hearing aids and who completed communication programs. Interestingly, higher action-stage scores were associated with greater reduction in self-reported hearing disability on the HHQ for participants who completed communication programs. Notably, greater hearing disability perceived by others and by oneself was associated with better outcomes on the International Outcome Inventory (IOI), and a greater reduction in self-reported hearing disability based on HHQ scores was noted for participants who obtained hearing aids than in those participating in rehabilitation programs.

Significant intervention uptake predictors were (1) application for subsidized hearing services, (2) higher socioeconomic status, and (3) greater communication self-efficacy. Interestingly, socioeconomic status, initial self-reported hearing disability, stage of change, self-efficacy, locus of control, hearing disability as perceived by others, and perceived communication program effectiveness accounted for 10% to 52% of the variance in intervention outcome 3 months postintervention. Focusing on hearing-aid uptake and outcome, greater initial self-reported hearing disability as measured by the HHQ was associated with a more successful intervention outcome, be it hearing aids or participation in a communication programs. This finding corroborates previous studies that identified hearing disability as a predictor of hearing-aid outcomes using the APHAB and the (Cox & Alexander, 1995; Saunders, Lewis, & Forsline, 2009). This finding is predictable, as those initially

reporting hearing difficulties clearly have more benefit to derive from an intervention, having started at a higher baseline. Further, the fact that persons with greater communication self-efficacy were less likely to obtain hearing aids confirmed the findings of Cox, Alexander, and Gray (2005a), who speculated that individuals who have greater cognitive, social, and behavioral resources have successfully found alternative ways to cope with their hearing impairment. The fact that adults with hearing impairment in the contemplation or action stage of change were more likely to pursue an intervention is consistent with the principles set forth in the transtheoretical stages of change model (Prochaska, DiClemente, & Norcross, 1992). They are prepared to compare and contrast the barriers to the benefits of pursuing an intervention and tend to be ready for a change in behavior in favor of seeking help. Finally, the fact that positive attitudes toward hearing aids and fewer cost concerns emerged as predictors of hearing-aid uptake and outcome is consistent with the work of previous investigators.

> **Pearl**
>
> Whereas the degree of hearing impairment is not a significant predictor of intervention uptake and outcomes in adults with mild to moderate self-reported hearing disability, the contemplation and action stages of change emerged as the most robust predictors of outcomes with hearing aids and communication programs (Laplante-LeVesque et al, 2012).

Cox, Alexander, and Gray (2005b) compared self-report data between DVA patients and private payers (PPs) in terms of the role of self-report data in the pre-fitting and subsequent outcomes with hearing aids. Participants had gotten hearing aids from one of 11 audiology clinics around the country, of which five were located in a DVA setting, and the remaining six were PP clinics, with one being a university clinic. Of the 213 participants, the majority were veterans. Participants had mild to moderately severe bilateral sensorineural hearing loss, with the average age of the DVA sample being 72 years and of the PP participants 75 years; 59% were first-time hearing-aid users and the remainder previous hearing-aid users. All participants completed the four pre-fitting questionnaires including the Medical Outcomes Study (MOS) Short-Form Health Survey (SF-36), a 36-item questionnaire that measures self-reported health status; the Expected Consequences of Hearing-Aid Ownership (ECHO); the HHIE, which was the measure of participation restrictions; and the APHAB, which was the measure of activity limitations. All participants were fitted with programmable devices that had wide dynamic range compression, and whenever possible fittings were bilateral.

Following 3 weeks of hearing-aid use, post-fitting disablement and satisfaction were measured using the HHIE, the APHAB, the Shortened Hearing-Aid Performance Inventory (SHAPIE), the Satisfaction with Amplification in Daily Life (SADL), and the ECHO. Health status differed across the PP and DVA samples. In short, the DVA hearing-aid patients self-assessed their health to be poorer on the mental health and physical health components of the SF-36. Age was a factor, such that veterans, older than 74 years of age self-rated their physical health to be poorer than PP hearing-aid patients, and

Characteristics of Amplification Tool (COAT)

Name: _____   Date: _____

Audiologist: _____

Our goal is to maximize your ability to hear so that you can more easily communicate with others. In order to reach this goal, it is important that we understand your communication needs, your personal preferences, and your expectations. By having a better understanding of your needs, we can use our expertise to recommend the hearing aids that are most appropriate for **you**. By working together **we** will find the best solution for you.

Please complete the following questions. Be as honest as possible. Be as precise as possible. Thank you.

1.   Please list the top three situations where you would most like to hear better. Be as specific as possible.

_____

_____

_____

2.   How important is it for you to hear better? Mark an X on the line.

Not Very Important   --   *Very Important*

3.   How motivated are you to wear and use hearing aids? Mark an X on the line.

Not Very Motivated   --   *Very Motivated*

4.   How well do you think hearing aids will improve your hearing? Mark an X on the line.

I expect them to:

Not be helpful   --   *Greatly improve my*
at all   *hearing*

5.   What is your most important consideration regarding hearing aids? Rank order the following factors with **1** as the most important and **4** as the least important. Place an **X** on the line if the item has no importance to you at all.

_____   Hearing aid size and the ability of others not to see the hearing aids

_____   Improved ability to hear and understand speech

_____   Improved ability to understand speech in noisy situations (e.g., restaurants, parties)

_____   Cost of the hearing aids

6.   Do you prefer hearing aids that: (check one)

_____   are totally automatic so that you do not have to make any adjustments to them.
_____   allow you to adjust the volume and change the listening programs as you see fit.
_____   no preference

Fig. 8.7 The Characteristics of Amplification Tool (COAT). [From Valente, M., Dunn, H., & Roeser, R. (2008). *Audiology treatment*. New York: Thieme.]

on the mental health components, veterans between 65 and 74 years self-rated their mental health to be poorer than PP hearing-aid patients. Further, the veterans had higher overall expectations than did the PP hearing-aid patients, and experience and gender did not moderate this difference in overall expectations. Specifically, the veterans were more optimistic than were the PP hearing-aid patients regarding dispenser ability and the merits of hearing aids. Veterans perceived themselves to have more problems with participation restrictions based on absolute HHIE scores than did PP hearing-aid patients,

7.　Look at the pictures of the hearing aids. Please place an X on the picture or pictures of the style you would **NOT** be willing to use. Your audiologist will discuss with you if your choices are appropriate for you – given your hearing loss and physical shape of your ear.

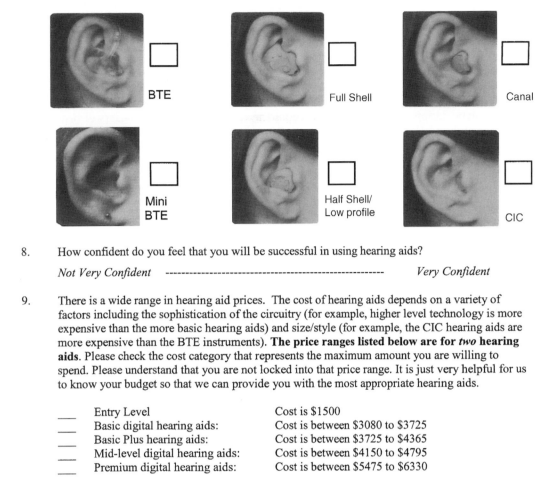

8.　How confident do you feel that you will be successful in using hearing aids?

Not Very Confident　---　*Very Confident*

9.　There is a wide range in hearing aid prices. The cost of hearing aids depends on a variety of factors including the sophistication of the circuitry (for example, higher level technology is more expensive than the more basic hearing aids) and size/style (for example, the CIC hearing aids are more expensive than the BTE instruments). **The price ranges listed below are for *two* hearing aids**. Please check the cost category that represents the maximum amount you are willing to spend. Please understand that you are not locked into that price range. It is just very helpful for us to know your budget so that we can provide you with the most appropriate hearing aids.

___	Entry Level	Cost is $1500
___	Basic digital hearing aids:	Cost is between $3080 to $3725
___	Basic Plus hearing aids:	Cost is between $3725 to $4365
___	Mid-level digital hearing aids:	Cost is between $4150 to $4795
___	Premium digital hearing aids:	Cost is between $5475 to $6330

Thank you for answering the questions.
Your responses will assist us in providing you with the best hearing healthcare.

Fig. 8.7　(*Continued*)

yet the only difference in terms of activity limitations in daily life was in the Background Noise subscale on the APHAB, where the veterans expressed more frequent problems.

Overall, the veterans and PP patients experienced significant benefit based on differences in pre- and post-fitting subscale scores on the HHIE and on the APHAB. Residual disablement was comparable across populations, and there were no differences between the groups in reported residual participation restrictions as measured on the HHIE and activity limitations as measured on the APHAB. Cox et al (2005b) calculated an overall benefit score, and differences emerged across PP and DVA hearing-aid users on the HHIE, wherein the DVA patients had higher mean benefit than the PP hearing-aid users. Again, gender was not a factor. As a positive effect, on the service and cost subscales of the SADL the veterans reported more satisfaction than did the PP patients. Finally, DVA and PP patients were comparable in terms of hearing-aid use time, which was about 8 hours per day. These findings shed light on some pre-fitting considerations. For example, the fact that PP patients were healthier suggests that hearing health may not be a priority for those paying out of pocket if they have competing health concerns. This underscores the importance of working with primary care physicians to screen for hearing loss in patients with comorbidities and to refer as appropriate, as managing hearing health status could improve quality of care and quality of life. The fact that DVA patients had higher expectations and overall were more satisfied suggested that audiologists in the private sector should make concerted efforts to counsel regarding expectations and perhaps should look to the DVA as a model for service delivery. An interesting finding which has implications for the pre-fitting is that the hearing aids of the PP patients had more high-tech features than did those of the DVA sample in that a higher proportion had digital processing and directional microphones, and the devices tended to be multi-channel. However, the PP patients did not emerge as experiencing as much absolute benefit as did the VA hearing-aid patients, and this may be due in part to poorer (higher) baseline scores in the VA population which is a consistent finding when using participants from a VA setting.

As part of a study of the role of pre-fitting counseling on hearing outcomes, Saunders et al (2009) explored the contribution of self-report data including pre-fitting expectations to hearing-aid benefit in a sample of older adults with a mean age of 69 to 70 years. Participants had mild to moderate sensorineural hearing loss typical of older adults seeking hearing-aid treatment and significant self-reported social and emotional handicap, but relatively few self-reported communication difficulties. A strong correlation between expectations as measured using the ECHO and benefit scores on the HHIE and the APHAB consistently emerged (Cox & Alexander, 2000), underscoring their role in the hearing-aid pre-fitting. Individuals whose aided benefit on the HHIE/Hearing Handicap Inventory for Adults [HHIA] exceeded the 95% critical differences (19 and 12, respectively) had significantly higher expectations scores than did those whose aided benefit did not exceed the 95% confidence differences (i.e. 95% CD refers to the change required to determine with 95% certainty that a true change in scores has occurred. This pattern emerged as well on the APHAB. Expectations were also related to satisfaction as measured using the SADL. Hence, self-report of expectations should accompany measurements of perceived activity limitations and participation restrictions.

The above studies confirm the findings of earlier investigators regarding the role of impairment and self-report data as pre-fitting considerations informing hearing-aid outcomes. Several investigators have explored the extent to which impairment versus self-report data inform decisions regarding hearing-aid candidacy. Newman, Jacobson, Hug, Weinstein, and Malinoff (1991) reported that in their sample of older adults, severity of hearing loss did not appear to affect benefit in the psychosocial domain. Specifically, persons with mild hearing loss derived the same amount of benefit from hearing aids as did individuals with severe hearing impairment. Benefit in their sample was defined according to the magnitude of reduction in self-perceived

hearing handicap following a short interval of hearing-aid use. Further, according to correlational analyses, hearing-aid benefit (difference between aided and unaided self-assessed psychosocial handicap) bears little relation to pure-tone hearing levels (Taylor, 1993). That is, pure-tone average (PTA) accounted for only a small proportion of the variability in psychosocial benefit. Swan and Gatehouse (1990) investigated factors that prompted individuals to seek audiological services. They noted that hearing-impaired individuals pursue hearing health care services because of self-perceived hearing disabilities and handicaps that often do not correspond to the degree of their hearing impairment. That is, most purchasers of hearing instruments are self-motivated because of communication problems (McCarthy, Montgomery, & Mueller, 1990).

Fino et al (1991) were among the first investigators to demonstrate that hearing-aid candidacy is directly linked to the pre-fitting score on a measure of self-perceived handicap, most notably the HHIE. Specifically, they found that the extent of self-perceived hearing handicap on the 10-item screening version of the HHIE (HHIE-S) is predictive of hearing-aid candidacy in that it reliably distinguishes between hearing-aid users and nonusers. At each hearing level category (e.g., mild, moderate, and moderately severe), persons who obtained hearing aids were more handicapped than those who did not. That is, of those with mild hearing loss, persons who obtained higher scores on the HHIE-S, indicative of greater self-perceived handicap, ultimately purchased a hearing aid (**Fig. 8.8**). Newman et al (1991) reported a link between handicap scores and hearing-aid use. They found that the average pre-fitting score on the HHIE-S was 18, irrespective of mean hearing level and mean word-recognition scores. Persons with mild and moderately severe hearing levels presented with comparable scores on the HHIE-S (i.e., 18). Similarly, persons with excellent and those with poor scores on a test of word recognition emerged with mean pre-fitting HHIE-S scores ranging from 16 to 18. **Figures 8.9 and 8.10** demonstrate the comparability of pre-fitting HHIE-S scores, irrespective of the severity of hearing loss or the severity of word-recognition problems. It is clear

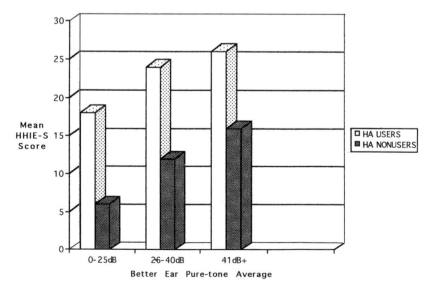

Fig. 8.8   Hearing Handicap Inventory for the Elderly, screening version (HHIE-S), scores as a function of hearing loss severity in hearing-aid (HA) users and nonusers. [From Fino, M., Bess, F., Lichtenstein, M., & Logan, S. (1991). Factors differentiating elderly hearing aid wearers and non-wearers. *Hearing Instruments, 43,* 6–10.]

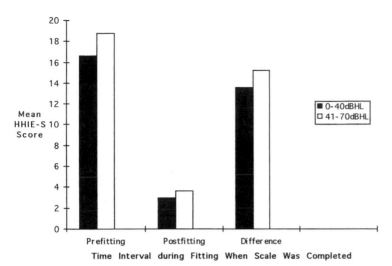

Fig. 8.9 Mean pre- and post-fitting HHIE-S scores on a sample of hearing-aid users with varying degrees of hearing loss (*N* = 91). Note: post-fitting took place 3 weeks after fitting. [From Newman, C. W., Jacobson, G. P., Hug, G. A., Weinstein, B. E., & Malinoff, R. L. (1991, Apr). Practical method for quantifying hearing aid benefit in older adults. *Journal of the American Academy of Audiology, 2*, 70–75.]

from the data of Newman and his colleagues and Fino and her colleagues that the degree of self-perceived hearing handicap is related to hearing-aid candidacy and uptake. Despite the emergence of data supporting the potential of self-assessment scales during the early stages of the rehabilitation process, most audiologists do not use formalized self-assessment inventories. As psychosocial factors explored through self-report scales help determine candidacy, rehabilitation programming, and benefit, especially with older adults, audiologists are encouraged to experiment with the large variety of tools available to the clinician (Cox & Alexander, 1999).

Special Consideration

Available findings suggest that self-reported handicap is predictive of hearing-aid benefit, yet most audiologists do not measure perceived handicap.

Physical Factors

The primary physical factors that may affect hearing-aid candidacy include vision status, manual dexterity, ear/ear canal variables, and overall health status. In general, the high prevalence of vision problems in older adults is an important factor in favor of pursuing amplification in the form of hearing aids, hearing assistance technologies (HATs), or a cochlear implant.

Vision Status

Pearl

Loss of one sense heightens the importance of the other senses to ensure an individual's safety and independence. Severity and nature of the vision problem should affect the choice of hearing-aid arrangement, hearing-aid style, and type of signal processing.

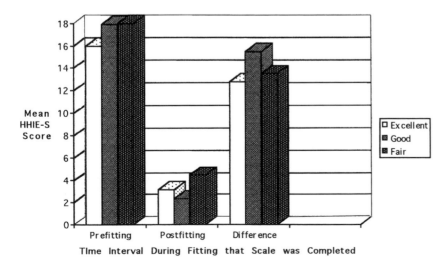

Fig. 8.10 Mean pre- and post-fitting HHIE-S scores on a sample of hearing-aid users as a function of word-recognition (*N* = 91). Note: post-fitting was 3 weeks following the fitting. [From Newman, C. W., Jacobson, G. P., Hug, G. A., Weinstein, B. E., & Malinoff, R. L. (1991, Apr). Practical method for quantifying hearing aid benefit in older adults. *Journal of the American Academy of Audiology, 2*, 70–75.]

The hearing-aid controls should be relatively visible, the wax loop and wax guards as easy as possible to maneuver, the hearing aid large enough to see and manipulate, and the battery size and battery door opening and locking should be as easy to see and deal with as possible. Older adults with vision impairment can benefit from hearing aids that are adaptive in terms of signal-processing capabilities; however, with regard to the "T-coil," an adaptive telecoil is not compatible with hearing loops and increasingly this is an important consideration. For older adults with low vision and manual dexterity problems, additional time should be spent during the hearing-aid orientation with special accommodations made to facilitate manipulation of the various controls. As discussed shortly, during the orientation the lighting should be adequate, and a magnifier available to help visualize the controls. When using visual speech mapping to review the audiogram and for hearing-aid verification, make sure that the computer monitor is visible and free of any glare and that contrast is set to optimize viewing. Given the importance of visual status, I recommend including a visual acuity measure of fine detail vision and of contrast sensitivity, which assesses the ability to detect edges under low-contrast conditions. Audiologists can adapt strategies to compensate for decrements in visual acuity and to provide edge-contrast sensitivity when orienting older adults to their hearing aid(s), HATs, or implantable devices. The fact that many older people do not wear glasses or wear glasses with outdated prescriptions and may not be aware of their declining vision underscores the importance of using visual aids during the orientation and of encouraging older adults to schedule an appointment with their eye-care provider, as this will promote successful use of amplification technologies and communication strategies (Lord, 2006).

Otological Considerations

The primary otological concerns that have impact on hearing-aid candidacy relate to conditions in the ear that may preclude hearing-aid use or may render a particular style or arrangement inappropriate. With regard to the outer ear, the presence of active infection, unusual growths, atresia, or stenosis of the external ear canal may influence the recommended options including consideration of a BAHA. If an ear has been surgically altered, a decision regarding the optimal way to proceed with the fitting should be made in consultation with a physician. Inability to obtain a sufficiently deep impression may contraindicate a completely-in-the-canal (CIC) hearing aid that must be custom made to fit and remain seated in the ear canal. A narrow canal may increase the likelihood that an open fit is the preferred option with attention paid to retention. Individuals with abnormal skin sensitivity in the area of the ear canal and persons experiencing excessive cerumen accumulation may not be candidates for the Lyric hearing aid. The balance between the skin lining the ear canal, the sebaceous oils, and the glands involved in the production of ear wax is affected in an unpredictable manner by age. Hence, older adults at risk for dermatological problems, wax blockage, and excessive wax buildup may be better suited for a receiver in the hearing aid rather than a receiver in the canal. With mini-BTEs, the domes and the tubing are prone to wax blockage and must be changed

Table 8.5 Medical Conditions Listed by the Food and Drug Administration (FDA) that Preclude Waiving Need for Medical Clearance in Persons 18+

1. Visible congenital or traumatic deformity of the ear
2. History of active drainage from the ear within the last 90 days
3. History of sudden or rapidly progressive hearing loss within the last 90 days
4. Acute or chronic dizziness
5. Unilateral hearing loss of sudden or recent onset within the previous 90 days
6. Audiometric air–bone gap equal to or greater than 15 dB at 500 Hz, 1000 Hz, and 2000 Hz
7. Visible evidence of earwax (cerumen) or any foreign body in the ear canal
8. Pain or discomfort in the ear

Note: Prospective user must sign a statement such as the one that follows: I have been advised by _____ _____ (Audiologist) that the Food and Drug Administration has determined that my best health interest would be served if I had a medical evaluation by a licensed physician (preferably a physician who specializes in diseases of the ear) before purchasing a hearing aid. I do not wish a medical evaluation before purchasing a hearing aid.

regularly. Replacing the domes and attaching securely must be emphasized and requires practice.

To make a determination regarding candidacy and the appropriateness of a particular style unit (e.g., the Lyric hearing aid), the audiologist must examine the shape and dimensions of the external canal to ensure compatibility with the features of the hearing aid. Older adults with the tendency toward excessive accumulation of cerumen should be acquainted with options for controlling cerumen so that it does not interfere with the operation of hearing instruments. Options include an adhesive wax guard positioned at the end of the hearing aid or mold, a wax stick to remove and replace the wax guard, or a brush and loop to clean the debris. As cerumen contamination compromises the reliability of hearing instruments (especially the Lyric and when selected wax guards are used), and hearing-instrument reliability relates to customer satisfaction, audiologists are urged to consider wax guards for older adults.

Middle ear problems such as active infection or persistent effusion may contraindicate hearing aid use. Patients should be fully informed about the recommendation for a medical examination to be sure that certain medical conditions are not present, but they can sign a waiver obviating the necessity for medical clearance, as required by the Food and Drug Administration (FDA). Any individual with significant warning signs or potential medical conditions must see a physician prior to the hearing-aid fitting. If any of the medical signs listed in **Table 8.5** are present, older adults should be referred to a physician rather than sign a medical clearance. According to FDA regulations, the audiologist must inform the user that exercise of the waiver is not in their best interest. Finally, older adults with significant medical problems such as diabetes or AIDS should receive medical clearance, for taking an earmold/hearing-aid impression can pose a problem in selected individuals at risk for infection.

Manual Dexterity

Although many features on today's digital hearing aids are adaptive, the miniaturization of hearing aids and their components is a challenge for many older adults. Specifically, older adults with manual dexterity problems, compromised wrist or finger mobility, reduced fine motor coordination, or diminished sense of touch or pain may have compromised function. Audiologists should attempt to ensure, prior to completing the sale, that the hearing-aid user or a partner or caregiver is able to manipulate, insert, remove, and adjust hearing-aid components. When deciding on hearing-aid candidacy, a dexterity check and an assessment of tactile sensation in the fingers can be helpful. Persons with hearing loss who because of a medical condition compromising sensory function lack sensation in the fingers may not be candidates for certain hearing-aid styles unless a partner or caregiver can be of assistance. Manual dexterity can be assessed formally using the Nine-Hole Pegboard Test, which evaluates fine-motor coordination and finger dexterity, or the Purdue Pegboard (manufactured by Lafayette Instrument Company), which measures gross movements of the hands, fingers, and arms as well as finger dexterity. Further, the Semmes-Weinstein Monofilaments Test can help to distinguish between light touch, diminished light touch, diminished protective sensation, loss of protective sensation, and deep pressure sensation. As clinical experience suggests that visual-motor coordination and touch recognition may affect successful use of amplification, audiologists are urged to experiment with the above measures. These tools are easily accessible through occupational or physical therapy departments or professionals. If formal measures of dexterity are not feasible, informal tests of wrist, hand, and finger motion and dexterity should be pursued. Watching an older adult attempt to remove and insert a wax guard and physically manipulate controls is an excellent informal screening test that will shed considerable light on fine hand function, including dexterity, range of motion, and strength. When assessing manual dexterity formally or informally, make sure the person with hearing loss uses the preferred or dominant hand to change/insert the battery.

Pearl

Older adults with arthritic or rheumatoid disorders, paralysis, or developmental disabilities are most prone to movement impairments that may interfere with hearing-aid manipulation, and thus may be more suitable candidates for HATs that have larger controls and can be manipulated independently.

Overall Health Status

Health-related quality of life (HRQOL) or the burden of chronic disease is gaining widespread acceptance as a factor to consider at the pre-fitting thanks to the work of investigators over the past 25 years. The SF-36 and the Sickness Impact Profile, a multidimensional indexes of generic quality of life, are widely used to assess the physical, emotional, and social dimensions of health (Chia et al, 2007). Using the SF-36 as their generic measure of HRQOL, Chia and colleagues assessed the impact of hearing impairment in a representative sample of community-based older adults living in Australia. All subjects underwent air- and bone-conduction testing and hearing handicap assessment, and they completed the SF-36. The average age of the

2431 participants was 67 years; 49% were male; 51% reported hearing problems (13% had unilateral hearing impairment, and 31% had bilateral hearing impairment); 33% owned hearing aids but only 26% reported habitually using them.

Overall, those with bilateral hearing impairment had lower SF-36 scores on each of the eight scales measuring the various dimensions of physical and mental health and social functioning than did those with unilateral hearing impairment or those without hearing impairment. Further, individuals with moderate to marked hearing loss had significantly poorer scores on the majority of dimensions of health measured and on the physical (PCS) and mental component scores (MCS). The dimensions of health on which those with moderate to marked hearing impairment had the poorest scores were in the sections measuring role limitations due to physical or emotional problems. Individuals with hearing loss across the frequencies were more disadvantaged than persons without hearing impairment and persons with high-frequency hearing loss. Interestingly, those with self-reported hearing problems had lower scores on the SF-36 than did those persons who did not report hearing problems. Further, means scores on the PCS and MCS were significantly lower in persons with self-reported hearing problems as compared with those without self-reported hearing problems. Finally, there was a trend for subjects who habitually used their hearing aids (26% of the sample) to have slightly better mean scores on the SF-36 than did those who did not own or use hearing aids, after adjusting for level of bilateral hearing impairment. The greatest difference in scores on the SF-36 between those who used hearing aids and those who did not emerged on the scales that assessed physical functioning and role limitations due to physical problems—dimensions contained in the PCS.

These findings support those of Dalton et al (2003), who found that scores on the PCS, MCS and on seven of the eight domains of physical and mental status correlated with increasingly severe hearing impairments. They also found that older adults with moderate to severe hearing loss were more likely than individuals without hearing loss to have impaired activities of daily living (ADL) and instrumental ADL. Chia and colleagues (2007) concluded that bilateral hearing impairment has an adverse effect on the social (e.g., intimate relationships, familial relations) and physical (e.g., managing medications, getting outside) domains of function and underscored that in light of the comorbidity of hearing impairment, physical conditions, and social issues, HRQOL must be considered in the design and implementation of therapeutic interventions. They suggested that given the differential relationship among self-reported hearing problems, measured hearing impairment, and SF-36 scores, it behooves audiologists to quantify and weigh all three domains of function when conducting hearing-aid fittings.

Pearl

Severe hearing loss has a significant association with decreased function in the mental and physical component scores of the SF-36 (Dalton et al, 2003).

The work of Chia and colleagues confirmed the data of Bess, Lichtenstein, Logan, Burger, and Nelson (1989), who were among the first investigators to relate HRQOL, otherwise known as functional health status, including poor general health, reduced mobility, and reduced interpersonal communication, to degree of hearing handicap, hearing impairment and hearing-aid candidacy. The mean scores on a measure of physical functional status, such as the Sickness Impact Profile (SIP), increased from 3.3 for older adults with no impairment to 18.9 among those with a hearing impairment in the better ear of 40 dB HL or more. When physical functional status appears to be reduced and independence is potentially compromised, the contribution of hearing status to the individual's condition should be considered and the possibility of audiological intervention pursued. In short, how a potential hearing-aid user scores in terms of sickness-related dysfunction can inform the decision to proceed with some form of hearing technology.

Dementia is a general term for mental deterioration that includes loss of memory and intellectual functioning. As discussed in previous chapters, it is a relatively common syndrome among older adults, and hearing impairment does appear to increase the likelihood of incident dementia. Although for some individuals dementia stands out as a health problem that may preclude successful hearing-aid candidacy, for selected individuals hearing aids or HATs, depending on the severity of the decline, have the potential to help maintain the residual assets/strengths and relieve emotional distress. In general, the more severe the dementing illness, the greater the cognitive decline and the less likely the individual is to use the hearing aid successfully. Persons with severe dementing illness are unlikely to be able to learn how to use new technology such as hearing aids and may refuse placement of hearing aids in their ears. For example, persons with more advanced stages of dementia may (1) have difficulty locating their head to position the unit in the ear, (2) be unable to maintain and adjust the hearing aid, (3) be unable to position and reposition the hearing aid, and (4) be confused by the amplified noise. Experienced hearing-aid users with advanced dementia are more likely to adjust and benefit from amplification than are new hearing-aid users with comparable degrees of dementing illness. For individuals who are not candidates for hearing aids, smartphone apps (e.g. FiRe, soundAMP R) HATs, especially hard-wired systems, should be considered especially for the homebound or persons in nursing homes. HATs promote communication among family members, can be used by physicians to aid in reaching a valid diagnosis of dementia, and can be used by nurses or social workers when conducting intakes. Alerting devices in the home are particularly important for this population, especially for persons who do not use hearing aids yet present with moderate to severe hearing loss. The use of these devices can help to optimize home safety. It is advisable that hearing-aid candidates complete a brief screening test of their cognitive abilities using the MMSE, which assesses orientation, word recall, attention and calculation, language abilities, and visuospatial ability (Folstein, Folstein, & McHugh, 1975). On the MMSE, scores in excess of 25 are traditionally considered normal, and scores less than 10 are indicative of severe impairment. Scores can inform decisions regarding choice of intervention and have potential as a benchmark against which to judge the impact of intervention on one' cognitive function.

> **Pearl**
>
> The audiologist is encouraged to explore the patient's mental status thoroughly prior to making a recommendation for a particular hearing technology and to monitor memory and cognitive function should a hearing aid be pursued.

Psychological Variables: Cognitive Status, Expectations, and Motivational Level

The psychological variables that have been identified by practitioners as potential determinants of hearing-aid candidacy and benefit include personality attributes, motivational level of the patient and caregiver, cognitive status, self-efficacy, coping strategies, expectations, and locus of control. Cox, Alexander, and Gray (2007) suggested that personality is in fact associated with outcome data obtained using selected self-report scales shedding light on an important role in the pre-fitting. They followed 205 hearing-aid users through their 6-month follow-up to ascertain how personality modulates hearing-aid outcomes. Participants in their study were individuals attending one of 11 audiology clinics around the country for the purpose of obtaining hearing aids; 139 of the subjects came from DVA clinics and 66 from non-DVA clinics. The average age of the men participating was 73 years, and that of women 75 years; and 42% of subjects were experienced hearing-aid users. Personality was assessed using the NEO Five-Factor Inventory (neuroticism, extraversion, and openness to experience [NEO]-FFI), which is a 60-item questionnaire that provides a measure of five personality traits: neuroticism, extraversion, openness, agreeableness, and conscientiousness. Expectations for the hearing-aid fitting were quantified using the ECHO scale developed by Cox and Alexander (2000). Finally, hearing-aid satisfaction was measured using the SADL, which quantifies satisfaction with aspects of the hearing-aid fitting including cost and competence of the audiologist (McCarthy & Schau, 2008).

Some interesting trends emerged, including the finding of a significant association between sound aversiveness and four of the five personality traits quantified using the NEO-FFI. As would be expected, those individuals whose neuroticism scores were higher were more likely to have a negative reaction to environmental sounds. In contrast, those whose scores were higher in extraversion, openness, and agreeableness were less likely to report that environmental sounds were unpleasant. This finding confirms that of Kochkin's (2007) who found that a major obstacle to hearing-aid adoption is that aids amplify background noise. Another rather interesting finding was that neuroticism accounted for 21% of the variance in scores on the HHIE, suggesting that higher neuroticism was associated with more participation restrictions or greater "hearing disablement." Neuroticism also accounted for 11% of the variance in scores on the sections of the APHAB, which measures activity limitations, and for 14% of the variance in responses to the aversiveness of environmental sound section of the APHAB. Personality did not relate to scores on the ECHO. Personality traits derived from the NEO-FFI and scores on the ECHO did not relate to any of the hearing-aid–fitting variables (e.g., soft sound audibility, match to target gain for conversational speech). Interestingly, the extent of the residual disability based on absolute scores on self-report measures after a period of hearing-aid use showed a pattern of association with both neuroticism and extraversion. Thus, for example, neuroticism and extraversion accounted for a significant proportion of the variability in aided scores on the HHIE, on global scores on the aided APHAB, and on scores on the sound aversiveness scale of the APHAB. The personal image (PI) scale of the SADL was the only satisfaction index that related to neuroticism, extraversion, agreeableness, and openness, suggesting that how hearing-aid users believe they are perceived by others does in fact relate to basic personality attributes. The relationship between selected personality attributes and residual disability (e.g., the difficulties that remain after 6 months of hearing-aid use) underscores the value of patient-specific or device-related counseling to help the patient better adapt to hearing-aid use.

The primary findings from the study by Cox et al (2007) relate to the pinpointing of pre-fitting variables that correlate with hearing-aid outcomes and to documentation that hearing-related self-report or patient-based variables are the most powerful predictors of outcome. Specifically, pre-fitting expectations were strongly related to device-related outcomes (such as overall satisfaction with the hearing aid, and feeling that it is worth the trouble and the cost), unaided HHIE scores accounted for 43% of the variability in the success component of outcome (no feelings of frustration and annoyance), and sound aversiveness and rating of degree of unaided difficulty accounted for 20% of variance in the acceptance component of outcome (not having difficulty in noise situations). In light of this finding, direct assessment of personality variables may not be necessary as long as practitioners administer self-report scales that correlate with patient personality attributes.

Cox et al (2005a) explored the personality of older adults seeking hearing aids, in an attempt to understand factors beyond those that are accepted (e.g., greater hearing loss, greater self-reported disablement associated with a given impairment) as contributing to decision making. Participants purchased hearing aids from a variety of clinics including five DVA medical centers and five private practice clinics. Average age of the DVA sample was 72 years, and average age of those purchasing hearing aids from the private practice clinics was 75 years; 59% of participants were acquiring hearing aids for the first time, whereas 41% were previous hearing-aid users. The personality of participants was assessed using the NEO-FFI. Participants also completed the Locus of Control (LOC) measure and the Coping Strategy Indicator, a 33-item scale that quantifies strategies for coping with stressful situations based on performance on three scales: problem-solving ability, support seeking, and avoidance.

Personality as defined by scores on the NEO-FFI did not relate to severity of hearing loss. Interestingly, new and experienced hearing-aid users did not differ in terms of personality traits; however, hearing-aid seekers displayed lower neuroticism and openness scores than the general adult population based on normative data on the NEO-FFI. The authors found that individuals who score low in openness are more conventional and cautious than are those who score high. Hence, they speculated, it is possible that these patients chose amplification because they have not been successful in formulating

strategies for compensating for the "disablement" associated with mild to moderately severe hearing loss. Further, hearing-aid seekers obtained higher scores than the general older adult population in their belief system regarding internal control as measured on the LOC scale. That is, they felt they were responsible for what happens to them and saw the need to take control of the situation to achieve a given outcome. Most interesting was the finding that hearing-aid seekers scored lower than the general population on all three scales that measure strategies for coping with stressful circumstances. For example, hearing-aid seekers reported less use of problem-solving coping strategies, less use of social supports for coping, and less use of avoidance coping than did the general elderly population. The fact that hearing-aid seekers use these three coping strategies less often than does the general older population suggests that we must emphasize these strategies during communication strategies training and counseling with hearing-aid users and their communication partners.

Saunders et al (2009) explored the link between pre-fitting counseling regarding expectations and hearing-aid outcome, given evidence that suggests that preconceived notions regarding hearing aids affect the hearing-aid use experience. Mean hearing levels of participants were consistent with a mild to moderately severe sloping bilateral loss. All subjects were new hearing-aid users who were ultimately fit with binaural digital hearing aids. The mean age of participants was 70 years, and the mean three-frequency PTA was 38 dB HL. Participants had considerable psychosocial handicap because of their hearing loss but minimal communication difficulties based on self-reports. The counseling offered was traditional, which included verbal discussion of what to expect from hearing aids in terms of listening difficulties in adverse listening situations, and in terms of benefits to be expected in quiet situations. Counseling entailed verbal discussion combined with auditory demonstration of real-world listening situations. The authors administered the ECHO to assess the expected hearing-aid outcomes, and the Psychosocial Impact of Assistive Devices Scale (PIADS) developed by Day, Jutai, and Campbell (2002) to assess competence with hearing aids, self-esteem, and adaptability.

The results were remarkable in that between 18% and 28% of the variance in aided response scores on the APHAB and SADL were accounted for by pre-fitting expectations. Further, those subjects who experienced significant benefit had higher expectation scores regarding psychosocial outcomes than did those in the low-benefit group. A similar trend was noted using the APHAB as the outcome measure, such that those participants experiencing high benefit had high expectation scores in terms of psychosocial outcomes. Expectations of this sample of new hearing-aid users were rather high from the outset, unrealistically so for hearing-related outcomes, according to the authors. The pre-fitting hearing-aid counseling regarding potential difficulties in adverse listening situations and benefit in quiet situations did alter expectations regarding listening in background noise and in adverse conditions. Thus, approaching the hearing-aid fitting with positive expectations for improvements in quality of life and psychosocial well-being yields better outcomes. Further, there is a relationship among pre-fitting expectations of quality-of-life improvement, self-image and outcomes. The authors also concluded that unrealistic expectations regarding hearing-aid outcomes

I am successful in this situation...

Goal (list in order of priority)	Hardly Ever	Occasionally	Half the Time	Most of the Time	Almost Always
1.					
2.					
3.					
4.					
5.					

C = how the client functions currently (pretreatment or with current technology/strategies)

E = how the client expects to function post intervention (HA, ALD, strategies, etc.)

√ = level of success that the audiologist realistically targets

A = how the client/family actually perceives level of success postfitting

Fig. 8.11 Patient Expectation Worksheet (PEW). [From Valente, M., Dunn, H., & Roeser, R. (2008). *Audiology treatment*. New York: Thieme.]

should be addressed at the pre-fitting in such a way that the patient remains motivated to try hearing aids despite possible shortcomings.

Palmer, Lindley, and Mormer (2008) described the Patient Expectation Worksheet (PEW), which is similar to the COSI and is quite easy to use. As shown in **Fig. 8.11**, the patient rates the current level of hearing ability unaided (C), the expected level of ability following intervention (E), and the actual level of difficulty post hearing aid fitting (A). The clinician then discusses with the patient realistic expectations regarding functioning in selected listening conditions, given the audiometric data and the technology options. Using the PEW at the pre-fitting assists the patient in forming realistic expectations and can help the patient decide on fitting options. Some general suggestions for helping the patient hone in on situational needs include demonstrating performance in quiet versus noise, the audibility of soft and loud sounds, audibility of environmental sounds, and intelligibility of media including television and cellular phones.

> **Pearl**
>
> Higher psychosocial expectations result in better outcomes (Saunders et al, 2009).

Cognitive Status

Cognitive status is an increasingly important factor to consider in the fitting of hearing aids especially for older adults who experience considerable difficulty in complex listening environments, where a variety of cognitive resources are enlisted to disambiguate the message. For purposes of this discussion, cognitive processing refers to how people acquire, store, manipulate, and use information. It involves listening, compre-

hending, remembering what has been heard, and communicating. The storage and processing resources in complex working memory function or the ability of the brain to hold and manipulate information in immediate memory (recall of complex sentences, repeating a list of words while holding other information in memory) is what affects hearing-aid success to a considerable degree (Rudner, Foo, Rönnberg, & Lunner, 2007). Working memory entails attending, inhibiting, storing, planning, and manipulating information, and it includes dual-processing schemata, namely auditory and visual working memory with each having a limited capacity (Mayer & Moreno, 1996). Individuals must retain relevant information in each working memory storage bin, as the bins are independent of each other, and must make connections between the information in each storage bin to process speech input, which typically makes use of auditory and visual modalities. Lunner (2010) suggests that auditory working memory for speech understanding involves a phonological loop responsible for the manipulation of speech-based information and a visuospatial sketchpad responsible for manipulating visual images. The phonological loop holds speech-based input in memory for 1 to 2 seconds. The sketchpad displays and manipulates information held in long-term memory.

As regards speech perception, working memory holds information that is derived from sensory inputs (auditory and visual) and information that has been represented and retrieved in long-term memory (phonological and semantic) (Baddeley, 1986). To understand speech, we must be able to recognize the speech input (phonological loop) and integrate it with previously learned words and with stored knowledge of semantics, the lexicon, phonology, and syntax. When the capacity limits of working memory are exceeded, because perhaps processing is too demanding, as in complex listening environments, understanding will be compromised as working memory becomes overloaded. As processing becomes more effortful, the system slows down (Pichora-Fuller, 2003). The working memory system is especially taxed when the speech signal is degraded either by an impairment or by external distortions such as noise or reverberation. For these reasons, assessment of working memory is an important part of the pre-fitting.

> **Pearl**
>
> Signal processing features that are designed to improve speech understanding may have both positive and negative consequences, with the effects depending in part on individual working memory capacity (Lunner, Rudner, & Rönnberg, 2009).

The major complaint of hearing-aid users is that they often miss information in acoustically demanding everyday listening environments. They find that they must guess and fill in words in order to interpret the message correctly. This cognitively demanding processing task, and the effectiveness with which individuals function, is dependent on working memory capacity and verbal information-processing speed. That is, because cochlear damage indirectly draws resources from working memory in effortful listening situations, the listener's overall working memory capacity will likely affect auditory performance indirectly (Lunner, 2003). Tests of working memory and executive function, wherein individuals are asked to shift attention from one speaker to another, challenges working memory and executive function, and can inform our understanding of how older adults function in adverse listening conditions (Rudner, Rönnberg, & Lunner, 2011). According to studies in cognitive psychology, working memory resources are considerably challenged when the auditory input is degraded and when persons with hearing loss are communicating in challenging and complex listening environments. Hearing loss introduces distortions into the sound input, and older adults with age-related hearing loss [ARHL] have to devote working memory resources to understanding speech when they are focusing on too many things at once (e.g., target message in the presence of multiple speakers) or when they are distracted by informational maskers (Lunner, 2010). For some, speech perception in noise will not decline with age if cognitive capacity is maintained, yet for others it will, and for hearing-aid–fitting audiologists should measure cognitive capacity, as clients with low cognitive capacity will have unique needs.

> **Pearl**
>
> Working memory is active storage used to hold information that is being manipulated. It is important for speech understanding in noise, as it sheds light on how people cope with different types of noise. Working memory is important in modulated noise and in unfavorable SNR unaided or with fast-acting compression (Rudner et al, 2011).

Our goal is to find the appropriate hearing aid for an older adult that will introduce as few distortions as possible. We know that hearing aids with nonlinear signal-processing schemes (e.g., gain regulation systems using wide dynamic range compression) may distort the input by insufficiently amplifying weak speech sounds that perhaps may contain important cues for understanding. We know that slow hearing instrument settings give less distortion of the speech signal than do fast settings, thus allowing better opportunity for phonological analysis or matching of the input with that which is represented in long-term memory (Lunner, 2010). Lunner (2003) found direct evidence to suggest a relatively robust correlation ($r = -0.61$) between performance on the reading span test (a test of working memory) and aided speech understanding in noise using the HINT. In part the reason for the shared variance is that, like speech-in-noise testing, the reading span test is a dual task that taps parallel memory storage and semantic processing capacity (Foo, Rudner, Rönnberg, & Lunner 2007). Presenting words in the presence of noise modulation is the best way to uncover the link to working memory, as this type of noise is designed to simulate real-life conversational interference of speech recognition with noise level variation throughout testing, such that some words are obscured by noise and other words are not and can be clearly perceived. When simultaneous storage and processing abilities are low, as indicated by poor performance on the reading span test, the ability to cope with a fast hearing instrument setting is also low; when the hearing instrument setting is fast, the speech signal is distorted, which places further strain on semantic processing.

> **Pearl**
>
> Cognitive slowing and age-related memory constraints are of special importance for auditory performance in elderly adults (Wingfield, 1996). Cognitive factors (e.g., effective use of linguistic context) can both enhance and limit auditory performance (Pichora-Fuller, 2003; Pichora-Fuller et al, 1995).

Motivation and Stage of Readiness

Motivation and stage of readiness are among the most important variables that affect adaptation to disability, rehabilitation candidacy, and rehabilitative potential (Kemp, 1990). They explain why behavior is initiated, why behavior persists, and why behavior is attenuated. These psychological processes influence an older adult's resolve regarding hearing-aid use. Specifically, motivation is a multivariate process that refers to self-directed behavior. It is defined by the perception of (1) what one wants from an intervention, (2) what one expects or believes can be achieved with a given intervention, (3) the relevance of the rewards associated with a given intervention, and (4) associated costs of pursuing an intervention (Kemp, 1990). Motivation to pursue intervention is optimal when people know what they want, expect it can be attained, and believe that the rewards are meaningful and occur at a reasonable cost.

Motivation influences one's capacity to overcome adversity, and one's desire to participate in social activities and to improve function (Kemp, 1990). One of the greatest challenges to a dispensing audiologist is determining motivational level and then motivating an older adult to purchase and use hearing aids. The aging process affects one's motivational level espe-

Table 8.6 Basic Questions Regarding Stage of Readiness for Hearing Intervention and Possible Recommendations

Please check the statement that best describes your perspective:
1. I do not think I have a hearing problem, and therefore nothing should be done about it. (If checked, audiologist should recommend an annual evaluation.)
2. I think I have a hearing problem. However, I am not yet ready to take any action to solve the problem, but I might do so in the future. (If checked, audiologist should recommend hearing-assistance technology.)
3. I know I have a hearing problem, and I intend to take action to solve it soon. (If checked, audiologist should recommend hearing aids.)
4. I know I have a hearing problem, and I am here to take action to solve it now. (If checked, audiologist should recommend hearing aids.)

cially as regards the purchase of rehabilitation services. Some of the age-related changes that may inhibit one's motivational level for pursuing amplification include the desire to maintain the status quo, fear of risk taking, and fear of failure. It is incumbent on the audiologist to recognize those variables that undermine an individual's motivation to pursue audiological rehabilitation, and to counsel the older adult regarding these fears and concerns. An understanding of motivational dynamics, as described in Chapter 7, can help the audiologist to ensure that lack of motivation does not preclude hearing-aid use and benefit. Often some motivational counseling at the time of the audiological evaluation or the pre-fitting will be necessary to convince a person with hearing impairment of the value of hearing aids. When motivating older adults to pursue amplification, it is important to instill realistic expectations, as often client expectations are unreasonably high, thus interfering with success (Schum, 1999). Asking basic questions during the hearing-aid fitting regarding stage of readiness can help the audiologist assess motivation, and can inform decisions regarding targeted interventions. A sample set of questions is listed in **Table 8.6**.

Sociological Variables

The primary sociological variables to be considered when selecting candidates for hearing aids include lifestyle, familial support, life events, and financial factors. One's lifestyle (e.g., engagement in physical activities, social interaction, and work-related activities) and the environment in which the individual functions must be explored prior to making any decisions regarding intervention. This exploration will help in the selection of a device that will optimize communication in the individual's specific social environments. In addition to impacting on a decision about candidacy, an appreciation of the physical and social environment and life events may affect decisions regarding hearing-aid style, hearing-aid features, hours of hearing-aid use, and need for hearing assistance technologies to supplement the hearing aid. The audiologist should explore lifestyle from the perspective of the hearing-impaired individual and should seek input from communication partners and formal caregivers. If responses to a formal or informal interview reveal that the individual has a limited social network, then the advantages of part-time hearing-aid use should be discussed, the advantages of early intervention emphasized, and HATs considered.

Kricos et al (2007) explored the link between life events, assessed using a checklist that quantified them, and hearing-aid adjustment in a sample of adult hearing-aid users and non-

users with a mean age of 73.2 years. Interestingly, different life events emerged as decisive in the decision to buy hearing aids. Some of the factors that were influential in the decision to seek amplification included a new life experience, such as change in hearing, the desire to hear people better, the birth of a grandchild, and a new marriage, whereas factors that deterred people from using hearing aids included change in job status, death of a spouse or partner, and the need for increased dependence or assistance in performing ADL. The authors concluded that major lifestyle changes or losses (e.g., retirement, death of a spouse) and increased dependence had more of a negative impact on hearing-aid use than did health-related life events. The findings that motivation to hear better (e.g., desire to understand others better) increased hearing-aid use among respondents, whereas loss or malfunction of a hearing aid discouraged hearing-aid use, have implications for candidacy.

> **Pearl**
>
> When appropriate, part-time hearing-aid use should not be discouraged, as ultimately new users gradually come to understand the benefit of hearing aids and increase their use to include several listening situations.

Availability of familial support will influence the appropriateness of hearing aids and the sophistication of hearing aids recommended. For example, if an individual is relatively independent and does not wish to rely on a family member or a formal caregiver for hearing-aid insertion or operation, then a hearing aid that is easier to insert and manipulate is appropriate (e.g., some people think in-the-ear units are easier to insert as there are fewer steps involved). With regard to financial factors, a recent study by Ramachandran, Stach, and Becker (2011) sheds some new light on why this variable is important. They demonstrated that full insurance coverage for bilateral hearing aids does play a significant role in the decision to purchase hearing aids. Interestingly, the average age at which hearing aids are purchased is younger and the hearing level at which persons will acquire hearing aids tends to better for those with full-coverage. Hence, it is important to explore possible third-party coverage, as some individuals may not be aware of what their health insurance covers. Interestingly, inability to pay for a hearing aid does not affect benefit and thus should not affect candidacy (Newman, Hug, Wharton, & Jacobson, 1993). Hearing-aid candidates should understand that persons who pay for hearing aids and those who obtain third-party coverage appear to derive comparable benefit based on improvement in perceived psychosocial handicap. Thus, rather than determining candidacy, financial factors may influence decisions regarding the style of hearing aid to purchase, the fitting arrangement, and the technological sophistication of the recommended unit.

Environmental Factors

According to the ICIDH classification system, one's environment and the context in which one lives will influence adaptation to the communication deficit and the intervention to be pursued. Older persons with a significant hearing impairment who live alone are ideal candidates for either hearing aid(s) or HATs because of the threat to safety and security posed by unremediated hearing loss. The audiologist must explore with them and their communication partner their needs relative to their environment, as this will inform the decisions to be made. Typically, homebound older adults do not see the importance of hearing alerting signals when living alone, nor do they care if the television volume is high. The art of counseling is very relevant in these situations, as once the difficulties are uncovered, the audiologist and person with hearing impairment can work together to decide on targeted solutions. It is important that older adults understand the threat to safety posed by an unremediated hearing loss, including inability to hear the smoke alarm, the fire alarm, the doorbell, or a burglar. They should be counseled about the importance of hearing technologies to alert them to potential danger in the physical environment.

Older adults who ultimately do purchase hearing aid(s) should be encouraged to wear them at home, especially when alone, to ensure that they can hear warning signals. A recent home visit demonstrated to me how important this is. Thus, during the pre-fitting stage, audiologists should consider visiting homebound individuals or people who live alone. For older adults who are active and not "technophobic," wireless streamers (e.g for use with TV and telephone) available as proprietary accessories for hearing aids can be invaluable in the home. Wireless functionality (e.g., pairing a streamer with a phone box or an iPod) enhances the experience of talking on the telephone (wireless or landline), watching television, listening to music, or using a computer. Using a remote microphone in the home when family members visit ensures that older adults are part of the conversation. According to anecdotal reports, while streamers are costly, "connectivity" adds to the quality of life of many hearing-aid users. The manufacturer sites have excellent videos of how the different wireless accessories interface with telephones and a range of entertainment systems and audio sources. Note that some of the remote controls and digital wireless accessories require manual dexterity, so user friendliness should be a priority. Be sure to consider the home environment, lifestyle, and physical variables when making recommendations.

In summary, a host of audiological and nonaudiological variables combine to determine candidacy and feasibility of hearing-aid use, and feature selection. The audiologist must be mindful of all variables that will determine the appropriateness of a given intervention to ensure satisfaction, benefit, and improved quality of life.

◆ Considerations in the Hearing-Aid Fitting Process

After completing the pre-fitting process, which entailed identifying the candidate for a hearing aid and documenting the person's audiological profile and communicative needs, the next step is the hearing-aid fitting. The goal here is to collaborate with the patient to identify the hearing-aid style and features that will meet the electroacoustic, physical, communication, and cosmetic needs of the patient.

The purpose of the fitting is to identify the most appropriate hearing-aid style or type of technology, and to determine the electroacoustic characteristics most likely to optimize performance. Persons with hearing loss want a hearing aid that provides physical comfort; makes soft sounds audible, loud sounds comfortable, and speech intelligible in quiet and in adverse listening situations; and meets their communication needs and expectations (Palmer et al, 2008). Audiologists rely on prescriptive strategies designed to restore normal loudness across frequency bands using either a loudness normalization or a loudness equalization rationale, yet the audiologist must ensure that the settings meet the real-world needs of the person with hearing impairment. Although the various prescriptive strategies share similar goals—(1) maximize audibility, (2) make some degree of speech audible without exceeding the listener's loudness discomfort level, (3) restore the normal loudness relations for speech and other environmental sounds, (4) improve speech recognition, (5) provide good sound quality, and (6) allow for natural sound to the users voice—the extent to which a particular strategy optimizes communication and reduces activity limitations and participation restrictions remains unknown, thus underlining the importance of verification and validation of the fitting (Blamey & Martin, 2009; Cox, 1995). Further, first-time users versus experienced users and cognitive and auditory status are critical considerations, and data from field and laboratory measures are integral to the fitting process (Smeds, 2004).

Prescriptive fitting of digital hearing aids using preexisting algorithms to determine soft sound audibility, to match to target gain for conversational speech, and to determine the appropriateness of output remains an important part of the programming and verification process (Cox et al, 2007; Ricketts & Mueller, 2009). According to best practices fitting guidelines, clinicians should use a validated prescriptive fitting method as a starting point for decisions about gain and output and as part of the verification process (Ricketts & Mueller, 2009). The most popular fitting strategies include the desired sensation level (input/output) version 5 (DSL [i/o], the NAL-nonlinear (NAL-NL1), the Cambridge method for loudness equalization [CAMEQ], and the Cambridge method for loudness restoration [CAMREST], (Palmer et al, 2008). In general, the methodologies differ in terms of the amount of amplification provided and the underlying fitting rationale (e.g., DSL, loudness normalization). With the goal being to achieve accurate fittings and to maximize speech intelligibility for specified input levels (provide different prescriptive targets as a function of input level), the NAL-NL1 fitting procedure is one of the most widely used methods for fitting adults with compression hearing aids (Aazh & Moore, 2007; Ricketts & Mueller, 2009).

Based on my review of the literature, it is clear that probe-microphone measurement methods have an important role to play in everyday practice. Real ear techniques help to customize the fit to relevant audiometric data, to help differentiate a good fitting of advanced digital devices from a bad fitting, and to judge the adequacy of the adaptive features, including directionality and telecoil efficiency. The following findings of Ricketts and Mueller (2009) and Aazh and Moore (2007) should drive practice in this arena. When conducting real ear measurements of gain (real ear insertion gain [REIG] measures), the clinician must decide on a correct fitting strategy (Ricketts & Mueller. 2009). For example, is the prescriptive goal to maximize audibility, optimize speech understanding, or provide the best quality sound? Similarly, the criterion to be used to determine closeness or adequacy of fit must be selected. Ricketts and Mueller suggest that it is wise to consider adjusting the high frequencies, namely 3000 to 4000 Hz, separately should patients raise concerns about high-frequency sounds. The higher frequencies often require the most adjustment to meet the target. Also, fine tuning will be necessary on occasion to bring as many frequencies as possible to within ±10 dB of the insertion gain targets. The greater the number of gain handles, the better the likelihood of meeting prescriptive gain targets at all frequencies (Aazh & Moore, 2007). Using target spectrums for speech allows the clinician to be less concerned about frequency-specific targets, which is very important in older adults. Finally, for clients who are music lovers, the fitting should include quality ratings for music.

Palmer et al (2008) caution that the targets should merely provide a benchmark for verifying audibility within the important constraints of user comfort, and the audiologist must expect that changes will be made as field testing and experiences will inform patient perspectives. The conclusions from a study by Smeds (2004) are quite relevant to the discussion of overall gain and selected features provided to older adult hearing-aid users. Participants had mild to moderate bilateral, symmetric, sensorineural hearing loss; their ages ranged from 54 to 83 years, with a mean age of 75 years. Participants who were first-time hearing-aid users were fit binaurally with digital, wide dynamic range compression (WDRC), behind-the-ear hearing aids equipped with feedback suppression systems, directional microphones, and noise-reduction systems. In general, participants preferred the prescriptive formula, which provided lower gain values and had lower compression ratios. These new hearing-aid users did not like restoration of normal overall loudness as they felt they were being overamplified by this approach. Interestingly, speech-recognition ability was not affected by the different prescriptive formulas. The authors concurred with the thinking of others that although experienced hearing-aid users may prefer higher listening levels, thanks in part to acclimatization, new or inexperienced users tend to prefer less gain than prescribed by many of the formulas (Humes, Wilson, Barlow, & Garner, 2002; Smeds, 2004).

Smeds (2004) speculated that the severity of the hearing loss may be a factor in gain settings, such that those with more severe hearing loss may tolerate higher loudness levels (OSPL90 settings) to possibly achieve improved speech understanding. The authors cautioned that, based on their observations, the gain prescribed by many of the widely used prescriptive strategies, including DSL [i/o], NAL-NL1, and CAMEQ,

may overestimate gain for new hearing-aid users with mild to moderate sensorineural hearing loss. Hence, the work of Smeds and of others underscores that ensuring loudness comfort is an essential part of the fitting, either by using a prescriptive approach as a starting point for determining initial maximum output settings, or by basing maximum output on unaided loudness measures. Loudness validation using high-intensity signals and aided output verification is integral, as well. This protocol ensures that average real-ear saturation response (RESR) does not substantially exceed average LDLs (Mackersie, 2007). Aided loudness discomfort should be evaluated in a systematic manner given its real-world relevance. Output verification is critical to ensure that hearing-aid user's threshold of discomfort (TD) is not exceeded. Specifically, the OSPL90 should not exceed the patient's TD to ensure comfort and to reduce exposure to potentially damaging input levels. Every effort should be made to ensure as wide a dynamic range as possible (Hawkins, 2011).

For the most part, the rules and strategies used with younger adults pertain to older adults. Simply put, the goal is acoustic accuracy. As discussed above, optimal hearing-aid fitting is one that makes speech audible without exceeding the listener's loudness-discomfort level, restores the normal loudness relations for speech and other environmental sounds, and, above all, enhances speech intelligibility in a variety of listening situations (Cox, 1995). Tests of speech recognition have considerable promise as part of the hearing-aid fitting. Routine tests of aided versus unaided speech understanding using monosyllabic words or sentence materials presented in quiet or noise and at conversational level can be used to document aided benefit. Speech tests such as the QuickSIN can provide an estimate of the amount by which the hearing aid reduces the negative effects of noise. Results of the speech intelligibility in noise test when speech is presented at soft to moderate levels can serve as the basis for the fine tuning of the gain and frequency response and again can provide useful for counseling regarding strategies for promoting successful communication.

Based on the work of Humes and others, the CST in the presence of multi-talker babble is a sensitive measure of hearing-aid benefit and of differences across technologies. According to Humes (2007a), 49% of variability in aided speech recognition performance can be accounted for by three predictor variables: unaided speech recognition, cognitive function, and age. Hence, if clinicians do not assess cognitive status at the prefitting, there is some assurance that cognitive status is taken into account at this stage. According to Humes (2007b) the higher the verbal cognitive ability as measured using the Wechsler Adult Intelligence Scale–revised (WAIS-R), the higher the unaided speech recognition score. The CST presented at a conversational level with multi-talker babble is an ideal tool for assessing aided speech recognition ability.

In their overview of studies on hearing-aid benefit, Humes, Kinney, and Thompson (2009) reported on the sensitivity of the CST as an outcome measure. The CST was presented at 65 dB SPL in quiet with the loudspeaker at a 0-degree azimuth. They presented the multi-talker babble from the CST at an SNR of +8 dB from a loudspeaker at 180 degrees azimuth. When hearing aids were well fit to prescriptive targets, irrespective of the technology or features (e.g., linear, directional), aided performance on the CST emerged as significantly better than unaided performance. Further, it was of interest that using the CST, superior performance in the aided condition emerged with directional technology over any of the other three technologies, namely WDRC, omnidirectional, or linear. Souza, Boike, Witherell, and Tremblay (2007) also found differences in aided speech scores emerge across technologies, emphasizing the value of aided speech testing.

Nabelek et al (2006) also demonstrated the value of aided speech recognition ability in the presence of background noise during the fitting. They assessed speech understanding in a group of part-time and full-time hearing-aid users with high-frequency sensorineural hearing loss fit with binaural hearing aids. Hearing levels of part-time users were slightly better than for full-time users (36 dB HL vs. 44 dB HL). They used the speech perception in noise (SPIN) test with speech babble presented at a +8 dB SNR. They too demonstrated a significant aided advantage over the unaided condition in both full- and part-time hearing-aid users. However, the aided-unaided ANL was comparable, confirming that ANL is not affected by use of hearing aids and is a pre-fitting measure rather than an index of outcome. The fact that unaided ANL is predictive of success with amplification underscores this notion. Nabelek and colleagues also noted that scores on the SPIN did not correlate with benefit or satisfaction, confirming the findings of Humes (2007a) that aided speech understanding is a unique dimension of outcome. With regard to amplified speech, the importance of ensuring that high-frequency information is sufficiently audible as a precondition to conducting aided speech tests, as this will help to maximize performance, cannot be overemphasized (Humes, 2007b). That is, restoration of audibility, prior to conducting aided speech tests, isolates the contribution of age or cognitive factors to aided speech understanding.

Pearl

The maximum output of the hearing aid must be set in a way that the functional dynamic range is as wide as possible, with the RESR as close as possible to the maximum output targets (Hawkins, 2011). Based on loudness scaling the output should be "loud but OK" rather than uncomfortably loud or comfortable.

Evidence-Based Consideration of Hearing-Aid Style and Features and Fitting Arrangement

Having first entered the market in 1987, digital hearing aids provide signal processing and features that theoretically provide advantages beyond those of strictly analog devices. Advances in digital technology have revolutionized hearing-aid design, increasing the array of options and dramatically expanding the fitting range of amplification (Kerckhoff, Listenberger, & Valente, 2008). Audiologists can now make decisions regarding product features that enable customization in terms of electroacoustics, communication, and lifestyle needs. In contrast to analog technology, digital hearing aids convert the waveform into a string of numbers, which allows for enhanced processing, unique features, and theoretically greater user comfort (Ricketts & Mueller, 2011).

The major communication difficulties expressed by the hearing impaired are understanding speech in noise, understanding in less than optimal listening situations, and using the telephone, especially cellular phones. The solution to many of these difficulties may be found through hearing-aid metamorphosis in the areas of directional microphone technology, WDRC processing, digital noise reduction, and wireless technology (Boothroyd, 2007). Additional features that may impact hearing-aid market penetration and user satisfaction are features that can promote device-related user satisfaction, including feedback suppression, power-on delay, low-battery indicator, and wax guards. A comprehensive pre-fitting helps the audiologist decide on the features most important to the consumer. Additional decisions to be made include the desirability of a binaural versus monaural fitting and hearing-aid style. What follows is an evidenced based discussion of features, fitting arrangement, and hearing-aid style. **Table 8.7** summarizes the features and options available in most present-day hearing aids, some of which are discussed below.

Digital Noise Reduction

Digital noise reduction (DNR), or noise suppression, algorithms were developed in an effort to improve listener comfort and sound quality in noisy environments and to decrease listener effort in challenging communication environments. In turn, DNR technology theoretically will enhance speech recognition in noise via one of several algorithms that have as their basis the difference in physical characteristics between noise and speech. DNR circuitry reduces ambient noise by analyzing the acoustic properties of noise and of speech, which differ. Noise tends to be more stable than speech and modulates at a different rate, whereas speech modulation varies in amplitude over time, and the acoustic properties of speech tend to be dynamic and frequency specific (Kerckhoff et al, 2008). Using DNR algorithms, the hearing aid will monitor input signals that are constant in frequency and amplify the parts of the speech input that are modulated (i.e., speech has a modulation rate that occurs between 3 and 10 Hz) or speech like. Although they differ across manufacturers, especially in terms of the SNR used, DNR algorithms generally sense whether or not a channel is dominated by noise, rather than separating speech from noise, and based on this determination a decision is made to reduce gain in each frequency channel based on the "modulation or lack of modulation of the unwanted noise signal and that of the desired speech signal" (Kerckhoff et al, 2008, p. 106).

The ideal DNR algorithm will recognize restaurant noise and traffic noise and will treat it differently from the speech signal, which needs to remain audible, and, by dint of the improved SNR, easier to understand. According to Sarampalis, Kalluri, Edwards, and Hafter (2009), by reducing the effort required to understand speech in a noisy environment via DNR, perhaps the hearing-impaired listener will be able to devote cognitive resources to understanding speech. Stated differently, one potential advantage of DNR is that it may reduce cognitive effort needed to understand sentences in challenging listening situations (e.g., situations wherein the SNR varies). Sarampalis et al demonstrated that participants perform better on a word-memory task and show quicker responses in visual reaction times when DNR is activated, which provides objective evi-

Table 8.7   Hearing-Aid Style, Features, Options, and Arrangements

Binaural versus monaural
Style
  Behind the ear (BTE), micro-BTE, in the ear (ITE), in the canal (ITC), completely in the canal (CIC)
Earmold
  Nonoccluding
  Receiver
  Receiver in the aid (RITA)
  Receiver in the canal (RITC)
  Fitting range of hearing aid
Features
  Type of microphone technology (e.g., directional, omnidirectional)
  Telecoil
  Digital noise reduction (DNR)
  Feedback suppression: digital feedback reduction (DFR)
  Low battery indicator
  Power on delay
  Wax guard
  Venting
  Volume control: manual, automatic
  Remote control
  Wireless routing technology: Bluetooth, FM
  Wind-noise management
  Data logging
  Side-to-side communication
  Trainable algorithms
  Frequency lowering
Gain processing considerations
  Compression type: compression vs. expansion
  Compression threshold (CT)
  Compression ratio: fixed, adjustable, or curvilinear
  Compression automatic volume control
  Compression time constants: attack/release
  Crossover frequency or frequencies between bands
  Number of programs; number of channels
Miscellaneous functions
  Hearing-aid on-off control
  Sleep circuit for reducing battery drain
  Options for use with telephone
  Remote controls: type of signal, size, number of parameters, ease of use
  Microphone: directional, omnidirectional, or both
  Extended high frequencies
  User-operated volume control

Sources: Adapted from Ricketts, T., & Mueller, G. (2011). *Today's hearing aid features: Fluff or true hearing aid benefit?* Paper presented at Audiology NOW, 23rd annual convention of the American Academy of Audiology, Chicago; and Rubinstein, A. (1997). Hearing aid fitting and management. *Seminars in Hearing, 18,* 87–101.

dence that perhaps DNR reduces listening effort and frees up cognitive resources for older listeners. The benefits of DNR in terms of improved speech recognition in noise remain elusive using standard laboratory measures; however, the ANL holds potential as a way of determining the value of DNR relative to acceptance of background noise, with the thinking being that smaller ANLs are associated with good acceptance of background noise.

Signal Processing Through Compression

The most common signal processing technique for providing audible signals across soft moderate and loud inputs is WDRC

(Palmer et al, 2008). Through nonlinear amplification, different amounts of gain can be applied to make weak sounds audible, average conversational speech comfortable, and intense sounds loud without being uncomfortable, based on the setting of basic parameters. The potential for increased audibility of sounds at given frequencies without discomfort resulting from high-intensity sounds is a huge advance for hearing-aid users (Preves & Banerjee, 2008). To accomplish the desired signal processing through WDRC, gain is adjusted according to the intensity of the input level (e.g., soft versus loud sounds); thus, the output is limited without distortion, there is increased intelligibility of soft sounds, and perception of loudness is restored and normalized. With improved audibility of soft consonants in ongoing speech and more normalized loudness perceptions for both low- and high-level sounds, theoretically speech understanding will improve (Cox & Xu, 2010).

It is helpful to understand the premises behind WDRC to select the appropriate parameters for older adults with ARHL. First, the most common complaint associated with hearing loss is difficulty hearing weak sounds. Next, average conversational speech is often inaudible and intense sounds are perceived as being louder, so different amounts of gain must be applied to make weak sounds audible, average conversational speech comfortable, and loud sounds loud without being uncomfortable. Further, older individuals require more favorable SNRs than do younger adults, and older adults lose their ability to respond to the temporal aspects of speech, and thus they are susceptible to losing the cues that are important for speech understanding (Helfer & Vargo, 2009; Preves & Banerjee, 2008). Additionally, temporal deficits compromise understanding of speech, and hearing aids tend to distort the low-rate envelope, which provides cues to vowel identity and consonant manner (e.g., "say" versus "stay") and voicing ("fuzz" versus "fuss"), and greater envelope distortion comes with more extreme compression parameters (e.g., short release time, high compression ratios) and is associated with greater envelope distortion (Jenstad & Souza, 2005; Souza & Arehart, 2009). To understand speech, older adults require longer gaps and larger differences in duration than do younger listeners with similar hearing thresholds (Gordon-Salant, Yeni-Komshian, Fitzgibbons, & Barrett, 2006; Snell & Frisina, 2000). Finally, according to emerging evidence, cognitive capacity (e.g., working memory and speed of processing) affects the benefit from WDRC such that compression processing release time is more critical for persons with lower cognitive abilities than for those with higher cognitive abilities (Cox and Xu, 2010; Gatehouse, Naylor, & Elberling, 2006a,b; Lunner & Sundewall-Thorén, 2007).

The setting of two basic parameters, namely attack time (AT) and release time (RT), affects the WDRC transition of the circuits in response to the intensity of the input level. AT is a measure of the speed at which device gain is decreased after the input sound level is raised, or the time it takes the hearing aid to stabilize in a state of reduced amplification after an abrupt increase in the input level (Rudner et al, 2011). RT is a measure of the time it takes for a hearing aid to return to a state of increased amplification after the input level is reduced. Most modern hearing aids use short/fast AT (10 to 20 milliseconds) so that sudden loud sounds will not be amplified to uncomfortably loud levels. According to Cox and Xu (2010), release times in the range of 10 to 100 milliseconds are generally considered to be short (fast), whereas release times greater than 500 milliseconds are generally considered to be long (slow). Short RTs provide for improved audibility of soft consonants in ongoing speech and more normalized loudness perceptions for both low- and high-level everyday sounds. Long release times have the advantage of helping to maintain the intensity relationships among speech sounds, thereby preserving their naturalness, intelligibility, and localizability. In contrast, a disadvantage of long RT is that the listener experiences brief intervals of very low gain during which important auditory events will be missed (Cox & Xu, 2010; Jenstad and Souza, 2005).

Fast-acting compression release time changes the shape of the temporal envelope of the speech signal, at times distorting it particularly in the presence of noise. When fast-acting compression is applied to a speech signal in noise, the extent to which the target and background acquire a common component of modulation affects speech intelligibility (Stone & Moore, 2007). Slow-acting compression release time (greater than 200 milliseconds) maintains a relatively constant output level and thereby does not distort the signal the same way that fast-acting compression release time does. However, a drawback with slow-acting compression RT is that a hearing aid that has just responded to a loud sound by decreasing amplification may under-amplify a following soft sound (Rudner et al, 2011). Fast-acting compression allows parts of the signal occurring during dips in noise to be amplified to an audible level. Several investigators have undertaken studies of the interaction between working memory and release time to determine the optimal parameters for speech understanding. Dr. Kerry Lynch, a former doctoral student of mine, completed a systematic review of speech recognition ability, cognitive factors, and release time. **Table 8.8** summarizes some of the most recent

studies in this area. Based on the results of a systematic review, and on the fact that the reading span test of working memory appears to be an excellent predictor of aided speech recognition in noise performance across speech material, noise type, and compression release time settings, the following conclusions can be drawn regarding release time settings and cognitive factors:

1. A decision as to the appropriate release time depends on several factors including cognitive ability and speech understanding.
2. Working memory capacity as measured using the reading span test is an important consideration when selecting appropriate RT during hearing-aid fitting and should be part of the armamentarium of audiologists (Cox & Xu, 2010).
3. Short-acting release time is better for individuals with low cognitive function (Cox & Xu, 2010).
4. According to self-ratings, a longer release time is better for comfort and a shorter release time is better for intelligibility; adults need context to extract meaning when short release times are prescribed (Cox & Xu, 2010).
5. Release time considerations are especially important for persons with low cognitive function; for persons with higher cognitive function, release time does not matter as much (Cox & Xu, 2010).
6. Individuals with higher cognitive scores perform better than those with lower cognitive scores on both short and long RT processing; individuals with lower cognitive ability perform significantly better with long RT (Lunner & Sundewall-Thorén, 2007).
7. The relationship between cognitive abilities and speech understanding with short and long RT processing depends

Table 8.8 Summary of Selected Studies on Working Memory, Speech Recognition, and Release Time Settings

Authors	Study Design	No. of Subjects	Mean Age (Years)	Hearing-Aid (HA) Characteristics	Type and Degree of Hearing Loss
Gatehouse et al, (2006a,b)	Within-subject, randomized, blind, crossover design	50	67.1 (range: 54–82)	New HA; monaural fitting; BTE*	Mild to moderate; sensorineural
Lunner & Sundewall-Thorén (2007)	Within-subject, randomized, blind, crossover design	23	65.6 (standard deviation [SD]: 12.8; range: 32–87)	Used participants own HAs; monaural and binaural fittings; BTE (N = 9) and ITE (N = 14)*	Mild to moderate; sensorineural
Foo et al (2007)		32	70.3 (SD: 7.7; range: 51–80)	Used participants own HA(s); monaural and binaural fittings; BTE and ITE*	Mild to moderate; sensorineural
Rudner et al (2009)		31	70 (SD: 7.7; range: 51–80)	Used participants own HA(s); monaural and binaural fittings; BTE and ITE*	Mild to moderate; sensorineural
Cox and Xu (2010)		24	71.8 (SD: 10.9; range: 41–89)	New HAs; binaural fitting; BTE*; signal processing more advanced than in previous studies	Mild to moderately-severe; sensorineural
Rudner, et al (2008)		32	70 (SD = 7.7)	Used own HAs; binaural fitting; BTE and ITE*	Mild to moderate; sensorineural

Abbreviations: BTE, behind-the-ear style hearing aid; ITE, in-the-ear style hearing aid; PTA, pure-tone average.
*Nonlinear, digital, dual-channel hearing aid(s).

on the characteristics of the speech materials (e.g., high- or low-context materials) (Cox & Xu, 2010).

8. The selection of appropriate RT during hearing-aid fitting should be an essential and systematic aspect of the protocol (Cox & Xu, 2010).

9. The majority of participants in the Cox and Xu (2010) study preferred the long release time settings because of the clarity, quality, and loudness of the input.

10. Modulated noise should be used to assess aided speech recognition ability in noise, as this type of noise has greater ecological validity and is more likely than unmodulated noise to reflect detriments and benefits of hearing-aid fittings and the contribution of cognitive ability (Lynch, 2011).

Digital Feedback Suppression Algorithms

According to Kochkin (2005), annoyance caused by feedback is a major factor associated with reduced satisfaction with hearing aids. With the advent of dynamic feedback management systems/digital feedback reduction (DFR), audible feedback oscillation does not pose the problem it had in the past. It is hoped that rejection of hearing aids due to annoying feedback is a thing of the past. Traditionally, hearing aids produce both mechanical and acoustic feedback. The solution to mechanical feedback, which results when mechanical vibrations from the receiver are picked up by the microphone of the hearing aid, is physical isolation of the microphone from the receiver and from the shell or case of the hearing aid (Preves & Banerjee, 2008). When mechanical feedback occurs, the hearing aid should be returned to the manufacturer, as this indicates a design flaw. Acoustic feedback or leakage arises when the output of the receiver leaks out of the ear canal via the vent or slit, and leaks around the edges of the hearing aid or earmold and is picked up by the microphone and then reamplified along with the other sounds picked up by the hearing aid. At times the feedback signal creates an audible oscillation that sounds like a whistle or a squeal and it can grow strong and be annoying. According to Preves and Banerjee, an ideal condition that breeds feedback is when the feedback signal is in the same phase as the input signal at the microphone. Hence, a theoretical solution is ongoing cancellation within the feedback path, accomplished in a variety of ways including phase cancellation and frequency shifting (Ricketts & Mueller, 2011). There are several theoretical advantages of DFR. First, with less feedback, more use-gain can be made available without venting alterations, especially for those with severe to profound hearing loss. Next, reduction of feedback potentially allows for open canal fittings on ears with greater degrees of hearing loss or the use of shells with larger vents. Further, the absence of feedback may increase hearing-aid use because the stigma and annoyance of the feedback is eliminated. Finally, certain types of feedback control adapt to changing environments such as when a telephone is placed on or close to the ear, which is a very appealing feature (Preves & Banerjee, 2008; Ricketts & Mueller, 2011).

Hearing-aid manufacturers use different feedback suppression systems, which vary in their effectiveness and limitations (Ricketts, Johnson, & Federman (2008). One major difference is the magnitude of available gain before feedback (AGBF). In many models, digital noise reduction processing interacts with the magnitude of gain, potentially affecting AGBF and contributing to variability across instruments. Ricketts et al's comparison of five commercially available hearing aids found large differences across units in terms of AGBF. Similarly, they noted that there was significant variability across individual listeners for each instrument in terms of AGBF despite the fact the instruments used the same feedback suppression (FS) algorithm, which suggests an interaction between the ear and the FS algorithm. Finally, it was notable that the feedback produced by the hearing aids once the hearing aids went into oscillation differed across instruments, and some of the feedback produced by the instruments upon oscillation was annoying. In light of the large AGBF range across instruments (0–15 dB) Ricketts and colleagues suggest that clinicians should take note of the AGBF when recommending hearing aids and should also ask patients directly about their reaction to any feedback produced by the instrument when first using it, as this could affect hearing-aid acceptance.

Although theoretically these systems are a wonderful advance, the primary shortcoming, namely gain limitation or reduction, is potentially problematic, especially because it tends to be in effect all the time. Interestingly, there is considerable variability in terms of the flexibility of the algorithms controlling gain reduction across hearing aids and in terms of the amount of gain before initial feedback occurs. As there are differences across models in the amount of automatic gain reduction before feedback, Ricketts and Mueller (2011) recommend measuring this feature. They found that the real-world benefit of feedback suppression is high given the popularity and preferences for RITE and receiver-in-the-aid (RITA) behind-the-ear units for both experienced and inexperienced hearing-aid users; however, AGBF is an important consideration and could be a detraction. When conducting real-ear measurements designed to check the feedback suppression option, this can be remedied it is important to disable the reference microphone thereby "forcing the real ear analyzer to use only the calibration of the sound field loudspeaker performed before the measurement to calculate the real ear aided gain (REAG)" (Frye & Martin, 2008). This will compensate for the fact that real-ear aided gain could be artificially high or low.

> **Pearl**
>
> The popularity of open canal fittings is attributable in large part to feedback suppression systems (Ricketts & Mueller, 2011). The advantages include pleasantness of the sound, naturalness of one's voice quality, comfort, and convenience.

Directional Microphone and Digital Signal Processing (DSP)

Directional microphone hearing aids (DMHAs) are an additional technology designed to amplify speech signals while reducing noise signals (i.e., improve SNR). They are designed to be more sensitive to signals coming from the front of the speaker (on-axis) and less sensitive to signals coming from behind the speaker (off-axis). The majority of directional microphones are automatic, in that the hearing aid will automatically switch to omnidirectional or directional depending on the listening environment. Hearing aids incorporating automatic system typically have preset decision rules determined by the characteristics of the acoustic environment (Wu, 2010). In twin microphone arrays, the hearing aid is adaptive in that the polar plot will change in response to the environment in an effort to minimize background noise and to maximize the speech signal, thereby enhancing the SNR in difficult listening situations (Ricketts & Mueller, 2011). The directional advantage experienced by the hearing-aid user varies with the amount of room reverberation, the distance between the speaker and the listener, the presence of frontal sound source, noise competition primarily behind the listener, and a high hearing-aid directivity index.

Wu (2010) explored the effect of age on directional microphone hearing-aid benefit and preferences. Older participants had mild to severe hearing loss and were a mix of experienced or new hearing-aid users. Subjects were fit with fully digital hearing aids that could be programmed to the omnidirectional or directional modes, which were programmed into the two memories of the hearing aids, and the participants were trained to identify listening environments and switch between the different memories by pushing the button on the faceplate to switch between the two microphone settings. That is, the automatic switch feature was disabled. Wu's findings were interesting, highlighting the role of laboratory and field tests in decisions regarding a recommendation for directional processing. Wu found performance on speech tests in noise were essentially comparable for older and younger adults. However, during the field trials older adults reported that DMHA did not work well for them, and they experienced smaller perceived benefit than did younger adults. Therefore, scores on laboratory tests did not predict the real-world benefit experienced by older adults. The fact that Wu did not assess preferences with automatic DMHA could be a variable, but it is clear from this study that the manual DMHA option may not be realistic.

Wu and Bentler (2010) explored the value of visual cues when using DMHA in a sample of adults in an effort to explore the role of environmental factors in the benefit from DMHA, their reasoning being that typically visual cues are available when the DMHA option is most effective, and that the acoustics of the listening environment will affect DMHA preferences, benefit, and the extent to which visual cues are used. The role of the environment and preferences for directionality were most interesting. The following environments were tested: talker-listener distance (3 feet versus 4 to 10 feet), noise-listener distance (3 feet versus 10 feet and 4 to 10 feet versus 10 feet), noise location (side versus all around and behind versus all around), SNR (favorable versus unfavorable and intermediate versus unfavorable), and reverberation (low versus high). The only significant finding was that participants preferred the omnidirectional mode in low reverberant environments. Further, visual cues did not impact preferences for microphone type, be it DMHA or omnidirectional. Further, despite the laboratory advantages of directional microphones, in the field DMHA did not emerge as the preferred option. Interestingly, participants preferred the omnidirectional microphone in many instances, stating that this setting provided for a louder signal, and there was a preference for the omni-

directional microphone as participants perceived less internal noise. Another interesting outcome was that people with good auditory-visual speech-recognition ability may derive more limited benefit from directional hearing aids; hence, expectations must be managed via counseling. Further, older adults in this sample indicated that speech sounded louder with the omnidirectional microphone and use of visual cues provided more benefit than did the benefit derived from directional microphones. The participants indicated that they did not find themselves in the optimal environment for benefiting from DMHA, which was an additional drawback to this technology.

According to Wu and Bentler (2010), the functionality of the directional microphone system needs to be verified frequently. Hearing-aid manufacturers tend to have difficulty with quality control of the directivity index of hearing aids with directional microphones, so directivity tends to both vary and decline over time for several reasons. According to Wu and Bentler, the average drift of a directional microphone is around 0.25 dB after 1 year of use, due to an accumulation of dirt and moisture in the microphone system's acoustic pathway. Clogged microphone ports generate frequency-dependent change in amplitude and phase, which has an impact on directivity and performance of speech recognition in noise (Wu & Bentler, 2012). Therefore, it is critical for clinicians to measure and monitor the directivity (i.e. attenuation of sounds arriving from angles other than in front of the listener) of directional hearing aids on a routine basis and a change in relative directivity (RD) of 30% suggests that microphone directivity in the hearing aid may be defective.

Pearl

With open-fit hearing aids, even with good directional hearing aids, directionality below 1500 Hz for many listening situations is limited (Mueller & Ricketts, 2006).

Johnson and Ricketts (2010) explored factors influencing dispensing rates of four universally available hearing-aid features: digital feedback-suppression processing, digital noise-reduction processing, directional processing, and the telecoil. It was notable that the amount of communication difficulty in listening environments or likelihood of acoustic feedback influenced the decision to recommend the above features. Despite the lack of evidence supporting the benefits of digital noise-reduction processing, hearing aids having this feature were dispensed significantly more often than the directional instruments and those with feedback-suppression processing. Interestingly, the largest variability among dispensers in terms of features dispensed was associated with the telecoil and directional processing. The price point of the hearing-aid feature, the audiologist-specific feature candidacy criterion based on patient need, and the audiologist's personal belief in the potential of a product feature explained the individual variability across audiologists in choice of features dispensed. Audiologists with reportedly younger patient populations dispensed the above four product features more often than did audiologists serving older patient populations. This is unfortunate, as most of these features work automatically, and the available evidence does not point to an age effect relating to benefit from these particular features. In my view, the low dispensing rate of the telecoil feature is problematic given the growth in interest in the use of induction-loop hearing assistance systems in public spaces in the U.S.

High-Frequency Amplification

Technological advances including feedback management, spectral shaping, wider band frequency response, and directional microphones have made it possible to provide substantial high-frequency amplification for those individuals with high-frequency hearing loss (Horwitz, Ahlstrom, & Dubno, 2008). However, evidence regarding the extent of benefit from high-frequency amplification for older adults with high-frequency hearing loss remains controversial. Some studies suggest that restored audibility does not improve speech understanding in quiet and that it is in fact deleterious, whereas other studies suggest that it is beneficial (Amos & Humes, 2007). Specifically, for those with moderate to severe high-frequency hearing loss, which is often associated with dead regions (inner hair cell is nonfunctional and activation of afferent fibers is not possible), amplification does not necessarily result in improved speech understanding. One negative consequence of high-frequency amplification may be a downward spread of masking, which reduces audibility of low-frequency speech information. Related to this is the fact that a threshold breakpoint may be 55 dB HL, such that above this level, delivering amplified speech energy to the receptor cells may be futile and even deleterious to speech understanding (Amos & Humes, 2007). Another negative consequence of high-frequency amplification is that it does not restore the contribution of the base of the cochlea to low-frequency cues (Horwitz, Ahlstrom, & Dubno, 2008). A major question is whether the benefit is different for understanding speech in noise versus quiet. Horwitz et al (2008) explored the contribution of high-frequency amplification to speech understanding in a sample of older adults with sloping high-frequency hearing loss with thresholds of 55 dB HL or greater above 2000 Hz. The study was prompted in part by theoretical evidence that listeners take advantage of binaural sound segregation cues (e.g., interaural acoustic differences in time of arrival or intensity level) to separate the speech from the competition, thereby improving speech reception. They found that the addition of high-frequency speech bands improved scores for tests of speech in noise, more so than for speech in quiet. They reasoned that the addition of the high-frequency information may have helped the listeners perceive voicing cues that were lost due to the presence of noise. While some investigators and clinicians believe that restoring the audibility of high-frequency information to persons with severe high-frequency sensorineural hearing loss provides significant benefit to speech understanding in noise overwhelmingly the hearing impaired do not express a preference for extended high-frequency bandwidth (Ricketts and Mueller, 2011).

The latter observation may in part be due to the presence of dead regions which may affect the ability to use high-frequency amplification. For example, Vickers, Moore, and Baer (2001) found that high-frequency amplification produced limited speech-understanding improvement in quiet for listeners with high-frequency dead regions, whereas listeners without dead regions derived substantial benefit from high-frequency amplification. Similarly, Baer, Moore, and Kluk (2002) observed similar results when subjects listened to nonsense syllables in the presence of background noise, confirming that listeners with cochlear dead regions benefit less from high-frequency amplification than do listeners without cochlear dead regions.

Frequency Lowering

The term *frequency lowering* (FL) refers to the use of technologies that take high-frequency inputs, such as speech, and deliver these sounds to lower frequencies. Originally designed for persons with severe to profound hearing loss, the theory behind frequency transposition is transforming of the amplified speech signal so that it is audible in a frequency region where the individual's hearing is better (Kerckhoff et al, 2008). Thus, FL is considered another approach to increasing the audibility of high frequencies. An additional premise underlying the introduction of FL into hearing aids is that this feature should provide improved awareness of environmental sounds, improved localization, and improved recognition for selected high-frequency sounds (Ricketts & Mueller, 2011). FL algorithms compensate for hearing loss in the high-frequency ranges where traditional hearing aids do not provide sufficient benefit. It has potential when extended high frequencies are not possible. An approach to FL adopted by some manufacturers is frequency transposition or frequency compression. In the former case, bands of high frequencies are shifted down by a fixed amount to a region audible to the hearing-aid user, whereas in the latter case the output frequency bandwidth of the signal is compressed by a fixed ratio (Ricketts & Mueller, 2011). According to Glista et al (2009), frequency compression compresses the output bandwidth of the signal by a specified ratio, thereby altering the positions of vowel formants in the frequency domain. Ideally, individuals who would benefit from FL are older adults who present with cochlear dead regions in the middle to high frequencies and those who have high-frequency loss, rendering inaudible the high-frequency sounds so important to intelligibility.

Evidence regarding the value of this technology is limited and equivocal. However, using a prototype instrument, Glista and colleagues (2009) did find that frequency compression improved high-frequency audibility and speech detection for high-frequency sounds (e.g., plural detection and consonant recognition) and speech-recognition ability in adults with high-frequency loss. They concluded that benefit observed from FL was attributed to the increased audibility of additional high-frequency energy, albeit presented in a lower frequency range. It is noteworthy that children in their sample were more likely than adults to express a preference for frequency compression. In summary, it is too early to conclude based on available evidence whether FL is beneficial for older adults. According to Ricketts and Mueller (2011), real-world benefit of FL technology has not yet been documented.

Self-Learning Features

Many hearing aids on the market today incorporate self-learning features wherein the hearing aid automatically adjusts the volume to settings typically used by the user. Primarily used to train overall hearing-aid gain, the technology for trainable hearing aids uses data logging to record volume control settings in the situations in which the hearing aid is being used. When set on automatic and turned on, the hearing aid automatically adjusts the start-up gain based on the volume control settings used previously. Hence, according to Mueller, Hornsby, and Weber (2008), this technology can be helpful in estimating preferred hearing-aid gain based on the end user. Mueller et al compared preferred gain settings with prescriptive gain settings established using NAL-NL1 targets in a sample of adults with a mean age of 64 years having mild to moderately severe sloping sensorineural hearing loss bilaterally. A secondary purpose of the study was to determine the effect of start-up gain on real-world preferred gain settings. Participants were experienced hearing-aid users who wore binaural hearing aids for at least 1 year prior to the start of the study. As part of the study they wore hearing aids with all special features activated including DNR, automatic directional microphone technology, data logging, and adaptive feedback cancellation, and the hearing instruments were linked to enable information sharing between instruments using electromagnetic transmission.

The results showed that start-up volume control setting had a significant impact on the preferred gain setting, and that when start-up gain deviated by +6 dB from the NAL target, the majority of participants preferred less gain, training their units down by about 3 dB. In contrast, when start-up gain was –6 dB from the NAL target, only 50% of participants chose to increase gain. Hence, if start-up gain was set below target, at least 50% preferred to stay below target and not adjust the volume control. The most favorable subjective ratings of loudness and satisfaction with loudness emerged when gain was set 6 dB below target. The findings that trained preferred gain differed significantly from NAL-NL1 targets and that preferred gain was influenced by start-up gain underscore the importance of field testing of the instrument and follow-up using data logging to help determine the prescriptive target that best meets the patient's needs. It is clear that setting hearing aids below target yields preferences in terms of satisfaction with loudness judgments. Because the participants were experienced, I would conjecture that preferred gain settings from the outset would deviate even further from target until hearing-aid users adjust to the newly audible information. The functionality of data logging should be explored thoroughly with older adults, as the ability to monitor volume control settings through data logging, setting-specific use, and use times can effectively inform post-fitting discussion during the hearing-aid orientation and discussion about communication strategies and the possible need to supplement hearing aids with HATs.

Connectivity and Wireless Technology

Hearing-aid users are fortunate to be part of the connectivity revolution, wherein via the telecoil switch and various Bluetooth-compatible devices on the market the hearing-aid user has a gateway to speakers in large rooms, in conference centers, and to external audio signals. Specifically, the term *connectivity* implies the ability to connect multiple sound sources seamlessly and wirelessly to personal hearing aids, navigation systems, telephones, television, MP3 players, computers, tele-

visions, and personal digital assistants (PDAs), thereby allowing individuals to be connected (Beck & Harvey, 2009). The principle behind the technology is the wireless reception of a sound from a remote source. The earliest example of wireless technology for hearing-aid users was the telecoil (T-coil), which is a tiny piece of metal wrapped tightly with copper coils, that is an option in hearing aids and is now built into cochlear implant processors (looped signals can be received by some bone-anchored hearing aids as well). The T-coil detects and converts magnetic energy into electrical energy, comparable to a microphone that converts acoustic to electric energy (Beck & Brunved, 2006). The T-coil allows for the pairing of hearing aids to several devices including a telephone handset, a neck loop, a hearing loop, and FM systems. Remote access to audio devices via wireless connectivity is a sustainable solution to the difficulty the hearing impaired experience in challenging acoustic environments associated with a combination of the effects of distance, reverberation, and room noise. In addition to improved SNR in noisy and reverberant rooms, other benefits of remote wireless microphones include maintenance of a constant speech input regardless of distance between speaker and listener, even when the speaker is moving around (Boothroyd, 2004).

Most technologies, be it hearing aids or HATs, rely on frequency-modulated (FM) or amplitude-modulated (AM) transmission or analog transmission via induction coils for connectivity (Kerckhoff et al, 2008). Bluetooth technology and newer methods of digital magnetic transmission of wireless technology enable the connectivity that is so important for older adults, and by improving access to audio signals and improving the interface with media devices we can effectively reduce the unnecessary isolation experienced by many hearing-impaired older adults. In my view the telecoil (T) (often thought of as a mini-antenna) is critical for older adults with moderate to severe hearing loss, and the ideal arrangement is a hearing-aid system that has both acoustic and inductive coupling options (e.g., acoustic coupling may be preferable for a quick telephone call; inductive may be preferable in noisy environments) (Citron, 2008). The option to recommend a hearing aid that switches automatically to T when the magnetic field is detected or requires switching is a matter to be discussed with the hearing-impaired consumer. The auto-T-coils have a magnetic reed switch (MRS) that is activated by a permanent magnet such as those found in the handset of most telephones (if it is not strong enough, some hearing-aid companies supply magnets that can be attached to the telephone); however, auto-T-coils cannot be activated by a magnetic induction field found in loop systems (Beck & Brunved, 2006). The advantages of the MT setting, especially when interfacing with a hearing loop, should be discussed as well.

If the hearing-aid user decides on a telecoil option, the audiologist should recommend a strong enough telecoil for the patient's needs, and should discuss accessories to consider, their purpose, the cost, the ease of use, and maintenance. A high-power telecoil, should be included to ensure adequate communication when speaking over a hearing-aid compatible (HAC) telephone and to afford auditory access to assistive technologies that transmit signals through wires such as induction loop systems or neck loops connected to FM receivers or using infrared (IR) light, FM radio waves, or an electromagnetic field. Also when ordering a hearing aid with the T option, to maximally receive a looped signal that typically is transmitted horizontally, request a T-coil oriented vertically when the hearing aid is worn in situ. Because optimal phone reception is with a horizontally placed T-coil, the hearing-aid user should be instructed to position the telephone to take full advantage of the " sweet spot" where reception is optimized. Given, the accessibility afforded by telecoils, some states, including Florida, Arizona, and New York, have laws that require audiologists and hearing instrument specialists to inform consumers about telecoils when purchasing hearing aids. As of this writing, only 67% of behind-the-ear hearing aids dispensed by audiologists include telecoils. Sadly, because of space limitations with miniaturization, many hearing aids do not or cannot include strong telecoils.

Telecoils enable the hearing-aid user to take advantage of accessories, such as neck loops or other add-ons, developed by both the phone industry (e.g., neck loops by Nokia and Motorola) and third-party manufacturers (e.g., CHAAMP by Audex, HAT S) to facilitate communication in selected situations. It is important to note that when a hearing aid with a T coil is recommended, its strength should be tested with the real ear. Finally, as part of the orientation, the hearing-aid user should be instructed in the proper use of the switching mechanism and in positioning the telephone relative to the hearing aid to find the magnetic signal or "sweet spot" where the signal is the strongest (Bentler & Mueller, 2009). Making sure to hold the phone close enough to trigger autocoils must be emphasized. Some older adults may still have older telephones in their homes and should be told that these phones may result in a weak or nonexistent signal. Instruction in the use of a magnet that often accompanies the hearing aid is indicated should this be necessary to augment the strength of the magnetic field. For older adults with dexterity problems, larger magnets may prove useful. I also recommend programming a separate frequency response for telecoil or acoustic coupling if the recommended hearing aid includes such a possibility (Citron, 2008). Audiologists should consider a dedicated program on the hearing aid that maximizes acoustic telephone reception (Beck & Brunved, 2006).

Pearl

As of this writing, automatic telecoils work with telephones but not with hearing loops. A manually operated telecoil may be preferable, but also may be more difficult for older adults to operate. To maximally receive a looped signal, it is best if the T-coil is positioned vertically in the hearing aid.

T-coil compatibility with FM systems that generate an electromagnetic field promotes speech understanding by compensating for the effects of background noise and distance in meeting rooms in group situations. Despite the value of these FM systems, older adults have not embraced them. However, I interface hearing aids with these systems on a regular basis so that older adults can experience the advantages of either a remote microphone or a desktop accessory microphone, which is excellent in small group settings.

Boothroyd (2004) explored the benefits and limitations of a remote FM microphone as an accessory to hearing aids in a sample of adults with mild to severe hearing loss with a mean age of 73 years (range 52 to 85 years). The mean better ear PTA in his sample was 48 dB HL. Participants were fit with behind-the-ear hearing aids with built-in FM receivers. It is important to note that the hearing aids were linear, single-channel analog units with adjustable compression limiting, so the generalizability to digital technology with its many features must be qualified. Interestingly, the better ear pure-tone thresholds at 2000 and 4000 Hz accounted for 87% of the variance in FM-assisted, hearing-aided phoneme recognition scores in noise over averaged input of 60, 75, and 80 dB SPL and 62% of the variance in hearing-aided phoneme recognition scores in noise averaged over inputs of 50, 55, and 60 dB SPL. However, thresholds at 2000 and 4000 Hz accounted for 84% of the variance in aided phoneme recognition in quiet averaged over inputs of 50, 55, and 60 dB SPL. Following a 2-week experience with the BTE FM system, participants expressed the greatest perceived benefit when listening to one person at a distance, be it in quiet or noise. The FM arrangement also proved beneficial when listening to one person in noise at a close distance. Close to half of the participants expressed benefit in meetings and while watching television. The participants' major complaint was of persistent noise when using the FM microphone, which picked up room noise. It is notable, also, that the perceived benefit declined with increasing age. Boothroyd reasoned that many of the older participants had adjusted their lifestyles to avoid difficult listening situations, diminishing the potential for actual benefit from an FM arrangement. Interestingly, as with the earlier study by Jerger, Chmiel, Florin, Pirozzolo, and Wilson (1996), participants indicated that they would be unlikely to purchase an FM system for a variety of reasons, including that it was too complicated to use, and the large size of the hearing aids was also a deterrent. Boothroyd concluded that additional counseling sessions are necessary if remote wireless microphones are to become an accepted accessory.

Although some present-day hearing aids include miniaturized personal FM systems, they are expensive and, as noted by Boothroyd (2004), extensive counseling to ensure adequate improvement in speech understanding is important. Chisolm, Noe, McArdle, and Abrams (2007) completed a study designed to explore real-world outcomes with FM systems with a sample of experienced hearing-aid users who were provided with considerable counseling, instruction, and coaching regarding FM use for a 6-week trial period. The subjects were veterans, with a mean age of 75 years, who had moderate adult-onset hearing loss, and many were dissatisfied with their hearing aids in at least one listening situation, making them eligible to benefit from an FM system. Some subjects were willing to try BTE hearing aids and were not currently using them. All subjects completed the CPHI and the COSI, and the responses were used to develop individualized treatment plans with the FM system. Overall satisfaction, satisfaction with the device characteristics, satisfaction in various listening situations with FM systems, and the quality of life attributable to the use of the FM systems were assessed. Subjects returned to the clinic for five visits with a significant communication partner for the fitting, verification of the FM response, instruction in the use of the BTE with the FM system, and role playing with the partner to facilitate adjustment.

The FM system coupled with the BTE hearing aids helped the participants achieve many of their listening goals, including improved communication in quiet, in noise, and in group situations; when listening to the television; and when speaking on the telephone. Responses on the CPHI confirmed that participants perceived improved communication performance with the FM system relative to the use of the hearing aid alone. Following the 6-week trial period, self-perceived quality of life, overall satisfaction, and satisfaction in selected situations were comparable with the FM system and with the hearing aid when it was used alone. Despite the perceived improvement in communication function, only 28% of participants would have been willing to pay for the hearing aid plus FM system, verifying that cost is a deterrent to the adoption of FM systems (Bloom, 2009).

Using a randomized crossover design, Jerger et al (1996) were among the first investigators to complete a study comparing FM systems to conventional analog hearing aids in their ability to enhance speech understanding in noise and to reduce the psychosocial handicap associated with hearing impairment. Subjects in the study were older adults with primarily high-frequency sensorineural hearing loss; 100 subjects were previous hearing-aid users and 80 were new hearing-aid users. The authors compared outcomes in four conditions: (1) hearing aid alone, (2) FM device alone, (3) hearing aid and FM device combined, and (4) no amplification. Subjects spent 6 weeks in each treatment condition, but instructions to facilitate the use of the FM systems were not extensive. The findings suggested that an FM system or an FM system coupled with a hearing aid provided dramatic improvements in speech understanding over and above that afforded by a programmable hearing aid. In contrast, hearing aids were comparable to the FM system in their positive impact on a self-perceived hearing handicap associated with the hearing loss. Similarly, despite the superiority of both the FM system and the hearing aid plus FM system on speech-recognition tasks, subjects overwhelmingly chose the conventional hearing aid as a system they would prefer to use in daily life. Interestingly, the hearing aid was used by subjects 11 hours per day, whereas the FM system was used 1 hour a day. The FM system was considered by most participants to be cumbersome and intrusive, obviating its routine use by older adults. The work of Chisolm et al (2007) corroborated the data of Jerger and colleagues, finding that the hearing impaired are not willing to embrace FM devices despite their benefits. The litmus test of "intent to acquire" continues to indicate a lack of acceptance on the part of adults with significant hearing impairment.

Bluetooth is a short-range wireless radio technology with a transmission range of 30 to 300 feet and operating within a frequency range of 2.4 to 2.5 GHz that is increasingly used to enable people to wirelessly connect to cellular phones (Bloom, 2009). Increasingly, wireless communication is tied to the Bluetooth protocol. Bluetooth accessories pair with Bluetooth devices to send the audio signal to the hearing aid via direct audio input, FM transmission, digital magnetic wireless transmission, electromagnetic relay, or an internal coil (Yanz, 2007). Bluetooth technology and newer methods of digital magnetic transmission hold a good deal of promise for hearing-aid users. Although the battery power requirements are a limitation, increasingly hearing-aid manufacturers are marketing hearing aids that embed a Bluetooth chip to facilitate a wireless connections (Bloom, 2009). However, the Bluetooth feature may increase the size of the hearing aids, so hearing-aid users must

choose between size and functionality (Sever & Abreu, 2009). Requiring a small antenna because of the high-frequency range and method of transmission, Bluetooth technology is used to pair hearing aids with a wide range of devices, including cellular phones, televisions, laptop computers, and audio devices such as the iPod. Unlike infrared transmitting devices, the Bluetooth originating device does not have to be in the line of sight, but rather within a network area, providing a huge advantage to potential users. In a typical setup, a microphone is placed within a few inches of the talker's mouth or an audio source such as a stereo system, and its output is carried by a wireless link to the listener, using Bluetooth technology. This arrangement is ideal for people who spend a good deal of time in their home and enjoy listening to their media devices. Baby boomers, who began turning 65 in 2011 and are relatively "tech" savvy, are ideal candidates for any of the devices, most of which are manufactured by the major hearing-aid companies so that the devices are compatible with the hearing aids (the proprietary nature of these systems is potentially problematic).

Bluetooth technology is limited in that it has the capability for one-to-one broadcast rather than point-to-multipoint broadcast, so that the use of this mode of transmission in places of worship, auditoriums, and schools is not feasible (Yanz, 2007). Battery drain is a huge issue as well with Bluetooth technology. Given some of these limitations, hearing-aid companies are experimenting with near-field magnetic induction (NFMI) and radiofrequency (RF) technologies (Schum & Sjolander, 2011). Several hearing-aid companies have embraced NFMI because the components are small, power requirements are low, and various levels of binaural signal processing can be used, wherein two hearing aids communicate with one another. These technologies use a gateway or intermediate device to transform the Bluetooth signal into either the NFMI or RF format. Although NFMI is in an early stage of application to hearing-aid technology, Schum and Sjolander (2011) contend that its use with a streamer allows patients to get the most from their residual hearing.

Connectivity has advanced well beyond the use of the T-coil, with significant developments in wireless transmission of audio signals to hearing-aid users. Schum and Sjolander (2011) summarized the advantages of connectivity: (1) higher quality and more intelligible speech signal; (2) increased comprehension of television sound and telephone conversation; (3) decreased mobility issues when multitasking, such as watching television and answering the telephone; and (4) fully integrated systems that are easier for those with manual dexterity problems to manipulate.

Pearl

A Bluetooth signal is more secure than an FM signal, as it incorporates adaptive "frequency hopping" to increase the robustness of a signal while at the same time minimizing interference (Lindley, 2007).

Hearing-Aid Arrangement: Monaural Versus Binaural

In addition to feature selection, a big decision the person with hearing impairment must make is whether to invest in one

Table 8.9 Ways in which Binaural Amplification Benefits Speech Recognition in Noise

1. Increases audibility of speech sounds
2. Improves directional hearing
3. Restores the availability of interaural level and timing cues, thereby improving spatial advantage
4. Provides for redundancy, as the listener is listening to the same signal delivered to both ears

Source: Adapted from Ahlstrom, J. B., Horwitz, A. R., & Dubno, J. R. (2009, Apr). Spatial benefit of bilateral hearing AIDS. *Ear and Hearing, 30,* 203–218.

or two hearing aids. The purported advantages provided by binaural amplification are listed in **Table 8.9** and include improved localization, binaural summation, improved ability to understand speech in noise, improved hearing at a distance, ease of listening, and a more natural/balanced sound. Although audiologists claim that people with bilateral hearing loss ultimately decide that two hearing aids are preferable to one, this is just anecdotal, and the evidence regarding whom to fit binaurally is lacking, as controversy remains regarding the perceived advantages of binaural versus monaural (Cox et al, 2011). Interestingly, however, clinically and in selected field trials there are always some proportion of hearing-aid users (21 to 46%) who prefer one hearing aid to two.

Cox et al (2011) explored pre-fitting variables that would predict preference for one rather than two hearing aids and approaches to the most cost-effective patient-centered solution to the fitting process. Hearing loss was not a predictor of preference for two hearing aids rather than one. In addition to meeting their communication needs, participants preferring a monaural fitting attributed this to comfort and quality. Hearing-aid users preferring two expressed a preference because of the restoration of balance, clarity of sounds, and comfort. This study shed light on the observation that binaural may be preferable for individuals having more daily problems, because of the binaural advantage and the reduction in the feeling of binaural imbalance. Based on their findings, Cox et al concluded that "bilateral aiding is not necessarily the patient-centered treatment for all adults with mild to moderate bilaterally symmetrical sensorineural hearing loss" (p. 194). Their findings suggested that, when asked, as many as 30 to 40% of potential hearing-aid users will decide on one hearing aid rather than two. Among those preferring one hearing aid over two, it seems that their preference may have been based in part on their lower tolerance thresholds for sound.

Cox et al (2011) describe a decision tree that may be helpful as part of a client-centered approach, with which prospective hearing-aid users are encouraged to consider the net benefit of binaural and the difference between treatment benefits (such as a decrease in symptoms of hearing loss) and treatment burdens (such as money, aggravation, stigma, and the discomfort of using two hearing aids). Another potential treatment benefit is the reduction of auditory deprivation effects associated with the use of two hearing aids (Silman, Gelfand, & Silverman, 1984). Cox and colleagues caution that benefits and burdens of treatment vary among users, and the treatment point at which net benefit is maximized is likely to vary as well. Accordingly, to facilitate decision making, they recommend doing a field trial, in which persons with hearing impairment

record their experiences in various settings and situations. The data-logging feature can be helpful here, especially if the hearing-aid users are asked to switch between one and two hearing aids. Cox and colleagues also confirm that laboratory measures are often not helpful in isolating the binaural advantage. In my view, clinicians should heed Cox et al's conclusions that "there is no accurate way to predict in advance the aiding preference for a particular individual," and "at this time, the most effective approach open to practitioners would be to conduct a candid unbiased systematic field trial comparing unilateral and bilateral fittings with each patient" (p. 195).

Ahlstrom et al (2009) explored the spatial benefit of bilateral amplification and the benefit of spatial separation for speech recognition in noise in a sample of older adult hearing-aid users. The goal of their study was to build on prior studies that suggest that older adults with hearing impairment may be deficient in the use of interaural difference cues to experience the binaural advantage, especially in noisy situations. The authors reasoned that if older adults are not as adept as younger adults in utilizing interaural difference cues provided by spatial separation, which helps to improve the SNR, then perhaps this could partly explain why older adults with hearing impairment experience difficulty understanding in noise. Participants had a mean age of 75 years, and had sloping high-frequency hearing loss. They were provided with commercially available bilateral digital hearing aids with WDRC. The hearing aids were programmed to match NAL-NL1 2-cc coupler targets with hearing-aid gain across frequency adjusted to within ±5 dB of target values of inputs of 50, 65, and 80 dB SPL. Participants wore the hearing aids for 3 to 6 months, after which outcomes were assessed, using the SSQ, in several domains: acceptable noise level, speech recognition in noise, and self-reported satisfaction and benefit. The SSQ was specifically designed to assess perceived binaural listening ability. Participants underwent a hearing-aid orientation following the fitting, even the experienced hearing-aid users, who comprised one third of the sample. The orientation included training in the use and care of hearing aids, including replacement of batteries and use of communication strategies.

Many of the findings were noteworthy and unexpected. In general, hearing-aid benefit for this sample was exceedingly small but present. One notable finding was that, using the HINT sentences with speech and babble spatially separated, the benefit from binaural hearing aids improved as a function of the high-frequency cutoff, with the most significant improvement occurring when the bandwidth increased from 1800 to 3600 Hz and not from 3600 to 5600 Hz. Further, listeners with higher ANL values without hearing aids who tolerated less babble reported more hearing-aid use, and participants who experienced more hearing-aid benefit based on performance on the ANL also reported more hearing-aid use. Listeners who achieved more spatial benefit with binaural hearing aids for speech recognition tolerated less favorable aided SNRs when speech and babble were spatially separated. In addition, and contrary to expectation, the ANL improved with hearing aids when aided speech and babble were spatially separated, with more babble tolerated when it was to the side of the listener rather than in front, which again has implications for counseling, especially regarding success with directional technology. No significant correlations were observed between hearing-aid benefit and cognitive deficits, even though it has been hypothesized that cognitive factors may account for individual differences in hearing-aid benefit once audibility is restored. Ahlstrom and colleagues speculated that the latter finding may be an artifact of the hearing-aid settings (very slow time constants) and the laboratory arrangement (12-talker babble). They concluded that older adults did not appear to take full advantage of the increase in audible speech information provided by binaural amplification, but they noted that this may be due to the fact that in some participants speech audibility was not restored across the full bandwidth of speech.

Summarizing to this point, binaural is often "better" because of the advantages it offers in terms of understanding in noise, localization, ease of listening and stabilization of word recognition scores; however, for some the disadvantages outweigh the advantages. For example, financial constraints and binaural interference as discussed in the next section are valid reasons for forsaking a binaural fitting. Note that when fitting binaurally, clinicians must avoid a "loudness percept that is too loud." Kuk (2008) recommends that the prescriptive targets for binaural and monaural fittings must be adjusted such that a gain that is 3 to 5 dB less is recommended. That is, the fitting target must be different from a monaural fitting, as a binaural fitting requires less gain. Finally, I would speculate that perhaps the preference for binaural hearing aids will be impacted by wireless connectivity between hearing aids introduced by some manufacturers. Although to date there is no evidence regarding the value of wireless technology that allows hearing aids in a binaural fitting to coordinate settings such as microphone mode and memories, the use of digital magnetic wireless communication has promise (Kerckhoff et al, 2008). Ear-to-ear wireless transmissions enable synchronization of gain, signal processing, and discrete pitch and amplitude cues between the ears thereby assisting in binaural hearing and understanding (Kerckhoff et al, 2008; Preves & Banerjee, 2008).

As noted above, the findings are mixed on the benefits of and preferences for a binaural fitting in selected older adults, and not all individuals with bilateral hearing loss benefit from binaural hearing aids. Some individuals experience binaural interference, whereby speech-recognition performance in the binaural hearing-aid condition is worse than performance in the best monaural condition. These individuals therefore function better with one hearing aid (monaural fitting) than two hearing aids (binaural fitting). Binaural interference should be viewed as a contraindication to a binaural hearing-aid fitting; hence, it should be assessed clinically using dichotic speech tests under earphones or in aided conditions. Chmiel and Jerger (1995) confirmed that elderly persons with central deficits (DSI-abnormal), as measured using dichotically presented sentences (the DSI), show significantly less improvement in self-reported handicap with amplification than did older adults without a central auditory deficit. Given the latter finding that a CAPD may prevent selected older adults from realizing the full potential of amplification, the hearing-aid selection process should include an estimate of central auditory processing ability to help in deciding on the fitting arrangement and the appropriate amplification system. For example, if a person has a speech-recognition score of 64% when the right

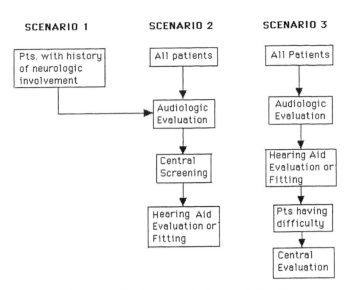

Fig. 8.12 Three scenarios demonstrating how central auditory assessment of hearing-aid candidates could be included in the overall evaluation of these clients. [From Valente, M. (2006). *Hearing aids: Standards, options, and limitations* (p. 434). New York: Thieme.]

hearing aid is worn and 84% when the left hearing aid is worn, then performance in the binaural hearing-aid condition should not be worse than 84%. If it is, then this is suggestive of probable binaural interference. Similarly, when experienced binaural hearing-aid users note a change in their everyday function, in addition to verifying hearing-aid performance with real ear or probe microphone measures, the audiologist must conduct speech-recognition testing (in quiet and in noise) with the hearing aid in the right ear, in the left hearing aid, and in both ears.

Using terminology from Musiek and Baran (1996), the audiologist should also test the ability to achieve a "fused binaural image." Musiek and Baran proposed three potential scenarios for incorporating tests of central auditory processing into the hearing-aid evaluation/process. As depicted in **Fig. 8.12**, one approach is to administer a central screening test for only those clients with a positive history of neurological involvement. A second approach is to administer a test of central auditory function for all hearing-aid candidates. A third approach is to conduct a central auditory screen on patients whose hearing aids have become ineffective over time. As noted above, the speech-recognition score in the binaural hearing-aid condition should be at least as good as the best monaural score. If not, then the hearing-aid user should discontinue with the binaural fitting and transition to wearing the hearing aid in the ear giving the better speech-recognition score. Binaural interference, a term coined by Jerger, Silman, Lew, and Chmiel (1993), is often the reason that older adults are not successful in using a binaural configuration.

Special Consideration

It is important to emphasize that it may take 6 to 12 weeks for an older adult to acclimate to binaural amplification, especially if one ear has been unaided for a lengthy period of time.

Despite the mixed results from laboratory and field studies regarding the documented benefits of binaural amplification and the phenomenon of binaural interference, which argues against a binaural fitting, the data on auditory deprivation are rather compelling. Arlinger et al (1996) defined auditory deprivation as a decrease in performance on auditory-based tests associated with the reduced availability of auditory information or deprivation due to lack of amplification in an ear.

Beginning in 1984, the research on auditory deprivation and recovery provided important evidence to be shared with patients regarding the value of binaural fittings when audiometrically, cognitively, and financially it is a viable option. Silman et al (1984) were among the first investigators to report on the concept of auditory deprivation associated with failure to amplify an ear with bilaterally symmetrical sensorineural hearing loss. Their findings suggest that when speech-recognition scores of subjects with bilateral sensorineural hearing loss who are fit monaurally are compared with those of a comparable group of subjects who are fit binaurally, speech-recognition scores in the unaided ear of the monaurally aided group decline dramatically over a 4- to 5-year period. Most encouraging are reports that some patients with auditory deprivation effects experience clinically significant albeit incomplete recovery following use of binaural amplification (Gelfand, 1995). These findings have been replicated by several investigators on a variety of populations, including older adults with presbycusis. Since the historic Eriksholm Workshop on Auditory Deprivation and Acclimatization, held in Denmark in August 1995, the functional plasticity of the auditory system has been established, especially in the context of hearing-aid use for those with at least a degree of hearing loss and, in some cases, when converting a monaural hearing-aid fitting to a binaural fitting (Arlinger et al, 1996). Functional plasticity refers to the system's ability to move from damaged to undamaged areas in order to function.

Silverman, Silman, Emmer, Schoepflin, and Lutolf (2006) conducted a prospective study on auditory deprivation in persons with asymmetric sensorineural hearing impairment. The mean age of participants in the unaided control group with asymmetric hearing loss and no history of hearing-aid use was 54 years, and that of the monaurally aided experimental groups with asymmetric sensorineural hearing loss was 55.7 years. Because the upper limit of the age range of participants was 77 years, I consider the conclusions from the study to be only somewhat applicable, as the entire sample was not composed of older adults. Participants had comparable pure-tone thresholds, spondee thresholds, and speech recognition scores at the start of the investigation. The experimental group was fitted monaurally with a hearing aid (of unspecified features) in the poorer ear. The findings, although subtle, were of considerable interest. Over a 2-year time frame, the spondee thresholds in the better and poorer ears did not change, even in the experimental group wearing a hearing aid in the poorer ear. Additionally, the change in pure-tone thresholds over time, which was slight, was comparable for the better ear of those in the experimental and control groups. Further, the PTA for the worse ear did not change significantly for participants in both groups. Differences in monaural word recognition scores (WRSs) over time were comparable in the better ear across both groups. However, changes over time in poorer ear WRSs were noteworthy for participants in the control and experimental groups. Specifically, change in the poorer ear of participants not receiving hearing aids was considerable as compared with the slight improvement in the poorer ear of those in the experimental group who received hearing aids. In fact, change in WRS was significant in 43.8% of the worse ears in the control group. I am guardedly optimistic regarding the clinical significance of the latter findings, in that the percent improvement in word recognition scores on the Central Institute for the Deaf W-22 word list in the aided ear was rather small (mean of 6%) after 2 years. Perhaps more convincing was the stability of scores, slight improvement, and lack of a decrement in scores over time in the aided ear of the experimental groups. **Figure 8.13** summarizes the differences in WRSs over time in the control and experimental groups (aided).

Based on the work of Silverman et al (2006), Gatehouse (1992), and others, the presence of late-onset auditory deprivation is a compelling reason for older adults who prefer a monaural fitting to consider a binaural fitting, especially in the presence of symmetrical or asymmetrical sensorineural hearing loss (worse ear aidable) and in the absence of binaural interference. If the phenomenon of late-onset auditory deprivation could be linked to decrements in quality of life or cognitive declines, it would provide even more powerful evidence for this fitting strategy. I concur with Gelfand (1995) that when financial considerations preclude binaural amplification, the possibility of alternating monaural amplification should be explored to minimize the potential for auditory deprivation effects to set in. In subjects who prefer a unilateral fitting, or when binaural interference argue against binaural fitting, the unaided ear should be monitored by pure tone and speech audiometry annually and use of an FM system or binaural fitting should be considered if signs of the deprivation effect occur.

Hearing Aid Coupling Considerations

With the renewed popularity of BTE hearing aids and the advent of the open-fit–mini/micro BTE hearing aids with slim tubes or receiver-in-the-canal products, audiologists once again must concern themselves with earmold/tubing modifications/selection, earmold guard or wax filter systems, and materials that can contribute to a successful fitting especially for the thin tube/thin-wire mini-BTE units (Taylor & Teter, 2009). The fundamental decisions to be made pertain to tubing size and length, venting, and parameters of the dome. With regard to earmold material, the choices remain acrylic, silicone, and soft silicone, with each having specific advantages/disadvantages for the elderly. Acrylic molds tend to be hard but durable and easy to fit and to modify, and silicone tends to be softer, and can expand to reduce possible slit leaks. Soft silicone is preferable for those with profound loss but is not typically the material of choice for the elderly. Regarding optimal vent diameters, Kuk and Baekgaard (2008) suggest using 500 Hz as the benchmark, so, for example, if a hearing-aid user has a hearing loss of 20 to 29 dB HL, the vent diameter should be 3 to 4 mm, whereas if the hearing loss is 50 to 60 dB HL, the vent diameter should be 0.5 to 1 mm. They emphasize that because the

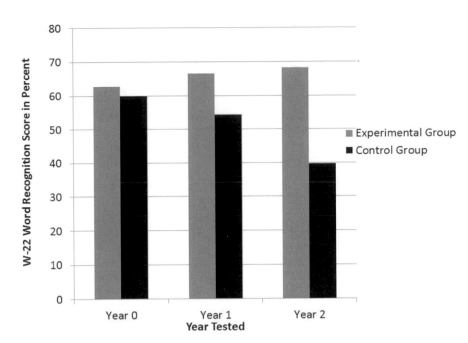

Fig. 8.13 Median word recognition scores on the W-22 word lists for the worse ear of the experimental aided group and worse ear of the control group at baseline (year 0), year 1, and year 2. [From Silverman, C. A., Silman, S., Emmer, M. B., Schoepflin, J. R., & Lutolf, J. J. (2006, Nov–Dec). Auditory deprivation in adults with asymmetric, sensorineural hearing impairment. *Journal of the American Academy of Audiology, 17*, 747–762. Reprinted by permission.]

vent effect reduces the output of hearing aids up to 2000 Hz, an occluding mold may be the only option for persons with significant hearing loss above 1000 Hz. Regarding decisions about tubing size, although thin tubing (inner diameter of 0.8 mm) is advantageous in terms of cosmetic appeal, it reduces high-frequency output as compared with standard No. 13 tubing, and audibility of the high frequencies is important for older adults. In the latter regard, Kuk and Baekgaard recommend standard No. 13 tubing when the hearing loss exceeds 65 dB HL.

With regard to open-canal fittings, the amount by which one wants to extend the low-frequency fitting range will impact the decision. The term *open-fit* or *open-ear* hearing aids typically refers to one of two arrangements: (1) a miniature BTE hearing aid coupled with a soft nonoccluding ear dome via a slim tube, leaving the ear canal open to take advantage of its natural resonance (RITA), or (2) a BTE hearing aid where the receiver is outside of the hearing-aid case and sits inside the wearer's ear canal (RIC/RITE). In RIC fittings, a thin wire that is insulated in a thin tube connects the receiver to the BTE case (Kuk & Baekgaard, 2008). Open canal hearing instruments are favored by clinicians and patients alike because of their small size and their ability to minimize occlusion, because they can fit a wide range of hearing levels, and because of their cosmetic appeal. They differ in several features, including method of sound delivery to the ear canal, distance between the microphone and the receiver, physical size of the devices, and bandwidth, with RIC aids using receivers with broad bandwidths, effectively extending their range. According to Kuk and Baekgaard, the wider bandwidth provides a richer and clearer sound; however, this receiver technology may only be appropriate for those with mild to moderate hearing loss. Regarding preferences for RITE/RIC or RITA, **Table 8.10** summarizes the conclusions from a variety of studies.

Kuk and Baekgaard described six basic BTE coupling options that differ according to the diameter of the tubing and the openness of the ear canal. In general, the choice of coupling method will be an open-ear versus an occluded-ear fit, and thin wire versus thin tube or standard No. 13 tube versus thin-tube fitting. Regarding the degree of occlusion, although individuals requiring gain up to 1500 Hz will be under-fitted with an open-fit hearing aid, an occluding mold may be uncomfortable and lead to nonuse, so I recommend a field trial with perhaps an occluding earmold (with vent) and possibly a double-dome fitting. Kuk and Baekgaard suggest that given the cosmetic appeal, audiologists should consider thin-tube fittings for open-ear and occluded-ear fittings.

Open, closed, and double domes can be used to close off the canal and allow varying amounts of low-frequency gain. The open dome provides the most reduction in gain at 500 Hz; the smaller the vent in a custom mold, the less low-frequency reduction, and a thin tube/wire coupled to a custom mold can extend the fitting range of mini-BTE units substantially (Taylor & Teter, 2009). Hence, open-dome fittings are most appropriate for hearing-aid users with mild to moderately severe loss, with closed-dome or double-dome fittings extending the fitting range considerably. One caveat regarding the closed-dome fitting is that there is some evidence to suggest that the ear canal is not sufficiently occluded to allow for significant low-frequency gain. The double-dome fitting may be slightly more occluding, allowing for a slight increase in low-frequency gain. Teie (2009) suggests that when prescribing a RITE hearing aid

Table 8.10   Preferences for Receiver-in-the-Ear (RITE) Versus Receiver-in-the-Aid (RITA) Hearing Aids

Style	Advantages	Disadvantages
RITE (RIC): receiver is in the ear canal	Smaller, less noticeable, than RITA; new users prefer this	Hard to remove dome and change wax guard
	Tubing does not get clogged	Hard to position RITE tubing
	Greater maximum gain at 4000 and 6000 Hz; more high-frequency gain before feedback than with RITA; preferable for those with significant high-frequency loss	Slightly more occlusion
	Better sound quality, higher satisfaction ratings and preferences in quiet	Receiver bulky and not comfortable
	Provides broader bandwidth and lower feedback risk due to shorter distance between microphone and receiver	Receiver is exposed to moisture and cerumen, and chance of damage is increased
	Receiver can easily be replaced by clinician, should damage occur, as the aid is modular in concept	
	Greater reserve gain before feedback at 4000 and 6000 Hz	
RITA: receiver is in the hearing aid	Easier maintenance and cleaning	Less occlusion than with RIC
	Comfortable in the ear and not too bulky	Cannot extend fitting range into the low frequencies effectively with closed domes or double domes
	Easier to position, easier to fit in ears with small canals, better retention in these cases	
	Less gain at 4000 and 6000 Hz	
	Less satisfactory in quiet	
	Better for persons not prone to cerumen buildup, as there is less maintenance and it is easier to maintain	

Sources: Adapted from Marcrum, C., & Ricketts, M. (2011). *Open canal hearing aids: Tips and tricks for the clinic.* http://www.myavaa.org/documents/JDVAC-2011-Presentations/Ricketts_HDVAC2011.pdf; and Alworth, L., Plyler, P., Rebert, M., & Johnstone, P. (2010). The effects of receiver placement on probe microphone, performance, and subjective measures with open canal hearing instruments. *Journal of the American Academy of Audiology, 21,* 249–266.

for persons with significant low-frequency loss, a custom mold option may be most appropriate. Real-ear measures are key due to the individual variability owing to the interaction between the shape of most ear canals (e.g., elliptical) and the shape of dome couplers (circular).

> **Pearl**
>
> Closed-dome or double-dome fittings extend the fitting range beyond that which is feasible with open-dome fittings. Using probe-tube measurements, Teie (2009) dramatically displays the differences in output especially in the low frequencies across open, closed, slim-tube, and double-dome fittings

When fitting older adults, always keep in mind that the important features are comfort, ease of operation, and the availability of features that will assist in their most difficult listening situations. It is critical that the consumer have the opportunity to judge the different signal-processing features and fitting options using real-life listening materials or in real-world conditions. It is often helpful to provide the hearing-aid user repeated opportunities to manipulate the controls and observe the ease or difficulty with which the individual approaches the task, as such trials can facilitate a decision regarding choice of a hearing aid that meets the many needs of the older adult.

An increasing number of older adults are demanding objective justification or verification of the value of their instruments relative to their cost and quality-of-life improvements. Audiologists are urged to involve the consumer in every aspect of the dispensing and decision-making process. Anecdotal reports suggest that the consumer finds this aspect of the fitting process clarifying, as often the benefits of selected features and a given technology become readily apparent. Objective verification of the adequacy of the hearing-aid performance and amplification targets using coupler measurements, probe microphone measurements, or sound-field measurements using speech and nonspeech stimuli is a precondition for any judgments regarding choice of a hearing aid that best meets the user's needs. Similarly, the person with hearing loss and the communication partner must be given the opportunity to validate performance change or benefit with the hearing aid. It is imperative that audiologists understand that, especially with older adults, verification of performance change using real ear measures, for example, does not necessarily translate into perceived hearing-aid benefit and satisfaction, and this is where the art and science of hearing-aid fittings must be reconciled.

Regarding post-fitting assessments, the data on acclimatization should inform the protocol used when assessing patients over time. Make sure to monitor changes in loudness perception associated with long-term hearing-aid use, and make sure that the binaural advantages are apparent for those persons purchasing binaural hearing aids. Audiologists must allow time for the hearing-aid user to acclimate to hearing aids, with the appropriate time for verification of the adequacy of the fitting ranging between 3 weeks and 3 months, depending on the outcome dimension assessed.

Acclimatization

It is critical to allow time for auditory and cognitive physiological and psychological acclimatization to hearing aids, especially when an ear or ears have been deprived of auditory input for an extended period of time or when transitioning from a monaural to a binaural fitting or from a binaural to a monaural fitting. As the typical older adult waits about 10 years between first noting a hearing loss and taking steps toward purchasing a hearing aid, the functional morphology of the auditory system may have been temporarily compromised by acoustic deprivation, necessitating a period of time for the process of adjustment associated with neural plasticity (Musiek & Baran, 1996). The term *auditory deprivation* is often conflated with the term *acclimatization,* which entails improvement in auditory performance over time and is associated with newly available acoustic information. Often mentioned when discussing acclimatization, the term *plasticity* entails an improvement in auditory function that has a physiological basis and is often a by-product of acclimatization. The term *acclimatization* was coined by Gatehouse (1992) and refers to how listeners with hearing loss require time to adapt to the new speech cues available through amplification, which is typically in the higher frequencies to restore loudness and audibility of sounds important for speech recognition. Gatehouse speculated that over time, due to brain rewiring and the need for the auditory system to accommodate to the high signal levels, which were previously inaudible, these levels can be processed by the auditory cortex as it begins to fill in the gaps from the previously unstimulated regions (Citron, 2008). Any change in auditory performance over time attributable to acclimatization cannot be linked to changes or modifications in acoustic information available to the hearing-aid user associated with adjusting electroacoustic features (Kuk, Potts, Valente, Lee, & Picirrillo, 2003).

Philibert, Collet, Vesson, and Veuillet (2005) explored whether the availability of acoustic information from hearing-aid use changed performance on auditory tasks that assess the peripheral auditory system. Participants had symmetrical sloping sensorineural hearing impairment and were first-time hearing-aid users. All hearing aids used digital technology. Participants were tested prior to hearing-aid use, as well as at 1, 3, and 6 months of hearing-aid experience. With the passage of time, the loudness ratings shifted such that the intensity was perceived as being less loud, especially at 2000 Hz. Interestingly, in the right ear the wave V latency was shortened, which the authors speculated was attributable to a possible increase in neural synchronization over time. Their finding that hearing-aid use may induce plasticity peripherally has support in the work of Munro and Trotter (2006), who looked at change in uncomfortable loudness levels (ULLs) over a period of 12 to 60 months of hearing-aid use. Participants had a symmetrical high-frequency sensorineural hearing loss. Mean age of participants who were fitted monaurally was 77 years. Participants used their hearing aids for a median of 5 hours per day. As was the case in the Philibert et al (2005)

study, there was an increase in tolerance levels for louder sounds, such that although the ULLs were similar in both ears before the hearing-aid fitting, they diverged considerably afterward, especially in the higher frequencies.

Munro and Lutman (2003) assessed acclimatization effects using word recognition measures, which in some studies were not successful in documenting these effects. Participants were 16 older adults with a mean age of 70 years who were first-time hearing-aid users with mild to moderate sloping high-frequency sensorineural hearing loss. They were fitted monaurally with digitally programmable BTE hearing aids, and were required to wear them 6 to 8 hours per day. The volume control was disabled so as not to interfere with the validity of the test results. Benefit based on change in speech recognition scores in noise over time was how acclimatization was assessed. Speech-recognition ability was assessed at increasing presentation levels over a period of 12 weeks in both the fitted and unfitted ears. There was little change in word-recognition scores in the control ear, which was not fitted with a hearing aid; however, there was a dramatic pattern of change in the fitted ear over time, which was influenced by presentation level. In short, there was an acclimatization effect, albeit small, in that at higher presentation levels word-recognition scores in the fitted ear gradually improved over time. The control or non-fitted ear did not display any change in benefit over time at any of the presentation levels. They found that after an extended period of hearing-aid use, individuals appeared to gain an increased tolerance for loud sounds. The findings on word-recognition scores are somewhat equivocal, but assessing speech-recognition ability at elevated presentation levels is sensitive to the effects of acclimatization.

The exact time frame for acclimatization also remains elusive, but new hearing-aid users should expect a 2- to 3-month adjustment period before their ear and brain acclimate to the newly audible sounds. Hilda Khakshoor, a former doctoral student of mine, conducted a systematic review of acclimatization using self-report questionnaires. Based on a systematic review of 15 studies, it appears that self-report measures are not sensitive to gradations of benefit over time. Although significant improvements in hearing-related quality of life are notable between 3 and 6 weeks following hearing-aid use, there is little recent evidence that self-report measures are sensitive to the gradual adjustments that the auditory system appears to make to amplification after 6 to 8 weeks of hearing-aid use.

Pearl

The acclimatization effect may in fact be due to "perceptual learning," wherein the hearing-aid user gradually adjusts to the newly audible speech cues such that the perceptual learning may translate into slight improvements in scores on selected outcome measures over time.

◆ Hearing-Aid Orientation

At the conclusion of the hearing-aid fitting, it is important to spend a considerable amount of time orienting the new hearing-aid user and the communication partner. The orientation is the audiologist's opportunity to supply information about (1) the hearing aid and its features, care, and maintenance; (2) instrument insertion and removal; (3) troubleshooting; (4) expectations/limitations; (5) a wearing schedule and situational uses; and (6) battery issues (Reese & Hnath-Chisolm, 2005). Information about device-related variables (instruction in use of technology), HATs, and patient-related information such as expectations are critical components of this part of the management process (Valente et al, 2006a). According to Boothroyd and colleagues (2007), there is ample evidence that hearing-aid usage is enhanced when device-related formal instruction takes place. It is well established that an effective orientation/consumer education program can reduce hearing-aid returns by half and promote hearing-aid satisfaction. The patient's primary communication partner, family member, or caregiver should be present during the orientation session to maximize success. Further, if the hearing-aid orientation can be conducted with one of the hearing aids in the patient's ear adjusted (by the patient) to a comfortable listening level, this would provide an opportunity to acclimate to the sound of his/her own voice while using the other unit for the orientation. When demonstrating the operation of the hearing aid, it is helpful to use a personal amplifier to ensure understanding if the hearing aid is not in the patient's ear. I also recommend a Lucite head with a plastic ear or ears, as these can be invaluable when instructing the person with hearing loss (PHL) about hearing-aid insertion. The hearing-aid orientation is considered complete when the patient is competent to handle the hearing aids(s) independently or with the assistance of a caregiver or communication partner who is well versed in care and maintenance (Valente et al, 2006a).

The typical orientation session lasts 45 minutes to 1 hour, depending on the hearing aid(s) dispensed and the consumer. There also should be booster sessions to ensure retention and carryover of the newly learned information. The amount of orientation time and the number of sessions required can vary significantly from one patient to the next. For individuals with cognitive problems, brief sessions over a period of a few weeks may be preferable because of their limited ability to concentrate or focus. Cognitive and auditory training using LACE is an important complement to the hearing-aid orientation. The importance of using multiple modalities including the visual and tactile senses, handouts, iPad or smartphone uapps, and instructional videos cannot be overemphasized. Magnifiers and adequate lighting is imperative as well. The self-efficacy model should inform the pacing of the orientation sessions. Self-efficacy is developed when individuals experience a sense of mastery over a particular task. The best way to master a skill is if the clinician begins with easier aspects before advancing to more difficult ones. Extensive practice and positive feedback is the optimal way to bolster self-efficacy (Smith & West, 2006).

During the orientation sessions, keep the following points in mind. Older adults require more and different reinforcement; they respond better to concrete goals that are immediate and affect daily functioning. **Table 8.11** includes some suggestions from Smith and West (2006) for incorporating self-efficacy principles into the hearing-aid orientation. Remember to reassure the patient as often as possible. Be sure to reward successes and keep reinforcement closely linked to the desired behavior (Kemp, 1990). Older adults often avoid difficult tasks because of anxiety associated with new or challenging tasks. Accordingly, the older adult should be given every opportunity to experience improvement or success, and should be encouraged to move from unaided to aided situations and from quiet to noisy situations gradually. When instructing the patient about the use and operation of the hearing aid, regular corrective feedback presented in a nonthreatening, supportive manner will go a long way toward reducing anxiety, sustaining continued involvement, and promoting motivation and a sense of success. Instructions should be repeated, and the audiolo-

Table 8.11 Self-Efficacy–Enhancing Strategies for the Hearing-Aid Orientation (HAO)

Strategy	Example
Work first with the simpler hearing-aid skills and then progress to more complicated skills. In addition to beginning with simpler skills to build user's confidence, this also reduces stress of new learning.	First distinguish between right and left hearing aid and then proceed to discussing the on-off switch.
Offer extensive practice with hearing-aid skills at different times during the HAO to encourage mastery experience.	Practice selecting hearing aid for each ear; practice hearing-aid insertion.
Patients should take home a checklist and practice newly learned skills to reinforce learning.	Identify hearing aid that goes in each ear.
Set clear goals for each session for learning to use and care for the hearing aids.	Patients should know that when they return for the follow-up, they will be expected to know how to insert the hearing aid in the correct ear.
Provide realistic and frequent feedback based on the patient's capabilities.	"Great, you inserted the hearing aid perfectly!"
Be positive when explaining a new skill so patient is not threatened.	"Many people are able to insert their hearing aids after a few trials like you are doing."
Make sure the learning environment is free of distractions.	Cell phones should be turned off; hearing-aid battery should be working.
Provide sufficient time for learning.	Make sure session is long enough for tasks to be learned.

Source: From Smith, S. L., & West, R. L. (2006, Jun). The application of self-efficacy principles to audiologic rehabilitation: A tutorial. *American Journal of Audiology, 15,* 46–56.

gist should verify that the patient has understood the information being conveyed. Revisiting topics that were difficult at an earlier session is critical. For example, if a patient was having trouble with accurate earmold insertion and with identifying the correct ear for insertion, then a goal that the audiologist may encourage is that the patient be able to insert the earmold accurately after 1 week of at-home practice. Providing mnemonics to remember that the unit with the red dot is for the right ear and the blue dot for the left ear is always helpful. An older person may have a different learning style. Learn what it is, use it, and respect it.

As Wingfield and Tun (2001) advise, a slower speaking rate may help to ensure adequate speech understanding for the older adult. However, it is important to avoid use of an overly slow rate of speech with an exaggerated tone that can be misconstrued as condescending. Keep in mind that older adults do not want sympathy from the hearing health care practitioner but do want to work with an empathic professional who understands the problems posed by hearing impairment. Empathy can develop if the clinician remembers that older adults with acquired hearing loss have spent the bulk of their lives with normal hearing. Only recently have they had to live with loss of signal perception at a time when they are experiencing decreased ability to cope successfully with a variety of problems.

The concept of a self-efficacy based hearing-aid orientation is key, given the relation between self-efficacy and outcomes (Smith & West 2006). Self-efficacy–based training is important, as the higher the self-efficacy, the more likely and willing the individual will be to try to learn challenging tasks, such as battery insertion and removal. Further, those with high self-efficacy will persist and will try hard to succeed even though a task is challenging. A caregiver or communication partner should attend the hearing-aid orientation sessions and learn the new skills, as this can help facilitate self-efficacy.

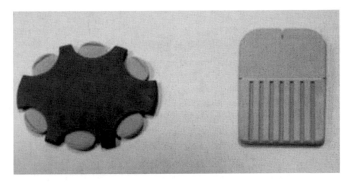

Fig. 8.14 Sample wax protection system.

should be discussed, including how and when to replace, clean, and remove obstructions. The effects of cerumen buildup on the receiver, the earmold, and in-the-ear and in-the-canal hearing aids, and proper cleaning techniques should be discussed. The wax guard option incorporated into the hearing aid should be discussed, as well as the symptoms of wax buildup and the various wax control options. **Figure 8.14** displays options available for protection from cerumen buildup; I find that older adults' manual dexterity and vision status are factors in their ability to effectively use this wax protection system. For those people who purchase Lyric hearing aids, the subscription arrangement, the life of the device (e.g., 120 days), frequency of return visits, replacement visits, and discussion of symptoms suggesting the need for a follow-up visit should be discussed.

The hearing-aid user should be familiarized with the function of each feature and switch, including microphone type and location of the sound inlet(s); volume control; on-off switch or two- or three-position switch (e.g., MT or M-T-O); multi-memory button; feedback managers; T and MT switches; power-on delay; removal handles; number of programs; windscreens; data logging (when applicable); direct audio input (DAI) and other input capabilities; and any wireless enhancements or sound-learning features. The detail with which each feature is discussed is dependent on several nonaudiological variables including the user's comfort level with technology, cognitive status, vision status, and physical or functional status. The more technologically savvy the user, the more detailed the instruction should be. The PHL and communication partner (CP) should know the features relevant to them, whether the switches adjust manually or automatically, and, when appropriate, how to operate the controls/switches. When discussing the features and controls, regularly make eye contact with the PHL to ensure that they understand your explanations and that they can adjust and operate the controls. Finally, persons fit with Lyric hearing aids should be familiarized with turning the device on and off, and adjusting the volume control, and any other settings. Compatibility with various ear inserts and headsets should be discussed, and it must be emphasized that the units must be removed before persons with hearing loss (PHLs) undergo an MRI scan, and that they should inform their physician before undergoing surgery, x-rays, or a CT scan. Finally, the PHL must understand that since the Lyric is water resistant, showering with it in the ear using proper precautions is fine, but swimming and diving are problematic.

> ### Pearl
>
> Older adults using hearing aids have better emotional and social well-being and greater longevity (Arlinger, 2003).

The hearing-aid orientation should begin with an overview of device-related information. With the informational brochure and other visual aids available, the discussion should include a review of hearing-aid components and features; battery issues; hearing-aid care (e.g., effects of water, perspiration, heat); insertion/removal; telephone use and telephone communication strategies; causes and prevention of feedback; and warranty information. Probably a good place to start the orientation is with an overall discussion of the hearing-aid components and landmarks. It is important to emphasize how to recognize the landmarks and how to remember which ear each unit is inserted in, based on the visible distinction between the units or the left/right indicator, if applicable. The hearing-aid user should be told the model number and manufacturer's name and where this information can be found on the units, and this information should be written in the informational brochure and on all paperwork accompanying the transaction. The PHL should be encouraged to keep the information in a safe place. For BTE units, the coupling system

Battery management and safety issues should be discussed with the hearing-aid users, their CP or caregiver. It is important to emphasize that the battery is the power supply for the hearing aid, and that it should be checked daily to ensure that it has an adequate charge, unless a battery indicator tone, which signals when the battery voltage is low, precludes the necessity of daily checks. PHLs should be familiar with the audible tone or hum that indicates battery voltage deterioration. When hearing aids use rechargeable batteries, recharging instructions should be discussed in detail. I give each patient a battery tester to check the power of the battery daily.

The battery size and corresponding voltage (e.g., 1.4 or 1.45 V) should be written down, and, given the standardization in the industry, it is helpful for patients to know the color associated with their battery number. The fact that the battery size limits the power and life of the battery should be emphasized, along with the factors that affect battery life, including selected hearing-aid features such as wireless applications and the use of Bluetooth for connectivity. **Table 8.12** gives the color for each battery size. Because size and color are standardized, you should encourage your patient to keep the color in mind if it is too hard to remember the battery number. The patient should know that the battery is air-activated and that the colored sticker keeps the battery inactive; removal of the sticker activates the battery. Hence, they should be instructed to remove the sticker only when they have to replace the battery. It is important to emphasize that the battery cannot be "deactivated" by replacing the sticker. The audiologist should distinguish between high-power and standard batteries. It should be emphasized that high-power batteries are appropriate only for the hearing aids that require the power to drive higher drain digital hearing aids with selected features.

A discussion of battery storage is important, as it can affect battery life; batteries should be stored in a cool, dry place, but not in the refrigerator, not near a cell phone, and not near metal objects that may cause the battery to drain (Citron, 2008). Patients should be told to store batteries in a safe place away from children or pets and not near medication bottles, as people with poor vision can confuse batteries and pills. It is important to emphasize that patients should dispose of spent battery cells immediately in a waste or recycling receptacle. It is a good idea to point out in the instructional brochure where they can find the phone number of the national button battery ingestion hotline. The length of time a single battery lasts and the shelf life of a battery packet is always important to discuss, along with tips on prolonging battery life. If the life cycle of the battery appears shorter than is typical, then the hearing aid may be malfunctioning, and the PHL should be encouraged to contact the audiologist. Specifically, once the tab is removed the cell will last about 60 days, whereas the shelf life of unopened packages is about 2 years (Citron, 2008). It might be worth telling patients that they can expect to use 30 to 50 batteries per year for each hearing aid so that they know what to expect in terms of cost (Strom, 2010). It is probably worth-

Table 8.12 Hearing-aid Battery Size and Color Codes

Tab Color	Size
Red	5
Yellow	10 or 230
Orange	13
Brown	312
Blue	675

while to give the PHL and CP an indication of how frequently they should expect to change the battery.

A great deal of time is often necessary when demonstrating and practicing battery insertion and removal. Hearing-aid users should be instructed that opening the battery compartment or removing the batteries from the hearing aid when it is not in use, especially at night, is an excellent way to save battery life. The PHL should know where the battery contacts are and should be encouraged to keep them clean, as poor contacts may mean a loss of power. A magnifier is sometimes useful to ensure that the patient can see the positive (+) and negative (–) on both the battery and battery compartment. Magnets for inserting and removing batteries should be demonstrated and recommended if they are helpful. It is also worth reassuring the patient that the battery door typically will not close easily if the battery is inserted upside down and that the hearing aid has a tamper-resistant locking battery compartment. Point out that the battery door typically will "click" when closed and that they should make sure to feel or listen for this. Make sure to emphasize and reiterate that the patient should never force the battery door closed. It is critical that you encourage the hearing-aid user to carry spare batteries at all times and always have a month's supply of batteries on hand. Patients should be given options for where to purchase batteries and what they might expect to pay. Patients often ask if there is a difference between brands in terms of battery performance, battery capacity, and dependability, so the clinician should be prepared to answer this question. **Table 8.13** is a sample handout that might be given to patients with their new hearing aid(s) that summarizes the important facts about the battery.

Hearing-Aid Preventive Care and Maintenance (Table 8.14)

Hearing-aid users should be encouraged to set aside a proper storage area for their hearing aids so that children or pets do not have access to them. Preferably, the hearing aid should be kept in a drawer in the bedroom so that it is associated with getting dressed for the day. The fact that extreme heat and cold, hairspray, water, or damage from being dropped can destroy a hearing aid must be emphasized. Hearing-aid users should be told not to attempt to dry a hearing aid, not to wear

Table 8.13 Hearing-aid Battery Checklist

- Hearing-aid battery size_____
- Hearing-aid battery color code____
- Store battery in a cool and dry area, but NOT in the refrigerator.
- Remove the battery or open the battery compartment when the hearing aid is not in use.
- Test the battery prior to inserting it into the hearing aid.
- Keep spare batteries at all times.
- Recharge the battery as appropriate (only applicable to hearing aids that are compatible with rechargeable batteries).
- Keep spare batteries in a safe place away from children and pets.
- Do not leave dead batteries in a place accessible to pets or children.
- Typical battery life ranges from 5 to 7 days.
- Open battery case door every night when you remove hearing aid.
- Lean on a nonslippery table when removing battery to avoid loss of battery.
- Ensure appropriate lighting when removing or inserting battery.
- Battery ingestion hotline phone number is as follows:

  _____

- Do not force the battery door closed; if it does not close, make sure to recheck the battery position and number.

it when drying or spraying their hair, and not to wear it when swimming or while in the shower. Audiologists should review how and when to clean the hearing aids and earmolds, and patients should be instructed on the steps to follow if ear wax accumulates in the wax guard or receiver tube, or if the tubing appears cracked or hard. Preventative maintenance should be discussed including the use of some-sort of DRI-AID kit or an appliance known as Dry and Store. Each of these options should be discussed as ways of removing moisture from the hearing aid or preventing moisture to build up in the hearing aid. Use of a forced–air earmold cleaner to dry the earmold after cleaning and to remove water droplets should be demonstrated. The availability of moisture-resistant tubing for those for whom moisture buildup is a problem should be mentioned. I think it is important to give each hearing-aid user a maintenance kit that includes a miniature battery tester, a small brush, a pack of extra batteries, a DRI-AID kit, a wax loop, wax guards, audio-wipes, Ad-Hear to protect the sound bore from wax, a brush, and a forced-air earmold cleaner. The audiologist should show how each of the tools in the kit are used and patients should be required to demonstrate their ability to use each tool independently. Emphasize that water resistant does not mean waterproof. For users of the Lyric hearing aid, the discussion about protecting the ear and unit from getting wet is especially important. If a hearing aid is water resistant, thereby allowing patients to use their instruments following strenuous exercise or rigorous labor, or when active outdoors in humid climates, or even when unexpectedly caught in the rain, this feature should be thoroughly discussed. Some manufactures suggest avoiding excessive perspiration to protect the hearing aid.

Sufficient time should be spent going through each step necessary to insert and remove the hearing aid/earmold in the correct ear and how to turn the unit on and off, if applicable. The patient should be given the opportunity to demonstrate competency in insertion and removal prior to the completion of the initial orientation session and at each successive management session. Use of a mirror is helpful so that the patient can see how a correctly inserted unit looks in the ear. The communication partner plays an important role in instrument insertion/removal, especially in the case of older adults with manual dexterity or cognitive issues. If patients are having dif-

Table 8.14   Tips for Proper Care and Maintenance of Hearing Aids

- Do not leave hearing aids on a radiator, near the stove, on an air conditioner, or in the bathroom where they can get wet.
- Avoid getting hearing aids dirty; make sure fingers are dry and clean before handling hearing aids.
- The hearing aid must be kept dry; do not wear in shower or while swimming.
- Do not use alcohol or cleaning fluid on the hearing aid.
- Do not expose the hearing aid to radiation from x-rays or to direct sunlight.
- Hearing aids are customized for each individual user, so do not use a hearing aid that belongs to someone else.
- Do not drop hearing aid on a hard surface; keep hearing aid away from children and pets.
- Do not adjust hearing-aid settings or programs if they are not user controlled.
- Remove hearing aid over a carpeted surface to avoid breakage, should it dislodge from the ear or fall out of hands.
- Place hearing aid in dehumidifier to remove moisture and keep hearing aid dry.
- Clean and disinfect your hearing aids regularly, but not with water.
- Remove hearing aid when applying hair spray or other personal care products as the fine particles can block the microphone inlet.
- To clean: spray hearing aid with a disinfectant/deodorizer made especially for hearing aids (including earmolds), then wipe down with a soft, dry cloth. Hearing aid and cleaning wipes that are premoistened can be used to remove wax and debris from hearing aids and earmolds.
- If the hearing aid appears to be malfunctioning, do not attempt to repair it; rather, schedule an appointment with the audiologist who dispensed the hearing aid.
- Gently wipe off earmold and aid when removed from the ear. Always check for earwax and gently remove it or replace the wax guard.
- Check hearing-aid opening for wax prior to reinserting it. If necessary, clean opening with a cerumen removal tool (e.g., a brush). Clean the hearing aid from below, as this will prevent particles of wax or dirt from getting inside the hearing aid. If wax buildup constantly occurs, contact a hearing health care professional for possible cerumen management. Use wax guards as appropriate.
- Check tubing/mold of behind-the-ear hearing aids for debris and clean on a weekly basis.
- Make sure mold is blown dry prior to reconnecting to the hearing aid if cleaning the mold with mild soap.
- Brush off hearing-aid microphone and receiver with small brush before insertion.
- Remove hearing aid when you are perspiring, especially when it is very hot or when exercising vigorously.

ficulty inserting and removing the earmold, I find it helpful to have them watch me as I place the hearing aid/earmold in my ear and to have them place it in my ear or in a plastic demonstration ear. Sensory memory and transference is helpful, so repeated attempts are important. It is important to provide tips so the patient knows and can be reassured when the hearing aid is sitting correctly in the ear. Consistent with the principles of self-efficacy, Citron (2008) recommends starting with instrument removal, as this is much easier than insertion. Color coding of the right and left ear instruments is often imperative, as it is easy to confuse the left and right ear units. The advantage of the power-on delay and the relationship to audible feedback should be discussed during instruction in insertion and removal. Specifically, regarding the power on delay feature, patients should know what it means when they hear the series of tones indicating that the hearing instrument is beginning to amplify sound. The audiologist should make sure that the delay is appropriate to the level of manual dexterity the patient demonstrates.

Even though the feedback interceptor/stopper has reduced the problem of feedback tremendously, a discussion about the causes and prevention of feedback is relevant. It is worth demonstrating that holding a hearing aid in one's hand and hearing the audible whistling indicates that the battery is working and the hearing aid is on. The nature of the volume control, if there is one, should be discussed, and the patient should understand how the sweep volume control or touch-and-release volume control works, including the number of possible positions and the number of beeping tones associated with a given position. For some older adults, a hearing aid with a simple volume control is preferable to one with numerous positions or indicators; the fewer controls, the better.

It is important to have patients practice using the telephone (landline and cell) with the hearing aids before they leave the audiologist's office. Hearing-aid users should understand that typically it is not necessary to remove the hearing aid when using the telephone even though feedback is often a problem, but adjusting the angle of the phone relative to the hearing-aid microphone can help to reduce this problem (Citron, 2008). Similarly, lowering the volume control on the hearing aid may reduce feedback. Patients should be afforded the opportunity to practice acoustic and inductive coupling of the hearing aid to the telephone. Activation of the telecoil and location of the "sweet spot" often takes considerable practice, but this is critical. Further, patients should have practice locating the program setting if the audiologist programs a separate frequency for acoustic or inductive coupling. It is a good idea to help patients locate the hearing-aid compatibility (HAC) rating of their cell phone by suggesting that it typically can be found on display in the store or in the manual accompanying the phone. They should be told that the higher the M rating (M3 or M4), the better the HAC and the clearer the conversation. Similarly, the higher the hearing-aid rating in the microphone mode or in the telecoil mode, the better the connection and the lower the noise interference. Finally, I encourage my patients to set the hearing aid for vibrating alerts when there is an incoming phone call, as often the ring tone will not be audible even when wearing hearing aids. Use of neck loops or silhouettes and the T-coil setting should be discussed if conversation remains difficult on the cell phone. Checklists such as the ones

displayed in **Tables 8.15** and **8.16** can ensure that all device-related features and information have been reviewed in the session and understood by the patient and the communication partner, and they should be given the checklists to take home. I recommend reviewing the information at the return visit.

> ### Pearls
>
> Patients experience more positive outcomes after they are trained to properly use and handle their hearing aids.
>
> The audiologist should measure outcome at the post-fitting booster session, because if residual difficulty remains, HATs and home-based rehabilitation (e.g., LACE) should be considered after it is determined that no additional hearing-aid adjustments are necessary.

Troubleshooting

Basic hearing-aid troubleshooting should be considered an integral part of the hearing-aid orientation. There are a variety of approaches to teaching patients to troubleshoot their hearing aids. I prefer a problem- or descriptor-based approach that includes identification of the complaint or problem, knowledge of potential causes, and procedures for testing each cause. Based on a survey of hearing-aid fitting problems conducted by Jenstad, Van Tasell, and Ewert (2003), the problems with which the hearing-aid user and family member should become conversant include (1) improper fit; (2) the presence of unwanted sounds, distortion, or feedback; (3) poor sound quality; (4) battery-related issues; and (5) difficulty handling the controls. I recommend reviewing each of the potential problems and offering specific solutions from the troubleshooting guide and checklist shown in **Table 8.16**. The most important piece of information to impart about troubleshooting is when to contact the dispensing audiologist because of a potential malfunction of one of the hearing-aid components. Patients should be encouraged to contact the audiologist if there is any change in how they are functioning with the hearing aid or if the hearing aid is malfunctioning. It is imperative that audiologists emphasize their availability to assist with problems that may arise with the hearing aid. The checklist shown in **Table 8.16** directs patients to contact the audiologist when they cannot resolve problems that may arise.

When the hearing-aid fitting is concluded, patients are given their supplies and selected handouts, as these materials will empower them to care for their hearing aids independently. The "goodies" might include a user brochure, daily log, wax guards, dehumidifier or drying kit, miniature battery tester, soft brush, and extra batteries. When patients return for a second post-fitting or booster session, the audiologist should begin by asking for a brief summary of their experiences and then conduct a quick check of their ability to remove the hearing aid, insert the battery, reposition the hearing aid, and adjust the units, thereby confirming that they are operating the aid correctly and that they remember the information reviewed during the previous session. The audiologist should make sure that they can manipulate the device independently, or that the partner or caregiver understands how to step in when necessary.

Table 8.15 Hearing Instrument Operation and Maintenance Checklist

			Check if no problem	Check if problem
Name and model of unit: _____	Serial number: _____	Right ear		
Name and model of unit: _____	Serial number: _____	Left ear		
Hearing-aid features				
Date: _____				
Locating landmarks:				
Match hearing aid to:				
R ear				
L ear				
Battery				
Knows how to insert battery				
Knows how to remove battery				
Knows how to open battery door				
Knows how to remove strip from battery before using for first time				
Knows battery size and type				
Knows how to recharge battery (if applicable)				
Knows battery life				
Controls (if applicable)				
Volume				
On-off switch				
Telecoil (self-activated?); hears with cell phone				
Microphone switch				
Programs: familiar with settings				
Programs: knows how to change/switch programs				
Remote control (if applicable)				
Power-on delay				
Data logging				
Feedback intercepter				
Cleaning and care				
Knows to keep hearing aid dry and away from heat and water				
Knows where to store hearing aid(s)				
Knows how to use wax loop				
Familiar with Dri-Aid kit				
Knows how to clean hearing aid				
Know how to replace wax guard when clogged				
Warranty Date: _____				
Knows when to call audiologist because of problem with hearing aid (familiar with policy regarding drop-ins for repairs or assistance with hearing aids)				
Insertion and removal of hearing aids				
Knows in which ear to place hearing aid				
Knows how to insert hearing aid				
Knows how to remove hearing aid				

Source: Adapted from Access wireless: http://www.accesswireless.org/Disability-Categories/Hearing.aspx.

Service policies should be discussed including warranty, loss/damage policies, and supplemental insurance policies. It is important to discuss state regulations regarding the trial period, the hearing-aid manufacturer's policy regarding the warranty, and a supplemental hearing-aid insurance policy against damage from fire, water, theft, or accidental breakage. The downside of placing hearing aids on one's homeowner's policy should be discussed as well. In the discussion of warranties, the three options—implied, express, and extended warranties—should be clarified (Ditzler, 2008). Implied warranty is the most basic type, guaranteeing that if the product does not perform up to the standard for which it is designed, the manufacturer will remedy the problem by either repair or replacing the product or providing the consumer with a full refund for the returned merchandise. The limited warranty varies by manufacturer in terms of coverage and length of time it is in effect.

The express warranty, required on hearing instruments in a large number of states, extends assurance to the consumer that the manufacturer will remedy any problems with performance or defects in the product. The terms and conditions of the express warranty are incorporated in the paperwork the patient is given at the time of purchase. Many hearing instrument express warranties include coverage for loss and accidental damage. This warranty often extends coverage to 3 years, especially on high-end instruments. The option to purchase an extended warranty or service contract that goes beyond the limited warranty offered by the manufacturer should be discussed, as some patients are interested in additional coverage for their hearing instrument. Finally, the audiologist's policy regarding scheduling drop-in or follow-up appointments in the event that a problem arises with the hearing aid should be discussed and given to the patient in written form.

Table 8.16 Troubleshooting Problem and Solutions Checklist

Problem	Sample Symptom and/or Solution
Physical fit	
Earmold or hearing-aid shell is too tight	Return to audiologist
Earmold or hearing-aid shell is too loose	Return to audiologist
Hearing aid is whistling	Return to audiologist
Hearing aid does not feel comfortable in the ear	Return to audiologist
Ear feels plugged	Return to audiologist
Ear canal is sore	Return to audiologist
Quality of voice/sound	
Own voice sounds too loud, unnatural, funny	Return to audiologist
Sounds are tinny	Return to audiologist
Sounds like you are in a tunnel or barrel	Return to audiologist
Sounds are distorted	Return to audiologist
Your voice echoes	Return to audiologist
Background noise sounds too loud	Return to audiologist
Hear static	Return to audiologist
Music sounds unnatural	Return to audiologist
Environmental sounds too loud	Return to audiologist
Hearing aid sounds noisy	Return to audiologist
Hearing aid has an echo	Return to audiologist
Hearing aid sounds hollow	Return to audiologist
Hearing aid buzzes	If there is a T switch, make sure it is on M
Hear distant sounds better than close sounds	
Cannot hear people from behind	
Sounds are too boomy	
Controls/battery/earmold	
Battery has to be replaced daily	Return to audiologist
Cannot hear sound or understand speech	Return to audiologist when hearing aids are in ear and battery is new
Hearing aid is pumping	Return to audiologist when hearing aids are in ear and battery is new
Hearing aid cuts in and out	Return to audiologist when hearing aids are in ear and battery is new
Hearing aid is weak	Check battery
Wax guard clogged with wax	Replace wax guard
Cannot hear on the telephone	Telecoil not activating, return to audiologist
Dried cerumen is present on the hearing aid	Wipe off with dry cloth or audio-wipe surface
Hearing aid does not work at all	If have volume control hearing aid, may not be turned on, tubing may be clogged; replace battery; return to audiologist
Hearing aid sounds scratchy	Battery contacts may be dirty
Feedback	
Inadequate gain before develop feedback	Audiologist should check fit of earmold/check vent size; check response of hearing aid; check tubing
People complain that hearing aid whistles	Audiologist should check fit of earmold/check vent size

Patient-Related Information: Expectations and Wearing Schedule

The goal of this part of the orientation is to ensure that realistic expectations are set regarding various aspects of hearing-aid function, features, fit, and outcomes. According to specialists in geriatric rehabilitation, how specific and realistic patients' expectations and goals are will help determine overall performance success (Kemp, 1990). In light of the Internet explosion and the easy availability of information, some "educated consumers" may have unrealistically high expectations regarding hearing-aid quality and performance. It is important for audiologists to gain an understanding of what PHLs and their CPs expect from their hearing aids and if necessary to place this information in context and to qualify some of the exaggerated claims so that expectations can be kept in check. The ECHO, which quantifies perceptions about hearing-aid use, can be invaluable as a starting point for discussion of expectations (Cox

et al, 2007). I find that information from the ECHO helps inform expectations and communication strategies counseling. Using the ECHO demonstrates that pre-fitting expectations relate to hearing-aid outcomes, including improved satisfaction and benefit.

Integral to the discussion of expectations is a review of the information that patients found online. PHLs and their CPs must understand that hearing aids will not restore hearing to normal. The audiologist should be clear that hearing aids can restore some degree of audibility, but some difficulty understanding in complex listening situations may remain due to the nature of age-related degenerative changes. The audiologist should underscore that PHLs can realistically expect to have a reduction in the degree of difficulty they have communicating, depending on the acoustics of the listening situation, and that use of communication strategies to compensate for the loss of auditory input is essential. Of utmost importance, the hearing-aid user must understand that despite many advancements, the adage that hearing aids are "not very smart" still rings true. Hearing-aid users must understand that it takes time to realize the potential benefit from hearing aids, and thus they should not become discouraged early on. As part of expectations counseling, the PHL and their CP should come to understand that the ear and the brain must become reeducated to hearing selected patterns of sounds that have only now become audible thanks to their hearing aids (Ross, 1996), and that, in a sense, they are now being bombarded with a world of sounds they may have forgotten existed. They must be encouraged to gradually use the hearing aids, to remain patient as they become reoriented to or acquainted with the location and source of these "new" sounds, and to gradually increase use in diverse listening environments. It is imperative to emphasize that while hearing aids have features that make noisy environments more tolerable, hearing aids cannot eliminate background noise completely. This discussion should also emphasize optimal positioning in relation to the directional microphone technology (e.g., positioning oneself with the signal of interest in the front and at a reasonable listening distance), and that the best way to maximize communication is by reducing the distance between the speaker and the listener. Make sure to reiterate that the hearing aid will not facilitate understanding when the speaker is in a separate room and that being able to visualize the speaker is critical. **Table 8.17**

summarizes appropriate expectations for persons with hearing impairment.

A personalized hearing-aid wearing schedule should be developed by the audiologist in consultation with the PHL and the CP. The PHL should be encouraged to use the hearing aid(s) for a brief time interval at first, gradually increasing hours of use and the variety of listening situations. The data-logging feature built in to the current generation of hearing aids can be very useful in verifying hours of use and situational usage and can inform follow-up orientation and counseling sessions. It is advisable that hearing-aid users wear their hearing aids in quiet situations at first. Palmer and Mormer (1997) recommended a "listening tour" of household sounds including water from the faucet, toilet flushing, and doorbell ringing. The PHL should be encouraged to use the hearing aid in quiet conversation at home, during quiet indoor activities, and when viewing the television or radio. Once PHLs feel accustomed to amplified sound at home and feel comfortable wearing the hearing aid, they should venture into new hearing situations (Ross, 1996). For example, the PHL should wear the hearing aid outdoors during quiet activities and during group conversation when dining with or entertaining visitors. The PHL should be encouraged to wear the hearing aid in group situations outside the home, in large listening areas such as a church or synagogue, and at work. Persons with mild to moderate hearing loss should

Table 8.17 Expectations Relating to Hearing-Aid Use and Communication

I. Self-efficacy expectations
   A. Your ability to use communication strategies in difficult listening situations will help promote improved speech understanding.
   B. Practicing the techniques relating to operation of the hearing aid will help you to use the hearing aid successfully.
   C. Increasing use time with hearing aids in the ears gradually over time, such that after several days or a few weeks you wear the hearing aid regularly, will make the hearing aid feel easier to handle and more comfortable to wear.
   D. If you wear the hearing aids on a regular basis, you can expect to achieve improved comfort and communication skills.
   E. Trying the hearing aid in a variety of situations and reporting back to the audiologist about your experiences will help address issues relating to hearing-aid use and overcome communication breakdowns.
II. Situational expectations
   A. Hearing aids make speech and soft sounds louder so they are easier to hear; however, they also make noise louder so you may continue to have some difficulty understanding in noisy or reverberant rooms.
   B. Hearing aids will enable you to hear sounds in the environment you may not have heard for a while including your clothes rustling and water running.
   C. Hearing aids will help you understand your communication partner when h/she is within 3 to 6 feet of you (i.e., in the same room!) when speaking.
   D. Hearing aids may make your voice and that of others sound different and this will require some adjustment.
   E. Hearing aids may make your own voice too loud or may make it sound as if your voice is in a barrel, and you should report this to the audiologist, who can make adjustments to the hearing aids to address this problem.
   F. When two or three people are speaking to you simultaneously, a good deal of information may be misunderstood, so facilitative strategies will be important; typically you will have difficulty deciding between the target and competing speakers.
   G. When competing speakers are talking, seeing the target speaker's face will be advantageous.
   H. Hearing aids will help to resolve the loss of audibility associated with sensorineural hearing loss by making cues and soft sounds that were previously inaudible more audible.
   I. Your voice will sound funny until you get used to the hearing aids.
III. Outcome expectations
   A. Hearing aids will make it easier to communicate in many situations.
   B. Hearing aids will not make you look feeble or weak.
   C. People will not treat you differently because you wear hearing aids.
   D. People will not make fun of you because you wear hearing aids.
   E. Hearing aids with noise reduction algorithms in combination with communication strategies will help accentuate the target speech at the same time de-emphasizing the noise.
   F. Hearing aids will make communicating less effortful.
   G. Hearing aids in combination with communication repair and instructional strategies will optimize speech understanding.

find their hearing aids useful in business meetings as long as they supplement the auditory information with visual cues, environmental modifications, and possibly a hearing loop or FM system with a desktop accessory. If PHLs complain that selected sounds produce an uncomfortably loud hearing sensation or interfere with their communication, they should be told to alert the dispensing audiologist at the follow-up visit, as a simple hearing-aid adjustment may resolve the problem. It is helpful for the PHL to keep a listening diary, noting the situations that are problematic, so that at the follow-up visit adjustments can be made to the hearing aid and strategies can be offered for coping with these situations (this can be used in tandem with the data-logging feature).

Patients should be encouraged to gradually increase their hearing-aid wearing schedules until they are worn for most of the day, as use time is correlated with benefit. Stark and Hickson (2004) found that improvement in scores on the HHIE varied with use time, such that those wearing their hearing aids more than 4 hours per day experienced more benefit than did those wearing their units less than 1 hour per day. Patients should be encouraged to wear their hearing aids at home, as this will enable them to hear alerting signals such as the doorbell or the smoke detector. Finally, it is important to emphasize that wearing the hearing aids can help promote plasticity and reduce the probability of decrements in speech understanding due to auditory deprivation.

Special Consideration

Listener comfort and ease of use are especially important features to older adults with impaired hearing.

◆ Post-Fitting Process: Outcome Validation and Verification

Following the fitting process, the PHL and CP return for the post–hearing-aid fitting 3 weeks to 3 months following the fitting. The post-fitting session has multiple goals. The audiologist checks to make sure that PHLs are utilizing their hearing aids correctly, and conducts an additional orientation session if it appears necessary, which is often the case with older hearing-aid users. Self-efficacy principles apply to the post-fitting session, so the audiologist should start with a review of the easier tasks (e.g., hearing-aid removal) and proceed to the more difficult ones. At the first post-fitting session, it is important to assess how the patient perceives the value of the hearing aids. That is, we want to determine objectively if the intervention is successful; whether the PHL's ability to function has been improved; how the outcomes we measure in the laboratory setting resonate with the experience of the PHL and the CP; and what is the reaction of PHLs to their purchase experience and the care they have received.

To answer the above questions, two essential goals of the post-fitting session are verification (e.g., determining whether a hearing aid's gain and output at various frequencies meet some predetermined goal) and validation (e.g., determining whether a hearing-aid fitting has resulted in benefit or patient satisfaction). We administer verification measures of hearing-aid performance to ensure that the hearing aid meets the targets chosen during the fitting (e.g., verify audibility through probe microphone measures) to make any necessary adjustments based on feedback from the PHL. Gain verification must be accomplished at each of the post-fitting visits to ensure that prescriptive targets are met and maintained. Small deviations from target gain are often desirable, and adjustments are often necessary as the patient acclimatizes to the hearing aid. Actual speech or a speech-like signal should be used in addition to tonal stimuli when attempting verification of prescriptive methods. Telecoil output should also be verified, and in-situ measures of directional efficacy and assessment of the feedback suppression circuitry are also recommended.

Pearl

Restoration of audibility through at least 4000 Hz is imperative if aided speech understanding is to be maximized (Humes, 2007b).

Using validation measures we must ascertain how the PHL and CP are functioning with the hearing aids. Integral to the validation phase is assessment of the domains of hearing-aid outcome. Based on the research conducted by Humes (2001), the independent dimensions of outcome to be quantified include speech recognition performance (aided and unaided, in quiet and in noise); hearing-aid usage; and subjective benefit and satisfaction from the perspective of the PHL and their communication partner. It is important when justifying the time taken to assess outcomes to keep in mind that laboratory measures of benefit using speech-recognition materials and self-report measures which assess participation restrictions and activity limitations complement and supplement probe microphone verification data (Taylor, 2009). The many outcome dimensions are summarized in **Table 8.18**. It is important to look at the correlation across and within the various outcome measures, as there will not be a one-to-one relationship. When verification measures suggest that hearing-aid performance is adequate yet validation measures suggest that function and communication are not optimized, this will set the stage for further hearing-aid feature/response modifications; discussion of HATs as a supplement or a complement; and the need for additional counseling and rehabilitation to resolve residual disabilities. The validation phase is multifactorial and should continue over a 6-month to 1-year time frame, as periodic visits will help to verify short-term, medium-term, and long-term benefits.

Kochkin's (2011a) findings are clarifying and humbling in terms of shedding light on how clinicians should interpret outcomes experienced and expressed by persons with hearing loss. There is a strong relationship among quality hearing health care, benefit, and quality-of-life improvements, such that the amount of reduction in hearing handicap dictates the quality-of-life improvements. Kochkin found that the majority of hearing-aid users he sampled experienced significant improvements in quality of life when they had a very dramatic (i.e., 70%) improvement in their hearing problem. Taking this one step further, those experiencing improvement in their

Table 8.18   Dimensions of Outcome

Performance Measures	Hearing-Aid Usage Measures	Benefit Measures (Disease-Specific and Generic Measures)	Satisfaction Measures
Speech-recognition performance in quiet (unaided and aided) at soft and normal conversational level Speech recognition in noise (unaided and aided) at various SNRs and presentation levels	Data logging (use by program; daily use) Battery use Diaries Report of daily hours of use Report of proportion of time hearing aid used in selected situations	Pre- and post-measures of activity limitations and participation restrictions (Hearing Handicap Inventory; APHAB; COSI; SSQ): PHL Pre-and post-measures: CP (Hearing Handicap Inventory–Spousal version) Residual activity limitations and participation restrictions (IOI-HA [Cox & Alexander (2002)], IOI-SP [Noble (2002)]); HAPI; GHABP) Expectations (ECHO) SF-36; SIP	SADL Satisfaction with sound quality, cosmetics, comfort, ease of use, dispenser factors, hearing-aid features; situational specific

Abbreviations: APHAB, Abbreviated Profile of Hearing-Aid Benefit; COSI, Client-Oriented Scale of Improvement; ECHO, Expected Consequences of Hearing-Aid Ownership; CP, communication partner; GHABP, Glasgow Hearing-Aid Benefit Profile; HAPI, Hearing Aid Performance Inventory; IOI-HA, International Outcome Inventory for Hearing Aids; IOI-SP, International Outcome Inventory; PHL, person with hearing loss; SADL, Satisfaction of Amplification in Daily Life; SF-36, Short-Form Health Survey; SNR, signal-to-noise ratio; SIP, Sickness Impact Profile; SSQ, Speech, Spatial & Qualities of Hearing Scale;
Sources: Adapted from Abrams, H. (2009). Outcomes measurement in the audiologic rehabilitation of the elderly. In L. Hickson (Ed.), *Hearing care for adults 2009—The challenge of aging. Proceedings of the Second International Adult Conference* (pp. 279–285); Abrams, H., & Chisolm, T. (2008). Measuring health- related quality of life in audiologic rehabilitation. In J. Spitzer & J. Montano (Eds.), *Adult audiologic rehabilitation.* San Diego: Plural; and Humes, L. (2001). Issues in evaluating the effectiveness of hearing aids in the elderly: What to measure and when. *Seminars in Hearing, 22,* 303–314.

hearing attributed this in large part to best-practice patterns. Kochkin developed a best-practice index that categorizes a practice on a scale ranging from minimalist to comprehensive. **Table 8.19** lists the components of the best-practice index, which I encourage audiologists to consider.

Pearl

Outcome measures serve to verify and validate whether the goals of the hearing-aid fitting are achieved. Are the variety of speech inputs to which the client is exposed audible, comfortable, and tolerable across as wide a frequency range as possible? Do the electroacoustic characteristics necessary to achieve target produce maximum speech recognition and sound quality? Have the communication and psychosocial handicaps associated with hearing loss been adequately addressed? The relationship among quality hearing health care, benefit, and quality-of-life improvements is very strong (Kochkin, 2011a).

Validation: A Primer on Subjective Self-Report Measures

The Office of Technology Assessment (1978) defines treatment efficacy as the "probability of benefit to individuals in a defined population from a medical technology applied for a given medical problem under ideal conditions of use" (p. 16). The term *treatment efficacy* addresses several questions related to quality (Are we meeting the client's expectations?), treatment effectiveness (Do hearing aids work?), and treatment effects (In what way does the use of hearing aids alter behavior?) (Olswang, Thompson, Warren, & Minghetti, 1990). Over the past decade increased attention in the area of treat-

ment efficacy has focused on HRQOL, an umbrella concept that includes dimensions of body, activity, and participation (Stark & Hickson, 2004). Hearing-aid benefit is inferred from scores on outcome measures (**Table 8.18**) that identify and quantify the overall advantage attributable to the intervention in terms of activity limitations and participation restrictions. Subjective benefit must be expressed with respect to a frame of reference (e.g., baseline information) and relative to a specific significance level (e.g., 95% critical differences for a true change).

The success of interventions with hearing aids, implantable devices, hearing assistance technologies, and audiologi-

Table 8.19   Components of Hearing-Aid Fitting Best-Practice Index Developed by Kochkin

Use sound booth
Verification using real-ear measures
Subjective validation
Objective validation
Customer satisfaction survey
Loudness discomfort measurement
Auditory retraining software
Audiological rehabilitation group
Self-help book, video, or referral
Achieved sound quality
Hearing health care professional skill set
Quality of office staff
Number of visits required to fit hearing aids
Total time spent on counseling
Hearing-aid comfort
Satisfaction with fit

Source: From Kochkin, S. (2010). Marke-Trak VIII: Customer satisfaction with hearing aids is slowly increasing. *Hearing Journal, 63,* 19–20, 22, 24, 26, 28, 30–32.

cal rehabilitation in general can be accomplished by using the WHO-ICF (WHO, 2001), which defines the effects of hearing impairment and describes how clinicians should assess the effects of treatment in terms of improving hearing functions (Valente et al, 2006a). Within the ICF framework, treatment outcomes can be measured based on the extent to which an intervention improves the HRQOL or the generic quality of life. HRQOL implies nonacoustic benefits of hearing aids, including the effect on cognitive function, well-being, and daily functioning. In contrast, generic measures of HRQOL assess the degree to which one's improvement in hearing status associated with hearing-aid use or use of implantable devices affects disease-specific measures of hearing and communication. The generic measure quantify reductions in participation restrictions (e.g., withdrawal from social situations) and activity limitations (e.g., understands conversations) relative to the baseline. Because environmental and personal (i.e., internal) factors influence the effect of the impairment on function, most HRQOL measures including those shown in **Table 8.18** embed these factors in the questions. Given the link between social isolation and hearing loss and social isolation, morbidity and mortality, I am currently exploring the effect of hearing aid use on social isolation which I believe has promise as an outcome indicator.

Pearl

Humes (2007a) has adopted the term benefaction as a combination of the terms benefit and satisfaction. According to the work conducted in his laboratory, the three outcome domains, namely self-reported benefit and satisfaction, hearing-aid usage, and objective measures of speech recognition, account for close to 75% of the variance in benefaction. Aided speech understanding bears very little relationship to scores on measures of benefaction and usage, and usage and benefaction share very little variance, so each domain of function should be assessed to gain insight about the outcome experienced by hearing-aid users.

By using sensitive subjective outcome measures of benefit, and considering the high cost of hearing-aid technologies, clinicians are increasingly accountable to PHLs regarding the value of an intervention as demonstrated by short-, medium-, and long-term HRQOL outcomes with hearing aids. Chisolm et al (2007) conducted a systematic review of studies of HRQOL associated with hearing-aid use. Of the 16 studies evaluated, 15 included participants over the age of 60 years and involved new hearing-aid users. All the studies were published before August 2004, so most participants were fit with analog hearing aids, and the studies did not specify the type of fitting or the verification procedures. Nine outcome measures were used, some of which were generic and others were disease specific. Most of the studies provided evidence at level 3, with two at level 1 and one at level 2. Interestingly, several studies demonstrated that hearing aids have impact on generic HRQOL. Specifically, Joore, Potjewijd, Timmerman, and Auteunis (2002) demonstrated reduced anxiety and depression, and greater social functioning post–hearing-aid fitting, and Mulrow, Tuley, and Aguilar (1992b) and Mulrow and colleagues (1990) found significantly reduced states of depressions. However, Stark

and Hickson (2004) did not note changes in general health or emotional and mental health status following hearing-aid fitting.

Using disease-specific instruments, significant improvements in participation restrictions and social and emotional functioning were associated with hearing-aid use. Chisolm et al (2007) found that using data from the level 1 and level 2 studies, it was clear that hearing aids have a robust effect on HRQOL using these instruments. Although the authors did not discuss the time frame over which the benefit was assessed, most of the studies assessed the short-term benefit, namely 3 to 6 weeks after the hearing-aid fitting. It is notable that 70 to 80% of participants in most of the studies experienced benefit, defined as the difference between aided and unaided performance (Malinoff and Weinstein, 1989; Newman et al, 1991; Primeau, 1997). Most of the studies that documented disease-specific benefit used the HHIE or HHIE-S score as the dependent variable. Based on the systematic review and metanalysis they conducted, Chisolm et al concluded that hearing-aid use improves HRQOL by promoting the psychological, emotional, and social well-being of adult hearing-aid users with sensorineural hearing loss. Further, they suggested that audiologists have a robust arsenal of disease-specific instruments available to assess subjective hearing-aid benefit.

Ivory, Hendricks, Van Vliet, Beyer, and Abrams (2009) recently conducted a retrospective study of subjective outcomes on a sample of more than 4500 veterans receiving hearing-aid treatment for hearing impairment. The majority of participants were first-time hearing-aid users with mild to moderate sensorineural hearing loss. Hearing aids were dispensed at either no cost or at most a $50 copayment per visit. All styles and sizes of hearing aids and all levels of technology available in 2004 and 2005 were used. The Self-Assessment of Communication, revised version (SAC-Hx), a hybrid self-report tool made up of items that assess activity limitations was used by the investigators. The items were culled from other widely used self-report tools. The SAC-Hx was administered twice at the initial assessment and at 4 to 6 weeks post-fitting. Similar to the systematic review above, the majority of participants (84.3%) demonstrated an improvement in function after being fitted with hearing aids. Functional improvements were noted across all hearing-level categories.

Pearl

Audiology treatments provided through hearing aids, HATs, or implantable devices is successful in addressing the negative consequences of hearing impairment on bodily function. The importance of incorporating standardized and psychometrically sound outcome measures into routine clinical practice and matching the measures to the treatment goals cannot be overemphasized.

McArdle, Chisolm, Abrams, Wilson, and Doyle (2005) conducted a large multi-site study of the benefits of hearing aids using the generic WHO Disability Assessment Scale (WHO-DAS-II) and disease-specific HLQOL measures, namely the HHIE and APHAB. The WHO-DAS-II is a health-status instrument that measures dimensions of disability and health status. Communication and participation are two of the domains that the tool taps. Participants were 380 veterans eligible to receive hearing aids at no cost through the DVA's hearing-aid program. They were randomized upon recruitment into an immediate treatment (IT) group and a delayed treatment (DT) group. Veterans were fit with in-the-ear, digitally programmable, analog or fully digital hearing aids. Short-term (2 week) and long-term benefit was assessed. Along with the APHAB and the HHIE, the WHO-DAS-II instrument was responsive to hearing-aid treatment effects. Overall, hearing-aid use improved scores on the generic measure and on the two disease-specific measures. Treatment effects were more pronounced for the disease-specific measures than for the generic measure after 2 months of hearing-aid use. Notably, hearing-aid efficacy was maintained after 12 months of hearing-aid use on the HHIE, the APHAB, and the communication domain scale on the WHO-DAS-II. Beneficial treatment effects were sustained after 6 months on the participation domain scale of the WHO-DAS-II. Projecting from the number of individuals exhibiting change scores exceeding 90% critical differences for true changes in scores, McArdle and colleagues suggested that for clinical purposes, disease-specific instruments are more useful than the generic indices of HRQOL.

It is notable that Mulrow et al (1990) and Humes (2001) also reported that subjective benefit is maintained after 1 year of hearing-aid use. Regarding critical differences, Malinoff and Weinstein (1989) noted that on the HHIE, nearly 80% of subjects in their study had mean scores differing by more than 18%, the value that reflects the 95% critical difference for a true change attributed to intervention (Weinstein, Spitzer, & Ventry, 1986). Similarly, using the HHIE-S and a 10-point cutoff as the 95% critical difference for computing a true change in HHIE-S scores, Newman et al (1991) found that 78% of participants demonstrated a true change/reduction in perceived hearing handicap, whereas 7% of subjects did not reach the criterion for a significant change in handicap. The remaining proportion of subjects (i.e., 15%) had total handicap scores that were less than the confidence interval of 10, and thus were not eligible to be included in this computation. Similarly, using the HHIA-S, Primeau (1997) noted that after 6 weeks of hearing-aid use 77.7% of participants experienced a significant reduction in self-perceived handicap. Primeau found that young and older adults and new and experienced hearing-aid users were comparable in terms of the magnitude of perceived benefit in the psychosocial domain.

Stark and Hickson (2004) explored the impact of hearing-aid use on persons with hearing loss and on their communication partner using hearing-specific and generic measures of HRQOL. The mean age of participants who were fitted with digitally programmable hearing aids was 71 years and the mean age of the communication partner was 64 years. The majority of participants had mild to moderate hearing impairment. The SF-36, a measure of physical functioning, general health, and mental, social, and emotional function, was used to quantify generic HRQOL. Three months after the initial hearing-aid fitting, participants completed the generic and disease-specific measures to which they responded at the baseline fitting. Mean pre-fitting HHIE scores of participants was 43%, suggesting significant self-perceived hearing handicap. The mean post-fitting HHIE score was 23%, suggesting a statistically and clinically significant reduction in hearing handicap post-fitting. Notably, the situations that were most problematic were hearing a whisper, understanding television and radio, understanding in restaurants, and feeling left out in group situations. Individuals with more severe hearing impairment experienced the greatest reductions in HHIE scores, and those who wore hearing aids for more than 4 hours experienced the most benefit or greatest reduction in hearing handicap. Communication partners indicated the most common problems associated with hearing loss to be difficulty watching television, difficulty conversing in noisy environments, annoyance, and frustration. On the spousal version of the Quantified Denver Scale (QDS-m), there was a significant reduction in mean scores following hearing-aid use (however, the reliability of this instrument is unknown). With the exception of a decrement in score on the General Health subscale (i.e., deterioration in general health) of the SF-36 among participants with greater hearing loss, no significant changes emerged following hearing-aid use. The fact that in general little improvement in HRQOL on a generic measure emerged is consistent with most other studies in this area.

Pearl

The critical difference for a true change in HHIE scores using a face-to-face administration is 18%, whereas it rises to 36% when using a paper-pencil administration.

Humes, Halling, and Coughlin (1996) followed a sample of 20 older adults with mild to moderately severe, bilaterally symmetrical, high-frequency sensorineural hearing loss with various hearing-aid use histories (e.g., some subjects were new users, some were experienced). Subjects were fitted with binaural multiple-memory in-the-ear (ITE) hearing aids. A close match to the NAL-R target was achieved, and verified over time, for the majority of subjects, with NAL targets reduced by 5 dB at all frequencies for both ears to allow for binaural loudness summation. Subjects completed the Hearing Aid Performance Inventory (HAPI) and the HHIE at 20, 40, 60, 80, and 180 days post-fitting. The HAPI is considered a measure of auditory disability and the HHIE is considered a measure of psychosocial handicap. Overall, subjects experienced significant amounts of benefit in the disability and handicap domains following even a brief interval of hearing-aid use, namely 2 to 3 weeks post-fitting. It was notable that short-term benefit was comparable to long-term benefit, suggesting little acclimatization with the multiple-memory hearing aids.

Saunders et al (2009) explored medium-term benefit from hearing aids in a sample of older adults who were fitted with digital hearing aids. Mean hearing levels of participants were consistent with a mild sloping to moderately severe bilateral loss. Participants had significant social and emotional handicap associated with hearing loss based on a mean baseline score of 41 (standard deviation [SD] = 21.8) on the HHIE and of 48 (SD = 19.8) on the HHIA. All subjects were new hearing-aid users who made four visits to the clinic for the pre-fitting; the fitting; the post-fitting to determine if the hearing aids were fitting properly and to ensure that the patient understood how to insert and maintain hearing aids and to make necessary frequency gain and output level adjustments to the hearing aids; and 8- to 10-week follow up to check hearing-aid output using real-ear measures and to complete self-report measures to determine aided listening benefit, quality-of-life outcomes, and satisfaction. The extent of the activity limitation based on responses to the APHAB and the magnitude of participation restrictions based on responses to the HHIE decreased dramatically with hearing-aid use; 28 to 38% (excluding AV scale on the APHAB) of participants' scores on the APHAB and 48 to 56% of participants scores on the HHIE/HHIA improved significantly based on the 95% critical differences for a true change. The difference in outcome on the two questionnaires was consistent with reports of the participants at the start of the study. Most participants reported considerably greater emotional and social impact than communication difficulties.

Vuorialho, Karinen, and Sorri (2006) evaluated the benefit of hearing-aid use in a sample of Finnish older adults using a quality-of-life measure and a disease-specific instrument. The study was driven by the fact that people in need of audiological rehabilitation comprise 6% of the study population, and to win funding, evidence of the beneficial effects of hearing aids is necessary. The mean hearing level of the 98 subjects who were fitted with hearing aids was 48 dB HL (range 34 to 65 dB HL), and the mean baseline HHIE-S score was 28.7, suggesting that subjects were experiencing hearing-related activity restrictions. Six months after the hearing-aid fitting, 58% of patients were using their hearing aid for at least 2 hours a day (regular users), and 32% were using the hearing aid for less than 2 hours per day (occasional users). The majority of subjects were fitted monaurally with a behind-the-ear hearing aid; 57% of the hearing aids were of the digital signal processing (DSP) type. It was noteworthy that prior to the fitting, 70% of subjects felt handicapped and limited by their hearing loss. Six months following the fitting, the number of subjects who felt handicapped had decreased significantly, and mean HHIE-S scores overall decreased significantly to 12.7, suggesting that there was little residual difficulty following hearing-aid use. It was noteworthy that users of analog and DSP units experienced dramatic reductions in hearing handicap as did occasional and regular users. Interestingly, self-reported health status improved dramatically for regular hearing-aid users and for women.

Williams, Johnson, and Danhauer (2009) expanded on the work of Chisolm and colleagues and used the International Outcome Inventory for Hearing Aids (IOI-HA) to assess benefit and satisfaction of a sample of users of multichannel digital hearing aids with automatic dynamic directional microphones. The frequency gain response of the hearing aids was verified using real-ear insertion gain for soft, average, and loud inputs. Approximately 3 months after the hearing-aid fitting, 160 subjects were mailed the IOI-HA and a practice-specific questionnaire developed for the study; 40% completed and returned the questionnaires (34 men and 30 women). Of these, approximately half were new users and half were experienced users. The mean age of respondents was 73 years. The hearing loss of the sample was bilateral, sensorineural, and predominantly moderate sloping to severe in the high frequencies. Overall, mean satisfaction ratings and overall quality of life ratings were high for this sample. It is encouraging that participants in the Williams study were satisfied and experienced significant improvement in quality of life as they used their digital hearing aids.

Smith, Noe, and Alexander (2009) evaluated the efficacy of multiple-memory, multiple-channel, DSP hearing aids worn by a sample of veterans with a mean age of 74 years who had mild to severe bilateral hearing loss. Subjects had worn their hearing aids for at least 6 months and no longer than 2 years. Mean scores on the IOI-HA showed that veterans using DSP hearing aids with advanced features including directional microphones, noise-reduction algorithms, and multiple memories experienced positive outcomes in the domains of benefit, hours of use, quality of life, and satisfaction. Smith and colleagues concluded that clinicians who fit veterans with advanced technology hearing aids should use their norms for the IOI-HA when assessing hearing-aid outcomes.

Chang, Tseng, Chao, Hsu, and Liu (2008) explored age effects on subjective benefit from hearing aids in a sample of older adults. Participants were fitted with digital, multichannel, compression hearing aids between 2005 and 2007. The young old (55 to 80) and the older sample (>80 years) were comparable in terms of baseline HHIE-S scores, speech reception thresholds [SRTs], MCLs, and word-recognition scores. Following 4 months of hearing-aid use, mean improvement in spondee thresholds and word-recognition scores was significant and comparable across age groups. Further, mean scores on the HHIE-S improved dramatically for both groups, suggesting significant reductions in handicap associated with hearing-aid use. The benefit experienced by both groups was comparable, as was the residual disability that remained. Satisfaction rates and daily usage of hearing aids was comparable across age groups as well. Affirming the differences between the domain of satisfaction and benefit (mean benefit was clinically and statistically significant for both groups), satisfaction levels for this sample were not that high, with 46% of those in the older group and 56% of those in the younger group reportedly satisfied with their hearing aids. Improvement in scores on the COSI was comparable for both groups as well.

The most comprehensive, randomized-controlled clinical trial of the time course of HRQOL outcomes with hearing aids was an early study conducted on a sample of 194 older male veterans with mild to moderately severe sensorineural hearing loss (Mulrow et al, 1990). Half of the subjects were assigned to a hearing-aid group and the other half to a waiting-list group. Each group was matched on important demographic and clinical characteristics. Ninety-eight percent of individuals in the hearing-aid group received monaural ITE hearing aids. Hearing-aid benefit was defined as a multidimensional phenomenon, according to the amount of improvement in scores on a variety of quality-of-life measures of the social, emotional, cognitive, physical, and psychological domains of function. Responses to items on the disorder-specific HHIE provided data on the perceived emotional and social effects of hearing loss. The other disorder-specific outcome measure was the Denver Scale of Communication Function (DSCF), which provided an estimate of perceived communication function. Subjects completed each of these disorder-specific quality-of-life measures at baseline and at 6-week and 4-month follow-up visits. Mean scores on each of these measures were comparable at baseline between subjects in the control (waiting list) and experimental (hearing-aid recipients) groups.

Hearing-aid treatment effects were noted on each of the disorder-specific quality-of-life outcome measures for the experimental group at both the 6-week and 4-month follow-ups. Although dramatic improvements in social and emotional function as assessed by the HHIE emerged in the hearing-aid group, mean scores for the control group remained the same. Similarly, the hearing-aid group demonstrated significant improvement in communication function as measured on the DSCF, whereas no change in communication function was noted for the waiting-list group. Of interest was the finding that benefit, according to the difference between unaided and aided responses to items on the HHIE and the DSCF, emerged 6 weeks after receipt of the hearing aid and was sustained at the 4-month follow-up (Mulrow et al, 1990). That is, hearing-aid benefit at 4 months following hearing-aid use was comparable to that obtained as early as 6 weeks following the initial fitting. The authors concluded that their study established that hearing aids do in fact improve the quality of life of persons with hearing loss and that short- and medium-term effects are most pronounced when using disorder-specific quality-of-life instruments. In this study, psychosocial acclimatization was not evident. This may be because of the time intervals at which benefit was measured, namely 6 weeks and 4 months following the initial hearing-aid fitting.

In summary, it is clear from the studies cited above that positive outcomes with hearing aids emerge soon after the initial fitting. The next studies to be reviewed suggest that benefit over time may vary. Some studies show changes in benefit scores in either a positive or negative direction over time, whereas others show no change in benefit over time. The variability in benefit may reflect the timing at which outcomes were measured or subject factors such as the magnitude of initial benefit derived from the hearing aid.

An early study of satisfaction by Bridges and Bentler (1998) foreshadowed some of the conclusions from Kochkin's (2010) study using the best-practice index. The focus of their study was the perceived value based on the relationship among well-being, hearing status, and hearing-aid use in a sample of 251 older adults who completed and submitted a questionnaire that was sent to about 1000 individuals; 30% of respondents were men, 70% were women, and the majority lived by themselves or with a spouse in a private home. Respondents ranged in age from 53 to 93 years. The questionnaire included items about depression (Geriatric Depression Scale [GDS]) and life satisfaction (Satisfaction with Life Scale [SWLS]) along with a personal data form. Interestingly, half of respondents reported a hearing loss, and the other half indicated that they did not feel they had hearing difficulties. Only 21% of respondents reported using hearing aids successfully, and 95% wore contact lenses or eyeglasses. Of the subjects who owned hearing aids, 78% considered themselves to be successful users. It was noteworthy that subjects reporting success with their hearing aids exhibited higher ratings of life satisfaction than those who currently wore hearing aids but did not report success. Also of interest was the observation that the mean score on the GDS for respondents who had worn hearing aids but do not wear them successfully now was higher (more depressed) than the mean score for individuals wearing hearing aids successfully now. Although this study was only a survey, and the subjects' audiometric data were not available, I think the findings are

valuable to audiologists who find themselves having to justify hearing aids to their clients or to managed care agencies. The data can certainly be used to suggest that "hearing aids are necessary, not only for improved communication, but also for enhanced sense of well-being" (Bridges & Bentler, 1998, p. 44).

The data from the 1999 National Council on Aging study confirm that hearing-aid use has a positive impact on quality of life, including a reduction in affective symptoms. That is, higher rates of depression, anxiety, and anger were found among older adults who do not use hearing aids yet have comparable self-reported hearing loss than among those who do use hearing aids (Kirkwood, 1999).

Humes et al (2002) conducted a longitudinal study of outcomes with hearing aids using measures of hearing-aid satisfaction and usage. Their results underscore the importance of long-term follow-up and the need for possible booster sessions to help resolve issues that arise over time among individuals using hearing aids, as the participants were followed for 1 or 2 years. The 134 older hearing-aid users who participated had bilaterally symmetrical sensorineural hearing loss. Mean high-frequency PTAs suggested that participants, who had a mean age of 72 to 73 years, had moderate hearing loss (1- and 2-year groups, respectively) and had mean HHIE scores of 38 and 35 (1- and 2-year groups, respectively). Participants wore hearing aids with linear circuits with output-limiting compression and Cass D amplifiers. All instruments were in-the-ear devices with a telecoil on at least one unit. Participants were satisfied with their hearing aids over the time interval studied. Although some aspects of satisfaction decreased over time, for the most part satisfaction levels remained stable. Specifically, over a 1-year period, device-related satisfaction declined slightly as did satisfaction in selected listening situations as measured on the Glasgow Hearing Aid Benefit Profile. Similarly, device-related satisfaction decreased over the 2-year follow-up as did satisfaction with the dispenser. Interestingly, hours of hearing-aid use declined slightly over the 1-year participants. However, on average, participants used hearing aids for more than 8 hours a day, which suggests that they perceived the value of the aids. Satisfaction and usage were partially correlated, confirming the connection between the two domains but underscoring the importance of looking at both usage and satisfaction.

One of the most important findings that has implications for counseling is that those with high satisfaction ratings 1 month post-fitting maintained the high rating, and they were more likely to remain satisfied than participants with lower satisfaction ratings. The same finding occurred for hearing-aid usage. This underscores the importance of holding a counseling session 1 month post-fitting, especially for those with low satisfaction ratings. These individuals would likely benefit from a discussion regarding expectations and perhaps may benefit from computer-assisted home-based rehabilitation to promote long-term satisfaction.

Takahashi et al (2007) conducted a follow-up study of subjective outcome with hearing aids using responses of 164 participants in the original sample participating in the NIDCD/DVA study. Perceived benefit from and satisfaction with hearing aids was assessed after 6 years of hearing-aid use. The mean age of participants was 73 years, with 76% of subjects being male veterans. Most hearing-aid users reported using their hearing aids at least 1 hour a day, with 51% of respondents using the original hearing aids dispensed. Hearing aids were 6 years old in 51% of the cases. Forty-four percent of subjects had new hearing aids, which were of the in-the-ear variety in 86% of the cases. Hearing-aid use rate was 85%, indicating a high level of acceptance. Participants reported significant subjective benefit and satisfaction after 6 years of hearing-aid use. Specifically, according to responses to the Hearing Aid Status Questionnaire (HASQ), which assesses hearing-aid use across different listening situations, the majority of respondents used their hearing aids in quiet, in noisy situations, in the car, and when listening to the television and radio. An equivalent number of subjects indicated either always or never using their hearing aids with the telephone. Interestingly, 23% of respondents indicated that they use their hearing aids infrequently because of difficulty understanding at a distance, in the presence of noise, and with certain speakers. Also presence of feedback, inconvenience, and loudness discomfort were cited as reasons given for no longer using hearing aids, lending support to the potential value of the features available in present-day digital hearing aids. The majority of respondents indicated that they used their hearing aids full-time and that their units were of great help in noise, quiet, and group situations.

It was of interest that participants reported considerable residual difficulty when using the hearing aid during television viewing, when listening in the presence of background noise, and in group situations. Responses on the IOI-HA revealed that more than 60% of participants used their hearing aids full time. More than 85% of respondents indicated that their hearing aids were quite helpful, over 80% indicated that their hearing aids were worth the trouble, over 80% felt that others were rarely bothered by their hearing difficulties, and more than 90% indicated that "their hearing aids made their enjoyment of life quite a lot better or very much better" (Takahashi et al, 2007, p. 342). Similarly, 80% indicated that they felt that hearing aids were "very much" worth the trouble. The authors compared outcomes on the IOI-HA between subjects with perceived mild to moderate difficulty and those with perceived moderately severe to severe difficulty. Participants with more perceived hearing difficulty used their hearing aids more often, reported more benefit, were more satisfied with their hearing aids, and perceived their hearing difficulties to have more of an impact on others. The findings that stand out as being particularly relevant are as follows: (1) participants experienced less aided benefit in more difficult listening situations as compared with easy listening conditions; (2) hearing aids did not appear to make much of a difference in the most difficult listening situations, including speech in noise, understanding speech at a distance, understanding different speakers, and listening on the telephone; and (3) despite ongoing listening difficulties in challenging situations, hearing-aid users achieved long-term benefit and satisfaction from their hearing aids. The findings of this study have significant implications for the hearing-aid pre-fitting in terms of feature selection, counseling regarding expectations, communication strategies, and the role of possible cognitive-based auditory training to help resolve residual disabilities typically not resolved in adverse listening conditions.

Some early studies on long-term hearing-aid benefit are noteworthy. Newman and Weinstein (1988) were among the first investigators to assess the efficacy of the HHIE as an index of long-term hearing aid benefit in the psychosocial domain. Eighteen male veterans with ages ranging from 66 to 84 years and a mean PTA of 43 dB HL in the better ear and 56.6 dB HL in the poorer ear were fitted with hearing aids. Subjects responded to the HHIE at baseline and 1 year following the fitting. Their significant others also responded to the significant others version of the HHIE (HHIE-SO) prior to and 1-year following hearing-aid use. Differences between scores on the initial and follow-up administration of the HHIE and HHIE-SO were statistically significant on the total, emotional, and social/situational subscales. The mean difference score on the HHIE was rather large (27.7), exceeding the 95% confidence interval that defines a clinically significant change due to the intervention.

Using a randomized controlled clinical trial, Mulrow et al (1990), Mulrow, Michael, and Aguilar (1992a), and Mulrow, Tuley, and Aguilar (1992c) documented that the benefit of hearing aids can be sustained up to 1 year following the initial fitting. Subjects were new hearing-aid users with sensorineural hearing loss. Half were assigned to the experimental group and fitted with monaural ITE hearing aids, and the other half comprised the control group. Groups were matched for hearing loss, age, physical status, and educational level. At 4-, 8-, and 12-month follow-up, the majority of subjects in the experimental group reported wearing their hearing aids for more than 4 hours a day. In general, 70 to 80% of the 162 subjects reported being quite satisfied with their units over the 1-year period during which they were followed. Mean scores on the HHIE improved after 6 weeks of hearing-aid use and were sustained at 4, 8, and 12 months, so the authors concluded that the benefits of hearing aids in the psychosocial and communicative domains of function are sustainable over a period of 1 year. The absolute and relative benefit in the psychosocial domain at 6 weeks was comparable to that at 4 months, 8 months, and 1 year.

Special Consideration

The longitudinal studies on benefits associated with hearing-aid use underline the importance of following hearing-aid users over time, as problems seem to arise that can be remedied through counseling or hearing-aid modification.

In summary, based on my synthesis of the literature on HRQOL outcomes the following conclusions can be drawn for older adults using hearing aids: (1) beneficial treatment effects from hearing aids emerge as early as 3 to 6 weeks after the initial fitting; (2) the benefit of hearing aids is demonstrable and sustainable in the handicap domain throughout a 1-year period; (3) accommodation or adaptation to hearing aids may take about 3 months and can be sustained out to 1 year; (4) nearly 70 to 80% of older adults appear to experience significant reductions in psychosocial handicap associated with hearing-aid use; (5) the audiological variable that appears to influence the magnitude of benefit is central auditory processing ability; and (6) age does not appear to influence hearing-aid benefit.

◆ Part 2: Cochlear Implants, Bone-Anchored Hearing Aids, and Hearing-Assistance Technologies

◆ Cochlear Implants

Over the past decade, there have been considerable improvements in speech-processing strategies used with cochlear implants (CIs), so that they are now a realistic option for healthy, older adults with severe to profound hearing loss for whom hearing aids are not conferring enhanced quality of life in important social environments. There are 300,000 older adults suffering from non–age-related profound hearing loss for whom CIs are a viable option, and patients in their eighth and ninth decades of life are realizing benefits from CIs (Rossi-Katz & Arehart, 2011). Cochlear implantation is a cost-effective option for older adults who qualify audiometrically and are considered good surgical candidates. Given increases in longevity, the number of older CI candidates is expected to increase, as is their mean age at presentation (Friedland, Runge-Samuelson, Baig, & Jensen, 2010).

Cochlear implant candidacy criteria vary considerably across insurance carriers, be it private or Medicare, and across implant manufacturers (Gifford, 2011). Whereas bilateral severe to profound sensorineural hearing loss was the criteria initially established for candidacy, presently Medicare and Cochlear Americas specify bilateral moderate to profound sensorineural hearing loss as the audiometric criterion. Speech-recognition testing without visual cues is the gold standard in terms of candidacy. Gifford emphasizes that the majority of implant manufacturers and Medicare specify that to counteract variability in stimuli, speech-recognition testing must be conducted using recorded stimuli. Regarding performance on speech-recognition tests, Medicare specifies that individuals with sentence-recognition scores up to 40% correct are considered candidates for CIs. As the audiogram is not predictive of functional communication performance, patients' self-report of social engagement and communication competence is an important criterion for CI candidacy.

Present-day CIs enable older adults to detect speech sounds within a normal range of hearing, experience improved speech recognition, and communicate over the telephone. In part, technological advances in CI systems have expanded the base of CI candidates. Technological advances include the availability of electrode arrays of various lengths, sizes, and configurations; improvements in surgical techniques and implant design, which have decreased the amount of trauma associated with placement of the electrode array in the scala tympani; and external input ports that allow for coupling with FM systems and personal music players (Zwolan, 2008). Relaxing candidacy criterion has also expanded the pool of individuals eligible for implants, such that persons with a moderate hearing loss in the low frequencies and profound hearing impairment in the middle to high frequencies are eligible as are those considered to be limited in terms of their benefit from hearing aids. The FDA's revised definition of limited benefit includes a sentence-recognition score of 50% or less on the ear to be implanted and a score less than or equal to 60% correct in the best aided listening condition (Huart & Sammeth, 2009;

Zwolan, 2008). Available evidence suggests that CIs provide improved access to verbal communication, environmental sounds, enhanced telephone communication, and enjoyment of music (Leung et al, 2005) for those adults not succeeding with well-fitted hearing aids. The impact of cochlear implant use on cognitive function is a fruitful area requiring exploration.

Interestingly, residual speech recognition carried higher predictive value for success than did the age at which an individual received an implant. Orabi, Mawman, Al-Zoubi, Saeed, and Ramsden (2006) assessed the benefits of cochlear implantation in a sample of postlingually deafened older adults who were implanted at Manchester Royal Infirmary from 1989 to 2002. The mean age of subjects was 69.8 years, and all subjects had a severe to profound sensorineural hearing loss at the time of implantation. The median duration of hearing loss was 11 years, but there was a wide range. For example, four subjects were profoundly deaf for more than 30 years. Thirty-four subjects were implanted in one ear, two had a bilateral implantation, and two subjects had a reimplantation. All received a multichannel implant. Outcome measures included performance on word and sentence tests, and self-report questionnaires of functional and quality-of-life benefits. Postoperative performance on speech testing revealed improved speech understanding using open-set word lists in quiet and noise relative to preoperative scores, with most of the benefit presenting within the first 9 months postimplantation. According to responses on the preimplantation expectations profile, the perceived improvement in hearing postimplantation significantly exceeded the subjects' initial set of expectations in the following areas: ability to hear sounds that allow for easy lipreading, ability to understand family and friends without lipreading, ability to detect sound, and self-confidence. According to respondents, quality of life and general health as measured on the Glasgow Health Status Inventory Questionnaire improved substantially.

Gifford, Dorman, Shallop, and Sydlowski (2010) conducted a retrospective study of postoperative speech perception performance in a sample of CI recipients with a mean age of 64 years (range 32 to 82 years). They looked at Medicare and FDA preoperative candidacy criteria and outcomes, and based on their findings they recommended that clinicians consider variables "beyond the audiogram," because similar ranges of audiometric threshold do not necessarily yield similar levels of postoperative performance. Specifically, they found little correlation between pure-tone levels and outcome with CIs, and between performance on preoperative standard speech tests used to assess candidacy and postoperative performance with either the CI alone or in the bimodal condition. Interestingly, they found that the mean improvement provided by the CI alone over the best preoperative-aided score was 27%, whereas the mean improvement provided by the combination of the implant in one ear and a hearing aid in the contralateral ear over the best preoperative score was 41%. They reported that 22 subjects would not have been eligible for CIs based on the candidacy criteria for one device despite the substantial benefit achieved. They argued that a low speech-recognition criterion score necessary for candidacy may ensure both a high hit rate but a high miss rate, which is unfortunate from the point of view of the quality-of-life benefits derived from hearing implants. Their finding of the advantage of bimodal over electrical-stimulation-only performance is quite important, as it provides further evidence of the importance of an appropriately fitted hearing aid to be used in combination with electrical stimulation. Encouragement of continued hearing-aid use with a CI is important from a counseling perspective.

Friedland et al (2010) conducted a retrospective analysis of medical record of adults implanted at age 65 years of age or older to isolate factors predictive of success. Then, in their own study, they compared postimplantation performance of older adults to that of a younger sample implanted between 18 and 65 years of age. Preimplant and 1-year postimplant performance on the HINT was compared, and factors that could account for any differences across groups were explored. Participants were implanted between 1999 and 2008. Mean age at implantation of participants 65 years of age or older was 74 years, with duration of deafness ranging from 1 to 74 years, with no participants self-reporting prelingual deafness (mean duration of deafness = 15.75 years). Preimplant hearing levels ranged from 60 to 120 dB HL. Irrespective of age, better preimplant scores on the HINT in quiet conditions was predictive of higher postimplant scores on consonant-nucleus-consonant [CNC] words, the HINT in quiet (HINT-Q), and the HINT in noise (HINT-N). Then, in another study, the authors compared postimplantation performance of a cohort of older adults to that of a younger sample. Mean age at implantation for those 65 years of age or older was 73 years, and mean age of those under 65 years was 46.7 years. Preimplant performance on the HINT-Q was comparable for both groups (i.e., 22 to 23). Mean postimplant scores on the HINT-Q and the HINT-N revealed significant benefit for both groups; however, benefit was greater in quiet than in noise, and the younger adults derived more benefit than the older adults (**Table 8.20**). Although not shown in the table, it is notable that 55 of 56 participants benefited from implantation. Interestingly, postimplantation performance was statistically significantly poorer for the elderly cohort than for the younger group on HINT–Q and on the CNC test. Comparing performance of the younger and older participants on the HINT-Q and the CNC test, the younger patients showed higher performance scores 64% of the time, and on the HINT-N, the younger patients showed higher performance scores 52% of the time. Age did not influence the odds that a younger participant would outperform an older participant.

Friedland et al concluded that although 1-year postimplantation scores of elderly recipients improved significantly, when controlling for preimplantation HINT-Q scores and duration of deafness, elderly patients would not be expected to perform as well as younger adults with similar preimplantation characteristics. This observation has implications for counseling elderly patients regarding expectations from CIs and also for

rehabilitative intervention postimplant, especially for those not predicted to do as well as a younger cohort. Audiologists should use the preimplantation scores on the HINT-Q to guide and gauge expectations counseling. One explanation posited for the differences may be that elderly patients may have inherent limitations in processing the high-rate stimulation paradigms used in current CIs. Further, cognitive and physical factors may account in part for differences in performance of this population of elderly patients.

Pearl

Individuals 65 years of age and older with severe hearing loss receive quality-of-life benefit from cochlear implantation comparable to the benefit that individuals with mild hearing loss receive from hearing aids (Cohen, Labadie, Dietrich, & Haynes, 2004).

It is well accepted that CI candidacy criteria are more relaxed than they were in the past, such that individuals with considerable residual hearing are being implanted, and an increasing number of those who are being implanted have enough residual hearing to benefit from amplification in the nonimplanted ear. In light of this trend, Dunn, Tyler, and Witt (2005) explored localization ability and speech perception in a sample of adults electrically stimulated in one ear and using acoustic stimuli in the other ear (i.e., hearing aids). Eleven of 12 adult participants wore behind-the-ear hearing aids and six were implanted with a Nucleus CI-24 Contour internal device; five of the 12 were implanted with the Clarion High-Focus internal device and one participant was implanted with the Clarion 1.0 internal device. Only three hearing aids were equipped with directional technology, and these participants were asked not to use the directional microphones during the study.

In general, the hearing aid alone provided the participants with little or no benefit on the speech perception tasks; however, the majority of participants (83%) obtained significantly higher scores on the CNC word lists in quiet when using the CI alone as compared with performance with the hearing aid alone. Only one third of the participants scored significantly higher when both the CI and hearing aid were used together. In contrast 84% of participants scored significantly higher on the City University of New York (CUNY) sentence lists presented in noise when the CI and hearing aid were used together, as compared with the CI or the hearing aid alone. It is notable that 60% of participants did show significant improvement in sentence perception with the hearing aid alone. Inter-

---

Table 8.20 Preimplantation and One-Year Postimplantation Performance on Speech-Recognition Tests in a Sample of Older and Younger Adults (*N* = 28 years)

Mean (Standard Deviation [SD]) Age at Implantation (Years)	Mean (SD) Preimplant HINT-Q Score	Mean (SD) Postimplant HINT-Q Score	Mean (SD) Postimplant HINT-N Score	Mean (SD) Postimplant CNC Score
73.3 (6.7)	22.4 (22)	70.4 (25.9)	58.3 (27.6)	38.1 (23)
46.7 (13.4)	23 (23)	83.2 (23.9)	65.2 (25.6)	52.8 (21.6)

Abbreviations: CNC, consonant-nucleus-consonant; HINT-N, Hearing-in-Noise Test in noise; HINT-Q, Hearing-in-Noise Test in quiet.
Source: Adapted from Friedland, D. R., Runge-Samuelson, C., Baig, H., & Jensen, J. (2010, May). Case-control analysis of cochlear implant performance in elderly patients. *Archives of Otolaryngology–Head and Neck Surgery, 136,* 432–438.

estingly, when the noise was presented opposite the CI, there were fewer decrements in speech perception performance than when the noise was facing the CI. That is, speech perception scores were better in the CI condition alone and in the combined condition when the noise was presented ipsilateral to the implant rather than from the front.

Regarding localization ability, the results were marked by considerable variability that precludes drawing conclusions due to the small sample size. But for most participants, a bilateral advantage emerged in at least one condition; however, clearly it is difficult for persons wearing a hearing aid in one ear and a CI in the other to integrate information from both ears so as to improve speech understanding in noise and localization ability. Dunn et al speculated that perhaps fitting CIs and hearing aids at the same time could maximize the ability to integrate the acoustic and electrical signals. As of this writing, the advantages of bimodal versus bilateral cochlear implant use in adults have not been isolated (yet some evidence suggests bimodal performance may be better), so it is premature to draw evidence-based conclusions (Cullington & Zeng, 2011).

The concept of interfacing remote microphone (RM) systems with CI processors has recently been explored in a sample of adults first implanted in adulthood (ages ranging from 43 to 71) with the goal being to enhance the SNR and ultimately speech understanding in suboptimal listening situations (Fitzpatrick, Séguin, Schramm, Armstrong, & Chénier, 2009). The 15 persons who participated in the study had profound hearing loss bilaterally and had used a speech processor for an average of 3.6 years (range 0.8 to 6.4 years). All subjects had high level open-set speech-recognition abilities. The goals of the study were to assess the speech-recognition benefits of RM technology (i.e., FM and infrared ALDs for television viewing) when listening to sentences in noise and to measure improvement in speech understanding during television viewing. For the purposes of the study, the RM devices were connected to the CI speech processor using interface cables provided by the CI manufacturer. When assessing speech understanding in noise, the CI system was coupled to a Sennheiser FM 2015 system. The RM device used either FM or infrared technology.

The results were promising in that participants understood more information when viewing television with an RM device that with their CI alone, and they reported that they perceived that the experience required less listening effort and resulted in improved comprehension. The same pattern occurred when listening to open-set sentences in noise. Performance, both objective and perceived, was better with a personal FM system coupled to the CI than with the implant alone. It is important to underscore the individual variability in benefit across subjects, emphasizing the need to quantify the listening requirements and experiences of each patient to prescribe an intervention that will maximize communication in important listening situations. The findings are of interest in that they mirror the findings of Chisolm et al (2007), which demonstrated the value of hearing aids combined with FM systems in adults. The investigators focused on the effort required to understand television, the amount of information understood with the CI alone and in combination with RM technology, and the confidence with which participants felt they understood television with the CI alone and in combination with the RM technology. Audiologists should consider gathering such information when working with CI patients to maximize their communication in varied situations.

Rossi-Katz and Arehart (2011) surveyed audiologists working in CI centers to determine practice patterns in their provision of CI services to older adults. Although the response rate was low (15%), the findings are of relevance to audiologists working with older adults who are considering or who use CIs. Typically, older adults required the same number of sessions as younger and middle-aged adults to determine CI candidacy—generally two sessions. Speech testing in quiet was routine for older and younger participants, and 58% of respondents were administered speech-in-noise tests, with candidate age not a factor in the decision to administer the tests. Remarkably, very few audiologists assessed cognitive status. An interesting difference emerged in terms of counseling practices used with older versus younger CI candidates, with emphasis placed on the possible impact of central auditory processing on outcomes as well as the effects of duration of deafness. Respondents suggested that the factors most predictive of successful CI use for younger and older adults included motivation, realistic expectations, availability of social supports, and duration of deafness. Those respondents noting a difference suggested that the ability to tolerate change and the availability of a support network were important considerations for older adults. Interestingly, time from implantation to activation was 4 weeks for older and younger adults, with a mode of one session. Age did not appear to influence the number of postoperative visits, which tended to vary across individuals, nor did it influence the nature of the rehabilitation sessions. The fact that practice patterns did not differ for older adults is unfortunate, given the cognitive, sociological, physical, and psychological factors that impact intervention outcomes with older adults. Given the low response rate, however, it is difficult to draw definitive conclusions. But this survey should serve to raise awareness of adapting practice patterns when working with older adult CI candidates.

In light of the series of studies documenting improvements in most domains of function with limited complications in those considered a candidate from a medical and psychological risk perspective, audiologists should consider discussing the possibility of cochlear implantation with hearing-impaired older adults with residual hearing within the fitting range who are not realizing adequate benefit from hearing aids or FM systems. Medicare and 90% of private insurance companies or commercial carriers cover the cost of cochlear implantation, and some insurers cover bilateral CI surgery for older adults meeting the candidacy criteria (Huart & Sammeth, 2009). In the case of the latter, older adults who present with existing medical or psychosocial problems and diminished cognitive capacity and communication skills may remain ineligible despite expanding audiometric criteria (Orabi et al, 2006).

◆ Bone-Anchored Hearing Aids

A viable option for older adults with unilateral severe-to-profound sensorineural hearing loss, the bone-anchored hearing aid (BAHA), an osseointegrated auditory prosthesis, can also be used by persons with conductive hearing loss, particularly those with chronically discharging ears, and persons with complete or near-complete single-sided deafness

(SSD), which means deafness in one ear (Valente, Valente, & Mispagel, 2006b). Ideal candidates should have normal hearing in the unaffected ear. In contrast to a CI, a BAHA is a titanium fixture that is surgically implanted into the skull (mastoid bone) behind the hearing-impaired ear. It works on a principle similar to that of bone-conduction hearing aids worn by individuals with chronic middle ear disease or external and middle ear deformities that preclude the use of traditional air conduction hearing aids, as sound is conducted directly to the cochlea via direct stimulation of the skull, bypassing the outer and middle ears. The sound vibration delivered to the skull transfers sound from the bad ear to the good ear.

The BAHA has three components: a titanium implant that is surgically implanted into the skull just behind the affected ear, which over time naturally integrates into the cranium; an external abutment that serves as a link between the titanium implant and the sound processor; and a sound processor with a microphone that picks up the sound, shapes it, and changes it into a vibratory stimulus that is passed through the abutment and titanium implant to vibrate the cochlea in both ears. The sound processor is either head worn or is worn on the body like a body hearing aid with a cord and receiver that snaps onto the abutment. Older adults with SSD who have not experienced much success with hearing aids should consider consulting with an otolaryngologist to determine candidacy. A unique feature of the BAHA is that prior to proceeding with the surgical procedure, individuals can try the a demonstration model, which includes a headband to affix the transducer to the skin, to gain a feel for the experience of hearing via bone conduction and the potential benefit. The trial can be attempted immediately or over a series of visits. In the appropriate candidate, the surgery, which is done on an outpatient basis, takes 30 minutes and has very few risks. However, as some older adults may have very sensitive skin, local wound care may be necessary when skin irritation or inflammation arise. Surgery can be performed under local anesthesia with sedatives when indicated. Medicare does include coverage of implantable hearing devices such as the BAHA, but about 75% of private insurance carriers cover BAHA surgery (Sorkin, 2007).

Recent reports suggest that BAHAs have successfully reduced the emotional and social handicap experienced by persons with SSD from a variety of etiologies. Although sound localization remains a challenge with the BAHA, individuals with SSD report improved function in everyday situations, including driving. Another interesting advantage of the BAHA is that it can be used with an FM system in difficult listening situation. The BAHA FM receiver simply plugs directly into the signal processor without the necessity of an extra adaptor (Christensen, 2009). Newman, Sandridge, and Oswald (2010) point out that establishment of realistic expectations regarding BAHA implantable technology is critical to success and therefore integral to any rehabilitation protocol.

Pearl

The implant is to be fully integrated with the mastoid bone before the processor can be attached.

◆ Hearing Assistance Technologies (HATs)

Given the high proportion of non–hearing-aid users among the hearing impaired, and hearing-aid owners who do not use hearing aids, use of hearing assistance technologies (HATs) should be encouraged to help facilitate reception of speech and nonspeech sounds and to reduce the activity limitations and participation restrictions associated with hearing loss. Specifically, despite technological advances in the hearing-aid industry, for some individuals with hearing impairment, hearing aids alone are insufficient to access auditory events in selected listening situations due most likely to a combination of peripheral, central, and cognitive factors. Further, in accordance with the transtheoretical stages of change model, many hearing-impaired individuals do not feel that their communication difficulties warrant investing in hearing aids or that hearing aids can be effective in overcoming their communicative breakdowns and attendant consequences. Encompassing technologies used by individuals with hearing impairment and processing problems to optimize communication, HATs have proven invaluable in overcoming some of the environmental barriers to successful communication without hearing aids and when coupled with hearing aids or CIs. For some hearing-aid users, amplification systems fall short, especially when they are not wearing their hearing aids in the home environment and in situations where the SNR is unfavorable. Similarly, communication partners and health care professionals often encounter obstacles when communicating with persons with hearing impairment, so HATs can prove exceedingly effective. For those not ready to pursue amplification, HATs should be seen as a point of entry or a targeted intervention that can enable the audiologist to match situational needs with a specific technology. Recall that our goal as audiologists is to ensure that we have been responsive to patients' expressed needs and can help them maintain a lifestyle conducive to their well-being.

In contrast to hearing aids, where the microphone is located at the ear of the listener, HATs take advantage of remote microphone technology that picks up the speech signal and transmits it directly to the listener's ear without attenuation or interference by noise. In short, HATs bridge the distance between speaker and listener, improving SNRs, and promoting an optimal environment for communication. Approximately 50% of dispensers reported selling assistive technologies for the television and telephone in 2006, with 47% indicating that they sold personal FM systems (Johnson, 2007). Included in the American Speech-Language-Hearing Association (ASHA) Preferred Practice Patterns (PPPs) for the professional of audiology and in the American Academy of Audiology (AAA) guidelines for audiological management of hearing impairment, it is now recognized that hearing aids, communication strategies training, and HATs are ideal holistic approaches to maximizing communication (ASHA, 2006; Thibodeau, 2009; Valente et al, 2006a). Audiologists must take the time to integrate HATs in their practice by educating patients and health care professionals working with the hearing impaired about their value. The quality of health care can truly be improved when physicians, psychologists, nurses, and physical therapists are able to easily communicate with hearing-impaired persons using HATs. I should note that smartphone apps such as FiRe or soundAMP R, coupled to a directional microphone (e.g. Apo-

Table 8.21 Categories of Hearing Assistance Technologies (HATs)

Categories	Situational Uses	Transmission Modes
Speech-enhancement devices	Telephone at place of employment, at home, and for recreational use	Relay system, Bluetooth, texting, Cap-Tel, TDD, telecoil, cellular
	Entertainment (e.g., television/radio/MP3 player)	Infrared, FM, Bluetooth, NFMI, Closed Caption
	One-to-one communication	Hardwired, Infrared, FM
Non–speech-enhancement devices	Group communication (group tours, meetings)	Hardwired, Infrared, FM, Bluetooth
	Telephone alerts (ring indicator, text message alert)	Visual (e.g., flashing light) Auditory (Loud ringer), Tactile (vibrator)
	Environmental alarms (e.g., baby cry, smoke detector, alarm clocks)	Auditory (low frequency alerts, hearing dogs), Visual (flashing lights), Tactile (vibrators, shaker)

Abbreviations: NFMI, near-field magnetic induction; TDD, telecommunications device for the deaf.

gee) and high quality earphones make for wonderful easy to use assistive devices, as well.

Hearing assistance technologies address four distinct and interrelated communication needs: (1) face-to-face communication (2) broadcast and electronic media, (3) telephone communication, and (4) alerting/environmental signals. Hence, within the general categories of speech and nonspeech enhancement devices shown in **Table 8.21,** four categories of HATs can be described: media devices, telecommunication devices, alerting systems, and personal listening systems. The decision as to which system(s) to recommend is made with a communication needs assessment of both the hearing-impaired patient and the communication partner that taps into the aforementioned situations (Chisolm et al, 2007). The assessment should help determine the best match between the patient's expressed needs, readiness for change, locus of control, self-efficacy, and available listening and alerting technologies, and ideally to interface personal hearing aids, CIs, and BAHAs with HATs (e.g., cellular phones, remote MP3 players) (Thibodeau, 2009). The devices are categorized as speech enhancing or non–speech enhancing (e.g., television-enhancement technology/media devices).

The patient's hearing ability is assessed in several specific listening situations to determine the need for HATs in lieu of or to supplement hearing aids. Despite technological advances, the successful use of hearing aids by older adults can be hampered by audiological and nonaudiological variables. The major audiological variables that might lead an audiologist to suggest HATs are central auditory processing problems and a cognitive decline that hinders speech understanding, espe-cially in suboptimal environments. The nonaudiological variables that contraindicate hearing-aid use in the elderly and argue in favor of HATs include cognitive impairments such as dementia, financial factors, manual-dexterity problems, psychological factors, and lifestyle considerations. **Table 8.22** is a needs assessment that incorporates some of the information Thibodeau (2009) includes in the "telegram" program designed to assess a variety of areas of difficulty ranging from telephone use, to recreation, to group communication. This should be administered during the routine audiological evaluation to determine the appropriate rehabilitation strategies, prior to the hearing-aid fitting to determine the interfaces to include with hearing aids, or after a brief interval of hearing-aid use to determine if it is providing adequate assistance in listening situations for the person with hearing impairment and the communication partner. It is imperative that the audiologist ask specific questions about hearing-related difficulties to elicit specific problems the patient is experiencing (Ross, 1996).

Sound-enhancement technologies all require similar components to function (Bankaitis, 2008). **Table 8.23** summarizes these components, including audio sources, the mode of signal transmission, and the coupling methodology for routing the signals from the receiver to the ear. Note that the transmitter and receiver (i.e., the mode in which the receiver directs the signal to the listener) rely on compatible technologies to work together; hence, an FM transmitter must be paired with an FM receiver in order for the system to work. Although a common audio source involves an individual speaking into a microphone (high quality microphone is key), increasingly the audio source involves a cellular telephone, television, iPAD, smart-

Table 8.22 Needs Assessment for Non–Speech-Enhancement Devices and the Telephone*

Do you have difficulty:	With a hearing aid.		Without a hearing aid.	
	Yes	No	Yes	No
1. Communicating over the telephone?				
2. Hearing the telephone when it rings?				
3. Hearing when someone knocks at the door or rings the doorbell?				
4. Hearing the alarms or alerting signals such as a smoke alarm or carbon monoxide detector when it sounds at home?				
5. Hearing alarms or alerting signals such as carbon monoxide or smoke detector when it sounds in a hotel?				
6. Hearing the alarm clock?				

*Web sites for resources for hearing assistance technologies are as follows: www.harc.com; www.oaktreeproducts.com; www.assistedaudio.com/applications/visual-alert-hearing-devices.

Table 8.23 Components of Hearing Assistance Technologies(HATs)

1. Audio source
    - Television, iPod, MP3 player
    - Telephone
    - Remote microphone worn by speaker (hand-held, lapel, head-worn)
2. How signal is transmitted from audio source to receiver
    - Hard-wired systems
    - Wireless systems: FM radio waves, infrared (IR) light waves, electromagnetic energy (induction pick-up), Bluetooth (BT)
    - Direct connection (hard wire or cable)
3. How signal can be delivered to ear (coupling method)
    - Auditory mode (e.g., earphones, earbuds)
    - Neck loop or silhouette inductor
    - Direct audio input (DAI)
    - Silhouette inductor

phone, or MP3 player. Regarding the manner in which the audio source is routed from the receiver to the ear, neck loops connect with many HATs and transmit the signal from the HAT in the form of an electromagnetic signal directly to the telecoil of a hearing aid. Worn around the neck, a neck loop is similar to a hearing loop. It can be plugged into a variety of audio devices, including an MP3 player and a computer, and in turn it transmits the audio signal directly to the hearing-aid telecoil, obviating the need for headphones. Alternatively, FM systems interface with hearing aids using induction or direct audio input, or the signal can be transmitted to a headphone worn by the person with hearing loss.

The least expensive way to route the sound source to the listener is via a hardwire connection using a wire or cable. In contrast, the signal can also be broadcast from the speaker to the listener wirelessly via radio waves (FM systems), infrared (IR) systems, or an induction loop. These modes of transmission are more costly, but the signal clarity is excellent. FM systems use broadcast technology and operate on frequency bands that are divided into different channels and are assigned by the Federal Communications Commission (FCC). Use of higher frequency bands, such as 216 to 217 MHz, as opposed to lower frequency bands, such as 72 to 76 MHz, tends to reduce distortions and interference (Bankaitis, 2008). IR systems transmit sound from the speaker to the listener via IR light waves using subcarrier frequencies that are not prone to interference such as 2.3 or 2.8 MHz. Maximum response with IR systems requires that users are positioned directly in front of the transmitter.

Induction loop systems or hearing loops use an electromagnetic field to deliver sound. A wire that circles a room and is connected to the sound system, the hearing loop is permanently installed and is connected to a microphone used by the speaker that includes an electromagnetic field in the area. The T-coil on the hearing aid or a CI picks up the electromagnetic signal and feeds it directly to the hearing-aid user (Bloom, 2009). In essence the telecoil functions as an antenna, relaying sounds from a microphone wirelessly directly into the ear free of background noise. Hence, using a telecoil is seamless and unobtrusive. According to Sterkens (2011), when listening in a hearing loop it is best if the telecoil is located vertically in the hearing aid, and audiologists should be aware that they can program the telecoil by increasing or decreasing the gain of

the microphone and the telecoil relative to each other. Although the U.S. is far behind other countries in the use of hearing loops, thanks to a campaign known as "Get in the Hearing Loop," sponsored by the Hearing Loss Association of American and the AAA, induction loop systems are increasingly being installed in people's homes for television viewing, in public spaces, in airports, and in houses of worship. They are also being installed in taxis, trains, and ticket windows at sports arenas. Some cities, including New York City, have used federal stimulus money to loop subway information booths. Nissan recently announced that more than 10,000 New York City taxis that are to be phased in will be equipped with hearing loops.

Increasingly, hearing aids have either a telecoil setting that eliminates background noise or a Mic-Telecoil (MT) setting that allows the hearing-aid user to hear ambient sounds. This setting is ideal when watching television via a hearing loop, as it allows the hearing-aid user to hear the television broadcast via the loop, converse with others in the room, and hear the telephone ringing. According to Sterkens (2011), the degree of hearing loss and the loop application, be it a home or a meeting room, will dictate how the audiologists program the hearing aid relative to the telecoil setting. She recommends a "telecoil only" program for individuals with open-canal fittings for situations that only demand listening, and an MT setting to be used when watching television and talking with friends and family. With the MT setting, which is typically a stronger setting, the hearing-aid user can hear others talking in the same room. For persons with severe hearing loss and closed earmolds, Sterkens also recommends a program that includes a blended MT program, and a program for telecoil only. She noted that to reduce interference from background noise she may program each hearing aid differently. For example, experience has taught her that it is best to program MT on the "direct speech listening" side, and T on the opposite ear that may be facing the noise or is away from the sound source. By doing this, the listener will not experience as much interference from background noise. A state-by-state listing of public buildings in the United States that are looped can be found at http://www.hearinglosshelp.com/loopedbuildingsbystate.htm. The *Washington Post* published an excellent article on hearing loops on April 9, 2012 (http://www.washingtonpost.com/national/health-science/how-hearing-loops-can-help/2012/04/09/gIQAvhEb6S_print.html).

Pearl

Whereas telecoils require no additional power, Bluetooth requires significant battery power, entails an unacceptable amount of battery drain, and has a limited range.

Personal listening systems are ideal for one-to-one or small group situations when distance or noise makes communication difficult. Personal listening systems such as the Pocketalker (**Fig. 8.15**) rely on a hard-wired connection, whereas the Hearing Helper utilizes an FM signal (**Fig. 8.16**). Hardwired systems that use a direct electrical connection in the delivery of the signal are commercially available, relatively inexpensive ($200 to $250), portable, and versatile, have good sound quality, and are ideal in one-on-one situations such as in a physician's of-

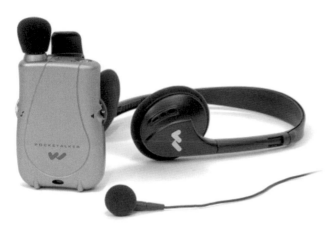

Fig. 8.15 The Williams Sound Pocketalker. (Courtesy of Williams Sound Corp.)

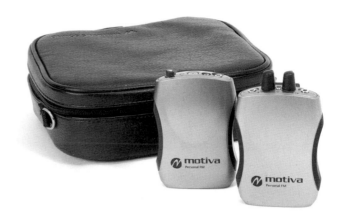

Fig. 8.16 Motiva personal FM System Hearing Helper with accessories. (Courtesy of Williams Sound Corp.)

fice, nursing home, or assisted-living setting, or when a nurse or social worker is taking a case history or conducting an intake. In addition to being invaluable in small group settings, hardwired personal listening systems can be used in a car with the television or radio. The major limitation is that the speaker has to be tethered to the listener. The basic system, as shown in **Fig. 8.15,** has a base that includes the microphone, tone and volume controls, and an input for an earphone connection. Most systems come with an extended cord to increase the flexibility of these devices (increases the distance between audio source and person with hearing impairment). Personal listening systems are easy to operate: the speaker speaks into the microphone, which is placed close to the mouth, and the message is delivered directly to the listener. When I am conducting in-service workshops for nurses, nursing aides, physical therapists, or speech-language pathologists, I distribute printed instructions to ensure that they understand earphone placement and use of the power and volume control switch.

A more versatile technology for improving the SNR and speech understanding in small group settings is a personal FM system such as the Motiva shown in **Fig. 8.16** along with coupling options shown in **Fig. 8.17**. The personal FM system con-

sists of a microphone worn by the speaker, which is connected wirelessly to a transmitter, and a receiver worn by the listener, which delivers the signal to the listener's ears via headphone, a sound-field speaker, or an interface (e.g., neck loop) with a hearing aid equipped with a telecoil. Personal FM systems can also be used with implantable hearing devices. The transmission range of personal FM systems is from 15 to 100 feet, and the speaker and listener are not limited to the confines of a room. FM systems are ideal for one-to-one and group settings. In a group setting, the speaker can talk to multiple listeners using a system equipped with multiple receivers and headphones. The Williams Sound Personal PA® FM Tour Guide system is shown in **Fig. 8.18**. FM systems have several distinct advantages that may make them worth the financial investment. They can facilitate speech understanding in large and small group situations, and in the presence of a background of noise such as in restaurants, at lectures, or at noisy receptions. FM systems can be used outdoors, when the speaker and listener are in different rooms, and with radio or television. When an older adult is on a trip or at a lecture, the speaker can use the microphone/transmitter of the personal FM system, enabling the person with hearing loss to follow the entire discus-

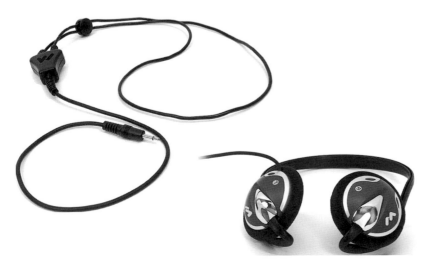

Fig. 8.17 Neck loop and headphone options for the Pocketalker. (Courtesy of Williams Sound Corp.)

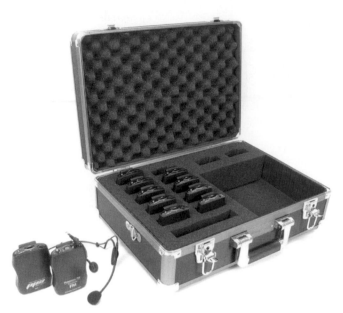

Fig. 8.18 Personal PA® FM Tour Guide System (TGS PRO 737). (Courtesy of Williams Sound Corp.)

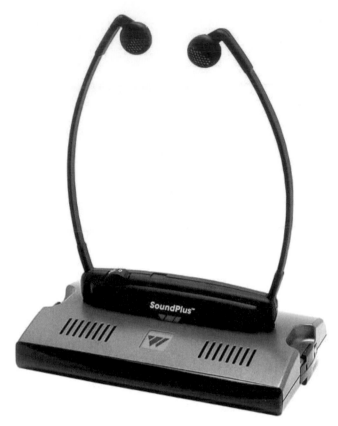

Fig. 8.19 Infrared System—Sound Plus TV Listening System. (Courtesy of Williams Sound Corp.)

sion. I find this indispensable in a variety of settings, including nursing homes, assisted-living facilities, and when speaking one on one with clergy.

◆ Media/Television Devices

For some older adults, the television is their only link to the outside world, and they often complain of difficulty hearing it, difficulty transitioning from one type of program to another, and difficulty understanding when other signals are present (Sever & Abreu, 2009). A frequent complaint of family members is that persons with hearing loss raise the volume on the television to an uncomfortably loud level, and hence they do not necessarily consider themselves to have difficulty understanding the television! Even when wearing hearing aids, older adults still find that the signal is not sufficiently amplified (Pichora-Fuller, 1997). The difficulty lies in the fact that extraneous noise in the environment, the distance between the TV and the viewer, and reverberation combine to distort the sound signal. Media devices that enhance the SNR for the listener are ideal for home or apartment use. Several amplification devices are available for television, each delivering the auditory signal to the listener's ear in a different way: (1) IR systems, (2) FM systems, (3) hardwired systems, (4) TV loop systems, and (5) the Bluetooth streamer. Although devices differ in how the sound source from the television is delivered to the listener's ears, they each effectively reduce the impact of distance, noise, and reverberation on the intelligibility of the signal.

The IR systems are wireless; they utilize invisible IR light beams to transmit the TV sound signal. They are commercially available, portable, easy to install, and have excellent sound quality. They work best for persons with mild to moderately severe hearing impairment. As shown in **Figs. 8.19 and 8.20,**

IR systems consist of a transmitter that plugs directly into the sound source, be it a television, VCR, or DVD player equipped with standard output jacks. The transmitter sends the signal to a receiver headset via invisible light waves. For many models including the one shown in **Fig. 8.20,** the transmitter serves as the recharging base for the headset. The battery life is approximately 8 hours and typically it takes about 3 hours to recharge the battery. The person with hearing impairment wears a receiver (available in several varieties) that uses a detector that decodes the signal from the emitter/transmitter, amplifies it, and directs it to the listener's ears (Davis, 1994). The person wearing the receiver must be in the same room and must always face the light emitting diodes. Further, the path between the transmitter and receiver must be uninterrupted, as light rays do not travel through solid surfaces. As shown in **Fig. 8.19** receivers are battery powered and lightweight, with one of the most common ones being the Stethoset receiver with an output jack for attaching additional HATs or neck loops. The IR system allows the TV to be heard at the desired volume by everyone in the room, and the person with hearing impairment merely adjusts the volume on the receiver to a comfortable listening level. In light of their value, many TV listening solutions are now commercially available online at audio vendors and in retail stores such as Costco, Target, and Radio Shack. Persons with hearing loss should be encouraged to use them as an adjunct to hearing aids or when television understanding poses a challenge. Positive experiences with TV

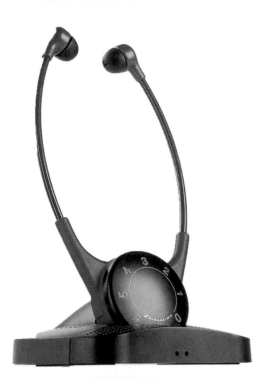

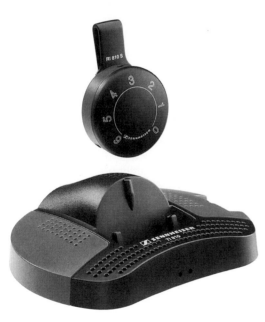

Fig. 8.20 Sennheiser Infrared System with under-the-chin headphone and with a special receiver designed to connect to a neck loop. [From Valente, M., Dunn, H., & Roeser, R. (2008). *Audiology treatment*. New York: Thieme.]

listening devices can provide a positive experience with amplification, which can be generalized to hearing aids for persons not ready to purchase them. Note that persons with hearing loss can use their personal receivers with systems in public facilities, but they will only be compatible with an IR transmitter of the same frequency.

The FM systems are also wireless, easy to install, portable, and battery powered. The listener does not have to be con-

fined to the same room for listening; signals can be transmitted a long distance. The systems can be used indoors and outdoors, and people with all levels of hearing impairment can benefit (Davis, 1994). The FM system contains a transmitter, microphone, receiver, and a device to couple sound to the listener's ears. It works in much the same way as the IR system; however, the transmitter, which is attached to the microphone, transduces the audio signal that is picked up from the TV and transmits it through the room as a frequency-modulated signal. The receiver picks up the signal, demodulates it, and delivers it directly to the ear. The receiver directs the sound to the ear via a neck loop, earbud, headphone, silhouette, or direct audio input. The volume of transmission can be controlled at the television or at the FM receiver (Davis, 1994; Pichora-Fuller, 1997).

Hardwired systems are portable, easy to install, battery-operated, and relatively inexpensive. However, the listener is tethered to the wire, thus limiting their mobility, and the sound quality is not as good as with the IR or FM systems. Personal hardwired systems consist of an amplifying unit with a microphone placed near the television speaker. The signal from the television is picked up by the microphone, which rests close to the audio source, changed into an electrical signal, amplified, and changed back into sound that is delivered via an earpiece to the listener. The earpiece is typically a headset or an earbud, yet some people who wear BTE hearing aids may choose to connect their hearing aid to the TV by direct audio input, wherein a wire connected to the television plugs into the hearing aid. With direct audio input, the television connection can be wired so that viewers without hearing problems can hear the signal from the TV loudspeaker (Pichora-Fuller, 1997). The hard-wired connection is the least flexible but most inexpensive way to couple HAT to the television to optimize the listening experience.

The TV loop systems do not have some of the advantages inherent in the FM or IR systems in that they are not as portable; they require some installation (taking approximately one hour), and transmission distance is limited to within or close to the loop. Sound quality depends on the listener's location relative to the loop; signal strength is strongest when the listener is closest to the loop wire and weakest when the listener is in the center of the looped area (Davis, 1994). As discussed above, use of the MT setting is preferable when using an audio loop for television viewing, as this will enable the person with hearing loss to carry on a conversation or hear alerting signals while watching television. With these systems, sound is picked up by a microphone at the television, converted into an electrical signal, amplified, and directed to a wire that is looped around the listening area. The receiver is typically a hearing aid with a T-coil that converts the electromagnetic signal from the wire loop back into sound. For persons not having a hearing aid with a T-coil, the signal can be picked up through a compatible headset receiver.

Present-day hearing aids that are Bluetooth compatible utilize a transmitter to communicate between the television and the streamer. Bluetooth-compatible television sets come straight from the factory and have expanded the technology for the hearing impaired. Bluetooth technology offers hearing-aid users the ability to connect with the television and can be a tool for motivating the hearing impaired to consider purchasing hearing aids (Sever & Abreu, 2009). An increasing number of hearing aids are equipped with Bluetooth, allowing for gateway devices that enable digital audio streaming from Bluetooth devices directly to the hearing aid or CI.

Induction-loop systems that use the principle of electromagnetic induction can be used by hearing-aid wearers to transmit the television signal. A Bluetooth neck-loop amplifier is available from Williams Sound. It creates a wireless link to a telecoil-enabled hearing aid and is ideal for listening to mobile phones, computers, or other Bluetooth-enabled devices with one's hearing aid. It has a limited range (35 feet), as with most Bluetooth devices, and the battery life provides up to 6 hours of talk time.

Finally, some older adults may not be able to understand the audio signal from the television even with the above technology, because of the severity of loss or auditory-processing difficulties. Closed captioning of printed text strings is an important consideration for older adults, as they tend to watch more television than do younger adults, and they tend to rely on the television rather than the Internet for news; for some, streamers or television accessories and assistive technologies are not an option (Gordon-Salant & Callahan, 2009). The U.S. Congress passed the Television Decoder Circuitry Act in 1990, which mandated that closed captioning must be included in all televisions having a screen size exceeding 13 inches. Then in 2010 Congress passed the Twenty-First Century Communications and Video Accessibility Act, which requires broadcasters to add closed captions to rebroadcasts of older programs that previously aired before closed captioning was begun. This bill enables persons with hearing impairment to participate in the Internet age, as it ensures captioning of television programs on the Internet, a closed captioning button on television remote controls, and hearing-aid compatibility for Internet, telephone, and communication equipment. According to President Obama, this legislation will make it easier for people who live with a hearing impairment to do what many of us take for granted, that is, navigating a TV or DVD menu to sending an email on a smart phone (http://www.whitehouse.gov/the-press-office/2010/10/08/remarks-president-signing-21st-century-communications-and-video-accessib). Specifically, Sec. 203, Closed Captioning Decoder and Video Description Capability of the Twenty-First Century Act states the following:

(a) AUTHORITY TO REGULATE—Section 303(u) of the Communications Act of 1934 (47 U.S.C. 303(u)) is amended to read as follows:
(u) Require that, if technically feasible—(1) apparatus designed to receive or play back video programming transmitted simultaneously with sound, if such apparatus is manufactured in the United States or imported for use in the United States and uses a picture screen of any size—
(A) be equipped with built-in closed caption decoder circuitry or capability designed to display closed-captioned video programming. (http://www.gpo.gov/fdsys/pkg/PLAW-111publ260/pdf/PLAW-111publ260.pdf)

Table 8.24 highlights some features of this act related to television viewing.

Gordon-Salant and Callahan (2009) compared the benefits of closed captioning versus hearing-aid use for TV viewing in a sample of older adults who had worn hearing aids for at least

Table 8.24 Highlights of the Twenty-First Century Communications and Video Accessibility Act that Pertain to Television Viewing

- Increases access to the Internet through improved user interfaces for smart phones
- Provides for the ability to watch new TV programs online with the captions included
- Mandates that remote controls have a button or similar mechanism to easily access the closed captioning on broadcast and pay TV
- Makes TV program guides and selection menus accessible to people with vision loss
- Enables Americans who are blind to enjoy TV more fully through audible descriptions of the on-screen action. For low-income Americans who are both deaf and blind, providing up to $10 million per year to purchase communications equipment to access the telephone system and the Internet so these individuals can more fully participate in society.

Source: From the National Association for the Deaf (http://www.nad.org/news/2010/10/nad-applauds-congress-increasing-access-technology-and-internet)

2 months (mean age 74.5 years) who had their vision corrected to 20/20 by contact lenses or glasses. Their findings have considerable implications for counseling regarding TV viewing in that without the use of a hearing aid or closed captioning, close to 70% of participants understood very little of the spoken message. Further, binaural hearing-aid use alone did not provide any advantage in terms of recognition of information on the television. However, closed captioning alone and close captioning plus hearing-aid use yielded similar recognition scores across all types of programming ranging from drama and game shows to news programming. Interestingly, despite the limited advantage of hearing aids, the majority of participants wore their hearing aids when viewing the television, but close to 90% of participants rarely used closed captioning despite the objective advantage. Given the importance of television viewing in the lives of older adults, during the counseling session, the audiologist should demonstrate the complete array of technologies available for television viewing, and discuss the advantages and disadvantages of the different options.

◆ Telecommunication Technology

The telephone is a necessity, especially for older adults, as it is the best way to remain in contact with friends and relatives who have moved away. Telecommunication technologies provide for auditory enhancement of the signal. There are numerous options depending on such variables as hearing loss severity, hearing-aid use, and auditory processing abilities. **Table 8.25** summarizes some of the telecommunication options in terms of auditory or visual enhancements. The first option is an amplified telephone such as the corded or wireless phones shown in **Figs. 8.21, 8.22, and 8.23**. Clarity, a division of Plantronics, has an excellent Web site that categorizes their amplified phones according to the listener's severity of hearing loss, as amplified phones tend to vary in terms of the gain provided. The phones can be corded or cordless and there is considerable variability in terms of the style, ranging from Trimline phones to phones with a built-in answering machine, and

Table 8.25   Telecommunication Options

Amplifying the system through:
    Amplified telephones
    Handset amplifiers
    In-line amplifiers
    Portable couplers
    Interpersonal listening devices
    Strap-on amplifiers
    Caption-enabled telephones
Visual representation of the signal through:
    Computers
    Fax
    Teletypewriter (TTY) or TDD
    Voice carryover telephone (Captioned phones)
    Internet-protocol relay (IP)
Wireless transmission:
    Bluetooth

Source: From Sandridge, S. (1995). Beyond hearing aids: Use of auxiliary aids. In P. Kricos & S. Lesner (Eds.), *Hearing care for the older adult.* Boston: Butterworth-Heinemann.

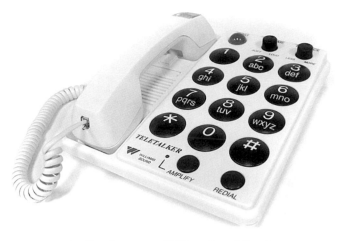

Fig. 8.21   Teletalker. (Courtesy of Williams Sound Corp.)

some are combination phones that are amplified and have large keypads for persons with low vision (**Fig. 8.21**). Amplified phones can increase the incoming sound between 20 and 50 dB of amplification, depending on the listener's hearing loss severity. Most amplified phones are equipped with an adjustable incoming volume control, a visual ring indicator, an adjustable tone control, visual ringers in the handset and base, and an adjustable ringer. Most are hearing-aid compatible and many are T-coil compatible.

There is considerable variability in the phones' features. Persons with hearing impairment who prefer low technology can find amplified phones with low feature density, whereas those who prefer high-tech phones can find many features density, caller ID, bed-shaker accessories, panic buttons for ease of use when in distress, or adjustable tone controls (Bankaitis 2008). But phones with more features are more expensive. Audiologists should familiarize patients with the options and factors to consider when they purchase a phone. Individuals

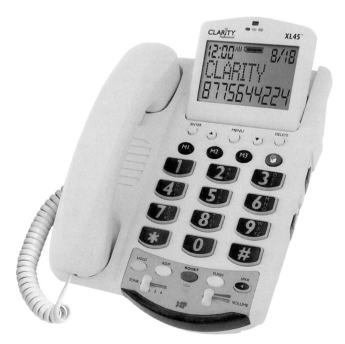

Fig. 8.22   Clarity Professional XL45™ corded caller ID telephone, featuring Digital Clarity Power™. (Courtesy of Clarity.)

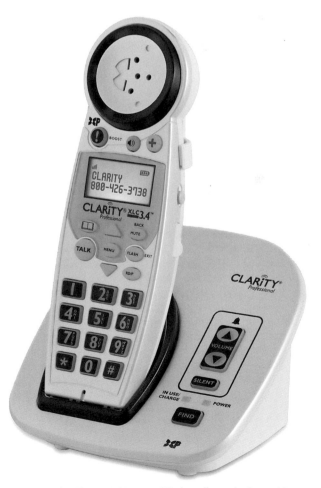

Fig. 8.23   The Clarity XLC3.4 amplified cordless telephone. (Courtesy of Clarity.)

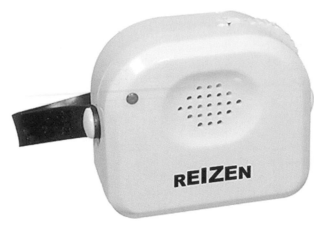

Fig. 8.24 Reizen strap-on amplifier. [From Valente, M., Dunn, H., & Roeser, R. (2008). *Audiology treatment.* New York: Thieme.]

with milder hearing loss may only need a phone with an adjustable audible ringer, whereas persons with severe hearing loss should be advised to purchase phones with the bed-shaker accessory. Similarly, persons with manual dexterity problems often associated with arthritis should know that some companies manufacture phones that are easy to use because they incorporate a contoured headset shape and Soft-Touch keypads with buttons that have generous spacing between them. Recently, some manufacturers have included innovative digital hearing-aid technology in their phones. For example, Clarity has a feature based on digital signal process-

ing technology built into hearing aids, known as Digital Clarity Power™, which makes soft sounds audible while keeping loud sounds within a comfortable range. Phones equipped with this feature can identify and amplify the human voice, while at the same time eliminating extraneous noise including echoes (http://clarityproducts.com/about-clarity/the-digital-clarity-power-difference/.

A variety of telephone amplifiers are available for persons not interested in purchasing an amplified phone. Portable amplifies are used with existing phones and simply amplify the voice of the caller (Bankaitis, 2008). They come in two distinct categories: strap-on amplifiers and in-line amplifiers. Designed to strap onto the earpiece of a telephone handset (**Fig. 8.24**), strap-on amplifiers are available in two varieties: acoustic couplers or inductive couplers. Acoustic couplers, which are available for use on a variety of phones, attach to the receiver of the handset by an elastic or detachable strap. Strap-on amplifiers, which amplify signals from 20 to 30 dB, may pose difficulties for older adults with poor manual dexterity because of the need to attach and remove the coupler each time the phone is used. Also, older adults may forget to turn the battery off, thus draining it and necessitating its replacement, which can become costly. Strap-on amplifiers are inexpensive, with some costing less than $15. Persons with hearing impairment should also be made aware of the availability of universal telephone amplifiers that convert any corded phone into an amplified phone. Some of these amplify the incoming voice by as much as 45 dB. Some also incorporate digital sound processing, thereby eliminating extraneous noise and echo. **Figures 8.25 and 8.26** display a variety of telecommunication options.

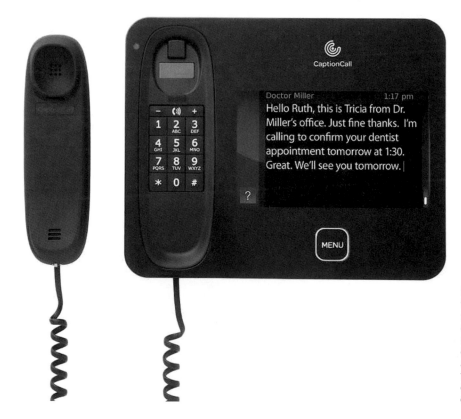

Fig. 8.25 Caption Call Phone. It has the following features: large text—7-inch display screen with adjustable text makes it easy to read every word of every call; location flexibility—set up the phone anywhere in the home with a wired or wireless Internet connection; customizable audio—easily adjust ringer or handset volume and frequency as the listener prefers; telecoil loop connection—for hearing aids with a telecoil option.

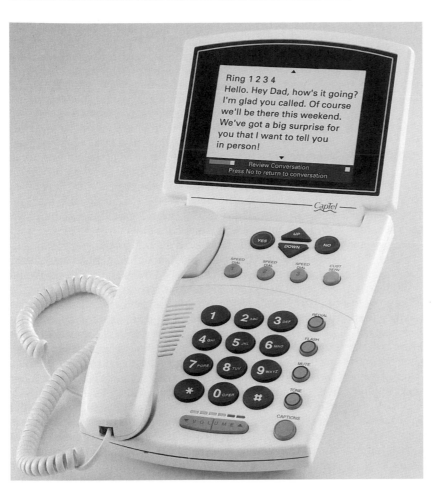

Fig. 8.26 Hamilton CapTel 800i Captioned Telephone. (Courtesy of Oaktree Products.)

Pearl

Older adults rely on the telephone to communicate with family members and friends, to make contacts with health professionals, and to make emergency contacts. Therefore, it is imperative that older adults with hearing aids who continue to have difficulty using the phone be made aware of the available options.

In-line amplifiers are interfaced between the body of the telephone and the handset. They are placed between the base and the receiver so that telephone processing can take place at the phone's base (Bankaitis, 2008). In order for in-line amplifiers to work, the telephone's signal processing must take place prior to the incoming voice being amplified by the telephone amplifier. Incompatible with cordless phones, the amplifiers attach to a corded telephone and amplify the volume of the incoming voice. In-line amplifiers do not work with corded phones on which the dial pad is built into the receiver. In-line amplifiers may amplify the incoming signal by 18 to 40 dB depending on the model and user settings. The 9-V battery that drives in-line amplifiers lasts between 6 and 12 months depending on use. Amplified telephones and telephone amplifiers may not provide adequate amplification for individuals with severe to profound hearing loss or for persons with extremely poor speech-recognition ability. Telecommu-nications Relay Services (TRS) enable individuals with a hearing impairment to communicate via a variety of visual systems, thereby promoting telephone access. Telecommunication options include facsimiles (fax) machines, electronic mail (e-mail), text messaging, voice carryover (VCO) telephones and teletypewriters (TTYs).

The VCO phones transmit incoming calls as text, thereby providing the hearing impaired the ability to read what the caller is communicating. VCO is an option for older adults who can speak clearly, but due to a severe hearing loss and/or processing difficulties, they have difficulty understanding conversations over the telephone. Using VCO relay and a specially designed telephone with a text display, a VCO user speaks directly to the other person over the telephone. A communication assistant (CA) types what is spoken by the other person for the VCO user to read. Providing a more natural flow of conversation, an enhanced option is a two-line VCO that allows users the option of using one telephone line for speaking and one for receiving typed messages from the CA who relays the message. Distinct from TTY devices, the VCO user does not have to type to communicate over the telephone. Individuals selecting this option must own a VCO telephone or a text telephone (TTY). Some amplified telephones incorporate VCO technology, allowing the hearing impaired to speak into the telephone while reading the words of the other person that are coming across the built-in screen.

The TTY devices transmit visual signals over the standard telephone line. TTYs consist of a keyboard, a modem, a display screen, and a cradle for the handset. Like VCO phones, TTYs look very much like a standard phone, except that they include a typewriter-style keyboard, a screen for displaying text, and a paper printout that enables the user to record the conversation. Relying on a sound-based coding system (e.g., Baudot), the TTY converts text into audible beeps that are then transmitted over the telephone line, and the written message appears as text across the TTY display screen (Bankaitis, 2008). When two parties are using a TTY, they take turns typing in their messages using a special text-code system. If one member of a party has a TTY, then the phone conversation is facilitated by a relay operator who types in a message, which is displayed across the listener's TTY. The non-TTY user communicates verbally with the CA (i.e., the relay operator) and the operator verbally communicates the message from the TTY user. The telephone company provides the relay service free of charge for persons wishing to speak with a TTY user. At present, local relay services may be contacted by dialing 711. VCO users can communicate with TTY users, and tele-Braille calling allows persons who are deaf and blind to use a special Braille keyboard to type and read their relay calls. With the appropriate software, the hearing impaired can make their computers work like a TTY. Audiologists should inform patients with significant hearing loss and difficulty communicating over the phone about the telecommunication relay services.

An alternative to TRS, Internet protocol (IP) relay, allows persons with hearing impairment to communicate through their telephone systems using a computer and the Internet, rather than a TTY and a telephone, obviating the need to invest in a TTY. The first leg of an IP relay call goes from the caller's computer, or other Web-enabled device, to the IP relay center via the Internet. The center is usually accessed via a Web page. The second leg of the call is from the CA to the receiving party via voice telephone through the public switched telephone network. Effective November 2009, IP relay users must be registered with a default IP relay provider. Some advantages of IP relay are that it permits much faster typing by the person with hearing impairment, it allows users to see much more of the conversation on their computer screens than is possible with a TTY, and the transmission quality may be faster. The FCC has an excellent fact sheet on IP relay services available at http://transition.fcc.gov/cgb/consumerfacts/iprelay.pdf.

◆ Cellphone Compatibility

Difficulty hearing on the telephone is one of the more common complaints among hearing-aid users. Originally, hearing aids were designed to compensate for lack of access to acoustic signals in face-to-face listening environments (Mackersie, Qi, Boothroyd, & Conrad, 2009). But now daily communication increasingly takes place over the telephone, and hearing-aid users find that hearing aids do not capture as effectively as they would like the output of telephone receivers. Hence the linking together of the hearing aid and the telephone has gained increasing importance with advances in each arena influencing that of the other (Levitt, 2007). Prior to the widespread use of digital cellular telephones, the major complaints regarding

telephone communication included inadequate coupling between the hearing aid (landline) and the hearing aid, acoustic feedback, and electromagnetic interference associated with use of the telecoil (Mackersie et al, 2009). The former problems have been allayed to a certain extent, being replaced by the issue of electromagnetic interference and the fact that clarity on cell phones is compromised because they do not have the frequency shaping necessary to provide high-frequency information to people with hearing loss. The issue of hearing-aid compatibility (HAC) has gained increasing importance given the widespread use of digital cell phones and given the fact that the telephone conversation is transmitted over a wireless network using radio waves, and the speech signal is often reduced in intelligibility (Levitt, 2007; Sandrock & Schum, 2007). The FCC defines HAC as being based on two parameters: radio-frequency (RF) emissions and telecoil coupling. A 2006 mandate from the FCC requires manufacturers of cell phones to offer handset models that meet ANSI HAC standards. Cell phones are tested to identify the extent to which they comply with the FCC definition of HAC and are assigned a rating according to their compatibility in terms of RF emissions and telecoil coupling. The Twenty-First Century Communications and Video Accessibility Act of 2010 ensures that telephone equipment used to make calls over the Internet is compatible with hearing aids. This act mandates hearing-aid compatibility for Internet telephones.

Referred to as RF, the radio waves generated by cellular phones create a strong electromagnetic field around the antenna of a cellular phone that can be picked up by the T-coil or the microphone of the hearing aid (Levitt, 2007). The result is a buzzing sound audible to the hearing-aid user. In addition to the electromagnetic interference generated by wireless telephones, telecoil users may experience another form of interference referred to as baseband, which is magnetic interference from the electronic elements of the cell phone including the backlighting, display, keypad, battery, and circuit board (Kozma-Spytek, 2006). The amount of interference experienced by the hearing-aid microphone generally depends on the degree of RF emission produced by the digital cell phone and how immune the phone is to these emissions. Much progress has been made in improving the immunity of hearing aids to the emissions, and considerable effort has been put into reducing the interference generated by wireless telephones (Levitt, 2007). Present-day hearing aids have a built-in immunity to cell-phone interference. Even though recent federal regulations are easing compatibility issues, as are developments in hearing-aid technology aimed at alleviating the coupling problems, it remains important to share with the patient information about hearing-aid compatibility (Mackersie et al, 2009). Mackersie and colleagues (2009) and Kochkin (2007) make a strong case that audiologists have a responsibility to discuss the appropriate use of cellular phones with the 70% of hearing-impaired people who do not use hearing aids.

The HAC rating and information about whether a wireless device is compatible can be found in one of three places: (1) on the display card next to the phone in retail stores, (2) on the package directly, or (3) on the package insert of the manual accompanying the telephone. Cell phones tested for their telecoil coupling compatibility or for their acoustic coupling compatibility will be assigned a rating of T3 or T4 in the case of the former and M3 or M4 in the case of the latter. The T stands for telecoil, which means that the phone has been tested and rated for inductive coupling purposes, and the M stands for compatibility when the hearing aid is set in the microphone mode while using the cellular phone. Cell phones that receive an HAC rating of M3 or M4 have met or surpassed the ANSI standard. The higher the M rating, the lower the RF emission level and the less likely the hearing-aid user will experience interference. Hence, cellular phones that have a high immunity rating are assigned a 3 or 4, whereas phones with a poor immunity rating will be assigned an M1 or T1. If one uses the cell phone when the hearing aid is in M mode, the M3 or M4 rating is important, whereas if one uses the cell phone when the hearing aid is in "T-coil" mode, then the T3 or T4 rating is important. Although the FCC does not have regulatory authority over hearing aids, the FCC has encouraged the hearing-aid industry to test, rate, and label hearing aids according to their level of RF immunity to cellular phones. As of this writing, most new digital hearing aids have an M2/T2 rating. Although not universal, many hearing-aid manufacturers have complied, so that a hearing aid with a rating of M4 or T4 is more immune to RF interference than is a hearing aid with a rating of M3 or T3. Most new digital hearing aids have immunity ratings of at least M2, so digital hearing aids have more immunity to interference than do conventional analog hearing aids and (Kozma-Spytek, 2006).

When fitting behind-the-ear hearing aids, audiologists should ensure that the hearing aid is equipped with a T-coil that is RF immune. Most new T-coils fall into this category. To determine whether a particular cellular phone will interfere with a hearing aid, the hearing aid and cell phone ratings should be combined. A sum of four indicates that the cellular phone and digital hearing aid can be used together, and the higher the combined the score the better the listening experience. Specifically, a hearing-aid rating of M2 and a cellular phone rating of M3 will yield a combined rating of M5, which is considered "normal" use, whereas a combined rating of M6 or more would suggest that the hearing-aid user can expect "excellent" performance with the cellular phone. Note that Andrews Worldwide Communication (http://www.andrews.com/cell-phones/hac/) lists all cell phones that have the M4/T4 rating, which suggests that they are free of interference. Audiologists should note that CI users should be encouraged to try the cellular phone before making the purchase and they should understand the rating system when purchasing their phones.

Pearl

The Federal Communications Commission (FCC) defines hearing-aid compatibility (HAC) for cellular phones in terms of radiofrequency (RF) emissions, the M (microphone) rating, and telecoil coupling, the T (T-coil) rating; only phones rated as 3 or 4 are allowed to be sold as HAC.

The immunity ratings for hearing aids and the HAC ratings for cellular phones should be discussed with the hearing impaired, and it is important to emphasize that the ratings do not guarantee performance. Another matter to discuss with the hearing-aid user is that the design of the handset may influence performance, such that the greater the separation between the hearing aid and the RF transmission components, the less the interference. Thus, the clam-shell or flip-up design is preferable, as in this case the only section of the phone that flips up is the speaker, which is used for listening (Kozma-Spytek, 2006). The ability to control backlighting, use of vibrating alerts, and a volume control can also help the hearing-aid user minimize the RF interference. **Table 8.26** presents issues to discuss with hearing-impaired patients when they consider purchasing a cellular phone or new hearing aids.

Signal-Alerting Technology

Signal-alerting technology refers to a system that warns, signals, or alerts a person with a hearing impairment to important sounds present in the environment. For the person with hearing impairment, the sound must be enhanced or conveyed through some other sense, be it tactile or visual. Specifically, devices to alert persons with hearing impairment to conditions in the environment substitute visual signals or tactile signals when warning signals are not audible. Virtually every sound-producing event used for signaling or warning purposes can be coded into a visual or vibratory stimulus for the benefit of persons with hearing impairment (Ross, 1996). Signal-alerting devices are commercially available and are invaluable to homebound hearing-impaired persons, to persons with cognitive impairments, and to residents of assisted-living facilities and nursing facilities who cannot hear external events due to hearing loss. These devices can be used with or without hearing aids, and since many older adults who live alone remove their hearing aids when they are in their homes, these technologies can be invaluable.

Independent alerting devices are available for alarm clocks, smoke alarms, carbon monoxide detectors, doorbells and door knockers, and the telephone. Devices to indicate that the telephone is ringing can be visual or tactile. Telephone ringers increase the loudness of the incoming ring. Many amplified telephones include extra loud ringers, vibrotactile signaling options, or bright visual ring indicators, placed in either the base or the handset, signaling an incoming phone call. Typical telephone ring signalers have adjustable volume controls and some have adjustable frequency settings that are helpful to persons with hearing loss at frequencies at which the ring would be inaudible (used by only 14% of non hearing aid users). Some have strobe flashers to alert persons with hearing impairment to an incoming phone call. Remote ringers can be set up so that the light will flash in an adjacent room. This is very helpful for older adults who complain of difficulty hearing the telephone ring when they are in an adjoining room (Sandridge, 1995). Telephone ring signalers are available separate from amplified telephones, and some ringers are combination doorbell and telephone signalers. Some companies manufacture ringers that signal an incoming call from a landline or a cell phone using a bright visible signal or a bed shaker that is often sold separately. Vibrating pads can be added to this combination for the visually impaired and for when persons with hearing impairment are asleep. Some telephone ringers come equipped with strobe lights and some will accommodate a bed shaker, which is important for persons with severe hearing loss. Older adults who travel should consider purchasing a portable tele-

Table 8.26 Considerations When Purchasing New Hearing Aids and New Cellular Phones

When patients are purchasing new hearing aids:

1. Inform patients about the hearing aid's "built-in" immunity to cell phone interference; contact hearing-aid manufacturer when it is not noted on the information brochure that accompanies the hearing aid.
2. Ask patients if they plan on using a cellular phone with the hearing aid; if so, recommend a hearing aid with a telecoil, as for some hearing aids telecoils are necessary to take advantage of selected accessories developed by cellular phone manufacturers.
3. Review written materials with patients that describes the hearing aid's anticipated performance with digital cellular phones.
4. Inform patients that the Hearing Industry Association mandates a 30-day trial period with new hearing aids to ensure patient satisfaction with performance when the hearing aid is coupled to a cellular phone.
5. Inform patients to look at the cellular phone and review the T and M ratings. Inform them that a T3 or T4 rating means the device is intended for use with hearing aids in the telecoil mode, and that the higher the rating, the more likely they will be able to use the hearing aid on the T-coil setting. Similarly, inform them that the M3 or M4 rating means the device is intended for use when the hearing aid is in the microphone setting, and the higher the rating, the more likely they will be able to use their hearing aid on the microphone setting with the phone. Explain to patients that adding up the M and T ratings for the cellular phone and hearing aid provide a combined rating that will best inform them about performance. For example, a combined rating of 6 is considered best or excellent and the combination considered highly usable with excellent performance.
6. Inform patients that because of the individual variability in hearing loss, the rating does not guarantee performance, so they should try the phone with their hearing aid at the store before making the purchase. They should try several phones with their hearing aid because of the variability in cellular phone performance.
7. Recommend that patients consider purchasing cellular phones where the only part of the phone that flips up when the phone is in use is the speaker, as this will ensure greater separation between the hearing aid and the components/electronics of the cell phone, which may cause the interference.
8. Inform patients about the conundrum with backlighting on the cellular phone. That is, they should try to purchase a phone where they can control the backlighting, as when the backlighting is on, it may interfere with performance when using the T coil to communicate. Let the patient know that interference from backlighting is not considered when determining hearing-aid compatible (HAC) ratings.
9. Recommend that patients look for a telephone with a vibratory alert, as they may have difficulty hearing the ring signaling.
10. Advise patients to look for an easy-to-use volume control on their cellular phone.
11. Inform patients that for "hands-free" driving, many companies sell accessories such as a neck loop or ear hooks for use when the hearing aid is set in telecoil or when the cochlear implant is set on telecoil mode. They should also consider use of the speaker phone function if using the hearing aid in the microphone mode. The Bluetooth accessory on the hearing aid and cellular phone is another option for hands-free use.
12. When patients have cellular phone handset models that do not meet hearing-aid compatibility standards, positioning the receiver of the cell phone closer to the microphone of the BTE hearing aid rather than against the ear improves reception.
13. The cellular phone must be Bluetooth-compatible, and the streamer requires close proximity to the hearing aid (about 3 feet).

Source: From Cellular Telephone Industry Association (CTIA). (2009). Welcome to access wireless.org. www.accesswireless.org.

phone ring signaler, although hotels should be equipped with signaling and warning devices that can be made available upon request. Smarphone alarms do have a vibrate setting and this should be discussed, as well. Finally, universal sound signalers that alert the hearing impaired to all sounds including telephones, alarms, and a baby crying are important options to be considered. Telephone ringers are commercially available, and Internet sites including Amazon sell alerting devices. All of this information should be shared with persons with hearing impairment as part of their hearing-aid orientation.

The ability to hear signals such as the fire alarm, a doorbell, the smoke alarm, a baby crying, or a carbon monoxide detector is quite important especially for older adults when they are asleep or home alone and not wearing hearing aids. Many signaling systems signal more than one sound such as the doorbell and telephone. It is important to note that a receiver that works with the various signalers must be mounted in the home, as it will receive the signal from the power line and in turn will alert the hearing impaired to the presence of one of many signals such as the smoke alarm or doorbell. Many receivers include white flashing strobe lights, as they have been found to be effective in alerting hearing-impaired persons who are asleep. Amplified smoke detectors provide audible signals that can be supplemented with a strobe signal. The hearing impaired should make sure to purchase and mount smoke detec-

tors with audible low-frequency signals (520 Hz) because many smoke detectors generate sounds at 3100 Hz, which is a problem for those who have middle- to high-frequency hearing loss. As with telephone devices, remote lights can be set up in various rooms with selected alarms that flash strobe lights when smoke is detected.

When purchasing a smoke detector, persons with hearing impairment should ask whether it meets the standard set by the National Fire Protection Association. Such standards attempt to ensure that the visual light system is bright enough and the audible signal is at the frequency most likely to awaken a sleeping deaf person. Special alarm clocks produce a vibrotactile, visual, or amplified auditory signal to awaken the hearing impaired. They are also available in travel models. There are also alarm watches that are ideal when traveling. Some companies manufacture alarm clocks that can also serve as a receiver (Bankaitis, 2008). Hearing-impaired persons may not be able to hear an alarm clock with an audio signal. A variety of options are available for home and travel. Most alarm clocks use either light or vibration to wake up the person from sleep. Alarm clocks that chirp loudly can be purchased by persons with milder hearing impairments. Small travel alarms or smartphones set to vibrate, when used as an alarm clock, can be placed under the pillow, to awaken the sleeping traveler. Most baby-monitoring systems are wireless, and the signal can be sent to multiple receivers throughout one's home. Devices that alert persons with hearing impairment to the ringing of the doorbell are available from selected dealers. As with the smoke alarm system, the ability to be alerted visually to the fact that someone is at the door generates a sense of security that is so important to older adults. The simplest solution for the home is installation of a light that flashes when the doorbell rings. It is important to inform patients that most signalers require a receiver that has a different strobe light sequence for each signal, so that the alarm clock, the telephone, and the baby monitor can be distinguished. A sonic house, which can be viewed at http://www.justbekuz.com/images/sonichouse.jpg, demonstrates how a receiver works with various signalers to alert the hearing impaired to a danger or a signal in the home.

Pearls

If several devices are needed, whole house alerting systems can be installed centrally, or combination systems may be preferable, although they are more costly. Comprehensive alerting systems are equipped with individual sensors for the different systems (e.g., radio alarm, smoke detector, etc.), each with its own response code.

Audiologists should consider becoming full-service hearing health care providers by including HATs as an integral part of the rehabilitative services being offered. This can help to ensure that all hearing-related difficulties are addressed, and the emotional and social challenges posed by hearing impairment confronted and overcome successfully.

◆ Conclusion

This chapter was lengthy because there is considerable information available on hearing aids, implantable devices, and HATs. These technologies enhance the communication function for older adults with handicapping hearing impairments. Hearing aids are effective treatments for the communication disabilities and psychosocial handicaps that attend ARHL. It is incumbent on audiologists to ensure that older adults are informed of the value of hearing aids/HATs in combination with audiological rehabilitation, in overcoming the communication difficulties that attend hearing loss, and of the importance of HATs and implantable devices in the context of audiological rehabilitation as adjuncts to hearing aids. Audiologists must remember to look beyond the technology at the individual and remember that the nature of the amplification system should be targeted and driven by the expressed needs of the older patient. The following important premises were enumerated by McSpaden (1996):

◆ Patients do not come into a dispenser's office because their audiogram is abnormal. They come in because their perception indicates a loss, a decrease in sensitivity, a change, or simply a social "failure" that they impute to their hearing.

◆ Patients do not care about numbers. What is important is their perception of what the numbers mean.

◆ To the extent that we improve the patient's communicative efficiency, what we have done will be worth it. If we do not improve communicative efficiency, yet achieve good aided thresholds and higher discrimination scores, whatever we have done is not worth it.

◆ No one listens to anything at threshold. Everyone wants to listen to everything at MCL without ever exceeding LDL. This is true for every signal.

◆ It is not about hearing any kind of signal; it is about understanding and decoding.

◆ The patient is the one with the symptoms.

◆ We must stop anthropomorphizing the audiogram. The audiogram is merely a graph of auditory behavior, elicited on a given day, at a given time. It is not the hearing-impaired person.

◆ Make every effort to meet the needs of the patient, and stop trying to make the patient's needs fit our understanding.

◆ It's about the patient!

Finally, and in conclusion, many persons with hearing loss are craving for connections. According to one of my wisest patients, inform your patients that their hearing loss and attendant consequences will disappear, if they utilize hearing technologies!

References

Aazh, H., & Moore, B. C. (2007, Sep). The value of routine real ear measurement of the gain of digital hearing aids. *Journal of the American Academy of Audiology, 18,* 653–664

Abrams, H. (2009). Outcomes measurement in the audiologic rehabilitation of the elderly. In L. Hickson (Ed.), *Hearing care for adults 2009—The challenge of aging. Proceedings of the Second International Adult Conference* (pp. 279–285).

Abrams, H., & Chisolm, T. (2008). Measuring health- related quality of life in audiologic rehabilitation. In J. Spitzer & J. Montano (Eds.), *Adult audiologic rehabilitation.* San Diego: Plural

Ahlstrom, J. B., Horwitz, A. R., & Dubno, J. R. (2009, Apr). Spatial benefit of bilateral hearing AIDS. *Ear and Hearing, 30,* 203–218

Alworth, L., Plyler, P., Rebert, M., & Johnstone, P. (2010). The effects of receiver placement on probe microphone, performance, and subjective measures with open canal hearing instruments. *Journal of the American Academy of Audiology, 21,* 249–266

American Speech-Language-Hearing Association (ASHA). (2006). *Preferred practice patterns for the profession of audiology.* http://www.asha.org/docs/html/PP2006-00274.html

Amos, N. E., & Humes, L. E. (2007, Aug). Contribution of high frequencies to speech recognition in quiet and noise in listeners with varying degrees of high-frequency sensorineural hearing loss. *Journal of Speech, Language, and Hearing Research, 50,* 819–834

Arlinger, S. (2003, Jul). Negative consequences of uncorrected hearing loss—A review. *International Journal of Audiology, 42*(Suppl 2), S17–S20

Arlinger, S., Gatehouse, S., Bentler, R. A., Byrne, D., Cox, R. M., Dirks, D. D., et al. (1996). Report of the Eriksholm Workshop on auditory deprivation and acclimatization. *Ear Hear Suppl, 17,* 87S–98S

Baddeley, A. (1986). *Working memory.* Oxford: Clarendon

Baer, T., Moore, B. C. J., & Kluk, K. (2002, Sep). Effects of low pass filtering on the intelligibility of speech in noise for people with and without dead regions at high frequencies. *Journal of the Acoustical Society of America, 112*(3 Pt 1), 1133–1144

Bankaitis, A. (2008). Hearing assistive technologies. In M. Valente, H. Hosford-Dunn, & R. Roeser (Eds.), *Audiology treatment* (2nd ed.). New York: Thieme

Beck, D., & Brunved, P. (2006). *T-coils: Beyond the telephone.* http://www.oticonusa.com/oticon/profesional_resources/library/news_from_oticon_t-coils_beyone-the-telephone.html

Beck, D., & Harvey, M. (2009). Traditional and nontraditional communication and connectivity. *Hearing Review, 16,* 30–33

Bentler, R., & Mueller, G. (2009). Hearing aid technology. In J. Katz, L. Medwetsky, R. Burkard, & L. Hood, (Eds.), *Handbook of clinical audiology* (6th ed.). Philadelphia: Wolters Kluwer

Bess, F. H., Lichtenstein, M. J., Logan, S. A., Burger, M. C., & Nelson, E. (1989, Feb). Hearing impairment as a determinant of function in the elderly. *Journal of the American Geriatrics Society, 37,* 123–128

Blamey, P. J., & Martin, L. F. (2009, Apr). Loudness and satisfaction ratings for hearing aid users. *Journal of the American Academy of Audiology, 20,* 272–282

Bloom, S. (2009). Connectivity: Early steps point the way toward wireless wonders to come. *Hearing Journal, 62,* 17–20

Boothroyd, A. (2004, Feb). Hearing aid accessories for adults: The remote FM microphone. *Ear and Hearing, 25,* 22–33

Boothroyd, A. (2007). Wireless technology is driving a hearing aid metamorphosis. *Hearing Journal, 60,* 11

Boothroyd, A., Fitz, K., Kindred, J., Kochkin, S., Levitt, H., Moore, B., and Yanz, J. (2007). Hearing aids and wireless technology. *Hearing Review* http://www.hearingreview.com/issues/articles/2007-06_05.asp

Bridges, J., & Bentler, R. (1998). Relating hearing aid use to well-being among older adults. *Hearing Journal, 51,* 39–44

Chang, W. H., Tseng, H. C., Chao, T. K., Hsu, C. J., & Liu, T. C. (2008, Jun). Measurement of hearing aid outcome in the elderly: Comparison between young and old elderly. *Otolaryngology–Head and Neck Surgery, 138,* 730–734

Chia, E. M., Wang, J. J., Rochtchina, E., Cumming, R. R., Newall, P., & Mitchell, P. (2007, Apr). Hearing impairment and health-related quality of life: The Blue Mountains Hearing Study. *Ear and Hearing, 28,* 187–195

Chisolm, T. H., Johnson, C. E., Danhauer, J. L., Portz, L. J., Abrams, H. B., Lesner, S., et al. (2007, Feb). A systematic review of health-related quality of life and hearing aids: Final report of the American Academy of Audiology Task Force on the Health-Related Quality of Life Benefits of Amplification in Adults. *Journal of the American Academy of Audiology, 18,* 151–183

Chisolm, T. H., Noe, C. M., McArdle, R., & Abrams, H. (2007, Jun). Evidence for the use of hearing assistive technology by adults: The role of the FM system. *Trends in Amplification, 11,* 73–89

Chmiel, R., & Jerger, J. (1995, Apr). Quantifying improvement with amplification. *Ear and Hearing, 16,* 166–175

Christensen, L. (2009). New bone-anchored amplification options for children. *ASHA Leader* http://www.asha.org/publications/leader/2009/090714/090714g.htm

Citron, D. (2008). Counseling and orientation toward amplification. In M. Valente, H. Hosford-Dunn, & R. Roeser (Eds.), *Audiology treatment* (2nd ed.). New York: Thieme

Cohen, S. M., Labadie, R. F., Dietrich, M. S., & Haynes, D. S. (2004, Oct). Quality of life in hearing-impaired adults: The role of cochlear implants and hearing aids. *Otolaryngology–Head and Neck Surgery, 131,* 413–422

Consumer Reports. (2009, Jul). Hear well in a noisy world. Hearing aids, hearing protection, and more. *Consumer Reports*

Cox, R. (1995). Page ten: A hands-on discussion of the IHAFF approach. *Hearing Journal, 48,* 39–44

Cox, R. M., & Alexander, G. C. (1995, Apr). The abbreviated profile of hearing aid benefit. *Ear and Hearing, 16,* 176–186

Cox, R. M., & Alexander, G. C. (1999, Aug). Measuring satisfaction with amplification in daily life: The SADL scale. *Ear and Hearing, 20,* 306–320

Cox, R. M., & Alexander, G. C. (2000, Jul–Aug). Expectations about hearing aids and their relationship to fitting outcome. *Journal of the American Academy of Audiology, 11,* 368–382, quiz 407

Cox, R. M., & Alexander, G. C. (2001, Apr). Validation of the SADL questionnaire. *Ear and Hearing, 22,* 151–160

Cox, R. M., & Alexander, G. C. (2002, Jan). The International Outcome Inventory for Hearing Aids (IOI-HA): Psychometric properties of the English version. *International Journal of Audiology, 41,* 30–35

Cox, R. M., Alexander, G. C., & Gray, G. A. (2005a, Feb). Who wants a hearing aid? Personality profiles of hearing aid seekers. *Ear and Hearing, 26,* 12–26

Cox, R. M., Alexander, G. C., & Gray, G. A. (2005b, Dec). Hearing aid patients in private practice and public health (Veterans Affairs) clinics: Are they different? *Ear and Hearing, 26,* 513–528

Cox, R. M., Alexander, G. C., & Gray, G. A. (2007, Apr). Personality, hearing problems, and amplification characteristics: Contributions to self-report hearing aid outcomes. *Ear and Hearing, 28,* 141–162

Cox, R. M., Alexander, G. C., Johnson, J., & Rivera, I. (2011a, May–Jun). Cochlear dead regions in typical hearing aid candidates: Prevalence and implications for use of high-frequency speech cues. *Ear and Hearing, 32,* 339–348

Cox, R. M., Schwartz, K. S., Noe, C. M., & Alexander, G. C. (2011b, Mar–Apr). Preference for one or two hearing AIDS among adult patients. *Ear and Hearing, 32,* 181–197

Cox, R. M., & Xu, J. (2010, Feb). Short and long compression release times: Speech understanding, real-world preferences, and association with cognitive ability. *Journal of the American Academy of Audiology, 21,* 121–138

Cellular Telephone Industry Association (CTIA). (2009). *Welcome to access wireless.org.* www.accesswireless.org

Cullington, H. E., & Zeng, F. G. (2011, Feb). Comparison of bimodal and bilateral cochlear implant users on speech recognition with competing talker, music perception, affective prosody discrimination, and talker identification. *Ear and Hearing, 32,* 16–30

Cunningham, L., & Friesen, L. (2005). Predicting hearing aid acceptance. *Audiology Today, 17,* 25

Dalton, D. S., Cruickshanks, K. J., Klein, B. E., Klein, R., Wiley, T. L., & Nondahl, D. M. (2003, Oct). The impact of hearing loss on quality of life in older adults. *Gerontologist, 43,* 661–668

Davis, D. 1994. Television amplification devices. In M. Ross (Ed.), *Communication access for persons with hearing loss.* Parkton, MD: York Press

Day, H., Jutai, J., & Campbell, K. (2002). Development of a scale to measure the psychosocial impact of assistive devices: Lessons learned and the road ahead. *Disability and Rehabilitation, 24,* 31–37

Dillon, H., James, A., & Ginis, J. (1997, Feb). Client Oriented Scale of Improvement (COSI) and its relationship to several other measures of benefit and satisfaction provided by hearing aids. *Journal of the American Academy of Audiology, 8,* 27–43

Ditzler, J. (2008). A primer on hearing aid warranties and insurance coverage. *Hearing Review* http://www.hearingreview.com/issues/articles/2008-04_03.asp

Dunn, C. C., Tyler, R. S., & Witt, S. A. (2005, Jun). Benefit of wearing a hearing aid on the unimplanted ear in adult users of a cochlear implant. *Journal of Speech, Language, and Hearing Research, 48,* 668–680

English, K. (2008). Counseling issues in audiologic rehabilitation. *Contemporary Issues in Communication Science and Disorders. 35,* 93–101

Fino, M., Bess, F., Lichtenstein, M., & Logan, S. (1991). Factors differentiating elderly hearing aid wearers and non-wearers. *Hearing Instruments, 43,* 6–10

Fitzpatrick, E. M., Séguin, C., Schramm, D. R., Armstrong, S., & Chénier, J. (2009, Oct). The benefits of remote microphone technology for adults with cochlear implants. *Ear and Hearing, 30,* 590–599

Folstein, M. F., Folstein, S. E., & McHugh, P. R. (1975, Nov). "Mini-mental state". A practical method for grading the cognitive state of patients for the clinician. *Journal of Psychiatric Research, 12,* 189–198

Foo, C., Rudner, M., Rönnberg, J., & Lunner, T. (2007, Jul–Aug). Recognition of speech in noise with new hearing instrument compression release settings requires explicit cognitive storage and processing capacity. *Journal of the American Academy of Audiology, 18,* 618–631

Friedland, D. R., Runge-Samuelson, C., Baig, H., & Jensen, J. (2010, May). Case-control analysis of cochlear implant performance in elderly patients. *Archives of Otolaryngology–Head and Neck Surgery, 136,* 432–438

Frye, K., & Martin, R. (2008). Real ear measurements. In M. Valente, H. Hosford-Dunn, & R. Roeser (Eds.), *Audiology treatment* (2nd ed.). New York: Thieme

Gatehouse, S. (1992, Sep). The time course and magnitude of perceptual acclimatization to frequency responses: evidence from monaural fitting of hearing aids. *Journal of the Acoustical Society of America, 92,* 1258–1268

Gatehouse, S. (1999). Glasgow Hearing Aid Benefit Profile. Derivation and validation of a client-centered outcome measure for hearing aid services. *Journal of the American Academy of Audiology, 18,* 80–103

Gatehouse, S., Naylor, G., & Elberling, C. (2006a, Mar). Linear and nonlinear hearing aid fittings—1. Patterns of benefit. *International Journal of Audiology, 45,* 130–152

Gatehouse, S., Naylor, G., & Elberling, C. (2006b, Mar). Linear and nonlinear hearing aid fittings—2. Patterns of candidature. *International Journal of Audiology, 45,* 153–171

Gatehouse, S., & Noble, W. (2004, Feb). The Speech, Spatial and Qualities of Hearing Scale (SSQ). *International Journal of Audiology, 43,* 85–99

Gelfand, S. A. (1995, Mar). Long-term recovery and no recovery from the auditory deprivation effect with binaural amplification: Six cases. *Journal of the American Academy of Audiology, 6,* 141–149

Gifford, R. (2011). Who is a cochlear implant candidate? *Hearing Journal, 64,* 16–22

Gifford, R. H., Dorman, M. F., Shallop, J. K., & Sydlowski, S. A. (2010, Apr). Evidence for the expansion of adult cochlear implant candidacy. *Ear and Hearing, 31,* 186–194

Glista, D., Scollie, S., Bagatto, M., Seewald, R., Parsa, V., & Johnson, A. (2009). Evaluation of nonlinear frequency compression: Clinical outcomes. *International Journal of Audiology, 48,* 632–644

Gordon-Salant, S., & Callahan, J. S. (2009, Aug). The benefits of hearing aids and closed captioning for television viewing by older adults with hearing loss. *Ear and Hearing, 30,* 458–465

Gordon-Salant, S., Yeni-Komshian, G. H., Fitzgibbons, P. J., & Barrett, J. (2006, Apr). Age-related differences in identification and discrimination of temporal cues in speech segments. *Journal of the Acoustical Society of America, 119,* 2455–2466

Hawkins, D. (2011, Nov–Dec). It's the output. *Audiology Today,* 66–67

Hearing Industries Association. (2010, Dec). *Quarterly statistics report.* Washington, DC: HIA

Helfer, K. S., & Vargo, M. (2009, Apr). Speech recognition and temporal processing in middle-aged women. *Journal of the American Academy of Audiology, 20,* 264–271

Hj Report. (2010). Hj Report. *Hearing Journal. 63,* 7–8

Hj Report. (2011). Hj Report. *Hearing Journal, 64,* 7

Hornsby, B., & Ricketts, T. A. (2004). *High-frequency hearing loss and frequency importance.* Paper presented at the annual meeting of the American Academy of Audiology, Salt Lake City, UT

Hornsby, B. W., & Ricketts, T. A. (2006, Mar). The effects of hearing loss on the contribution of high- and low-frequency speech information to speech understanding. II. Sloping hearing loss. *Journal of the Acoustical Society of America, 119,* 1752–1763

Horwitz, A. R., Ahlstrom, J. B., & Dubno, J. R. (2008, Jun). Factors affecting the benefits of high-frequency amplification. *Journal of Speech, Language, and Hearing Research, 51,* 798–813

Huart, S., & Sammeth, C. (2009). Identifying cochlear implant candidates in the hearing aid dispensing practice. *Hearing Review, 16,* 24–32

Humes, L. (2001). Issues in evaluating the effectiveness of hearing aids in the elderly: What to measure and when. *Seminars in Hearing, 22,* 303–314

Humes, L. (2007a). Hearing-aid outcome measures in older adults. In C. Palmer & R. Seewald (Eds.), *Hearing care for adults 2006* (pp. 265–276). Switzerland: Phonak AG

Humes, L. E. (2007b, Jul-Aug). The contributions of audibility and cognitive factors to the benefit provided by amplified speech to older adults. *Journal of the American Academy of Audiology, 18,* 590–603

Humes, L. E., Halling, D., & Coughlin, M. (1996). Reliability and stability of various hearing aid outcome measures in a group of elderly hearing aid wearers. *Journal of Speech and Hearing Research, 39,* 923–935

Humes, L. E., Kinney, D., & Thompson, E. (2009). Comparison of benefits provided by various hearing aid technologies in older adults. In L. Hickson (Ed.), *Hearing care for adults 2009—The challenge of aging. Proceedings of the Second International Adult Conference* (pp. 131–138).

Humes, L. E., Wilson, D. L., Barlow, N. N., & Garner, C. (2002, Aug). Changes in hearing-aid benefit following 1 or 2 years of hearing-aid use by older adults. *Journal of Speech, Language, and Hearing Research, 45,* 772–782

Hyde, M., & Riko, K. (1994). A decision-analytic approach to audiological rehabilitation. In J. P. Gagne & N. T. Murrary (Eds.), *Research in audiological rehabilitation: current trends and future directions. Journal of the American Academy of Rehabilitative Audiology, Monograph Supplement, 27,* 337–374

Ivory, P. J., Hendricks, B. L., Van Vliet, D., Beyer, C. M., & Abrams, H. B. (2009, Dec). Short-term hearing aid benefit in a large group. *Trends in Amplification, 13,* 260–280

Jenstad, L. M., & Souza, P. E. (2005, Jun). Quantifying the effect of compression hearing aid release time on speech acoustics and intelligibility. *Journal of Speech, Language, and Hearing Research, 48,* 651–667

Jenstad, L. M., Van Tasell, D. J., & Ewert, C. (2003, Sep). Hearing aid troubleshooting based on patients' descriptions. *Journal of the American Academy of Audiology, 14,* 347–360

Jerger, J., Chmiel, R., Florin, E., Pirozzolo, F., & Wilson, N. (1996, Dec). Comparison of conventional amplification and an assistive listening device in elderly persons. *Ear and Hearing, 17,* 490–504

Jerger, J., Silman, S., Lew, H. L., & Chmiel, R. (1993, Mar). Case studies in binaural interference: Converging evidence from behavioral and electrophysiologic measures. *Journal of the American Academy of Audiology, 4,* 122–131

Johnson, E. (2007). Survey finds higher sales and prices, plus more open fittings and directional microphones. *Hearing Journal, 60,* 52–58

Johnson, E. (2008). Despite having more advanced features, hearing aids hold line on retail price. *Hearing Journal, 61,* 42–48

Johnson, E. E., & Ricketts, T. A. (2010, Mar). Dispensing rates of four common hearing aid product features: Associations with variations in practice among audiologists. *Trends in Amplification, 14,* 12–45

Joore, M. A., Potjewijd, J., Timmerman, A. A., & Auteunis, L. J. (2002). Response shift in the measurement of quality of life in hearing impaired adults after hearing aid fitting. *Quality of Life Research, 11,* 299

Kemp, B. (1990). The psychosocial context of geriatric rehabilitation. In B. Kemp, K. Brummel-Smith, & J. Ramsdell (Eds.), *Geriatric rehabilitation.* Boston: College Hill

Kerckhoff, J., Listenberger, J., & Valente, M. (2008). Advances in hearing aid technology. *Contemporary Issues in Communication Sciences and Disorders, 35,* 102–112

Kirkwood, D. (1999). World of Hearing conference seeks to raise awareness of hearing loss, care. *Hearing Journal, 52,* 49–52

Kirkwood, D. (2009). Despite challenging economic conditions, practitioners in survey remain upbeat. *Hearing Journal, 62,* 28–31

Kirkwood, D. (2010). In troubled economic times, the hearing aid industry remains an island of stability. *Hearing Journal, 63,* 11–12, 14, 16

Kochkin, S. (2005). MarkeTrak VII: Hearing loss population tops 31.5 million. *Hearing Journal, 12,* 16–29

Kochkin, S. (2007). MarkeTrak VII: Obstacles to adult non-user adoption of hearing aids. *Hearing Journal, 60,* 24–50

Kochkin, S. (2009). MarkeTrak VIII: 25 year trends in the hearing health market. *Hearing Review. 16,* 12–31

Kochkin, S. (2010). Marke-Trak VIII: Customer satisfaction with hearing aids is slowly increasing. *Hearing Journal, 63,* 19–20, 22, 24, 26, 28, 30–32

Kochkin, S. (2011a). MarkeTrak VIII. Patients report improved quality of life with hearing aid usage. *Hearing Journal. 64,* 25–32

Kochkin, S. (2011b). MarkeTrak VIII: mini-BTEs tap new market, users more satisfied. *Hearing Journal, 64,* 17–18, 20, 22, 24

Kochkin, S. (2011c). MarkeTrak VIII: Reducing patient visits through verification and validation. *Hearing Review. 18,* 10–12

Kochkin, S. (2012). MarkeTrak VIII: The key influencing factors in hearing aid purchase intent. *Hearing Review, 19,* 12–25.

Kochkin, S., Beck, D. L., Christensen, L. A., Compton-Conley, C., Kricos, P. B., Fligor, B. J., et al. (2010). MarkeTrak VIII: The impact of the hearing healthcare professional on hearing aid user success. *Hearing Review, 17,* 12–34

Kozma-Spytek, L. (2006, October 9). Hearing aid compatibility for digital wireless phones. Audiology Online. http://www.audiologyonline.com

Kricos, P. B., Erdman, S., Bratt, G. W., & Williams, D. W. (2007, Apr). Psychosocial correlates of hearing aid adjustment. *Journal of the American Academy of Audiology, 18,* 304–322

Kuk, F. (2008). Fitting approaches for hearing aids with linear and nonlinear signal processing. In M. Valente, H. Hosford-Dunn, & R. Roeser (Eds.), *Audiology treatment* (2nd ed.). New York: Thieme

Kuk, F., & Baekgaard, L. (2008). Hearing aid selection and BTEs: Choosing among various "open-ear" and "receiver-in-canal" options. http://www.hearingreview.com/issues/articles/2008-03_02.asp

Kuk, F. K., Potts, L., Valente, M., Lee, L., & Picirrillo, J. (2003). Evidence of acclimatization in persons with severe-to-profound hearing loss. *Journal of the American Academy of Audiology, 14,* 84–99

Laplante-LeVesque, A., Hickson, L., & Worrall, L. (2012). What makes adults with hearing impairment take up hearing aids or communication programs and achieve successful outcomes? *Ear and Hearing, 33,* 79–93

Leung, J., Wang, N., Yeagle, J., Chinnici, J., Bowditch, S., Francis, H., & Niparko, J. K. (2005). Predictive modes for cochlear implantation in elderly candidates. *Archives of Otolaryngology–Head and Neck Surgery, 131,* 1049–1054

Levitt, H. (2007). Historically, the paths of hearing aids and telephones have often intertwined. *Hearing Journal, 60,* 20–24

Lindley, G. (2007). Accessing the "far world": A new age of connectivity for hearing aids. *Hearing Review, 14,* 54–59

Lord, S. (2006). Visual risk factors for falls in older people. *Age and Ageing, 35 (Suppl 2),* ii42–ii45

Lunner, T. (2003, Jul). Cognitive function in relation to hearing aid use. *International Journal of Audiology, 42*(Suppl 1), S49–S58

Lunner, T. (2010). Designing hearing aid signal processing to reduce demand on working memory. *Hearing Journal, 63,* 30–31

Lunner, T., Rudner, M., & Rönnberg, J. (2009, Oct). Cognition and hearing aids. *Scandinavian Journal of Psychology, 50,* 395–403

Lunner, T., & Sundewall-Thorén, E. (2007, Jul-Aug). Interactions between cognition, compression, and listening conditions: Effects on speech-in-noise performance in a two-channel hearing aid. *Journal of the American Academy of Audiology, 18,* 604–617

Lynch, K. (2011). *The role of cognition in aided speech recognition in noise performance in older adult experienced hearing aid users using different compression release time settings: A systematic review.* Capstone Project, Graduate Center, CUNY

Mackersie, C. L. (2007, Jun). Hearing aid maximum output and loudness discomfort: Are unaided loudness measures needed? *Journal of the American Academy of Audiology, 18,* 504–514

Mackersie, C. L., Qi, Y., Boothroyd, A., & Conrad, N. (2009, Feb). Evaluation of cellular phone technology with digital hearing aid features: Effects of encoding and individualized amplification. *Journal of the American Academy of Audiology, 20,* 109–118

Malinoff, R. L., & Weinstein, B. E. (1989, Dec). Measurement of hearing aid benefit in the elderly. *Ear and Hearing, 10,* 354–356

Marcrum, C., & Ricketts, M. (2011). Open canal hearing aids: Tips and tricks for the clinic. http://www.myavaa.org/documents/JDVAC-2011-Presentations/Ricketts_HDVAC2011.pdf

Mayer, R., & Moreno, R. (1996). A split attention effect in multimedia learning: evidence for dual processing systems in working memory. *Journal of Educational Psychology, 90,* 312–320

McArdle, R., Chisolm, T. H., Abrams, H. B., Wilson, R. H., & Doyle, P. J. (2005). The WHO-DAS II: Measuring outcomes of hearing aid intervention for adults. *Trends in Amplification, 9,* 127–143

McCarthy, P. A., Montgomery, A. A., & Mueller, H. G. (1990, Jan). Decision making in rehabilitative audiology. *Journal of the American Academy of Audiology, 1,* 23–30

McCarthy, P., & Schau, N. (2008). Adult audiologic rehabilitation: A review of contemporary practices. *Contemporary Issues in Communication Science and Disorders, 35,* 168–177

McSpaden, J. (1996). Thirty-six hearing premises. *Hearing Review, 3,* 8–10

Moore, B. C., Huss, M., Vickers, D. A., Glasberg, B. R., & Alcántara, J. I. (2000, Aug). A test for the diagnosis of dead regions in the cochlea. *British Journal of Audiology, 34,* 205–224

Mueller, H. G., Hornsby, B. W., & Weber, J. E. (2008, Nov-Dec). Using trainable hearing aids to examine real-world preferred gain. *Journal of the American Academy of Audiology, 19,* 758–773

Mueller, H. G., & Ricketts, T. A. (2006). Open-canal fittings: Ten take-home tips. *Hearing Journal, 59,* 24–37

Mulrow, C. D., Aguilar, C., Endicott, J. E., Tuley, M. R., Velez, R., Charlip, W. S., et al. (1990, Aug). Quality-of-life changes and hearing impairment. A randomized trial. *Annals of Internal Medicine, 113,* 188–194

Mulrow, C., Michael, T., & Aguilar, C. (1992a). Correlates of successful hearing aid use in older adults. *Ear and Hearing, 13,* 108–113

Mulrow, C. D., Tuley, M. R., & Aguilar, C. (1992b, Apr). Correlates of successful hearing aid use in older adults. *Ear and Hearing, 13,* 108–113

Mulrow, C. D., Tuley, M. R., & Aguilar, C. (1992c, Dec). Sustained benefits of hearing aids. *Journal of Speech and Hearing Research, 35,* 1402–1405

Munro, K. J., & Lutman, M. E. (2003, Jul). The effect of speech presentation level on measurement of auditory acclimatization to amplified speech. *Journal of the Acoustical Society of America, 114,* 484–495

Munro, K. J., & Trotter, J. H. (2006, Dec). Preliminary evidence of asymmetry in uncomfortable loudness levels after unilateral hearing aid experience: Evidence of functional plasticity in the adult auditory system. *International Journal of Audiology, 45,* 684–688

Musiek, F., & Baran, J. (1996). Amplification and the central auditory nervous system. In M. Valente (Ed.), *Hearing aids: Standards, options and limitations.* New York: Thieme

Nabelek, A. K., Freyaldenhoven, M. C., Tampas, J. W., Burchfiel, S. B., & Muenchen, R. A. (2006, Oct). Acceptable noise level as a predictor of hearing aid use. *Journal of the American Academy of Audiology, 17,* 626–639

Newman, C. W., Hug, G. A., Wharton, J. A., & Jacobson, G. P. (1993, Aug). The influence of hearing aid cost on perceived benefit in older adults. *Ear and Hearing, 14,* 285–289

Newman, C. W., Jacobson, G. P., Hug, G. A., Weinstein, B. E., & Malinoff, R. L. (1991, Apr). Practical method for quantifying hearing aid benefit in older adults. *Journal of the American Academy of Audiology, 2,* 70–75

Newman, C., Sandridge, S., & Oswald, L. (2010). Relationship between expectations and satisfaction for BAHA implant system in patients with single-sided deafness. *Seminars in Hearing, 31,* 15–27

Newman, C. W., & Weinstein, B. E. (1988, Apr). The Hearing Handicap Inventory for the Elderly as a measure of hearing aid benefit. *Ear and Hearing, 9,* 81–85

Noble, W. (2002, Jan). Extending the IOI to significant others and to non-hearing-aid-based interventions. *International Journal of Audiology, 41,* 27–29

Office of Technology Assessment. (1978). *Assessing the efficacy and safety of medical technologies.* Washington, DC: Congress of the United States, Office of Technology Assessment, OTA-11-75

Olswang, L., Thompson, R., Warren, S., & Minghetti, N. (1990). *Treatment efficacy research in communication disorders.* Rockville, MD: American Speech-Language-Hearing Foundation

Orabi, A. A., Mawman, D., Al-Zoubi, F., Saeed, S. R., & Ramsden, R. T. (2006, Apr). Cochlear implant outcomes and quality of life in the elderly: Manchester experience over 13 years. *Clinical Otolaryngology, 31,* 116–122

Palmer, C., Lindley, G., & Mormer, E. (2008). Hearing aid selection and fitting in adults. In M. Valente, H. Hosford-Dunn, & R. Roeser (Eds.), *Audiology treatment* (2nd ed.). New York: Thieme

Palmer, C., & Mormer, R. (1997). A systematic program for hearing aid orientation and adjustment. *Hearing Review, High Performance Hearing Solutions Supplement, 1,* 45–52

Philibert, B., Collet, L., Vesson, J., & Veuillet, E. (2005). The auditory acclimatization effect in sensorineural hearing-impaired listeners: Evidence for functional plasticity. *Hearing Research, 205,* 131–142

Pichora-Fuller, M. K. (1997). Assistive listening devices for the elderly. In R. Lubinski, & D. Higginbotham (Eds.), *Communication technologies for the elderly.* San Diego: Singular

Pichora-Fuller, M.K. (2003). Cognitive aging and auditory information processing. *International Journal of Audiology, 42 (Suppl 2),* 2S26–2S32

Pichora-Fuller, M. K. (2006). Perceptual effort and apparent cognitive decline: Implications for audiological rehabilitation. *Seminars in Hearing, 27,* 284–293

Pichora-Fuller, M. K., Schneider, B. A., & Daneman, M. (1995, Jan). How young and old adults listen to and remember speech in noise. *Journal of the Acoustical Society of America, 97,* 593–608

Preminger, J. E., Carpenter, R., & Ziegler, C. H. (2005, Sep). A clinical perspective on cochlear dead regions: Intelligibility of speech and subjective hearing aid benefit. *Journal of the American Academy of Audiology, 16,* 600–613, quiz 631–632

Preves, D., & Banerjee, S. (2008). Hearing aid instrumentation signal processing and electroacoustic testing. In M. Valente, H. Hosford-Dunn, & R. Roeser (Eds.), *Audiology treatment* (2nd ed., pp. 1–35). New York: Thieme

Primeau, R. (1997). Hearing aid benefit in adults and older adults. *Seminars in Hearing, 18,* 29–36

Prochaska, J. O., DiClemente, C. C., & Norcross, J. C. (1992, Sep). In search of how people change. Applications to addictive behaviors. *American Psychologist, 47,* 1102–1114

Ramachandran, V., Stach, B., & Becker, E. (2011). Reducing hearing aid costs does not influence device acquisition for milder hearing loss, but eliminating it does. *Hearing Journal, 64,* 10–18

Reese, J. L., & Hnath-Chisolm, T. (2005, Jun). Recognition of hearing aid orientation content by first-time users. *American Journal of Audiology, 14,* 94–104

Ricketts, T., Johnson, E., & Federman, J. (2008, Nov-Dec). Individual differences within and across feedback suppression hearing aids. *Journal of the American Academy of Audiology, 19,* 748–757

Ricketts, T., & Mueller, G. (2009). Whose NAL-NL fitting method are you using. *Hearing Journal. 62,* 10–14

Ricketts, T., & Mueller, G. (2011). *Today's hearing aid features: Fluff or true hearing aid benefit?* Paper presented at Audiology NOW, 23rd annual convention of the American Academy of Audiology, Chicago

Ross, M. (1996). You've done something about it! Helpful hints to the new hearing aid user. *SHHH Journal, 17,* 7–11

Rossi-Katz, J., & Arehart, K. H. (2011, Dec). Survey of audiologic service provision to older adults with cochlear implants. *American Journal of Audiology, 20,* 84–89

Rubinstein, A. (1997). Hearing aid fitting and management. *Seminars in Hearing, 18,* 87–101

Rudner, M., Foo, C., Rönnberg, J., & Lunner, T. (2007, Dec). Phonological mismatch makes aided speech recognition in noise cognitively taxing. *Ear and Hearing, 28,* 879–892

Rudner, M., Foo, C., Rönnberg, J., & Lunner, T. (2009, Oct). Cognition and aided speech recognition in noise: specific role for cognitive factors following nine-week experience with adjusted compression settings in hearing aids. *Scandinavian Journal of Psychology, 50,* 405–418

Rudner, M., Foo, C., Sundewall-Thorén, E., Lunner, T., & Ronnbei, J. (2008). Phonological mismatch and explicit cognitive processing in a sample of 102 hearing-aid user. *International Journal of Audiology, Suppl 2,* S91–S98

Rudner, M., Rönnberg, J., & Lunner, T. (2011, Mar). Working memory supports listening in noise for persons with hearing impairment. *Journal of the American Academy of Audiology, 22,* 156–167

Sandridge, S.(1995). Beyond hearing aids: Use of auxiliary aids. In P. Kricos & S. Lesner (Eds.), *Hearing care for the older adult.* Boston: Butterworth-Heinemann

Sandridge, S., & Newman, C. (2006). *Improving the efficiency and accountability of the hearing aid selection process using the COAT.* Article archives www.audiologyonline.com

Sandrock, C., & Schum, D. (2007). Wireless transmission of speech and data to, from, and between hearing aids. *Hearing Journal, 60,* 12–16

Sarampalis, A., Kalluri, S., Edwards, B., & Hafter, E. (2009, Oct). Objective measures of listening effort: Effects of background noise and noise reduction. *Journal of Speech, Language, and Hearing Research, 52,* 1230–1240

Saunders, G. H., Lewis, M. S., & Forsline, A. (2009, May). Expectations, prefitting counseling, and hearing aid outcome. *Journal of the American Academy of Audiology, 20,* 320–334

Schneider, M., & Pichora-Fuller, M. K. (2000). Implications of perceptual deterioration for cognitive aging research. In F. Craik & T. Salthouse (Eds.), The handbook of aging and cognition (2nd ed.). Mahwah, NJ: Lawrence Erlbaum

Schum, D. J. (1999, Jan). Perceived hearing aid benefit in relation to perceived needs. *Journal of the American Academy of Audiology, 10,* 40–45

Schum, D. (2009). Advanced technology fittings-customizing features. *Audiology Online*

Schum, D., & Sjolander, L. (2011). The impact of connectivity for the older patient. *Hearing Journal. 64,* 44–50

Sever, C., & Abreu, C. (2009). Bluetooth: The great connector. *Advance for Audiologists, 11,* 22–23

Shi, L. F., Doherty, K. A., Kordas, T. M., & Pellegrino, J. T. (2007, Jun). Short-term and long-term hearing aid benefit and user satisfaction: A comparison between two fitting protocols. *Journal of the American Academy of Audiology, 18,* 482–495

Silman, S., Gelfand, S. A., & Silverman, C. A. (1984, Nov). Late-onset auditory deprivation: Effects of monaural versus binaural hearing aids. *Journal of the Acoustical Society of America, 76,* 1357–1362

Silverman, C. A., Silman, S., Emmer, M. B., Schoepflin, J. R., & Lutolf, J. J. (2006, Nov-Dec). Auditory deprivation in adults with asymmetric, sensorineural hearing impairment. *Journal of the American Academy of Audiology, 17,* 747–762

Smeds, K. (2004, Apr). Is normal or less than normal overall loudness preferred by first-time hearing aid users? *Ear and Hearing, 25,* 159–172

Smith, S. L., Noe, C. M., & Alexander, G. C. (2009, Jun). Evaluation of the International Outcome Inventory for Hearing Aids in a veteran sample. *Journal of the American Academy of Audiology, 20,* 374–380

Smith, S. L., & West, R. L. (2006, Jun). The application of self-efficacy principles to audiologic rehabilitation: A tutorial. *American Journal of Audiology, 15,* 46–56

Snell, K. B., & Frisina, D. R. (2000, Mar). Relationships among age-related differences in gap detection and word recognition. *Journal of the Acoustical Society of America, 107,* 1615–1626

Sorkin, D. (2007). A BAHA for Maxi. *Volta Voices. 14*, 48–49

Souza, P., & Arehart, K. (2009). Hearing aid features: Do older people need different things. *Hearing Care for Adults. Proceedings of the Phonak Conference.* http://www.phonakpro.com/content/dam/phonak/b2b/Events/conference_proceedings/chicago_2009/proceedings/25_P69344_Pho_Kapitel_14_S139_144.pdf

Souza, P. E., Boike, K. T., Witherell, K., & Tremblay, K. (2007, Jan). Prediction of speech recognition from audibility in older listeners with hearing loss: Effects of age, amplification, and background noise. *Journal of the American Academy of Audiology, 18*, 54–65

Stark, P., & Hickson, L. (2004, Jul-Aug). Outcomes of hearing aid fitting for older people with hearing impairment and their significant others. *International Journal of Audiology, 43*, 390–398

Sterkens, J. (2011). *20Q: What is old is new again—Why hearing loops are back to stay.* http://www.hearingloss.org/sites/default/files/docs/20q_whatisoldisnewagain_hearingloops.pdf

Stone, M., & Moore, B. (2007). Quantifying the effects of fast-acting compression on the envelope of speech. *Journal of the Acoustical Society of America, 121*, 1654–1664

Strom, K. (2010). A market update and the top-50 trends in hearing care, Part 1. *Hearing Review.* http://www.hearingreview.com/issues/articles/2010-05_01.asp

Swan, I. R., & Gatehouse, S. (1990, Jun). Factors influencing consultation for management of hearing disability. *British Journal of Audiology, 24*, 155–160

Takahashi, G., Martinez, C., Beamer, S., Bridges, J., Noffsinger, D., Sugiura, K., et al. (2007). Subjective measures of hearing aid benefit and satisfaction in the NIDCD/VA follow-up study. *Journal of the American Academy of Audiology, 18*, 323–349

Taylor, B. (2009). Measuring quality in your practice: First rate clinical practices = unsurpassed business success. *Audiology Online Continuing Education Course*

Taylor, B., & Bernstein, J. (2011). The red flag matrix hearing aid counseling tool. *Audiology Online Continuing Education Course.* http://www.audiologyonline.com/articles/article_detail.asp?article_id=2380

Taylor, B., & Teter, D. (2009). Earmolds: Practical considerations to improve performance in hearing aids. *Hearing Review. 16*, 10–14

Taylor, K. S. (1993, Dec). Self-perceived and audiometric evaluations of hearing aid benefit in the elderly. *Ear and Hearing, 14*, 390–394

Teie, P. (2009). Ear-coupler acoustics in receiver-in-the aid fittings. *Hearing Review, 16*, 10–16 http://www.hearingreview.com/issues/articles/2009-12_01.asp

Thibodeau, L. (2009). Hearing assistance technology systems as part of a comprehensive audiologic rehabilitation program. In J. Montano & J. Spitzer (Eds.), *Adult audiologic rehabilitation.* San Diego: Plural

Valente, M. (2006). *Hearing aids: Standards, options, and limitations.* New York: Thieme

Valente, M., Abrams, H., Benson, T., Citron, D., Hampton, D., Loavenbruck, A., et al. (2006). *Audiologic management of adult hearing impairment (American Academy of Audiology Task Force).* Staff publications, paper 2. http://digitalcommons.wustl.edu/audio_fapubs/2.

Valente, M., Dunn, H., & Roeser, R. (2008). *Audiology treatment.* New York: Thieme

Valente, M., & Valente, M. (2008). Earhooks, tubing, earmolds and shells. In M. Valente, H. Hosford-Dunn, & R. Roeser (Eds.), *Audiology treatment* (2nd ed.). New York: Thieme

Valente, M., Valente, M., & Mispagel, K. (2006). *Fitting options for adult patients with single sided deafness.* http://www.audiologyonline.com/articles/article_detail.asp?article_id=1629

Ventry, I. M., & Weinstein, B. E. (1982, May-Jun). The hearing handicap inventory for the elderly: A new tool. *Ear and Hearing, 3*, 128–134

Vickers, D. A., Moore, B. C., & Baer, T. (2001, Aug). Effects of low-pass filtering on the intelligibility of speech in quiet for people with and without dead regions at high frequencies. *Journal of the Acoustical Society of America, 110*, 1164–1175

Vinay & Moore, B.C., (2007, Apr). Prevalence of dead regions in subjects with sensorineural hearing loss. *Ear and Hearing, 28*, 231–241

Vuorialho, A., Karinen, P., & Sorri, M. (2006, Jul). Effect of hearing aids on hearing disability and quality of life in the elderly. *International Journal of Audiology, 45*, 400–405

Walden, T. C., & Walden, B. E. (2005, Sep). Unilateral versus bilateral amplification for adults with impaired hearing. *Journal of the American Academy of Audiology, 16*, 574–584

Weinstein, B. E., Spitzer, J. B., & Ventry, I. M. (1986, Oct). Test-retest reliability of the Hearing Handicap Inventory for the Elderly. *Ear and Hearing, 7*, 295–299

Williams, V. A., Johnson, C. E., & Danhauer, J. L. (2009, Jul-Aug). Hearing aid outcomes: Effects of gender and experience on patients' use and satisfaction. *Journal of the American Academy of Audiology, 20*, 422–432, quiz 459–460

Wingfield, A. (1996, Jun). Cognitive factors in auditory performance: context, speed of processing, and constraints of memory. *Journal of the American Academy of Audiology, 7*, 175–182

Wingfield, A., & Stine-Morrow, E. A. L. (2000). Language and speech. In F. I. M. Craik & T. A. Salthouse (Eds.), *Handbook of cognitive aging* (2nd ed., pp. 359–416). Mahwah, NJ: Lawrence Erlbaum

Wingfield, A., & Tun, P. A. (2001). Spoken language comprehension in older adults: Interactions between sensory and cognitive change in normal aging. *Seminars in Hearing, 22*, 287–301

World Health Organization (WHO). (2001). *International Classification of Functioning, Disability, and Health.* Geneva, Switzerland: WHO

Wu, Y. H. (2010, Feb). Effect of age on directional microphone hearing aid benefit and preference. *Journal of the American Academy of Audiology, 21*, 78–89

Wu, Y. H., & Bentler, R. A. (2010, Feb). Impact of visual cues on directional benefit and preference: Part II—field tests. *Ear and Hearing, 31*, 35–46

Wu, Y., & Bentler, R. (2012). Clinical measures of hearing aid directivity: assumption, accuracy, and reliability. *Ear and Hearing, 33*, 44–56

Yanz, J. (2007). Assessing the feasibility of Bluetooth in hearing rehabilitation. *Hearing Journal. 60*, 52–60

Zwolan, T. (2008). Recent advances in cochlear implants. *Contemporary Issues in Communication Science and Disorders, 35*, 113–121

Chapter 9

Health Promotion and Disease Prevention for Older Adults

No one would suggest that the quality of life of all old deaf people can be improved by the most comprehensive audiological service, but large-scale screening would undoubtedly reveal very large numbers of people who could be helped.

—*Cochrane (1991)*

In view of its negative impact on elderly patients, it is worthwhile for doctors to actively and routinely screen for the problem using an easy-to-administer and culturally relevant questionnaire, which should include a question on patient's self-perception of the problem.

—*Wu, Chin, and Tong (2004, p. 84)*

Two benefits of a hearing screening program for older adults are to provide information on the condition and to raise awareness.

—*Walden, 2011*

◆ Learning Objectives

After reading this chapter, you should be able to

- state the epidemiological principles underlying health promotion activities;
- explain the reasons for screening older adults for the presence of handicapping hearing loss;
- utilize the approaches available for screening older adults for handicapping hearing impairment;
- utilize the approaches available for screening older adults for vestibular function associated with falls;
- provide primary care physicians and nurses with tools for screening older adults for otological functional impairments; and
- design and conduct hearing screening programs that will in the long term improve the health-related quality of life of older adults.

◆ Overview

As older adults continue to remain in their homes as they age, promoting health and preventive health care are emerging as areas of active concern in community-based care. Older adults are frequently the target of health-promotion activities geared toward preventing accidents, psychosocial illness, iatrogenic

problems, disease, and frailty (Pacala, 2010). Optimizing the health of those living in the community is an important goal of these activities. Further, if preventive activities targeted modifiable or acquired factors known to increase the risk of functional decline, they would help reduce the cost of caring for persons burdened by disabilities (Markle-Reid, Keller, & Browne, 2010), and several medical and governmental agencies have highlighted the need for improved and more efficacious hearing screening programs.

This chapter provides a context for health-promotion and disease-prevention activities designed to identify older adults with otological functional impairments including handicapping hearing impairment and tinnitus. It also discusses strategies for health-promotion and disease-prevention activities designed to identify and alleviate treatable conditions so as to improve or maintain function, health status, and quality of care.

Pearl

Global economic and demographic changes have led to an emphasis on empowering individuals to manage their health through preventive and health-promotion activities, with the goal being to reduce the burden of adverse conditions, including hearing impairment and associated conditions.

Healthy People (HP) 2000, a government initiative, provided a comprehensive roadmap of health-promotion and disease-prevention initiatives aimed at improving the health of Americans NCHS (2001). HP 2010, 10-year agenda for improving the nation's health, included 467 evidence-based disease-prevention and health-promotion objectives within 28 focus areas that were to be achieved over the first decade of the new century (Healthy People, 2010). The overarching goals of HP 2010 include (1) increasing the span of life and years of healthy life for Americans (quality of life), and (2) reducing health disparities across different segments of the population. Secondary goals include (1) achieving access to preventive services for all Americans, and (2) promoting the health of people with disabilities. Specifically, in keeping with the goals of primary prevention, two important objectives are increasing social participation and life satisfaction among those with disability, and removing environmental barriers to good health. Steps to ameliorate these environmental barriers include modifications to

Table 9.1 Strategies for Achieving the Health-Promotion and Disease-Prevention Agenda

- Community initiatives
- Collaborations among private sector, health care groups, and insurance companies
- Cooperation among policy makers to ensure investment in disease-prevention and health-promotion activities
- Health-promotion activities to empower citizens to make healthy choices
- Federal and state policies that emphasize prevention

Source: From Healthy People. (2010). *Healthy People 2010 final review.* http://www .cdc.gov/nchs/healthy_people/hp2010/hp2010_final_review.htm.

reverberant rooms and noisy ventilation systems so as to increase the capacity for older adults to use residual hearing (Crews and Campbell, 2004). In an effort to achieve the goals of a longer and healthier life for all Americans, four integral components or "pillars" of HP 2010 to be addressed by the various focus areas are physical fitness, nutrition, prevention, and making healthy choices. HP 2010 specifies that to realize the goals, a public–private partnership is necessary. **Table 9.1** lists the partnerships that were recommended to achieve the ambitious goals of the HP initiative.

According to the final review of HP 2010, the findings were mixed in terms of meeting or achieving the many ambitious goals set forth by the panel of experts. In the case of eight focus areas, including educational and community-based programs, environmental health and health communication, and heart disease and stroke, more than 70% of the objectives moved toward or achieved their targets (Healthy People, 2010). However, more than 30% of objectives could not be assessed for access to quality health services, disability and secondary conditions, educational and community-based programs, environmental health, and mental health and mental disorders. In light of the achievements of HP 2010, Healthy People 2020 builds on its strengths with a focus on attaining high-quality and longer lives that are free of preventable disease and disability, and the promotion of healthy behaviors across the life span.

Pearl

As chronic conditions and comorbidities become more prevalent with advancing age, the opportunity for preventive activities becomes more important.

Audiologists have an important role to play if progress toward each of the goals is to be achieved given the global burden of disease of hearing loss among adults, which often goes undetected. For example, progress toward an increase in the quality and length of life can be achieved if chronic conditions such as hearing impairment are ultimately associated with an increase in the number of years free of activity limitations or participation restrictions.

To achieve the overarching goals of increasing quality and years of healthy life, the team conducting the HP 2010 midcourse review emphasized that priority must be given to implementing effective health-promotion and disease-prevention

interventions among people in different geographic regions, in persons with and without disabilities, and in people of all races, education levels, and income groups. Vision and hearing were included as focus area 28 in the original document. As pertains to older adults, rehabilitation for hearing impairment, hearing examination, evaluation and treatment referrals, hearing protection, and noise-induced hearing loss in adults were delineated as particular objectives. In general, the goals relating to older adults include the following:

◆ Increase the number of deaf or hard-of-hearing people who use rehabilitation services and adaptive devices, such as hearing aids or cochlear implants. Technological devices are available now that can help children and adults who are deaf or hard-of-hearing be successful in society and the workplace.

◆ Increase the number of adults and children who schedule periodic hearing examinations.

◆ Increase the number of people who are referred by their doctor for a hearing evaluation and, if needed, treatment. The referrals depend on several factors, including the type of hearing loss, the age at which hearing loss occurs, the services available in a community, and a family's preferences.

◆ Increase the use of ear protection devices and equipment, such as earplugs or earmuffs. Noise-induced hearing loss (NIHL) is one of the most common occupational injuries and the second most self-reported type of occupational illness or injury. Industries that have high numbers of workers exposed to NIHL include agriculture, mining, and construction

The objectives focus on interventions designed to reduce or eliminate disability from hearing impairment by fostering health-promotion and disease-prevention activities and by bringing the primary care physician in as the professional responsible for conducting the screenings (**Table 9.2**). Indirectly, there is also a focus on broader issues, such as improving the availability and dissemination of health-related information (e.g., about hearing) via screening activities as well. Each objective had a target for specific improvements to be achieved by the year 2010, but targets were rarely specified for the hearing objectives.

Preventive activities are at the heart of HP 2010 (**Fig. 9.1**). They can be primary (prevent or inhibit illness from occurring in the first place), secondary (detect disease in an early stage, thereby minimizing its consequences), or tertiary (prevent the progression of disease and promote management so it does not impact the course of treatment) (Woolf, Jonas, Lawrence, & Kaplan-Liss, 2008). The goals include promoting healthy behaviors and protecting health. Primary and secondary preventive efforts have as their focus early identification and treatment of risk factors so that functional declines are averted, and the introduction of information about the value and availability of hearing interventions and communication strategies (**Table 9.3**) (Markle-Reid et al, 2010). A key underpinning of a goal-driven approach to prevention is matching preventive activities and recommendations with the individual's condition. In my view and that of HP 2010, the primary care physician in the community is a key player in health-promotion and disease-prevention activities because the majority of older adults increasingly receive care from generalists or primary care

Table 9.2 Hearing-Related Objectives in Focus Area 28

Hearing rehabilitation services	• Increase access by persons who have hearing impairments to hearing rehabilitation services and adaptive devices, including hearing aids, cochlear implants, or tactile or other assistive or augmentative devices
Hearing examinations	• Increase the proportion of persons who have had a hearing examination on schedule
Evaluation and treatment referrals*	• Increase the number of persons who are referred by their primary care physician (PCP) or primary care clinician (PCC) for hearing evaluation and treatment
Hearing protection*	• Increase the use of appropriate ear-protection devices, equipment, and practices
Noise-induced hearing loss	• Reduce adult hearing loss in the noise-exposed public
Preventive care and access to health services	• Increase the proportion of persons appropriately counseled about health behaviors

*Hearing screening focus.

physicians rather than from geriatricians (Eleazer & Brummel-Smith, 2009). Disease prevention and health promotion are also gaining momentum for economic and demographic reasons. In terms of economics, the health care system has had to invest substantially in caring for people with complications from chronic conditions/diseases that, if identified early, would not require such intensive medical and surgical intervention. In terms of demographics, the baby boom generation began to reach 60 years of age in 2006, resulting in a swelling of the ranks of older adults who will experience a host of chronic conditions, including hearing loss, for which interventions are available (Woolf, 2009). Promoting health and preventing or reducing the severity or impact of chronic disabling conditions by screening for the condition is at the heart of hearing-related tertiary prevention activities. These activities are especially important among the disadvantaged and minority populations, where disproportionate gaps in preventive care already exist.

Identifying individuals with a hearing loss that typically goes underreported, despite its often interfering with their daily life and its introducing potential diagnostic artifacts, is the basis for preventive activities targeting older adults with handicapping or disabling hearing impairments. For tertiary prevention to be successful, health care professionals must be educated about the chronic conditions to which older adults are susceptible that are associated with a hearing impairment so that they can become partners in detection activities (Pacala, 2010). Hence, for older adults who are healthy or who have chronic conditions, hearing screening is indicated, although the goals and intervention options may differ. In the case of the frail elderly, physicians should be sensitive to the presence of hearing loss so that they can make sure to engage the patient in the decision making using hearing assistance technologies coupled with communication strategies to promote understanding (e.g., use a Pocket Talker, reduce television volume when speaking to patients in the hospital). In short, screening programs can help alleviate the global burden of hearing disorders by identifying those with undetected hearing loss and matching their needs to available intervention strategies. However, the economic value added advantages remain to be determined (Rob et al, 2009).

Pacala (2010) describes an interesting model for prioritizing preventive activities by matching them with the patient's condition. For example, he suggests that in healthy older adults

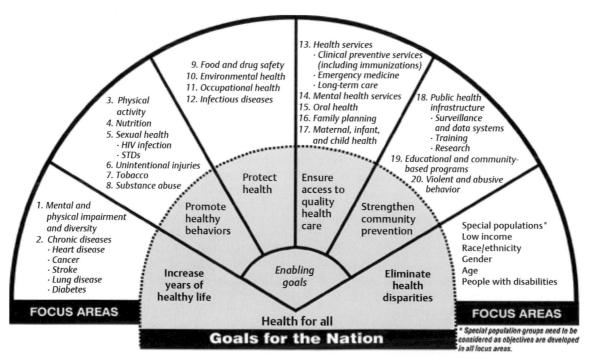

Fig. 9.1 Healthy People 2010: goals for the nation. (From http://www.csupomona.edu/~jvgrizzell/best_practices/goal2010.html.)

Table 9.3 Categories of Preventive Care

Primary	Secondary	Tertiary
Removal of risk factors for disease or functional decline	Avert the potential of individuals progressing through various stages of functional and cognitive decline	Activities for those who exhibit some type of functional decline or comorbidities; target high-risk groups
Ideal for asymptomatic adults and for healthy adults who are working or active retirees	Ideal for individuals who display some evidence of impairment and slight word-recognition difficulties; provide counseling regarding interventions and communication strategies	Interventions are aimed at limiting progression of disease, functional decline, and loss of independence
Ideal for those free of clinical evidence of the health condition or targeted disease	Tailor the intervention and follow-up to the individual's risk	Tailored interventions designed to maximize function and optimize health

Source: From Markle-Reid, M., Keller, H., & Browne, G. (2010). Health promotion for the community-living older adult. In H. Fillit, K. Rockwood, & K. Woodhouse (Eds.), *Brockelhurst's textbook of geriatric medicine and gerontology* (7th ed.). Philadelphia: Saunders Elsevier.

with no evidence of disease or functional decline, primary and secondary prevention should be the focus, whereas in individuals with chronic conditions or comorbidities, the preventive priority should be tertiary prevention, accident prevention, and promotion of quality of care and patient engagement.

> **Pearl**
>
> Hearing loss is the 15th most serious health problem in the world, and its prevalence in the United States is predicted to rise significantly. There is concern that we may be facing an epidemic of hearing impairment (Agrawal, Platz, & Niparko, 2008)

An important goal of HP 2010 was to maintain health and quality of life in older adults into the 21st century. Improving the functional independence, not just the length of life, is seen as an important element in promoting the health of individuals over 65 years of age. According to the HP 2010 report, chronic problems such as arthritis, osteoporosis, and vision and hearing impairments are priority areas because of their significant impact on daily life. Each of the HP documents emphasizes that primary health care providers are necessary partners in the maintenance of good health and functional independence. The role of health care providers is threefold: to structure and conduct appropriate multicomponent screening, to make multifaceted and tailored referrals and intervention recommendations, and to contact the failures via email or telephone to ensure their adherence with recommendations.

Healthy People 2020 builds on HP 2010 and HP 2000 with the goals being of considerable relevance especially in the design of preventive activities. The new objectives include (1) increase the proportion of older adults with one or more chronic health conditions who report confidence in managing their conditions; and (2) increase the proportion of older adults with reduced physical or cognitive function who engage in light, moderate, or vigorous leisure-time physical activities. Regarding multiple chronic conditions, the data from the Second Supplement on Aging (SOA–II) study, in which 30% of respondents aged 70 or over presented with hearing rated to be good and fair, hearing loss was prevalent in individuals with diabetes, arthritis, heart disease, and depression (Crews & Campbell, 2004). Individuals with hearing loss had higher

rates of comorbid and secondary conditions than did those without hearing loss, and individuals with both vision impairment and hearing loss had even higher rates. Similarly, data accumulated using participants in the National Health and Nutrition Examination Survey (NHANES) conducted between 1999 and 2004 revealed that hearing loss prevalence increases with age among individuals who smoke, are exposed to noise, or have cardiovascular risk factors such as diabetes mellitus and hypertension. Interestingly, increases in bilateral hearing loss prevalence occurred at an earlier age among those with modifiable risk factors such as smoking, noise exposure, and cardiovascular risk (Agrawal et al, 2008). Agrawal et al (2008) concluded that addressing some of the modifiable risk factors could result in reductions in the prevalence of hearing loss. Similarly, an updated guideline for the prevention of falls urged routine screening of older patients by primary care physicians for conditions that place them at risk for falls, which includes hearing impairment (American Geriatrics Society, 2009; Kuehn, 2010). Specifically, Rubenstein (2006) acknowledged that age-associated impairments of vision, hearing, and memory tend to increase the number of falls and stumbles among older adults, further underscoring the importance of hearing screening.

The U.S. Preventive Services Task Force (USPSTF) is a leading independent panel of private-sector experts in prevention and primary care that reviews the scientific evidence of the effectiveness of a broad range of clinical preventive services, including screening, counseling, and preventive medications, and then makes recommendations that are considered the "gold standard" for clinical preventive services (USPSTF, 2009). The USPSTF (2012) recently updated its guidelines regarding screening for hearing loss in adults 50+ years. In the 1996 guidelines, it recommended screening older adults for hearing impairment by periodically asking them questions about their hearing, counseling them about the availability of hearing-aid devices, and making appropriate referrals for abnormalities. This constituted a grade B recommendation (USPSTF, 1996).

Chou et al (2011) conducted a comprehensive evidence-based review of screening for hearing loss in primary care settings in adults 50+ years of age. The specific goal was to ascertain the benefits and harms of screening for hearing loss, to determine if the available evidence supports the need for screening rather than not screening, and to determine the benefits of treatment based on screening outcomes. The authors reviewed well over 20 studies that evaluated the diagnostic accuracy of a variety of screening tests, such as clinical tests, the watch-tick test, the whispered-voice test, a single question screen, hand-held audiometric devices, and questionnaires. Participants came from population-based studies, primary care or community-based settings, Veterans Administration hospitals, or settings with individuals having a high prevalence of hearing.

The authors set out to answer four key questions based on the data reviewed. First, does screening of asymptomatic adults of 50+ years of age lead to improved health outcomes? Second, how accurate are the hearing loss screening methods used by the various investigators conducting studies in the area? Third, how efficacious are the treatments in improving health outcomes of those participants detected by the screening as having hearing loss? Fourth, what are the adverse effects of hearing-loss screening in adults 50+ years of age? Fifth, what are the adverse effects of treating those participants 50+ years of age who were identified by the screening as having hearing loss? These answers to these questions are the basis for the USPSTF decision to recommend screening for a given disorder. In my view, the most important of the task force's conclusions was twofold: First, there is a lack of sufficient evidence linking screening outcomes to beneficial health outcomes, despite the findings of Mulrow and colleagues (1990) confirming the short-, medium-, and long-term benefits of amplification based on scores of veterans on a variety of disease-specific and generic quality-of-life measures. Second, there is a lack of evidence regarding the adverse effects of hearing screening activities in adults 50+ years of age. In light of these findings, Chou and colleagues (2011) concluded that "additional research is needed on the effectiveness of screening in typical primary care settings, the optimal age at which to start screening, and the severity of hearing loss that is likely to benefit from hearing aids to help define optimal screening test thresholds and methods" (p. 354).

Based on the evidence, including a review by Chou et al. (2011), the USPSTF (2012) concluded that there was insufficient evidence to understand the effects of screening as compared to no screening in terms of health outcomes. Hence, while their risk assessment suggested that increasing age is the most important risk factor for hearing loss, the USPSTF (2012) issued a grade of "I" for hearing screening concluding there was inadequate evidence to determine the balance of benefits and harms of screening for hearing loss in adults aged 50 years or older. They emphasized that the recommendations apply to adults 50 years of age or older who show no signs or symptoms of hearing loss, rather than to those seeking treatment for hearing problems. The consumer fact sheet prepared by the USPSTF (2012) (http://www.uspreventiveservicestask force.org/uspstf11/adulthearing/adulthearfact.pdf) is invaluable and I do recommend sharing it with patients and health care professionals. In this document an important distinction is made between what is meant by insufficient evidence (e.g., not enough information on screening for hearing loss to determine potential benefits and harms) and asymptomatic adults (e.g., people who have not noticed changes in their hearing or people who are not already visiting a health care professional about hearing loss). Audiologists have a responsibility to edu-

cate older adults about signs and symptoms of hearing loss to raise awareness about this prevalent condition.

Despite the conclusions of the USPSTF (2012) various task forces do recommend routine screening for conditions for which hearing loss is a considerable risk factor and for which validity of screening will be threatened without knowledge of hearing status. Specifically, the New York City Department of Health recommends that adults should be assessed for medical conditions that can cause depression, and we know from the literature that hearing loss is linked to depression either in heightening the risk or in terms of direct causality. For example, in the case of depression screening, which received a grade of B, the formal screening tools require adequate hearing status for valid responses, as positive screening tests trigger full diagnostic interviews using standard diagnostic criteria. If the older adults' response to one of the following two questions is yes, the screen is likely positive for depression:

Over the past two weeks, have you been bothered by:
   Little interest or pleasure in doing things?
   Feeling down, depressed, or hopeless?

Further, according to a recent article by Weinstein (2011), the American and British Geriatrics Societies recommend that physicians conduct a multifactorial risk assessment of community-dwelling older persons who report recurrent difficulty with gait or balance, or seek medical attention because of a fall. As available data suggest that hearing loss qualifies as a risk factor for falls based on correlations among pure-tone levels, dizziness, and sense of balance, screening older adults for hearing impairment is justified. Although screening for hearing status and risk of falls is seen as a low priority, the threats to quality of care and quality of life are significant, and therefore these conditions should not be overlooked (Johnson, Newman, Danhauer, & Williams, 2009).

◆ Principles of Screening

Health promotion serves an empowerment function, as it enhances independence, autonomy, and problem-solving skills and provides a context for protocols and interventions (Markle-Reid et al, 2010). The most successful health-promotion activities share the characteristics listed in **Table 9.4**.

An operational definition of screening is a necessary foundation for discussing health-promotion activities (Whitlock, Orleans, Pender, & Allan, 2002). Screening is the presumptive identification of an unrecognized disease or condition, wherein members of the general public are invited to undergo tests or examinations that can be administered rapidly and can readily differentiate individuals with higher and lower probabilities of having a disorder, with the former group then urged to seek medical attention for definitive diagnosis (Sackett, Haynes, & Tugwell, 1985; U.K. National Screening Committee, 2012). The greater the potential burden a disease represents to individuals and society, the greater the impetus to screen. Focusing on the immediate goal of identifying those at risk for a condition or identifying those at risk for developing a condition is an immediate goal of screening efforts, rather than the alleviation of symptoms (Krist & McCormally, 2008).

Table 9.4 Characteristics of Successful Health Promotion Programs for Older Adults

Target social, physical, and psychological determinants of health
Target those individuals who are most likely to benefit, that is, individuals who are interested and motivated to change their behavior
Multiple sectors—individual clinician, health care system, interdisciplinary team—must be engaged to foster collaborations
Function-based models of care from the patient perspective rather than the disease perspective
Economic analysis is key: cost-benefit analysis showing quality-of-life and quality-of-care benefits of the investment in prevention

Source: From Markle-Reid, M., Keller, H., & Browne, G. (2010). Health promotion for the community-living older adult. In H. Fillit, K. Rockwood, & K. Woodhouse (Eds.), *Brockelhurst's textbook of geriatric medicine and gerontology* (7th ed.). Philadelphia: Saunders Elsevier.

For a screening program to be successful, there must be a clear and measurable definition of the condition one is attempting to identify. In the case of adult-onset hearing loss, health care providers should screen to identify persons who are willing to seek and adhere to recommendations that will lead to successful outcomes. Screening protocols are designed with varying philosophies that will affect the sensitivity and specificity of the test protocols. A screening protocol that has high sensitivity yields a high proportion of individuals who actually have the disorder; a screening protocol that has high specificity yields a normal result in a high proportion of those who do not have the disorder (Sackett et al, 1985). In many cases the goal is to cast a wide net to ensure that few cases are missed or to identify those who might benefit from a diagnostic test to assist in management. Hence, it is critical from the outset that the purpose and goals are clearly stated (Krist & McCormally, 2008).

A set of common themes emerges from the literature on screening that also applies to screening for hearing loss. Specifically, screening is worthwhile if it leads to relief of distress or to improvement in the functions of daily living, and if it has high acceptability to patients and improves compliance with therapeutic recommendations (Mitchell & Coyne, 2010). For hearing-related dysfunction, the screening program, the target conditions for which preventive services are initiated, the screening tests, and the intervention strategies must meet the following criteria (Hickner & Solbert, 2008; Woolf et al, 2008; Yueh et al, 2010):

◆ The burden of illness must be substantial.
◆ The target condition should have serious consequences for the individual, the family, and possibly society.
◆ Prevalence and incidence rates should be high in the segment of the population targeted, and the incidence of the condition must be sufficient to justify the cost of screening.
◆ An intervention should be available to treat the disorder during the presymptomatic stage.
◆ The natural history of target condition must be such that adequate time is available for successful interventions to be instituted.
◆ The intervention should be effective, especially if implemented earlier than later; the intervention should improve function, quality of life, and quality of care.

◆ The screening test should not place the participant at risk of physical harm.
◆ Evidence of the effectiveness of preventive service should be based on health outcomes following interventions from well-conducted studies.
◆ Screening tests should be brief and easy to use, reliable, accurate, sensitive enough to identify high-risk groups, specific, have adequate predictive values (meaning that subjects with the disorder have an abnormal test result and subjects without the disorder have an abnormal test result [Sackett et al, 1985]), and accurately discriminate between levels of functional deficits.
◆ The screening test should be acceptable to the person undergoing the procedure.
◆ The screening process should be ethical and should not place participant at risk of physical harm
◆ Screening instruments should be appropriate for the segment of the older adult population being targeted.
◆ Screening instruments must be acceptable to the health care provider performing the assessment (Markle-Reid et al, 2010).
◆ The target population should be high risk and likely to adhere to recommendations and to benefit from interventions.
◆ Screening programs should be sustainable, and the likelihood that the person undergoing the screening will benefit from the outcome of the preventive measure, especially the intervention recommended, should be high (Chang, Burke, & Glass, 2009)
◆ Recommended interventions following the screening should enhance functional status or improve the ability to perform activities required to fulfill one's usual roles and maintain one's health and well-being.
◆ Screening activities should be associated with successful outcomes, including effectiveness data, cost-utility data, and data on patient acceptance.
◆ Effectiveness of the screening program should be demonstrated through randomized trials. The screening program can be considered effective only when available diagnostic and treatment services are used by the screened individuals, and when the treatment recommendations provided by the services are complied with (Sackett et al, 1985).
◆ Hearing screening programs should incorporate evidence-based compliance-improving strategies that are culturally appropriate.
◆ Compliance with evidence-based treatment recommendations is critical in light of the cost of mounting a screening program.
◆ Screening tests must be available at a reasonable cost to the patient, with reimbursement for preventive activities tied to effective outcomes.
◆ The screening protocol must include referral to community agencies and health care providers with the manpower necessary to provide the services, and the screening agency must follow-up with the patient to ensure that identified needs are met following referral (Markle-Reid et al, 2010).
◆ Screening protocols and interventions should be relevant to the population of interest; hence, cultural sensitivity is a key part of health-promotion activities (Frankish, Lovato, & Poureslami, 2007).

Table 9.5 Health Behavior Theories Underlying Successful Health-Promotion Activities

Social Learning Theories	Cognitive Theoretical Model
Behavioral capacity: participants must have the skills necessary for performing the desired behavior required to complete the screening Efficacy expectations: participants must have confidence in their ability to successfully carry out the recommended course of action Outcome expectations: participants must believe that adherence to recommended interventions will have desired effects, consequences, or actions; the expectation is that the action will contribute to further health and well-being	Health belief model: the inner world or motivational level of the participants influences their health-seeking behavior, and typically there must be a perceived incentive to take action Transtheoretical stages of change model: individuals progress through a sequence of discrete stages before embracing new behaviors

Sources: From Frankish, C., Lovato, C., & Poureslami, I. (2007). Models, theories, and principles of health promotion. In M. Kline & R. Huff (eds.). *Health promotion in multicultural populations*. Los Angeles: Sage Publications; and Glasgow, R., & Goldstein, M. (2008). Introduction to the principles of health behavior change. In S. Woolf, S. Jonas, & E. Kaplan-Liss (Eds.), *Health promotion and disease prevention in clinical practice* (2nd ed.). Baltimore: Lippincott Williams & Wilkins.

♦ A systems-based approach involving information technology, evidence-based guidelines, community involvement, and creation of appropriate incentives for preventive care is key to a successful screening effort (Pacala, 2010).

♦ The clinically preventable burden measured using the total potential health benefits from the service among both those who have received the service and those who have not yet received it should be high (Maciosek et al, 2006).

Pearl

Potential interventions resulting from screening must improve health outcomes for the USPSTF to assign a grade of A or B.

In addition to meeting the above conditions before launching a health-promotion program, there are theories of relevance that help to understand determinants of participant behaviors and motivations surrounding adherence to recommended interventions. These theories can be divided into two different categories (**Table 9.5**). These theories impact the approach to screening and the multicomponent interventions recommended following the screen. In addition, the five-A's framework (**Table 9.6**) plays a key role in the patient-centered

collaborative approach that has become a key part of health-promotion activities performed in primary care settings. For health behavior change to take place, that is for patient adherence to recommendations following screening, motivational interviewing on the part of the clinician conducting the screen should address the patient's perspective, provide empathy and emotional support for the decision regarding the most appropriate evidence-based intervention, and, in the case of a screening failure, must help patients succeed with the intervention they pursue (Miller & Rollnick, 2002). In this connection, the five-A's framework, which has been recommended for adoption by the USPSTF's Counseling and Behavioral Interventions Work Group, has considerable value both to facilitate behavioral change following screening and as part of counseling sessions associated with discussions about intervention options (Glasgow & Goldstein, 2008; Goldstein, Whitlock, & Depue, 2004).

According to the five-A's construct, the clinician should consider the steps listed in **Table 9.6**. It is incumbent on the audiologist when working with the health care provider doing the screening to ensure that any protocol includes instruction on the application of the five-A's framework, and the implementation plan must be customized to the physician's practice setting (Glasgow & Goldstein, 2008). When designing screening programs/interventions, the clinician must keep in mind

Table 9.6 The Five A's Approach to Behavior Change Counseling

Assess	Advise	Agree	Assist	Arrange
Patient's knowledge and past experience with any form of intervention for hearing deficits	Regarding possible interventions that target patient's symptoms, and for which evidence is available attesting to success with the recommended interventions The physician is in the most credible position to offer advice	Clinician and patient should collaborate and agree on next steps and on an intervention plan; if a hearing aid seems indicated, it can only help if the physician underscores its value	Identify environmental modifications and communication strategies that can be helpful as the patient moves toward intervention for the hearing deficit	Appointment with an audiologist or an ear, nose, and throat physician (depending on outcome of screen) and follow up to ensure adherence

that individuals are also more likely to seek evaluation and treatment for hearing loss when it is recommended by physicians, as they are considered the most credible source on health matters, and patients who are successful in changing behaviors credit advice from their physician as the motivating factor (Glasgow & Goldstein, 2008).

Pearls

Barriers to successful screening programs include the claim that health insurance does not cover screening, the fact that other medical problems are more important, or the fact that health care providers rarely express concern about hearing status (Jones et al, 2010).

Screening is most effective when high-risk groups are targeted and when the outcome initiates a chain of events leading to good treatment outcomes (Yueh et al, 2010)

Audiologists not only should be aware of strategies associated with successful preventive activities but also should be conversant with barriers to successful screening programs. Barriers are typically systemic or organizationally based but may be rooted in the screening protocol itself. One of the greatest barriers involves adherence to recommendations of the clinician following the screen. Often the patient fails to comply with follow-up tests recommended as an outcome of the screening because of (1) patient-related factors such as lack of interest, resistance, hearing health illiteracy, or financial factors; (2) clinician-related factors such as failure to communicate recommendations or lack of community resources to handle referrals; or (3) systemic problems such as results recorded in the patient's chart but never reviewed by the health care provider conducting the screen. The protocols to be discussed in the next section of this chapter have built-in mechanisms such as patient and clinician education modules that ensure that these barriers do not pose obstacles to hearing screening protocols. **Table 9.7** enumerates steps to build in to preventive services activities to overcome potential barriers to success.

Table 9.7 Steps to Include in Preventive Activities

1. Target individuals who have a high likelihood of complying with and benefiting from recommended interventions.
2. Discourage patients from purchasing interventions that are not of proven effectiveness.
3. Offer preventive services that have little potential for producing harm and considerable potential for being associated with beneficial outcomes.
4. Review the evidence that justifies the action (either referring for intervention or not referring for intervention).
5. Share decision making with patients to reflect their personal preferences.
6. Do not initiate preventive activities if the opportunity costs are high (uncertain balance between benefits and harms).

Source: From Guirguis-Blake, J., Calonge, N., Miller, T., Siu, A., Teutsch, S., & Whitlock, E.; U.S. Preventive Services Task Force. (2007, Jul). Current processes of the U.S. Preventive Services Task Force: Refining evidence-based recommendation development. *Annals of Internal Medicine, 147*, 117–122.

Proposed Screening Protocol

Here is a comprehensive hearing preventive services program that I recommend, based on my comprehensive review of the literature on health promotion and disease prevention and of studies on hearing screening in older adults that have been conducted since the early 1980s. It also grows out of the direction in which Medicare is moving with regard to components of a preventive service package. Historically, this package was a one-time comprehensive screening of selected systems paid for by Medicare Part B. The Initial Preventive Physical Examination (IPPE) covered a thorough review of health along with detailed counseling about preventive services for all new beneficiaries during their first 6 months of Medicare enrollment. Although Medicare now covers all the costs for a one-time, comprehensive "Welcome to Medicare" preventive visit during the first 12 months that a beneficiary has Part B, which does not include hearing screening, the Welcome to Medicare package was historic from the perspective of hearing health care benefits and is important for audiologists to be aware of (Medicare, 2012).

Several elements were mandated as part of the original preventive services package for new beneficiaries (Nicoletti, 2008). First, the visit had to be performed by a physician, a nurse practitioner, or a physician assistant. Second, a thorough medical history, including family history, medication history, and social history including activity level, was to be taken. Because of its prevalence and the burden of this illness, all patients were to be screened for the potential for depression using a screening tool that meets national standards. The Patient Health Questionnaire (PHQ-9) and the Beck Depression Inventory (BDI) are possible instruments. The USPSTF recommended two basic questions when screening for depression: (1) "Over the past month, have you felt down, depressed, or hopeless?" and (2) "Over the past month, have you felt little interest or pleasure in doing things?" (Nimalasuriya, Compton, & Guillory, 2009). These questions require auditory skills to comprehend, so a review of the patient's functional ability, hearing, and level of safety using a nationally standardized screening tool was recommended. The specific functions assessed included hearing impairment, risk of falls, activities of daily living, and home safety. The screening version of the Hearing Handicap Inventory for the Elderly and the screening version of the Dizziness Handicap Scale were recommended as scales designed to reliably and validly assess the first two functions.

Surprisingly, information about hearing and risk of falls was considered part of the patient's history, whereas the visual acuity screen was considered part of the physical exam along with height and weight. Also included in the physical exam was counseling about end-of-life planning and advance directives. Another important component of the preventive service package was education about the prevention of chronic conditions and counseling based on the results of the first five elements in **Table 9.8,** including a written plan and checklist given to the patient regarding follow-up and additional preventive services covered by Medicare. Although Medicare has done away with this one-time benefit, it is noteworthy that it was included, and it is hoped that it will once again be offered, considering the increased prevalence of hearing loss among older

Table 9.8 Selected Components of the Welcome to Medicare Part B Program, 2005

History
  Elements
  1. A review of the individual's medical and social history with attention to modifiable risk factors
  2. A review of the individual's potential risk factors for depression
  3. A review of the individual's functional ability and level of safety

Physical Examination
  Elements
  4. Check the individual's height, weight, blood pressure, visual acuity, and measurement of body mass index (a new requirement effective January 1, 2009)
  5. End-of-life planning (a new requirement effective January 1, 2009)

Counseling Patients
  Elements
  6. Education, counseling, and referral based on the results of the review and evaluation services described in the previous five components
  7. Education, counseling, and referral, including a brief written plan such as a checklist for obtaining the appropriate screening or other Medicare Part B preventive services
  8. Patient education is important as it has proven successful in altering compliance with therapeutic regimens (Mazzuca, 1982)

Source: From Milstein, D., & Weinstein, B. (2008). Hearing screening for older adults using hearing questionnaires. *Clinical Geriatrics.* http://www.clinical geriatrics.com/articles/hearing-screening-older-adults-using -hearing-questionnaires?page=0,0.

adults and the availability of beneficial treatments. Growing out of the above discussion of components of preventive services program, **Table 9.9** describes the elements included in the hearing-related preventive activities program I advocate.

Goals of Hearing Screening

The goal of health-promotion activities for hearing include: (1) to identify older adults who are at risk for hearing impairments and associated conditions that can impair the quality of care or can modify the course of treatment of comorbid conditions, and (2) to identify older adults who are willing to seek and are materially likely to benefit from and adhere to treatments that lead to successful outcomes (Gates, Murphy, Rees, & Fraher, 2003). Simply put, we must look at disabling hearing impairment and tinnitus in terms of the "clinically prevent-

Table 9.9 Considerations When Designing a Hearing Health Care Screening Program

Goal(s) of the screening?
Why bother screening for this condition?
Which health care provider conducts the screening and why?
Who and when to screen: what is the trigger?
Screening protocol
Outcome-based referral criteria
Recommendations and intervention plan
Patient and provider education

able burden" taking patient adherence into account (Maciosek et al, 2006). In this context, patient adherence refers to completion of follow-up treatments and making needed changes in behavior once an intervention is recommend.

With regard to the first goal listed above, older adults with multifactorial health conditions should be screened for hearing loss and tinnitus, as the accumulated effects of impairments of multiple systems render older adults vulnerable to situational challenges, and remediating hearing impairment may avert negative outcomes (Markle-Reid et al, 2010). Identifying older adults prepared to take the necessary steps to manage the activity limitations, participation restrictions, and psychosocial and cognitive correlates of hearing impairment and tinnitus is critical especially for the large number of healthy older adults who are living longer, postponing retirement, and engaging in voluntary and leisure activities.

Why Bother Screening for Hearing Loss and Tinnitus?

Hearing impairment and tinnitus are prevalent conditions that rarely occur in isolation but rather in the context of other physiological and psychosocial conditions (Crews & Campbell, 2004). Hearing loss is the most frequent sensory deficit worldwide, affecting more than 413 million people, with an estimated 255 million people suffering from disabling hearing loss which is moderate to profound (Mathers, Smith, & Concha, 2003). Presbycusis, the leading cause of adult-onset hearing loss, affects more than 50% of those over the age of 75 years and is the second leading cause of years living with a disability (YLD) at a global level, after depression (Mathers et al, 2002). Interestingly, there is evidence emerging that hearing loss does predict mortality with a relative risk (RR) of 1.17 (Mathers et al, 2009).

Despite the global prevalence of hearing impairment, hearing-aid use varies dramatically, with estimates ranging from 10 to 40% in developed countries and less than 1% in developing countries. Overall more than 95% of those with hearing loss could benefit from hearing aids (Kochkin, 2009; Mathers et al, 2009). The World Health Organization (WHO) estimates that only one tenth of the global hearing population in need of hearing aids actually receives them (WHO, 2004). Hearing loss is insidious and underrecognized, especially in persons with cognitive problems and chronic problems such as diabetes and heart disease, and older adults have reported that they would not have sought evaluation and treatment for hearing loss without screening intervention (Yueh et al, 2010). Additionally, a report by Crews and Campbell (2004) found that individuals with hearing loss have higher rates of comorbid and secondary conditions than do those without hearing loss, such that they are 1.7 times more likely to have experienced falls in the past year, 1.4 times more likely to report stroke, 1.7 times more likely to report heart disease, and have higher rates of hypertension. Similarly, older adults with both vision impairment and hearing loss have even higher rates of comorbid and secondary conditions (e.g., diabetes, hypertension) as compared with those without either sensory loss. They are three times more likely to have fallen in the past 12 months, 1.5 times more likely to report hypertension, two times more likely to have broken a hip, 2.4 times more likely to report heart disease, and more likely to have sustained a stroke (Crews & Campbell,

2004). We also know from the literature that hearing impairment and central auditory processing problems can be precursors to cognitive dysfunction, so it behooves clinicians to diagnose hearing impairment early.

A recent report by Lin et al (2011) found that hearing loss is independently associated with incident all-cause dementia. Specifically, in their prospective sample of 639 individuals undergoing audiometric testing, the risk of incident all-cause dementia increased log linearly with increases in severity of baseline hearing loss defined as hearing levels in excess of 25 dB HL. The hazard ratio (95% confidence interval) for incident all-cause dementia was 1.89 (1.00–3.58) for mild hearing loss, rising to 4.94 (1.09–22.40) for severe hearing loss. Finally, with the increased prevalence of chronic diseases such as diabetes among persons 20 to 79 years of age, co-occurring conditions such as hearing loss will also rise, once again underscoring the need to screen and identify hearing impairment so as to improve the quality of care and potentially reduce some of the consequences of the condition (International Diabetes Federation, 2012).

A recent report by the American and British Geriatric Societies recommended that all older adults be screened for conditions that may lead to falls, lending additional support to screening for hearing impairment due to the link between falls and hearing impairment. The hearing screening should include a tinnitus screen due to their co-occurrence, the high prevalence of tinnitus (estimates range from 4.5 to 8.5% in the United States and 9.7 to 19% worldwide), the functional and behavioral consequences of tinnitus, and the availability of treatments for tinnitus. Also, the National Commission on Prevention Priorities concluded that screening for hearing impairment with appropriate referral ranked 15th among those practices considered to be effective among persons over 65 years, with a priority greater than that assigned to diabetes and cholesterol screening, which tend to be targeted already (Maciosek et al, 2006). The criteria the commission used to prioritize conditions included clinically preventable burden (CPB), a measure of a service's health impact, and cost-effectiveness (CE), which is an index of a service's economic value. The team of researchers used the clinical preventive services (primary and secondary) recommendations of the USPSTF for an asymptomatic population and for persons at high risk of coronary heart disease. The fact that older adults are often asymptomatic when it comes to hearing loss is a key factor underscoring the need for hearing screenings to be conducted by physicians (of course this contrasts with USPSTF [2012] guidelines). In this survey, it is noteworthy that in terms of clinically preventable burden and cost-effectiveness, hearing loss remains under the radar in older adults.

Who Should Conduct the Screen?

It is commonly accepted that the physician, typically the primary care physician, is the gatekeepers for health care including medical and audiological services. In fact, 80% of the U.S. population make at least one visit to their physician annually, with older adults typically making multiple visits. According to a recent report, the average number of consultations with physicians for preventive care varies globally, with persons in Japan averaging 13.6 visits, persons in Germany 7.5 visits, and persons in the United States only 3.8 visits, so clearly visits to physicians are the rule rather than the exception (The Economist, 2009). In addition, physicians are considered the most credible source on health matters, and decisions about proceeding with recommended interventions are typically motivated by physicians (Glasgow & Goldstein, 2008). Despite the fact that physicians are the gatekeepers, they rarely screen for hearing loss in older adults, in part because of their limited knowledge, which underscores the importance of educating physicians about hearing screening. Furthermore, older adults rarely admit to hearing loss, so physicians need to include in their periodic health exams some form of hearing screening, and audiologists must develop and conduct educational outreach programs for physicians.

Wallhagen and Pettengill (2008) conducted a series of interviews of 91 older adults and their communication partners regarding recent conversations with their primary care provider about their hearing or about screening for hearing loss, independent of any complaints the participants with hearing loss may have expressed. Similarly, Johnson et al (2008) reported on the results of a survey of primary care physicians regarding their knowledge about and attitudes toward hearing/balance screening and referral. The survey was mailed to 710 physicians, and 95 responded, for a response rate of 13.7%. Fifty–one percent of respondents were in practice for more than 15 years, and half of the caseloads of respondents was composed of older adults. Only 3% of the respondents screened their elderly patients for hearing status on a regular basis, 5.7% screened for balance, and 10% screened for both. It was troubling that the most common screening method was the whisper test, despite its poor calibration and standardization. Nearly 90% of respondents indicated that they assessed balance by watching the patient's gait if the patient complained of or if the physician suspected that the patient was at risk for falls. Interestingly, 78% of physicians indicated that if they suspected a hearing loss, they would refer the patient to an audiologist without discussion of intervention objectives or suitability for amplification, again underscoring the need to educate physicians about intervention options and treatment adherence. It was paradoxical that the majority of respondents was aware of the implications of untreated hearing loss and believed in the importance of screening, yet close to 90% of respondents indicated that it was important to screen for hearing or balance problems only if there was a patient complaint. Here again, any screening program in which physicians participate must emphasize that older adults deny hearing loss, are loath to admit that a hearing loss might exist, or consider hearing impairment a normal concomitant of aging about which they would not complain. The results of the surveys conducted by Johnson and colleagues (2008) and by Danhauer, Celani, and Johnson (2008) underscore the role of the physician in hearing screening activities and the importance of educating physicians about hearing impairment (**Table 9.10**).

Who and When to Screen

Screening is necessary because older patients may be asymptomatic, in denial, or indifferent about their condition. Even if patients are symptomatic, physicians may be unable to recognize that a hearing impairment exists. Thus, a hearing screen-

Table 9.10 Hearing Screening by Physicians: What They Should Know

1. Physicians must be made aware of why they have a duty to screen older adults for hearing-related problems.
2. Audiologists must provide physicians with an overview and hands-on experience with instruments appropriate for screening for hearing-related problems.
3. Physicians must be aware of treatment options and the efficacy of each in terms of promoting quality of life and quality of care and reducing burden of disease.
4. Physicians must be instructed in how to recognize individuals at risk for or possessing hearing-related difficulties.
5. Physicians must be familiar with effective communication strategies.
6. Physicians must be instructed about the important role audiologists play in evaluating and treating older adults with hearing-related difficulties.
7. Evidence-based materials and approaches must be utilized for credibility purposes.
8. Physicians have considerable influence over the actions of their older patients and they are the gatekeepers of the health care system. Hence, their knowledge about hearing loss, its ramifications, and recognizing individuals with impaired hearing are key in terms of quality of care delivered from a diagnostic and management perspective is critical. Physicians are in the position of communicating with older adults the results of their medical exam including providing a medication list and a follow-up plan. If adherence is to be ensured, physicians must utilize communication strategies that will be effective with their hearing-impaired patients.
9. Physicians must discuss end-of-life and palliative care with the cognitively intact patient. It is important that physicians know how to overcome hearing impairment and speech-processing problems to ensure engagement of the patient. As part of the care plan, physicians are increasingly in the position of discussing home safety and approaches to averting dangers in the home, and communication is key.
10. Physicians are encouraged to conduct a depression and a cognitive assessment on older adults, and failure to control for impaired hearing prior to conducting the assessment may compromise the validity of the outcome.
11. Physicians have the ability to influence patients' efficacy expectations, readiness for change, and outcome expectations. A key component of patient-centered care is effective clinician patient dialogue, which requires that patients are able to hear and understand the physician (Glasgow & Goldstein, 2008). As suggested above, clinical outcomes associated with patient-centered care include diagnostic accuracy, effective management, and patient adherence to and satisfaction with recommended treatments. The patient's ability to hear and understand is crucial if physicians are to achieve the goal of a partnership in delivery of care. Sustainable relationship building skills, open-ended inquiry, empathy, and respect for the patient can only take place when the patient can hear and understand what the physician is saying.

ing should be conducted annually, especially during the periodic health examination, as an undetected hearing impairment can modify the course of treatment for other systematic and opportunistic conditions. Annual screening for hearing impairment is in keeping with the recommendations of the American and British Geriatric Societies, which in 2010 advocated screening all older adults annually for risk factors that might lead to falls. As preventive priorities must be matched to the patient's condition, two categories of patients should be considered for screening: those who are healthy and active with no evidence of disease or functional decline, and those who have multiple chronic conditions that place them at risk for hearing loss. Whether screening for hearing impairment for diagnostic and treatment purposes or to promote functional well-being, the protocol should be built in to the initial clinical encounter rather than patient initiated, wherein if the patient mentions a problem, then a screening is done.

As part of the history, physicians should consider including a questionnaire that assesses hearing loss and tinnitus. Physicians routinely examine the ear with an otoscope, so shifting to an Audioscope to visualize the ear and screen hearing at one or two frequencies should not be onerous. The hearing screen should probably take place early in the physical exam, so that if physicians detect a hearing problem, they can adjust their speaking volume accordingly and use some of the communication strategies discussed in earlier chapters. In addition, if the physician finds early on that the patient fails the pure-tone screen, then when proceeding to a depression screen or a cognitive screen, the physician should consider using a portable amplifier with a microphone and earphones (e.g., Pocketalker) to ensure that the patient's hearing impairment does not taint the test results. If physicians do not routinely engage in preventive activities, then they should screen if a family member reports a concern about hearing/understanding; if selected chronic conditions, such as diabetes or cardiovascular disease, place the patient at risk for hearing loss; if the patient takes ototoxic medications; or if the patient smokes or has a history of noise exposure. All of this information should be available from the routine history form that the patient completes prior to the office visit. Finally, if the patient is known to be depressed or to have a cognitive impairment, it would behoove the physician to conduct a hearing screen, as it may be that untreated hearing loss is a contributing factor.

After screening older healthy and active adults for hearing impairment, it is important to ensure that patients benefit from intervention to promote their functional well-being and are motivated to comply with the recommendation to pursue some form of follow-up. If intervention is recommended, they must experience enough benefit to adhere to treatment recommendations. Hence, as part of the screening keep in mind that those who are being screened must have the behavioral capacity to perform the screening task(s), must have confidence in their ability to carry out the recommended treatment plan (self-efficacy), and must believe in the outcomes that will derive from the recommended intervention (outcome expectations). The individual failing the screen also must be ready (in keeping with the Stages of Change Model) to make a lifestyle change that often comes with the decision to purchase hearing aids (Glasgow & Goldstein, 2008). In short, when screening healthy older adults, our goal is to identify those with a functional hearing deficit who have the intrinsic motivation and confidence necessary to overcome their sensory deficit. The Health Belief Model was described by Janz and Becker (1984) and the Stages-of-Change Model mentioned above was described by Prochaska, DiClemente, and Norcross (1992). Based on cognitive theories, the Health Belief Model was developed to predict participation in health-prevention programs (Becker, 1974). According to this model, health-related behaviors are determined and can be predicted by (1) perceived threat of disease or illness, (2) perceived benefits/barriers associated with engaging in particular behaviors, and (3) self-efficacy or the belief that one is capable of acting upon professional recommendations. These three behavioral determinants of the model should influence the design of any preventive-care protocol so that patients will comply with screening recommendations.

The Health Belief Model suggests that behavior is dependent on the value that an individual places on a desired outcome and the belief that if a behavior is performed it will result in a desired outcome (Noh, Gagne, & Kaspar, 1994). Perceived threat is a function of two interrelated perceptual components, namely perceived susceptibility and perceived severity. Perceived susceptibility refers to individuals' view regarding their risk of contracting a health condition such as a handicapping hearing loss. According to this model, the likelihood of engaging in appropriate health behavior increases as the level of perceived susceptibility increases. Thus, as pertains to screening outcomes, persons who fail a screen and have a positive diagnostic test are likely to agree to wear a hearing aid if they accept the diagnosis and recognizes that they can develop the devastating psychosocial and communication problems associated with hearing loss. Perceived severity refers to the subjective evaluation that if left untreated, a disorder, impairment, or disability will have devastating consequences, such as handicapping an individual or reducing the quality of life. Although perceived threat influences engagement in preventive health behavior in that it could influence a person to take action, the choice of behavioral options depends on the individual's perceptions of benefits. According to proponents of the Health Belief Model, patients' choice of behavioral options depends on their perceptions of the effectiveness of the intervention in reducing the consequences of the condition (i.e., benefits) and on the obstacles or negative outcomes associated with the available interventions (i.e., barriers such as cost). When perceived barriers outweigh benefits that may ensue from audiological intervention, compliance is impeded (Noh et al, 1994). So if, as a result of a positive screening, an individual is referred for an audiological evaluation and possible hearing-aid use, compliance may be increased if at the time of the screen the individual is made aware of the fact that hearing aids have proven useful in reducing the burden of disease. The information obtained at the screening may assist the patient in conducting an informal cost-benefit analysis (i.e., will the outcome with hearing aids outweigh some of the inconveniences of actually making the purchase such as the high cost and the need to make several return visits).

Special Consideration

In the context of audiological screening and audiological rehabilitation, the Health Belief Model holds that people must feel threatened by their condition (handicapping hearing loss), they must believe that there will be psychosocial and communicative benefits associated with engaging in a particular behavior (audiological evaluation, hearing-aid purchase), and they must feel competent to adjust to the demands of hearing-aid use (Noh et al, 1994).

Pearl

Knowledge that a clinical preventive service is effective is not a sufficient condition to set priorities for increasing the delivery of preventive care (Maciosek et al, 2006).

◆ Screening Protocol

The comprehensive approach to hearing screening that I am recommending was informed by my synthesis of the epidemiological literature, the literature on social learning (social cognitive) theory, and an informal meta-analysis of screening studies conducted on older adults over the past few decades. My synthesis of the epidemiological literature revealed that successful screening programs shared several important features. They were comprehensive and delivered by a skilled health care provider. Individuals who were targeted were either at risk for the health condition or were likely to benefit in terms of their self-efficacy and outcome expectations. The health promotion activities were integrated and coordinated across providers and settings, as multisector participation, especially in terms of referral agencies, is key. Further, the protocol was function rather than disease based, took into account the desire on the part of the patient to take action, and included tailored and multicomponent interventions (Markle-Reid et al, 2010). Additional keys to success included a protocol that was brief, easy to administer, acceptable to both the health care provider and the patient, accurately discriminated across varying levels of function, ethical, entailed follow-up mechanisms and community resources that were in place to handle referrals and monitor adherence, and most important included educational materials for the patient as part of the targeted intervention. These patient education materials are important because studies suggest there is a relationship between health literacy and rates of chronic health conditions. In short, individuals with inadequate health literacy have significantly higher rates of certain chronic conditions including arthritis and hypertension as compared with those with adequate literacy (Wolf, Gazmararian, & Baker, 2005). **Table 9.11** summarizes important features of successful screening programs.

Special Consideration

Screening protocols that do not include an educational component are associated with low compliance rates.

Table 9.11   Features of Successful Screening Programs

Resources: patient–clinician partnership
Collaborative goal setting
Patient-centered counseling, including discussion of functional impact of failure to act on patient behavior
Physician education
Patient readiness assessment
Financial incentives, the systematic use of patient and clinician reminder and recall systems, and better access to services

The multicomponent screening protocol includes the following components and features as shown in **Table 9.12**.

Hearing Health Risk Appraisal

The first step in the screening is completion of a risk profile assessment to identify potential risk factors for hearing impairment. **Table 9.13** is a sample hearing health risk assessment form with binary choices for the respondent. Responses to this brief questionnaire can help guide the physician in recommending an intervention. The conditions included in the risk profile assessment are those that have an apparent association with hearing impairment. For example, hearing impairment is significantly associated with depression, and the relationship is independent of age and socioeconomic status (Yueh, Shapiro, MacLean, & Shekelle, 2003). Further, hearing loss is common in individuals with diabetes, and thus diabetes is an independent risk factor for hearing impairment (Bainbridge, Hoffman, & Cowie, 2008). Comorbidities might place the respondent at risk for hearing impairment. If the individual with comorbidities fails the screen, this might influence the course of the medical examination or how the physician communicates with the patient during the examination. If patients are free of chronic conditions and appear to be relatively healthy but fail the physiological and self-report screen, this might lead to a discussion of intervention options to consider when they have their hearing tested. The hearing health risk appraisal form should be easy to score and available in mul-

Table 9.12   Multicomponent Screening Protocol

Protocol	Features and Components
HISTORY: Risk profile assessment	Assess comorbidities or multimorbidities
PHYSIOLOGICAL FUNCTION: Audioscope™/Otoscopic exam	COUNSELING ABOUT LIFESTYLE CHANGES
	Physician education materials: hearing tactics, communication strategies, tinnitus management options
	Patient education materials: hearing tactics, hearing-assistive technologies, hearing-aid orientation/counseling, tinnitus management, speech reading, Web-based auditory training materials
FUNCTIONAL DEFICIT: Self Report	Mechanisms for periodic follow-up

tiple languages depending on the caseload. As health risks change over time, it would be important for these forms to be completed annually.

Screen for Physiological Function

The screen for hearing impairment includes an otoscopic examination to rule out the presence of impacted cerumen and a pure-tone screen to determine risk for hearing impairment. When screening for hearing impairment, the setting is an important consideration. It is of utmost importance that the screening take place in a clinical or natural environment that is conducive to obtaining reliable and valid outcomes (American Speech-Language-Hearing Association [ASHA], 1997). Thus, the ambient noise levels should be low enough to allow for accurate screening. The Welch Allyn Audioscope™, a handheld otoscope with a built-in audiometer, is well accepted as a reliable and valid alternative to a portable screening audiometer (Yueh et al, 2010). Further, Liu, Collins, Souza, and Yueh (2011) demonstrated that a tone-emitting otoscope such as the Audioscope is a cost-effective approach to hearing screening along with being a practical and feasible approach to screening. The Audioscope depicted in **Fig. 9.2** is a miniature audiometer capable of delivering into the external auditory canal a 20, 25, or 40 dB HL tone at frequencies of 500, 1000, 2000, and 4000 Hz, but for older adults 40 dB HL is the recommended frequency. The Audioscope has a conditioning tone built in to allow for a trial period prior to the actual test. This is especially helpful with older adults, enabling the audiologist to verify that the patient knows what is expected. To use the Audioscope, an appropriate-size ear speculum is placed within the external auditory canal to achieve an adequate seal. The tympanic membrane must be visualized before the testing begins. A tonal sequence is presented by pushing a button on the Audioscope, and the patient merely raises a hand or finger to signify that the tone has been heard. When the tone stops the patient should quickly put the finger or hand down again to await the next signal presentation. Although the Audioscope and the portable audiometer have similar operating characteristics,

Table 9.13   Hearing Health Risk Appraisal Form

Health Condition	Yes*	No**
1. Do you smoke cigarettes?	1	0
2. Do you or a family member believe that you have difficulty hearing and understanding others?	1	0
3. Have you been told that you now have cardiovascular disease?	1	0
4. Have you ever been told that you now have diabetes mellitus?	1	0
5. Have you been told that you now have arthritis?	1	0
6. Are you taking aminoglycoside antibiotics, cisplatin, an antiinflammatory drug, or loop diuretics?	1	0
7. Have you had a fall within the past year?	1	0
8. Have you been told that you have low vision or blindness?	1	0
9. Have you been told that you are suffering from depression?	1	0

* 1 point
** 0 points

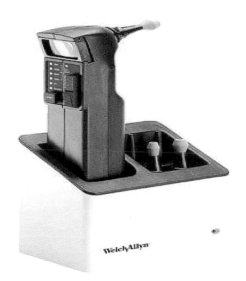

Fig. 9.2   The Audioscope™.

the Audioscope has some advantages. For example, it may be less costly than a screening audiometer, it is more portable, and it enables the clinician to view the external auditory meatus prior to the screening to determine whether cerumen is present, potentially invalidating screening adults. Additionally, an Audioscope screen can be completed in 33 seconds (McBride, Aguilar, Mulrow, & Tuley, 1990). The fact that the Audioscope must be calibrated on a regular basis should be communicated to the primary care physician engaged in screening.

The hearing impairment screen requires decisions regarding the frequency and intensity characteristics of the signal as well as the pass/fail criteria. Ventry and Weinstein (1983) were among the first investigators to suggest elevating the fence to 40 dB HL for community-based individuals 65 years of age or older. They offered two simple explanations for selecting 40 dB HL. First, 90% of older adults with hearing levels in excess of 40 dB HL perceive themselves as being handicapped by their impairment. Second, although some individuals with hearing levels less than 40 dB HL obtain hearing aids, the majority of older adults complying with the recommendation for audiological intervention (e.g., hearing aids and audiological rehabilitation) have hearing levels in excess of 40 dB HL. The epidemiological literature suggests that the higher compliance with audiological recommendations associated with the use of a higher fence is integral to defining the efficacy of any screening program. A third justification for a 40 dB HL screening level is that a failure indicates that an older adult with multiple comorbidities is likely to have a hearing impairment that may interfere with diagnosis and communication about medical findings and therefore requires adaptations on the part of the physician (Ventry & Weinstein, 1983; Weinstein, 1992).

With regard to decisions about the frequencies at which one should screen, 1000 and 2000 Hz have gained widespread appeal as 500 and 4000 Hz may lead to over-referrals due to contamination by noise or the very high rate of hearing impairment at 4000 Hz in older adults; 1000 and 2000 Hz are important frequencies because of the strong relationship be-

tween hearing level at these frequencies and speech perception. Further, anyone who fails a screening at 1000 and 2000 Hz will likely fail at 4000 Hz. The high prevalence of hearing loss at 4000 Hz substantially increases the risk of over-referrals (i.e., false-positives) (Gates, Cooper, Kannel, & Miller, 1990). Although 500 Hz may have some advantages as a frequency at which to screen, it is not typically included because of the confounding effects of ambient noise and because of the low incidence of middle-ear disease in older adults. Interestingly, screening specificity (using conventional audiometry as the gold standard) tends to be lowest at 500 Hz (ASHA, 1997).

One of the early studies designed to test the efficacy of pure-tone screening was conducted by Lichtenstein, Bess, and Logan (1988), who screened a large sample of older adults in a primary care setting using the Welch Allyn Audioscope, a handheld instrument with excellent between-location and between-subject reliability (Bess, 1995). In their study, screenings were conducted at 40 dB HL at 1000 and 2000 Hz. The sensitivity and specificity of the screen were judged against specific criteria for hearing impairment, namely the presence of a 40-dB hearing loss in both ears at either 1000 or 2000 Hz, or the presence of a 40-dB hearing loss in either ear at both 1000 and 2000 Hz. According to Lichtenstein et al (1988), the Audioscope performed quite well, with sensitivities ranging from 87 to 96% and specificities ranging somewhat lower, from 72 to 90%. Bienvenue, Michael, Chaffinch, and Zeigler (1985) also used a 25 dB HL screening level, and found that the Audioscope performed well against a hearing impairment criteria of ≥30 dB HL. In their sample of adults 51 to 81 years, sensitivities were as high as 93% and specificities were on the order of 70%. Frank and Petersen (1987) screened a large sample of older adults at 40 dB HL comparing the outcome on the Audioscope against hearing impairment criteria ≥45 dB HL at 500 to 4000 Hz. Overall sensitivity was high, on the order of 90%, as was the specificity of the Audioscope (i.e., 90%). Using thresholds ≥40 dB HL as the gold standard, McBride et al (1990) also reported high sensitivities and specificities with the Audioscope on a sample of older adults at Veterans Administration centers and community clinics.

◆ Functional Hearing Deficit: Self-Administered Questionnaires

Recommended by physicians, nurses, the American Geriatrics Society, and audiologists worldwide, the screening version of the Hearing Handicap Inventory for the Elderly (HHIE-S) shown in **Table 9.14** is the most widely researched and accepted self-report questionnaire for detecting older adults at risk for hearing impairment (Johnson, et al, 2008; Yueh et al, 2007). It contains 10 simple questions that query the respondent about the handicap or disability associated with hearing loss and taps into the emotional and social effects of hearing loss (Ventry & Weinstein, 1983). Its test-retest reliability is 0.84. The questions address situations related to hearing, and patients respond by stating whether the situation represents a problem. A "no" response is scored 0, "sometimes" is scored 2, and "yes" is scored 4. Total scores range from 0 to 40, with a score less than 10 indicating no handicap and a score greater than 24 indicating moderate to severe handicap (Mulrow & Lichten-

Table 9.14   Hearing Handicap Inventory for the Elderly–Screening Version

Instructions: The purpose of this questionnaire is to identify the problems your hearing loss may be causing you. Answer YES, SOMETIMES, or NO for each question. To obtain a total score add up the YES (4 points), SOMETIMES (2), and NO (0) responses. If your score is greater than 10, we recommend that you schedule a hearing test with a certified audiologist at a local hearing clinic.

	YES (4)	SOMETIMES (2)	NO (0)
E1. Does a hearing problem cause you to feel embarrassed when you meet new people?			
E2. Does a hearing problem cause you to feel frustrated when talking to members of your family?			
S1. Do you have difficulty hearing when someone speaks in a whisper?			
E3. Do you feel handicapped by a hearing problem?			
S2. Does a hearing problem cause you difficulty when visiting friends, relatives, or neighbors?			
S3. Does a hearing problem cause you to attend religious services less often than you would like?			
E4. Does a hearing problem cause you to have arguments with family members?			
S4. Does a hearing problem cause you difficulty when listening to TV or radio?			
E5. Do you feel that any difficulty with your hearing limits or hampers your personal or social life?			
S5. Does a hearing problem cause you difficulty when in a restaurant with relatives or friends?			

TOTAL SCORE: HHIE-S _____ **Refer if score >10**

---

stein, 1991). The probability of a hearing impairment is directly related to score on the HHIE-S according to a study conducted using an older primary care population. In short, a score of less than 10 indicates a 13% probability of hearing impairment, whereas a score of greater than 24 is indicative of an 84% probability of hearing impairment (Lichtenstein et al, 1988). The majority of studies using the HHIE-S as the screening instrument use a cutoff score of 10 as indicative of a positive screen for hearing impairment. Interestingly, 45% of a sample of older adults with HHIE-S scores ≥10 and with a 4 frequency pure-tone average ≥41 dB HL in the better ear, used or felt they required hearing aids, confirming 10 as a potential cutoff score (Chang, Ho, & Chou, 2009). The operating characteristics against pure-tone audiometry have been established for the HHIE-S. According to a study conducted using a sample of older adult community volunteers and the Ventry and Weinstein criteria of 40 dB HL, the likelihood ratio for hearing impairment ranged from 0.36 using a cutoff of 0 to 8 on the HHIE-S, rising to 12 when the cutoff was between 26 and 40 (Lichtenstein et al, 1988). The overall accuracy in identifying people with and without hearing impairment is 75%.

In addition to its well-described validity, depending on cutoff scores, with sensitivity ranging from 0.33 to 0.80 and specificity ranging from 0.67 to 0.77, the HHIE-S has several other strengths (Yueh et al, 2003). Completion of the questionnaire helps patients realize the social and emotional consequences of hearing loss, which may help them to seek audiological assistance especially if the physician underscores the value of audiological interventions. Further, a meta-analysis by Chisolm et al (2007) recently revealed that hearing aids have medium to large beneficial effects when the disease-specific HHIE-S is used to measure outcome. Individuals with scores in excess of 18 on the HHIE-S are likely to purchase and benefit from hearing aids. Similarly, according to Chang et al (2009), when administered to a sample of community-dwelling older adults residing in Taipei, Taiwan, scores on the HHIE-S are associated with higher rates of hearing-aid use especially among those with moderate to profound hearing loss. The same effect emerged in a meta-analysis of the benefits of counseling-oriented rehabilitation. Further, although less sensitive to early-onset hear-

ing impairment (50% of those with mild hearing impairment do not sense any consequences), it does identify individuals with moderate to severe hearing loss with activity limitations and participation restrictions. Finally, it is easy to administer and takes only 3 to 5 minutes to complete using computerized or paper-pencil administration (McBride et al, 1990).

Several investigators have explored the sensitivity of a global history measure such as "Do you have a hearing problem now?" or "Do you think you have a hearing problem?" to identify older adults with potential deficits (Gates et al, 2003; Yueh et al, 2010). Gates and colleagues (2003) compared responses to the global question as a subjective criterion of hearing loss to scores on the HHIE to see which question best correlated with their criterion level of handicapping hearing level, namely an audiometric screening threshold level of 40 dB HL or greater at 1000 and 2000 Hz. In their sample, 27% of participants had the criterion level of hearing loss noted above. The sample was somewhat limited in terms of range of hearing impairment (mean pure-tone average [PTA] in the worse ear for females was 28 dB HL and for males was 31 dB HL) and self-perceived hearing handicap, in that the mean HHIE-S score was 5.7 for males and 3.5 for females, yet between 35% and 48% claimed a hearing problem based on responses to the global question. Likelihood ratios, sensitivity and specificity values, and predictive values are shown in **Table 9.15** for the HHIE-S and the global question. The proportion of individuals referred for a hearing test differed dramatically, such that fewer people were referred based on a positive screen on the HHIE-S (10 or greater). The global measure was more sensitive, 71% versus 36%, in detecting the authors' criterion for hearing loss, yet the HHIE-S was more specific, such that it over-referred fewer (8%) false-positive cases than did the global question (28%). The authors did not view the over-referral rate as problematic, as they argued that most individuals who were referred could benefit from testing and counseling. Yueh and colleagues found that three quarters of the veterans in their sample felt they had a hearing impairment yet 18% screened positive for hearing loss using the Audioscope and 59% screened positive using a cutoff score of 10 on the HHIE-S. These authors also had a high rate of false-positive screens,

Table 9.15   Outcomes Comparing Global Screen to the Hearing Handicap Inventory for the Elderly–Screening Version (HHIE-S)

Sensitivity and Specificity for the HHIE-S and the Global Question: "Do you have a hearing problem now?"	Referred, %	Sensitivity, %	Specificity, %	LR+	LR–	PPV, %[1]	NPV, %[1]
HHIE-S[1]	15.2	36	92	4.7	0.70	63	80
Global Question	39.5	71	72	2.5	0.40	48	87
Both positive	14.2	34	93	5.0	0.71	65	79
Both negative	40.4	72	71	2.5	0.39	48	87

Abbreviations: LR+, positive likelihood ratio; LR–, negative likelihood ratio; NPV, negative predictive value (percentage with a negative screening test who did not have hearing loss); PPV, positive predictive value (percentage with a positive screening test who had hearing loss).
[1]Cutoff score of 0–8 vs. 10.
Source: Data from Gates, G. A., Murphy, M., Rees, T. S., & Fraher, A. (2003, Jan). Screening for handicapping hearing loss in the elderly. *Journal of Family Practice, 52,* 56–62.

and only 4.1% of veterans screened with the HHIE-S used hearing aids after 1 year and only 7% of those screened with the HHIE-S and pure tones used hearing aids after 1 year.

> ## Pearl
>
> For audiologists providing the training for primary care physicians, it is important to specify the hearing levels to be used (e.g., 25 dB HL versus 40 dB HL) along with the advantages and disadvantages associated with each.

Numerous attempts have been made to assess the efficacy of the HHIE-S as a screening tool, to compare the HHIE-S to the Audioscope as a screening tool, and to compare sensitivity of the global question to scores on the HHIE-S. In general, most of the validity studies used the presence of hearing impairment as the gold standard, with sensitivities, specificities, and predictive values varying as a function of the screening method, but a gold standard of hearing impairment is not as acceptable to the USPSTF as the long-term outcomes associated with the screening. In fact, according to my interpretation of the USPSTF guidelines, the gold standard against which to validate a screen should be the outcome associated with compliance with the recommendation, which is integrally intertwined with clients' internal perceptions about their condition and with their belief regarding the feasibility of remediating the condition for which they have undergone a screening.

A recent randomized-controlled trial by Yueh et al, (2010) is one of the first of its kind in audiology to tie screening to hearing aid use, so their data can inform our thinking about selecting a protocol. The primary objective of the study was to evaluate differences in the rate of hearing-aid use across control group (no screening) and three groups of veterans who underwent different screening protocols, which are described in **Table 9.16**. Participants were a sample of veterans 50 years of age or older considered to be eligible for audiology services including hearing aids in the Veterans Administration (VA) system. Experienced hearing-aid users were excluded, as were individuals who had undergone a hearing test within the 6 months prior to the screening. An unbalanced randomized strategy was used to assign participants to one of the four options including the control arm. All participants who screened positive were told that they might have a hearing loss and they

were given instructions regarding proceeding with a follow-up hearing evaluation at the VA hospital conducting the screen. Subjects who screened negative including those in the control arm were given the number of the Audiology Clinic if they wanted to schedule further testing. The clinic was not aware of the screening outcome.

All participants completed a series of baseline questionnaires including a health status questionnaire and this question about self-reported hearing loss: "Do you think you have a hearing problem?" The mean age of participants was 60 years, and 94% of participants were men. **Figure 9.3** displays the chain of referrals over 1-year period for participants who screened positively, with the primary outcome being that participants indicated that they continued to use hearing aids 1 year after the screening. As shown in **Fig. 9.3**, individuals with a positive screening outcome were asked to contact the audiology clinic for an audiological evaluation. Those who did were tracked for adherence (that is, keeping their appointment) and whether they were eligible audiologically for hearing aids. All participants were contacted after 6 months to ask about visits to the audiologist or otolaryngologist. Those participants receiving hearing aids were tracked to see if they felt the hearing aid was helping them, whether they were using the hearing aid after 1 year, and to determine subjective satisfaction with the hearing aid and the quality-of-life benefits of the hearing aids. The outcomes on the each of the screening tests are shown in **Table 9.17**.

It is evident that outcomes were different across screening groups in terms of proportion passing and failing the screen, proportion contacting the audiologist for follow-up testing, and adherence. In general, differences were small across the

Table 9.16   Screening Strategies in a Randomized-Controlled Trial of Veterans

Otoscopic	Questionnaire	Dual
Tonal otoscopic at 40 dB HL at 2000 Hz	HHIE-S	PT and HHIE-S
Positive screen: inability to hear tone	Positive screen: score of 10 or more	Positive screen on either tonal otoscopic or HHIE-S

Abbreviations: HHIE-S, Hearing Handicap Inventory for the Elderly–Screening version; PT, pure-tone.

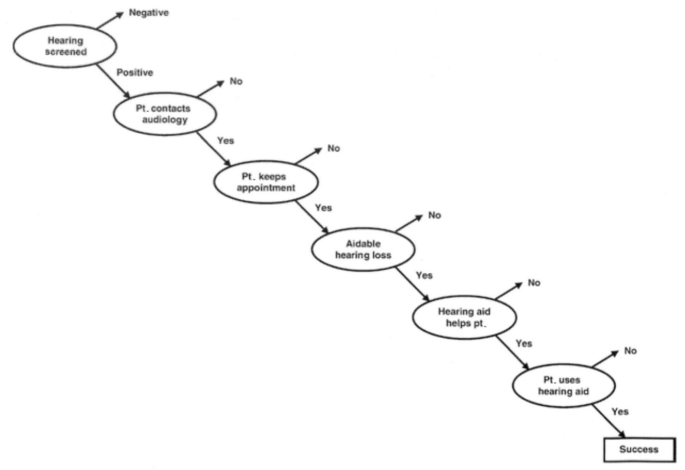

Fig. 9.3 Flow chart depicting the chain of events from screening through 1 year of hearing-aid use. [Adapted from Yueh, B., Collins, M. P., Souza, P. E., Boyko, E. J., Loovis, C. F., Heagerty, P. J., et al. (2010, Mar). Long-term effectiveness of screening for hearing loss: The screening for auditory impairment—which hearing assessment test (SAI-WHAT) randomized trial. *Journal of the American Geriatrics Society, 58,* 427–434.]

screening groups in terms of the proportion with correctable hearing loss and the proportion fitted with hearing aids and using hearing aids after 1 year. In general, the screening group that completed the HHIE-S or the HHIE-S and the Audioscope had more audiology visits and were more likely to keep their appointment with the audiologist. However, although more participants failed the questionnaire-only screen and the dual screening, the proportion of participants obtaining and using hearing aids after 1 year was comparable across screening arms,

with 7.4% of the dual-screen subjects using the hearing aid after 1 year as contrasted with 4% of the questionnaire-only subjects. This study is an excellent attempt at validating a screening approach to identifying and treating patients with hearing impairment. However, the proportion of participants who kept their audiology appointment (e.g., adherence) was low, as was the proportion of veterans who were using hearing aids after 1 year. This finding is in keeping with earlier studies on hearing screening in that typically a very small proportion of individuals who undergo follow-up audiological evaluations actually take the next step, namely, purchasing hearing aids. The more successful rates have occurred in studies where hearing evaluations or hearing aids were provided at no cost, yet the rates are still low.

My review of the literature revealed that low compliance with advice regarding interventions is due in part to the high cost of hearing aids, the lack of insurance coverage for the evaluation or for the hearing aid, myths about hearing aids (e.g., they amplify noise, are not appropriate for persons with sensorineural hearing loss), the belief that hearing aids call attention to the handicap (i.e., the stigma associated with hearing loss and the use of hearing aids), ageism (e.g., the belief that hearing loss is a normal concomitant of the aging process), and

Table 9.17   Screening Outcome and Follow-Up

Event	Audioscope Screen, %	HHIE-S Screen, %	Dual Screen, %
Screening positive	18.6	59	63.6
Scheduling an audiology evaluation	17.3	31	34.4
Patients using hearing aids after 1 year	6	4.6	7.6
Patients 65 years and older using hearing aids after 1 year	11.7	7.1	16.7

Screening for Functional Communication Impairments (SFCI)

Instructions: The purpose of this questionnaire is to identify any problems you are having which may relate to your ears—including hearing difficulties or tinnitus (ringing, buzzing, noises in your ears/head). Please circle either *Yes*, *Sometimes*, or *No* for each question. If you use hearing aids, please answer the way you hear without using the hearing aids. If you are not experiencing any hearing difficulties, please mark *No* for each item. Patient ID: ___ ___ ___ ___				

	Scoring Values for Each Item	4	2	0	NA
H-1	Does a hearing problem cause you difficulty when listening to the television or to the radio?	Yes	Sometimes	No	
MI-1	Is it important for your hearing problem to cause you less difficulty when listening to the television or radio?	Yes	Sometimes	No	
H-2	Does a hearing problem cause you difficulty when visiting friends, relatives or neighbors?	Yes	Sometimes	No	
H-3	Does a hearing problem cause you to feel frustrated when talking to members of your family?	Yes	Sometimes	No	
MI-2	Is it important for you to feel less frustrated by a hearing problem when talking to members of your family?	Yes	Sometimes	No	
MI-3	Is it important for a hearing problem to cause you less difficulty when visiting with friends, relatives, or neighbors?	Yes	Sometimes	No	
T-1	Do you feel that you can no longer cope with your tinnitus?	Yes	Sometimes	No	
T-2	Because of tinnitus, do you have trouble falling asleep or staying asleep at night?	Yes	Sometimes	No	
T-3	Do you feel that you cannot escape your tinnitus?	Yes	Sometimes	No	
S-E	How confident do you feel that you are ready to take the necessary steps to help you hear/understand better in difficult listening situations (Please circle number that applies)?	Not 0 1	Somewhat 2 3 4 5	Very 6 7	
	TOTAL SCORE				

In the box below, please circle the number that corresponds with: The severity of the problem Not at all severe Extremely severe	
Hearing Loss: 0 1 2 3 4 5 6 7	
Tinnitus: 0 1 2 3 4 5 6 7	

Fig. 9.4 Screening for functional communication impairments.

the false impression that hearing aids are not effective in remediating the psychosocial and communicative consequences of hearing loss. In my view there is a two-part remedy to low compliance: (1) recommendations following screening must be multifaceted and targeted to the individual's needs, and (2) the screening protocol must tap into the individual's readiness and confidence in his or her ability to change.

Summarizing to this point, screening programs are considered effective in terms of cost and benefit if large numbers of

patients who undergo the screening comply with the recommendation to pursue treatment and experience enough benefit to adhere to treatment. To this end, I have developed a brief, easy-to-administer questionnaire, shown in **Fig. 9.4**, that incorporates questions from reliable and valid parent instruments (e.g., Tinnitus Handicap Inventory and Hearing Handicap Inventory [HHI]) and builds on social learning theory principles. The Screening for Functional Communication Impairment (SFCI) contains 11 questions; three address social and emotional consequences of hearing impairment (H), three pertain to the experience of tinnitus (T), and the rest emphasize motivational interviewing (MI) strategies, specifically the person's belief in the importance of behavior change and the person's confidence or self-efficacy (SE) in taking action. The items borrowed from the HHI are those that rank high in terms of the proportion of people with hearing impairment or reporting difficulty in the particular problem areas based on the work of Gates and colleagues (2003), a pilot study in which I am engaged, and item analyses of the HHI. The scoring system has not yet been fully worked out but, based on the pilot, if T ≥4, a referral is indicated and if H + MI + SE >8, a referral is indicated based on the SFCI scores. Affirmative responses to MI 1, 2, and 3 suggest that respondents feel it is important to and they want to change their situation; affirmative responses to H-SE and T-SE suggests that respondents are confident that they have the skills to make a change and that the behavior change will result in beneficial outcomes. Affirmative responses to the items about hearing deficits and tinnitus suggest that the respondent perceives difficulty in the domains of function assessed by the particular items.

◆ Referral Guidelines and Multifaceted Interventions

Referral criteria following the multicomponent screen must relate back to the health risk appraisal form completed at the beginning of the encounter with the physician, as the health status of the patient coupled with the subjective report provide key information that determines whether a referral is necessary and the nature of the referral. For example, we are seeking to identify those healthy and active older adults who have a hearing loss that is associated with activity limitations and participation restrictions and who are motivated and confident that they want to purchase hearing aids that will enable them to communicate and remain independent. In contrast, in the case of a patient with compromised health status due to multiple comorbidities and a shortened life expectancy, we may recommend communication strategies and the use of assistive devices in small groups and when watching television so that they can continue to communicate with family members and their physicians and remain connected through media. **Table 9.18** presents referrals based on the health of the patient and screening outcomes that should be considered by the physician. For example, a chronically ill patient with multiple co-occurring health conditions who failed the pure-tone screen might be given an information packet on communication strategies and hearing-assistive technologies, with possible referral to an audiologist if necessary for medical management. The physician should adopt effective communication strategies that

enable him to communicate with the patient. As another example, the family members of a frail, homebound older adult who failed the pure-tone screen might be given tips to facilitate communication with the homebound patient. Further, tips for home safety should be distributed, including hearing-assistive technology that can be easily installed in the home and used by the patient.

If the individual owns but does not use a hearing aid, information about hearing-aid use might be given to the homebound patient and caregiver. In contrast, if the patient is a healthy older adult with at most one chronic condition, who screened positive on the self-report questionnaire and the pure-tone screen, he or she should be referred to the audiologist for a hearing evaluation and possibly a hearing aid. An information packet on hearing aids and hearing-assistance technologies might be distributed, and the physician should discuss the value of hearing aids, given the outcome on the screen, and should refer the patient to an audiologist. A written intervention plan might be given to the patient along with the hearing profile, including recommendations for behavioral interventions. The physician should schedule a follow-up session or telephone contact.

> **Pearl**
>
> Key components of patient behavior change are information and counseling; "more counseling tends to be better counseling, and any counseling, no matter how brief, is better than none at all" (U.S. Department of Health and Human Services, 1994, p. 29).

Audiologists are integral to the success of physician screening initiatives, and part of their role is providing the physician with literature to be distributed to the patient that will promote a patient–clinician partnership, which is integral to successful outcomes. The physician must know how to recognize patients who are hearing impaired, how to communicate with the hearing impaired, how to discuss options that are appropriate for the patient, and how to give advice that will guide the patient's actions. The physician must tell older patients that age is not a limiting factor for the hearing impaired to benefit from hearing aids and available hearing-assistive technologies. A physician "tool box" modeled after that used for preventive care for selected chronic conditions is highly recommended. The tool-box might include screening forms, the Audioscope referral criteria/options, communication strategies, and a Pocket-Talker. Further, audiologists should impart tips regarding how best to educate and counsel older adults, as their advice is critical.

Vogt and Kapp (1987) suggest the following patient education guidelines: (1) The physician should use terms the patient

Table 9.18 Targeted Referral Option Outcomes

Multiple co-occurring health conditions (multimorbidity)—chronically ill	Frail—homebound elderly	Healthy older adult (at most 1 co-occurring condition)
Positive on pure-tone screen	Positive on pure-tone screen	Positive on pure-tone screen, self-report, both
Information packet on communication strategies and hearing-assistance technologies; possible referral to audiologist	Tips for communicating, tips for home safety	Referral to audiologist, information packet on hearing aids and assistive technologies

can understand. (2) Patients generally remember only three or four points, so the physician should present only the important information. (3) The physician should be specific when giving instructions and explanations. (4) The physician should provide written information. (5) The physician should sit down when providing informational counseling, as this gives the perception that you are willing to take the time to explain all the important information. (6) The physician should reinforce or review the information presented to make sure it is understood and that the patient will act on it.

The components of patient education might include the following:

1. Screening for hearing-related issues and identifying hearing deficits can improve the quality of care and reduce the burden of illness associated with untreated hearing loss.
2. An encounter form or the risk-assessment appraisal form should be used (**Table 9.13**).
3. A checkup questionnaire such as the SFCI data collection sheet, a pure-tone screening, an otoscopic outcome, and the office policy for screening should address the patient's risk level.
4. Record the outcomes of the screening tests, and take into consideration the realities of the local medical resources, insurance coverage, and patient preferences. Physician recommendations are the single most important factor in a patient's decision about whether to pursue hearing health care interventions.
5. The patient–physician partnership agreement is signed by both as a step toward better managing a patient's condition and making recommendations.
6. A reminder system helps patients remember the actions or tests they need to complete as part of their agreement.
7. An office policy is needed regarding how to communicate with the hearing impaired, as an effective communication system fosters a positive outcome and patient satisfaction.

Patient education materials are critical as well, as health literacy is closely tied to utilization of the health care system and to lower mortality and morbidity. Promoting hearing health literacy may increase the ranks of first time hearing aid users, close the gap between self-ratings of hearing difficulty and measured hearing loss, and shorten the time span between the onset of hearing loss and the patient's seeking assistance. Audiologists are falling short in communicating the technologies and strategies that are available for the hearing impaired. Over the past 50 years, hearing-aid adoption rates have remained stable; in 1955, five million Americans needed hearing aids but only 1.2 million (24%) wore them, and in 2004, 24 million Americans needed hearing aids but only 6.2 million (26%) wore them (Kochkin, 2005). Thus, the use rate among those needing hearing aids remains almost the same. Audiologists must develop creative strategies to change the status quo via educational outreach to encourage the hearing impaired to try amplification earlier, so that they can continue to work productively, enjoy leisure activities, and contribute to society. The earlier individuals learn about the detrimental effects of hearing impairment and come to understand the physiological and psychosocial value of hearing aids, the sooner they will be ready to avail themselves of our services.

In my view, these educational materials should include a discussion about hearing-assistive technologies because when the hearing impaired are in the contemplation and preparation stage of readiness, successful use of such devices may help them modify their behavior and become more accepting of audiological interventions, including hearing aids and audiological rehabilitation. Perhaps through wellness programs and public service announcements about hearing loss, we can effectively move persons with untreated hearing loss into the preparation phase, at which point they will be ready to consider a hearing test and possible interventions. When it is clear, based on their own decisional balance sheet, that the benefits of targeted audiological interventions are equal to or exceed the cost, people with hearing loss will be prepared to take action. We can assume that they perform their own cost-benefit analysis, and it is our responsibility to make them aware of the benefits to facilitate their analysis. A more complete discussion of educational initiatives was developed in earlier chapters.

Special Consideration

One out of six Americans over 70 years has visual impairment; one out of four has hearing impairment (CDC/NCHS National Health and Nutrition Examination Survey [NHANES], 2009).

◆ Conclusion

Hearing loss is a global public health problem, and active screening programs can help increase case detection. The bulk of evidence suggests that it is reasonable to screen older adults for hearing impairment and related deficits, given their prevalence and given the availability of interventions and technologies to meet the variety of needs posed by impaired hearing and tinnitus (Mathers et al, 2003). Despite technological advances, less than 1% of hearing-impaired individuals in developing countries and between 10% and 40% of hearing-impaired individuals in developed countries use hearing aids. Preventive health care must be tailored to the patient in terms of the referral and follow-up guidelines and information dispensed. The most efficacious way to reach the majority of older adults is to involve primary care physicians, family practitioners, or geriatricians in the process (another way is through Web-based approaches). After all, medical professionals are the entry point into the health care system, and most older adults see a primary care physician on a regular basis, providing a natural opportunity for case finding. Further, older adults often prefer it if a physician rather than an audiologist performs the initial screen, as the recommendation of a physician is important in their view (Fujikawa & Cunningham, 1989). Adherence is improved if physicians are the ones making the recommendations, as they are considered the most credible sources for health matters. Formal screening is important, as older adults underreport or fail to report a hearing deficit, but provider education regarding screening protocols and the value of screening is important as fewer than 15% of physicians screen for hearing deficits, which are as one of the eight conditions missed in traditional medical exams. Audiologists are obligated to educate physicians about the value of hearing screening and about effective screening protocols.

Hearing deficits rarely occur in isolation, and the target of hearing screening activities should be older adults at risk for hearing impairment due to the presence of multiple comorbidities, and older healthy and active adults with functional hearing deficits who are likely to adhere to physician recommendations regarding treatment. Screening is considered successful when individuals comply with recommendations to pursue hearing health care services; hence, persons with functional hearing deficits must be ready to change their behavior and confident in their ability to do so. Therefore, the protocol being recommended is a departure from the traditional approaches, as the goal is to capture those who will pursue and benefit from intervention.

The protocols to be used, the referral criteria, the appropriate professional to do the job, and the value of hearing screening activities remain the subject of considerable debate. Education of older adults about hearing health care is an important component of any screening endeavor, as adequate health literacy fosters better access to health care and lower morbidity and mortality. Patient education about hearing impairment and its treatment is designed to place individuals in a better position to participate in their own health care, hence maximizing the potential therapeutic benefit (Mazzuca, 1982). Educational material should describe hearing impairment and related deficits, such as tinnitus and falls, should discuss the effect of untreated hearing deficits on psychosocial function and quality of care, and should describe the variety of interventions that are successful at alleviating hearing impairment and its consequences.

Patient education should be considered by audiologists as a process of "influencing patient behavior, producing changes in knowledge, attitudes and skills required to maintain or improve health. The process begins with the imparting of factual information, and includes interpretation and integration of the information in such a manner as to bring about attitudinal or behavioral changes which benefit the person's health status" (Vogt & Kapp, 1987, p. 273). This process is built into the protocol recommended, as the epidemiological literature underscores the integral role self-efficacy and outcome expectations play in successful preventive activities.

Over the past two decades, several screening protocols have been proposed for identifying older adults with hearing loss requiring some form of targeted intervention. Despite differences across protocols in terms of such variables as pass-fail criteria, hearing levels and frequencies for screening, choice of a self-report questionnaire, and adequate sensitivity and specificity data, older adults demonstrate poor compliance with recommended follow-up and intervention activities. Further, as currently designed, the efficacy of traditional screening programs in terms of health outcomes has not been documented. The multicomponent screening protocol described in this chapter is an attempt at overcoming the disadvantages of the existing approaches by incorporating models of health behavior change and social learning theory along with the philosophy of matching preventive priorities with the patient's health status. When selecting a screening protocol, the audiologist should always consider the goal of the preventive activity and the net benefit associated with the service, along with the certainty that benefit will accrue if the patient complies with the recommendations and perhaps that ignoring the issue could be harmful in terms of health status.

The importance of individualizing recommended interventions to the patient and the situation cannot be overemphasized (USPSTF, 2011). Screening programs can be considered effective only if available diagnostic and treatment services are utilized by those undergoing the screen and when the patient complies with treatment recommendations and the screen is linked to beneficial outcomes. Counseling and education are integral to health promotion and disease prevention activities, and a variety of resources including Web-based resources and social networking sites should be used to create a milieu that reinforces healthy behavior. It is my hope that the discussion in this chapter will encourage audiologists to collaborate with physicians in launching screening programs that will help to close the gap between the total number of hearing-impaired older adults and the number who purchase intervention services (e.g., hearing aids or hearing-assistance technologies) that improve the quality of life and quality of care.

References

Agrawal, Y., Platz, E. A., & Niparko, J. K. (2008, Jul). Prevalence of hearing loss and differences by demographic characteristics among US adults: Data from the National Health and Nutrition Examination Survey, 1999–2004. *Archives of Internal Medicine, 168*, 1522–1530

American Geriatrics Society. (2009). *Prevention of falls in older persons: AGS/ BGS clinical practice guidelines.* http://www.medcats.com/FALLS/frameset .htm

American Speech-Language-Hearing Association (ASHA) Panel on Audiologic Assessment. (1997). *Guidelines for audiologic screening.* Rockville, MD: ASHA

Bainbridge, K. E., Hoffman, H. J., & Cowie, C. C. (2008, Jul). Diabetes and hearing impairment in the United States: Audiometric evidence from the National Health and Nutrition Examination Survey, 1999 to 2004. *Annals of Internal Medicine, 149*, 1–10

Becker, M. (1974).The *health belief model and personal health behavior.* Thorofare, NJ: Charles B. Slack

Bess, F. (1995). Applications of the Hearing Handicap Inventory for the Elderly-screening version (HHIE-S). *Hearing Journal, 48*, 51–55

Bienvenue, G. R., Michael, P. L., Chaffinch, J. C., & Zeigler, J. (1985, Sep-Oct). The AudioScope: A clinical tool for otoscopic and audiometric examination. *Ear and Hearing, 6*, 251–254

Chang, H. J., Burke, A. E., & Glass, R. M. (2009, Dec). JAMA patient page. Preventive care for older adults. *Journal of the American Medical Association, 302*, 2722

Chang, H. P., Ho, C. Y., & Chou, P. (2009, Oct). The factors associated with a self-perceived hearing handicap in elderly people with hearing impairment—results from a community-based study. *Ear and Hearing, 30*, 576–583

Chisolm, T. H., Johnson, C. E., Danhauer, J. L., Portz, L. J., Abrams, H. B., Lesner, S., et al. (2007, Feb). A systematic review of health-related quality of life and hearing aids: Final report of the American Academy of Audiology Task Force on the Health-Related Quality of Life Benefits of Amplification in Adults. *Journal of the American Academy of Audiology, 18*, 151–183

Chou, R., Dana, T., Bougatsos, C., Fleming, C., & Beil, T. (2011, Mar). Screening adults aged 50 years or older for hearing loss: A review of the evidence for the U.S. preventive services task force. *Annals of Internal Medicine, 154*, 347–355.

Cochrane, A. (1991). Effectiveness and efficiency: Random reflections on health services. In C. Mulrow & M. Lichtenstein (Eds.), Screening for hearing impairment in the elderly: rationale and strategy. *Journal of General Internal Medicine, 6*, 249–258

Crews, J. E., & Campbell, V. A. (2004, May). Vision impairment and hearing loss among community-dwelling older Americans: Implications for health and functioning. *American Journal of Public Health, 94*, 823–829

Danhauer, J. L., Celani, K. E., & Johnson, C. E. (2008, Jun). Use of a hearing and balance screening survey with local primary care physicians. *American Journal of Audiology, 17*, 3–13

The Economist. (2009). *Reforming American health care.* http://www.economist.com/node/13899647

Eleazer, G. P., & Brummel-Smith, K. (2009, May). Commentary: Aging America: meeting the needs of older Americans and the crisis in geriatrics. *Academic Medicine, 84*, 542–544

Frank, T., & Petersen, D. R. (1987, Jun). Accuracy of a 40 dB HL Audioscope and audiometer screening for adults. *Ear and Hearing, 8*, 180–183

Frankish, C., Lovato, C., & Poureslami, I. (2007). Models, theories, and principles of health promotion. In M. Kline & R. Huff (eds.). *Health promotion in multicultural populations.* Los Angeles: Sage

Fujikawa, S., & Cunningham, J. K. (1989, Dec). Practices and attitudes related to hearing: A survey of executives. *Ear and Hearing, 10*, 357–360

Gates, G. A., Cooper, J. C., Jr, Kannel, W. B., & Miller, N. J. (1990, Aug). Hearing in the elderly: the Framingham cohort, 1983-1985. Part I. Basic audiometric test results. *Ear and Hearing, 11*, 247–256

Gates, G. A., Murphy, M., Rees, T. S., & Fraher, A. (2003, Jan). Screening for handicapping hearing loss in the elderly. *Journal of Family Practice, 52*, 56–62

Glasgow, R., & Goldstein, M. (2008). Introduction to the principles of health behavior change. In S. Woolf, S. Jonas, & E. Kaplan-Liss (Eds.), *Health promotion and disease prevention in clinical practice* (2nd ed.). Baltimore: Lippincott Williams & Wilkins

Goldstein, M., Whitlock, E., & Depue, J. (2004). Multiple health risk behavior interventions in primary care: summary of research evidence. *American Journal Preventive Medicine, 27 (Suppl 2)*, 61–79

Guirguis-Blake, J., Calonge, N., Miller, T., Siu, A., Teutsch, S., & Whitlock, E.; U.S. Preventive Services Task Force. (2007, Jul). Current processes of the U.S. Preventive Services Task Force: Refining evidence-based recommendation development. *Annals of Internal Medicine, 147*, 117–122

Healthy People 2010 Final Review. http://www.cdc.gov/nchs/data/hpdata2010/hp2010_final_review.pdf. Retrieved Sept. 7, 2012.

Healthy People 2020 (2010). http://www.healthypeople.gov/2020/Topics Objectives2020/pdfs/HP2020_brochure_with_LHI_508.pdf. Retrieved Sept. 7, 2012.

Hickner, J., & Solbert, L. (2008). How to organize the practice for improved delivery of clinical preventive services. In S. Woolf, S. Jonas, & E. Kaplan-Liss (Eds.), *Health promotion and disease prevention in clinical practice* (2nd ed.). Baltimore: Lippincott Williams & Wilkins

International Diabetes Federation (IDF). (2012), *Diabetes atlas* (5th ed.). http://www.idf.org/diabetesatlas/5e/the-global-burden

Janz, N., & Becker, M. (1984). The Health Belief Model: A decade later. *Health Education Quarterly, 11: 1-47 (1984).*

Johnson, C. E., Danhauer, J. L., Koch, L. L., Celani, K. E., Lopez, I. P., & Williams, V. A. (2008, Feb). Hearing and balance screening and referrals for Medicare patients: A national survey of primary care physicians. *Journal of the American Academy of Audiology, 19*, 171–190

Johnson, C. E., Newman, C. W., Danhauer, J. L., & Williams, V. A. (2009, Sep). Eye on the elderly. Screening for hearing loss, risk of falls: A hassle-free approach. *The Journal of Family Practice, 58*, 471–477

Jones, R. M., Woolf, S. H., Cunningham, T. D., Johnson, R. E., Krist, A. H., Rothemich, S. F., et al. (2010, May). The relative importance of patient-reported barriers to colorectal cancer screening. *American Journal of Preventive Medicine, 38*(5, Issue 5), 499–507

Kochkin, S. (2005). MarkeTrakVII: Hearing loss population tops 31 million people. *Hearing Review, 12*, 16–29

Kochkin, S. (2009). MarkeTrak VIII: 25-Year trends in the hearing health market. *Hearing Review. 16*, 12–31

Krist, A., & McCormally, T. (2008). What to do with abnormal screening test results. In S. Woolf, S. Jonas, & E. Kaplan-Liss (Eds.), *Health promotion and disease prevention in clinical practice* (2nd ed.). Baltimore: Lippincott Williams & Wilkins

Kuehn, B. M. (2010, May). Primary care screening and intervention helps prevent falls among elderly. *Journal of the American Medical Association, 303*, 2019–2020

Lichtenstein, M. J., Bess, F. H., & Logan, S. A. (1988, May). Validation of screening tools for identifying hearing-impaired elderly in primary care. *Journal of the American Medical Association, 259*, 2875–2878

Lin, F. R., Metter, E. J., O'Brien, R. J., Resnick, S. M., Zonderman, A. B., & Ferrucci, L. (2011, Feb). Hearing loss and incident dementia. *Archives of Neurology, 68*, 214–220

Liu, C. F., Collins, M. P., Souza, P. E., & Yueh, B. (2011). Long-term cost-effectiveness of screening strategies for hearing loss. *Journal of Rehabilitation Research and Development, 48*, 235–243

Maciosek, M. V., Coffield, A. B., Edwards, N. M., Flottemesch, T. J., Goodman, M. J., & Solberg, L. I. (2006, Jul). Priorities among effective clinical preventive services: Results of a systematic review and analysis. *American Journal of Preventive Medicine, 31*, 52–61.

Markle-Reid, M., Keller, H., & Browne, G. (2010). Health promotion for the community-living older adult. In H. Fillit, K. Rockwood, & K. Woodhouse (Eds.), *Brockelhurst's textbook of geriatric medicine and gerontology* (7th ed.). Philadelphia: Saunders Elsevier

Mathers, C., Smith, A., & Concha, M. (2003). Global burden of hearing loss in the year 2000 [Internet]. In World health report 2001. Mental health: New understanding. Geneva: World Health Organization. http://www.who.int/healthinfo/statistics/bod_hearingloss.pdf

Mathers, C., Smith, A., & Concha, M. (2009). *Global burden of hearing loss in the year 2000 [PDF-95 KB]. Health statistics and health information systems: the global burden of disease (GBD).* Geneva: World Health Organization

Mathers, C., Stein, C., Ma Fat, D., Rao, C., Inoue, M., Tomijima, N., et al. (2002). *The global burden of disease 2000 study (version 2): Methods and results (GPE discussion paper No. 50).* Geneva: Global Program on Evidence for Health Policy, World Health Organization

Mazzuca, S. A. (1982). Does patient education in chronic disease have therapeutic value? *Journal of Chronic Diseases, 35*, 521–529

McBride, W., Aguilar, C., Mulrow, C., & Tuley, M. (1990). Screening tests for hearing loss in the elderly. *Clinical Research, 38*, 707A

Medicare. (2012). *Welcome to medicare preventive visit.* http://www.medicare.gov/navigation/manage-your-health/preventive-services/medicare-physical-exam.aspx

Miller, W., & Rollnick, S. (2002). *Motivational interviewing: Preparing people for change.* New York: Guilford

Milstein, D., & Weinstein, B. (2008). Hearing screening for older adults using hearing questionnaires. *Clinical Geriatrics.* http://www.clinicalgeriatrics.com/articles/hearing-screening-older-adults-using-hearing-questionnaires?page=0,0

Mitchell, A., & Coyne, J. (2010). *Screening for depression in clinical practice: An evidence-based guide.* New York: Oxford University Press

Mulrow, C. D., Aguilar, C., Endicott, J. E., Tuley, M. R., Velez, R., Charlip, W. S., et al. (1990, Aug). Quality-of-life changes and hearing impairment. A randomized trial. *Annals of Internal Medicine, 113*, 188–194

Mulrow, C. D., & Lichtenstein, M. J. (1991, May-Jun). Screening for hearing impairment in the elderly: Rationale and strategy. *Journal of General Internal Medicine, 6*, 249–258

National Center for Health Statistics. (2001). Healthy People 2000 Final Review. Hyattsville, Maryland.

Nicoletti, B. (2008). Reimbursement for clinical preventive services. In S. Woolf, S. Jonas, & E. Kaplan-Liss (Eds.), *Health promotion and disease prevention in clinical practice* (2nd ed.). Baltimore: Lippincott Williams & Wilkins

Nimalasuriya, K., Compton, M. T., & Guillory, V. J.; Prevention Practice Committee of the American College of Preventive Medicine. (2009, Oct). Screening adults for depression in primary care: A position statement of the American College of Preventive Medicine. *Journal of Family Practice, 58*, 535–538

Noh, S., Gagne, J. P., & Kaspar, V. (1994). Models of health behaviors and compliance: Applications to audiological rehabilitation research. In J.P. Gagne & N. Tye-Murray (Eds.), Research in audiological rehabilitation: Current trends and future directions. *Journal of the American Academy of Rehabilitative Audiology, Monograph Supplement, 27*, 375–389

Pacala, J. (2010). Preventive and anticipatory care. In H. Fillit, K. Rockwood, & K. Woodhouse (Eds.), *Brockelhurst's textbook of geriatric medicine and gerontology* (7th ed.). Philadelphia: Saunders Elsevier

Prochaska, J. O., DiClemente, C. C., & Norcross, J. C. (1992, Sep). In search of how people change. Applications to addictive behaviors. *American Psychologist, 47*, 1102–1114

Rob, B., Vinod, A., Monica, P., Balraj, A., Job, A., Norman, G., et al. (2009). Costs and health effects of screening and delivery of hearing aids in Tamil Nadu, India: An observational study. *BMC Public Health, 9*, 135 http://www.ncbi.nlm.nih.gov/pmc/articles/PMC2695455/

Rubenstein, L. Z. (2006, Sep). Falls in older people: Epidemiology, risk factors and strategies for prevention. *Age and Ageing, 35*(Suppl 2), ii37–ii41

Sackett, D., Haynes, R., & Tugwell, P. (1985). *Clinical epidemiology: A basic science for clinical medicine.* Boston: Little, Brown

U.K. National Screening Committee. (2012). *U.K. screening portal.* http://www.screening.nhs.uk/screening

U.S. Department of Health and Human Services. (1994). *The clinician's handbook of preventive services.* Alexandria: International Medical Publishing

U.S. Preventive Services Task Force. (1996). Screening for hearing impairment in older adults. In *Guide to clinical preventive services* (2nd ed., pp. 393–405). Washington, DC: Department of Health and Human Services

U.S. Preventive Services Task Force. (2009). *Guide to clinical preventive services, 2009.* Agency for Healthcare Research and Quality Publication No. 09–IP006. Rockville, MD: AHRQ. http://www.ahrq.gov/clinic/pocketgd.htm

U.S. Preventive Services Task Force. (2011). *Focus on older adults.* http://www.uspreventiveservicestaskforce.org/tfolderfocus.htm#opp

U.S. Preventive Services Task Force. (2102). Screening for hearing loss in older adults. http://www.uspreventiveservicestaskforce.org/uspstf/uspshear.htm

Ventry, I. M., & Weinstein, B. E. (1983, Jul). Identification of elderly people with hearing problems. *American Speech-Language-Hearing Association, 25*, 37–42

Vogt, H. B., & Kapp, C. (1987, Mar). Patient education in primary care practice. Tips on planning a workable in-office program. *Postgraduate Medicine, 81,* 273–278

Walden, T. (2011). *Academy responds to USPSTF.* http://www.audiology.org/news/Pages/20111220a.aspx

Wallhagen, M. I., & Pettengill, E. (2008, Feb). Hearing impairment: Significant but underassessed in primary care settings. *Journal of Gerontological Nursing, 34,* 36–42

Weinstein, B. (1992). Hearing screening in the elderly: What to do? *American Speech-Language-Hearing Association Reports, 21,* 112–114

Weinstein, B. (2011). Screening for otologic functional impairments in the elderly: Whose job is it anyway? *Audiology Research, 1,* 42–48

Whitlock, E. P., Orleans, C. T., Pender, N., & Allan, J. (2002, May). Evaluating primary care behavioral counseling interventions: An evidence-based approach. *American Journal of Preventive Medicine, 22,* 267–284

Wolf, M. S., Gazmararian, J. A., & Baker, D. W. (2005, Sep). Health literacy and functional health status among older adults. *Archives of Internal Medicine, 165,* 1946–1952

Woolf, S. H. (2009, Feb). A closer look at the economic argument for disease prevention. *Journal of the American Medical Association, 301,* 536–538

Woolf, S., Jonas, S., Lawrence, R., & Kaplan-Liss, E. (2008). *Health promotion and disease prevention in clinical practice.* Philadelphia. Walters Kluwer/Lippincott Williams & Wilkins

World Health Organization. (2004). *WHO Guidelines for hearing aids and services for developing countries,* vol. 2. Geneva: World Health Organization

Wu, H. Y., Chin, J. J., & Tong, H. M. (2004, Feb). Screening for hearing impairment in a cohort of elderly patients attending a hospital geriatric medicine service. *Singapore Medical Journal, 45,* 79–84

Yueh, B., Collins, M. P., Souza, P. E., Boyko, E. J., Loovis, C. F., Heagerty, P. J., et al. (2010, Mar). Long-term effectiveness of screening for hearing loss: The screening for auditory impairment—which hearing assessment test (SAI-WHAT) randomized trial. *Journal of the American Geriatrics Society, 58,* 427–434

Yueh, B., Collins, M. P., Souza, P. E., Heagerty, P. J., Liu, C. F., Boyko, E. J., et al. (2007, May). Screening for Auditory Impairment-Which Hearing Assessment Test (SAI-WHAT): RCT design and baseline characteristics. *Contemporary Clinical Trials, 28,* 303–315

Yueh, B., Shapiro, N., MacLean, C. H., & Shekelle, P. G. (2003, Apr). Screening and management of adult hearing loss in primary care: Scientific review. *Journal of the American Medical Association, 289,* 1976–1985.

Chapter 10

Primary Care Physicians and Audiologists: Partners in Care

Your mom, Mrs. Jones, does not need a hearing aid. She is doing fine without it.

> *–Dr. Smith's response to family members who are concerned that their mother is no longer participating in family conversations*

Your dad appeared a little confused and at first he did not respond appropriately to the questions I asked regarding routine matters. I then used this little amplifier I recently read about and his responses were accurate. I suggest that you make an appointment with a hearing-aid specialist to see if he could benefit from one of the new technologies on the market.

> *—A primary care physician, in response to the question regarding to whom a family should take their father, suggesting that an audiologist would be good but a hearing instrument specialist would probably be fine as well*

The elderly. They are the future.

> *—Brooks (2010)*

The profound, pervasive, and enduring consequences of population ageing present enormous opportunities as well as enormous challenges for all societies.

> *—World Population Ageing 1950–2050 (2002)*

◆ Learning Objectives

After reading this chapter, you should be able to

- ◆ recognize the value of educating primary care physicians regarding hearing and balance problems in the elderly;
- ◆ prepare informative material to share with primary care physicians regarding how and why to screen for hearing, tinnitus, and balance problems in the elderly, and how to communicate with the hearing impaired; and
- ◆ understand the importance of sharing with the primary care physician signs and symptoms of hearing and balance problems in the elderly.

◆ Overview

Most physicians and health care professionals will be caring for older adults at some point, irrespective of their specialty (Eleazer & Brummel-Smith, 2009). Competencies in most practice areas and in the delivery of humane and compassionate care are critical to the delivery of services to older adults. Adequate and effective communication are at the heart of service delivery, and the audiologist plays a key role in this domain. Although good communication skills are essential when caring for older adults, several studies have shown that patients, especially those who are very ill, are not satisfied with their encounters with physicians, especially when it comes to communicating bad news, such as a diagnosis of cancer, or when discussing advanced directives and other sensitive issues (Bishop & Morrison, 2007).

Knowing how to communicate with older adults and focusing on prevention, including identifying conditions that threaten functional capacity, such as hearing loss and vestibular dysfunction, should be a priority for health care professionals. This chapter addresses the importance of working collaboratively with primary care physicians (PCPs), geriatricians, and others who work with older adults to ensure that they have the knowledge and skill set necessary to assist audiologists in identifying older adults at risk for hearing loss and for falls that are associated with vestibular dysfunction, so that we can reduce disability and promote healthy aging and well-being. I believe that collaborating with physicians will help remedy the findings that most adults wait ~10 years before pursing audiological intervention and that 25 to 40% of hearing-aid users stop using them. To this end, I first review some modern principles of adult learning that I believe should serve as a guide when developing curricula or hearing health care clinical practice guidelines for use by physicians.

◆ Adult Learning Principles

There are several approaches to teaching and learning that have an impact on a physician's knowledge base, attitudes, and skill set (Khan & Coomarasamy, 2006). In an effort to promote implementation of our educational interventions with physicians, let's begin by discussing a simple philosophy that can inform the educational strategies we use when working with adult learners such as physicians. Simply put, to ensure that physicians will apply the hearing health care knowledge and skills we hope to impart, they must adopt a positive attitude regarding the relevance of this information to clinical outcomes and patient health gains (Khan & Coomarasamy, 2006). Hence, we must always keep this goal in mind when developing an educational curriculum! Stated differently, the educational strategies we adopt should be dictated by our educational objectives, which include improvement of patient care and outcomes of care for older adults at risk for hearing impairment and falls. Borrowing from the medical literature (Grimshaw & Russell, 1994), our goal is to foster awareness, knowledge, and positive attitudes about these issues and to encourage physicians to address these issues in their practice. This might entail changing physicians' behavior (i.e., transferring learning to the workplace, applying new knowledge), and possibly changing guidelines for delivery of care to the elderly (e.g., face the patient when taking a history), which can result in improving the well-being of the patient (Khan & Coomarasamy, 2006).

But PCPs have busy practices and limited time, which means that the material we provide must be practical, concise, relevant, and goal oriented (Lieb, 2009). The educational activities we propose should enable physicians to be active participants, and the learning process should be interactive and learner centered, and should use multiple strategies. Thus, the key word is *participatory,* as interactivity helps to maintain interest and is proven to be an effective approach to continuing medical education (CME). I reviewed selected studies on the efficacy of interactive workshops and found that the evidence supports the idea that interactive workshops can improve education and patient outcomes (Khan & Coomarasamy, 2006). Ockene and Zapka (2000) suggest that our challenge is to balance the need to enhance knowledge and awareness about hearing health care, on the one hand, with attitudes and skills on the other hand, always keeping in mind that physicians have competing demands and time constraints. Clinically based E-learning modules can be used to effectively deliver complex and multilayered information to physicians. These modules should include clinical contexts, as the literature suggests that acquisition of knowledge and skills is enhanced using real clinical problems rather than hypothetical cases. Integrated interactive learning reinforces the acquired skills; can be done independently, allowing the users to set their own pace; and enables physicians to delve into the material as extensively as they wish. According to Khan and Coomarasamy (2006) elements of CME that enhance the value of learning and, ultimately, patient outcomes should be considered when designing courses on hearing health care. Some critical elements of learning are listed in **Table 10.1**.

We must consider cognitive issues and attitudes in fostering skill development (e.g., demonstrations and hands-on learning) to ensure that physicians absorb the information about hearing loss and falls and incorporate it into their practice, with the understanding that this new knowledge will help them in their efforts to promote quality of care and the well-being of their patients. Because of physicians' time constraints, educational outreach efforts must focus on important issues. Also, educational materials should use familiar language, so that extra reading and research is unnecessary, and should be delivered in a familiar context, such as a CME course or as part of grand rounds (Johnson et al, 2008).

Table 10.1 Critical Adult Learning Principles and Elements of Continuing Medical Education

Element	Importance
Motivation	Adults are only motivated to learn when they recognize the importance of the material to the work they do, and if they receive specific feedback or see a reward for learning the material (e.g., easier to communicate with the patient); learner needs must be taken in to account
Reinforcement	Positive reinforcement should be used during the practical hands-on sessions, as this is key to behavior change
Retention	The degree to which the adult learner will apply what is learned in class is directly related to how well they learned the material in the first place; clinical contexts, interactive approaches, and multifaceted strategies promote retention
Transference	The ability to use the information taught in the course in daily practice; physicians must see that the content of the course will benefit them pragmatically so they will readily incorporate the information into daily practice
Self-assessment	Courses should provide feedback and the opportunity to self-assess

Sources: Data from Lieb, S. (2009). *Principles of adult learning.* http://honolulu.hawaii.edu/intranet/committees/FacDevCom/guidebk/teachtip/adults-2.htm; and Khan, K. S., & Coomarasamy, A. (2006). A hierarchy of effective teaching and learning to acquire competence in evidenced-based medicine. *BMC Medical Education, 6,* 59.

Pearl

A nonstressful, nonjudgmental, engaging learning environment is key.

The Healthy People 2020 vision statement provides a framework for care of older adults with compromised sensory function. It addresses the health of the nation, with the goal being a society in which "all people live long, healthy lives" (Department of Health and Human Services [DHHS], 2008). An overarching element of Health People 2020 is health promotion and disease prevention activities aimed at reducing the likelihood that a condition will affect an individual and slowing down the progress of a disorder so as to minimize the potential disability. Here partnerships are key, with the goal being to reduce barriers to health care. Collaboration is important if persons at risk for chronic health problems are to be identified and treated early so that the burden of illness is reduced. Integral to the achievement of the goals set forth in Healthy People 2020 is effective communication between health care workers and patients and their families. Adequate communication is critical to accurate diagnosis and adherence to treatment. Interventions designed to promote health-related quality of life require that the patient partner with the health care system to achieve the desired outcomes. The patient's ability to hear and process what is being communicated is a key factor in successful interventions. Thus, audiologists have an important role to play in ensuring that untreated or unrecognized hearing loss does not compromise the goals of the intervention.

Be it in the office or at the bedside, effective communication figures prominently in the delivery of quality health care. Across the health care continuum, from diagnosis to treatment, from emergency room to palliative care, from the intensive care unit to the home, adequate communication is central to positive outcomes and patient compliance. The information that the PCP shares with the patient is lost if the patient is unable to process it. Not only do patient outcomes improve when barriers to communication are removed, but also physicians find that their job is easier and more fulfilling when the patient–physician interaction is improved. Hence, an important role for audiologists from the outset is advocacy and collaboration. To this end, this chapter discusses the essential information that audiologists should communicate to improve health equity for individuals with hearing and balance problems.

Facts to Share: Prevalence Data and Burden of Condition

Hearing impairment, the most frequent sensory deficit in humans, is a chronic condition recently recognized as a major public health problem. Over 250 million people worldwide are affected, with close to 10 million Americans over the age of 65 suffering from hearing impairment. As the population ages, the prevalence continues to increase, so that by the year 2030 nearly 21 million Americans over the age of 65 are projected to have some degree of hearing impairment (Stewart & Wingfield, 2009). Currently, 30% of the population over 65 years of age is hearing impaired, rising to 40 to 50% among persons older 75 years, and to more than 80% in persons over 85 years of age. Nearly half of the 76 million baby boomers (born between 1946 and 1964) in the United States have experienced some degree of hearing loss. The risk of experiencing a hearing loss increases dramatically with each additional decade. Self-reported hearing problems are less prevalent among persons of Asian and African descent than among whites or Native Americans. In addition to ethnicity and race, gender and baseline hearing thresholds play a role in hearing loss progression and severity (Kochkin & Marketrak, 2007). The high prevalence of hearing impairment among persons over 85 years has implications for home health care, nursing home care, and end-of-life care, as the majority of recipients of these types of care are over 85 years of age.

Risk factors for peripheral hearing loss include a history of stroke, cardiovascular disease, diabetes, smoking, and hypertension. Interestingly, there is evidence that the presence of hearing loss increases one's risk of falls, and an untreated hearing loss can exacerbate depressive symptoms and cognitive abnormalities. Dual sensory impairments are prevalent among older adults as well. Of persons over 70 years of age, 18% are reportedly blind in one or both eyes, 33% report experiencing hearing problems, and ~10% report concurrent hearing and visual problems (Lam, Lee, Gómez-Marín, Zheng, & Caban, 2006). Crews and Campbell (2004) found that the likelihood of comorbid and secondary conditions was greater in older adults with dual sensory impairment than in those with either a hear-

ing or a vision problem. Specifically, persons with dual sensory impairment were three times more likely to have fallen in the past month and were two times more likely to have broken a hip. Also, adult-onset hearing loss in excess of 40 dB HL contributes to the global burden of disease, such that it represents the second leading cause of disability worldwide, after depression (Mathers, Smith, & Concha, 2003).

Unstable balance and falls also increase in prevalence as people age (Agrawal, Carey, Della Santina, Schubert, & Minor, 2009; Johnson et al, 2008; Rubenstein, 2006). One third of community-dwelling adults 65+ years of age and 50% of adults 80+ years of age have fallen; 10 to 20% of these individuals have multiple falls, and up to 10% of community-dwelling elders suffer major consequences from falls, including fracture (e.g., hip fracture), head injury, severe laceration, and joint dislocation. Falls, occurring in 30 to 60% of older adults annually, contribute substantially to rates of mortality and to premature nursing home placement (Rubenstein, 2006). The leading causes of falls include environmental factors, gait/balance disturbance, and dizziness/vertigo, with the latter two having many etiologies and comorbidities including hearing loss (Rubenstein, 2006). Risk factors include individual deficits, cognitive impairment, confirmed hearing impairment, and impaired functional status.

As the sensation of dizziness, which often leads to falls, is highly prevalent among people over the age of 65 (it is present in 50% of older adults), it is not surprising that dizziness symptom accounts for 8 million PCP visits in the United States. Agrawal et al (2009) have noted a link between vestibular dysfunction and risk of falling, underscoring the importance of diagnosing vestibular deficits in older adults with the goal being to reduce the burden of fall-related injuries. As most falls are associated with identifiable risk factors (e.g., weakness, unsteady gait, dizziness) and because evidence suggests that detection and amelioration of risk factors can significantly reduce the rate of future falls, audiologists have an important role to play in educating physicians about risk factors and offering techniques for identifying those at risk for vestibular disturbance and falls (Rubenstein, 2006).

Tinnitus prevalence rates are in the range of 4 to 19% worldwide among older adults. The prevalence of tinnitus rises with age, and age-related hearing loss is a major predictive factor. The prevalence of tinnitus varies by gender, race, definition, and general physical well-being. Men are affected more often than women of the same age group and race. Tinnitus prevalence in hearing-impaired patients is 75 to 80%; 10% of adults were reported to suffered tinnitus for longer than 5 minutes; 1% were severely annoyed as a result of their tinnitus, and 0.05% suffered from the most extremely severe tinnitus that prevented them from leading a normal life (Ahmad & Seidman, 2004). Tinnitus is more often reported in Caucasians than in African Americans (9% versus 5.5%). Individuals with hearing loss have a higher prevalence of tinnitus than do those not reporting hearing loss, and military veterans experience tinnitus more often than do individuals in the general population, most likely due to the co-occurrence of noise exposure and corresponding hearing loss. Tinnitus of unknown origin has been observed to occur in patients suffering with comorbidities such as hyperinsulinemia, diabetes mellitus, and hyperlip-

Table 10.2 Medical Causes of Tinnitus

Noise-induced hearing loss
Hearing loss associated with the aging process (presbycusis)
Temporal mandibular joint (TMJ) dysfunction
Head injury: transverse or longitudinal fracture
Lightning strike
Diseases of the inner ear, including Meniere's disease, inflammatory disorders such as arthritis, metabolic diseases, and neurological disease such as multiple sclerosis or eighth nerve tumor
Diseases of the middle ear, including otosclerosis
Selected medications including antidepressants, salicylates, and antiinflammatory agents
Depression
Kidney disease

Table 10.3 Sequelae of Tinnitus in Older Adults

Sleep disturbance
Difficulty concentrating
Depression
Anxiety
Inability to relax
Interference with work
Inability to cope
Unhappiness, distress
Tension, stress
Irritability, nervousness
Fatigue
Reduced sense of control
Poor sleep, difficulty in everyday functioning, or a reduced quality of life
People who are depressed have high incidence of tinnitus
Medications trigger tinnitus

Source: Data from Meikle, M. B., Stewart, B. J., Griest, S. E., & Henry, J. A. (2008, Sep). Tinnitus outcomes assessment. *Trends in Amplification, 12,* 223–235.

idemia, and more so in population older than 40 years of age (Kaźmierczak & Doroszewska, 2001).

Tinnitus is a serious enough problem for close to 20% of sufferers that they seek medical attention. It is potentially debilitating in ~10% of people who experience it. Physicians should understand that tinnitus is a symptom of a variety of disorders, some serious, some transient, and the patient should not be dismissed without a complete evaluation (Nondahl et al, 2002). It is important for physicians to understand that there are a variety of ways in which patients describe tinnitus, ranging from ringing to hissing, buzzing, or crackling, and that often the description assists in the diagnosis. Thus, although the most common descriptors include a high-pitched ringing, physicians should ask the patient to describe the tinnitus carefully. Selected medical causes of tinnitus are listed in **Table 10.2.**

From the perspective of tinnitus sufferers, physicians should know that dismissing the symptoms without doing a thorough assessment and without making a referral, and saying there is nothing that can be done, is a cause for dismay. A referral to an audiologist as part of a diagnostic workup is an excellent way for physicians to partner with audiologists. The physician should be aware that audiologists can assist in diagnosis as well as management of tinnitus. Hence, audiologists should make sure physicians understand the approaches to diagnosis and management, with emphasis on evidence-based specific management strategies for tinnitus. Physicians should be informed that some audiologists work extensively with tinnitus patients, so it is incumbent on the audiologist to recommend these proven specialists. A possible inducement to encouraging physicians to make appropriate referrals when a patient complains of tinnitus should be a discussion of the evidence regarding advances in tinnitus management and corresponding improvements in treatment outcome. It is important to underscore that the extent of the benefit and the nature of the benefit will depend in large part on the nature of the tinnitus; thus, patients with chronic intractable tinnitus can expect only small clinical improvements, whereas those with tinnitus due to an underlying medical condition may experience complete resolution as a result of medical intervention. It is also important that physicians understand the multidimensional nature of tinnitus and that interventions are more likely to remedy the functional (e.g., inability to sleep) and emotional domains (e.g., inability to concentrate). **Table 10.3** lists some of the nega-

tive effects of tinnitus; this list should be shared with physicians to ensure that they do not minimize the patient's complaints (Meikle, Stewart, Griest, & Henry, 2008).

Pearl

With hearing or balance problems, it is critical that audiologists educate PCPs about hearing and balance problems, and their etiology, ramifications, and treatment, to promote quality of care. PCPs have a responsibility to identify and refer older adults.

Despite the high prevalence of hearing loss among persons aged 65 years or older, the accompanying symptoms, and the threat that unidentified and untreated otological conditions poses to effective communication, quality of life and care, the majority of PCPs do not screen older adults for hearing loss and balance function, nor do they typically refer for an audiological evaluation or for consideration of a hearing aid (Danhauer, Celani, & Johnson, 2008). While the U.S. Preventive Services Task force (2012ab) concluded that the current evidence is insufficient to assess the value of screening for hearing loss in asymptomatic adults aged 50 years or older and does not recommend performing in depth risk assessment with management of identified risks to prevent falls in community dwelling adults 65 years of age and older, I feel discussing screening with physicians is an obligation we have to our patients. Hence, in this chapter I propose an approach to screening older adults for otologic functional impairments which should be included in any curriculum geared to population of health professionals.

◆ Age-Related Changes in the Auditory System

Any in-service or pre-service training about hearing loss and vestibular dysfunction must include a basic primer on the parts of the ear, with emphasis on those systems most affected by the aging process. Accordingly, the outer and middle ears should receive less emphasis than the inner ear and auditory pathways. From the outset it is important to emphasize that although within the peripheral auditory system the inner ear and central auditory pathways are most vulnerable to aging effects, the outer and middle ear undergo alterations as well. It is important to emphasize that even though the latter changes do not have a dramatic effect on the transmission of sound energy, they are of relevance because of their functional implications. Other issues to emphasize, in addition to the basic anatomy and the functions of the outer and middle ear, are discussed below.

Outer and Middle Ear Functional Changes and Treatable Conditions: Factoids

The glandular structure within the ear canal, most notably the sebaceous and cerumen glands, lose some of their secretory ability. A decrease in the fat present in the ear canal and an increase in the thickness and length of hair follicles in the fibrocartilaginous portion of the canal are commonplace changes with age as well. Additionally, failure of the self-cleaning mechanism that automatically expels cerumen/earwax, a naturally occurring substance that cleans, protects, and lubricates the external auditory canal, is common in older adults and accounts in part for the high prevalence of cerumen impaction. Interestingly, cerumen impaction is also more common in those with cognitive impairment and in individuals in nursing homes (Rawool & Harrington, 2007). As a result of the above physiological changes, the skin in the external ear canal becomes dry, and prone to trauma and breakdown, and cerumen tends to become more concentrated, hard, and thus impacted. One of the functional implications of an excessive buildup of cerumen is that a common cause of hearing-aid malfunction is the physical obstruction of the tubing, dome, and earmold that deliver amplified sound to the ear. An additional consequence of gradual cerumen buildup is constriction of the ear canal, which leads to a blockage of the sound-conducting mechanism and is associated with a conductive hearing loss. More than 33% (estimates range from 19 to 65%) of adults over 65 years of age, close to 12 million people, present with excessive or impacted cerumen that requires removal (Rawool & Harrington, 2007; Roland et al, 2008).

Individuals with osteoarthritis and no family history of hearing loss, noise exposure, or chronic middle ear effusion had a higher prevalence of middle ear abnormalities and of sensorineural hearing loss (associated with degenerative changes in the inner ear) than did an age-matched control group without arthritis (Tinetti et al, 2008). As arthritis is a prevalent chronic condition for which potentially ototoxic medications are prescribed, it is important to emphasize that physicians should screen the hearing of individuals with osteoarthritis routinely after age 65, despite the fact that the U.S. Preventive Services Task Force does not recommend routine hearing screening of asymptomatic older adults. As pertains to the middle ear, aging may cause hardening or calcification of the cartilaginous portion of the eustachian tube and atrophy of the tensor veli palatine (TVP) muscle that attaches to the eustachian tube, which in turn may lead to eustachian tube dysfunction (ETD) in older adults.

Smoking, be it passive or active, increases the risk of ETD and possible otitis media with effusion. The propensity for dysfunction and disease is exacerbated by age. Radiotherapy for nasopharyngeal carcinoma may cause ETD. Also, PCPs must be alerted to the connection between ETD and middle ear effusion. Head trauma from a blow to the head sustained from a fall can result in longitudinal fracture of the temporal bone and resulting conductive hearing loss. Motor vehicle accidents, to which older adults tend to be susceptible, can also result in head trauma. Doctors should be reminded to ask patients who have fallen or sustained a blow to the head if they recall where they may have hit their head and, if they did, whether they noted bleeding from the ear, which is a symptom of a longitudinal fracture typically associated with conductive hearing loss, facial dysfunction/paralysis, and vertigo; therefore, it is important to emphasize that these patients should be referred to an otolaryngologist or audiologist to rule in or out hearing loss that has the potential to be treated medically.

The Inner Ear and Auditory Pathways: Anatomical Changes and Auditory Implications

The most critical risk factor for the auditory sense organ, namely the organ of Corti, is age-related histopathological changes. Specifically, the sensory, neural, vascular, and supporting synaptic and mechanical structures within the peripheral and central auditory systems are especially vulnerable to the aging effects. Accordingly, from the outset, it is imperative to emphasize that the inner ear is composed of several functional components that are responsible for both hearing and balance, as physicians often do not associate audiology with vestibular dysfunction and the attendant consequences. The discussion should include a distinction between the role of the peripheral auditory system (responsible for detecting, encoding, and transduction of acoustic stimuli), which is composed of the auditory brainstem pathways responsible for neural transmission feature extraction and perception, and the role of the cortex, which subserves the functions of information processing labeling, storage, and retrieval of information. It should be emphasized that various frequencies are registered in different parts of the cochlea, and that this is the basis for the tonotopic organization of the auditory system. A discussion about tonotopicity can help physicians understanding the effect of sensorineural hearing loss on speech reception and perception.

It is important to inform PCPs that histological studies of the peripheral and central auditory nervous system suggest that while in many individuals changes predominate throughout the periphery, along the auditory brainstem pathways, and in the auditory cortex, they are not universal across individuals, nor are they universal across the nuclei or tracts within the auditory brainstem. The implications of the changes within the central auditory nervous system are profound; most notably, speech understanding in less than optimal listening conditions is compromised. The locus of the degenerative changes determines the functional effects of the physiological changes. Simulations or demonstrations of hearing loss can be found on the Phonak Website (http://www.Phonak.com/us/b2c/en/hearing/understanding_hearingloss/how_hearing_loss_sounds.html), and a cochlear hearing loss simulator is included with hearing-aid fitting software (http://www.audioscan.com/webpages/innovation.thm); these simulations are helpful in that they provide a feel for the sounds that a hearing loss renders inaudible.

Physicians should understand the distinction among the peripheral, central, and cognitive hypotheses that attempt to explain the difficulties older adults' experience. In terms of the peripheral hypothesis, emphasis should be placed on the loss of audibility associated with cochlear pathology and decrements in hearing high-frequency sounds, which results in difficulty understanding speech in quiet and in the presence of steady-state noise. Central auditory processing dysfunction (CAPD) is prevalent among older adults, and peripheral hearing loss is not necessarily a predictor of central auditory processing challenges. CAPD implies that individuals will have substantial difficulty understanding in the presence of auditory stressors such as competing noise and reverberation. One example to use is the cocktail party effect, in which older adults have difficulty following one conversation when there are several competing conversations taking place (Gates, Anderson, Feeney, McCurry, & Larson, 2008). Emphasize that there is evidence that CAPD can compromise the benefit derived from hearing aids in a previously satisfied hearing-aid user, necessitating further testing and possible modifications to the intervention. Further, the fact that CAPD has been identified as a possible precursor to cognitive decline is being explored should be addressed (Gates et al, 2008).

Physicians should understand that cognitive processing refers to how people acquire, store, manipulate, and use information, and that age-related changes have an impact on selected aspects of cognitive function that are important for understanding, including memory, attention, and speed of processing. Specifically, age limits the amount of new information and the rate at which it is acquired (processing speed), stored, manipulated, and used. Age impacts the amount of information one can remember while communicating, the amount of information that can be processed, and the speed with which new information can be processed. Age also impacts attention, such that there is a decrease in attentional capacity and understanding in less than ideal listening environments when the message is degraded by the speaker or the listening environment. Hence, older adults have difficulty keeping up with rapid speech and degraded input, and this may or may not be associated with peripheral hearing loss. Providing the foundations regarding speech understanding can help physicians understand why they must modify how they communicate to ensure that their older patients absorb what is being communicated. The case scenario in Appendix 10.1 highlights some of the cognitive and processing problems that are the hallmark of hearing loss in older adults; audiological interventions can be designed to address the decrements in speech understanding that attend the changes throughout the auditory system.

Additional Causes or Risk Factors for Hearing Impairment in the Elderly

It is critical from the outset that physicians understand the distinction between presbycusic changes in hearing associated with age-related changes in the auditory system, which occur within the peripheral and central systems, and hearing loss due to ototrauma, such as noise or ototoxic medications. Physicians should also know the medical conditions so prevalent in older adults that tend to have an auditory component, including diabetes, kidney disease, cardiovascular disease, cognitive deficits, osteoarthritis, and depression (Bainbridge, Hoffman, & Cowie, 2008). Points to emphasize are the data suggesting that type 2 diabetics experience significant impairments in hearing sensitivity and speech understanding relative to age- and gender-matched nondiabetics. Further, hearing impairment is more prevalent among adults with diabetes, and the association is independent of such risk factors for hearing loss as noise exposure, ototoxic medication use, and smoking (Disogra, 2008). Specifically, the prevalence of hearing impairment is higher among persons with diabetes (21%) than in those adults who do not have diabetes (9%) (Bainbridge et al, 2008). Also, older adults with hypothyroidism experience impaired speech understanding and reductions in audibility for pure-tone signals.

Adverse drug reactions (ADRs) in the form of auditory or vestibular symptoms are quite prevalent among older adults and are known to be more severe among older adults (Agrawal, Platz, & Niparko, 2008). ADRs in older adults occur for a variety of reasons, including lack of compliance due to compromised understanding of the prescription attributable to hearing or visual problems or possibly because of confusion between two medications that might sound alike (e.g., Plavix or Paxil) to a hearing-impaired person or may look alike to a visually impaired older adult. Some of the auditory or vestibular side effects of medications frequently prescribed for older adults include dizziness, ear discomfort, lightheadedness, vertigo, bilateral hearing loss that is often profound and delayed in onset, and tinnitus. Similarly, performance on selected electrophysiological tests conducted by audiologists are affected by selected medications, so it is important to inform physicians that they much instruct patients to stop taking selected medications prior to vestibular studies. It is important to underscore that in light of the variety of medical conditions associated with hearing loss that are prevalent among older adults, individuals presenting with any of the above conditions should be screened for hearing impairment and associated tinnitus. Finally, highlight that affective disorders, such as depression, and cognitive disorders, such as senile dementia of the Alzheimer's type, are also associated with sensorineural hearing loss, and the prevalence of hearing loss is higher among persons with dementia than among those without it.

In addition, inattention or confusion related to depression or dementia may give the impression of significant hearing loss and should be considered in a systematic geriatric assessment. Physicians must understand that when conducting assessment of mental status of older adults prior to surgery or during an intake, they must eliminate hearing impairment as a confounding variable in the diagnostic process. Also, as vision impairment is common among older adults as well, resulting in dual sensory loss, it is critical to discuss the fact that decreased vision or hearing acuity can interfere with reception of the spoken message, leading to communication breakdowns and possibly tainted diagnose (Heine & Browning, 2002). **Table 10.4** lists the medical conditions associated with hearing impairment.

Pearl

Hearing loss should be ruled out in individuals being worked up for cognitive or affective disorder (Appendix 10.1).

Table 10.4 Summary of Medical Conditions Associated with Hearing Loss

1. Long-term or limited use of prescribed ototoxic or otoactive medications including:
   a. Aminoglycoside antibiotics for treatment of life-threatening illnesses; e.g., neomycin, kanamycin, dihydrostreptomycin, amikacin, tobramycin, sisomicin, chemotherapeutic agents such as cisplatin and carboplatin
   b. Diuretics for treatment of congestive heart failure, renal failure, cirrhosis, and hypertension
   c. Aspirin or salicylate-containing medications that are used as antiinflammatory agents for the treatment of arthritis (reversible with cessation of the salicylate)
2. Diabetes
3. Kidney disease
4. Head trauma
5. Thyroid dysfunction,
6. HIV/AIDS: hearing loss may be the effect of ototoxic meds and/or a direct result of the disease or the opportunistic infections and tumors associated with the disease; HIV/AIDS may affect central auditory processing, leading to difficulties understanding speech in noise
7. Noise exposure
8. Metabolic conditions such as lupus
9. Vestibular dysfunction and dizziness
10. Depression
11. Senile dementia

Vestibular Dysfunction and Dizziness

Dizziness is the third most common complaint among outpatients, and is a major cause of falls in the elderly. Age-related morphological changes that take place in the vestibular system must be emphasized (Tusa, 2009). The overall prevalence of vestibular dysfunction increases markedly with age, with the prevalence being greater in persons in the "other" race/ethnicity category, which includes "other Hispanic" and multiracial (Agrawal et al, 2009). As older adults accrue comorbidities with increasing age, the prevalence of falls increases, especially among those over 80 years of age. Vestibular dysfunction is especially important in older adults given the fact that it tends to increase the propensity toward falls, which in turn leads to a multitude of health problems and to hospitalization. The data of Agrawal and colleagues from the 2001–2004 National Health and Nutrition Examination Surveys suggest that the prevalence of vestibular dysfunction varies by risk characteristic, such that heavy tobacco users, hypertensives, and diabetics have higher rates of vestibular dysfunction. Heavy smoking was not a risk factor for vestibular dysfunction, but lower educational status seems to be. Individuals with more than a high school education had lower odds of vestibular dysfunction than did those who did not attending high school (Agrawal et al, 2009). Age is the most significant risk factor for vestibular dysfunction, with the likelihood of falling being 7-fold higher in persons 80 years and older as compared with persons in their 40s. The relationship between age and falling is mediated by vestibular dysfunction such that the likelihood of falls is reduced in older adults when controlling for vestibular dysfunction. Gender did not play a role in vestibular dysfunction. The authors concluded that diagnosis of vestibular

Table 10.5 Potential Causes of Dizziness

Vestibular dysfunction associated with benign paroxysmal positional vertigo (BPPV), 21%
Fear of fall and disuse, 18%
Migraine and motion sensitivity, 14%
Vestibular loss, 14%
Anxiety/depression, 11%
Cerebellar problems, 6%
Orthostatic hypotension, 2%
Medication: antidepressants, diuretics, β-blockers, chemotherapeutic, and muscle relaxants

Source: Data from Tusa, R. (2009). Dizziness. *Medical Clinics of North America*, 263–271.

dysfunction will help to increase the diagnosis of falls and possibly reduce the burden of fall-related injury, so it is critical that etiologies of vestibular dysfunction be discussed as part of any in-service training.

Although typically undetected and underreported, the rate of falls increases with age, and falls and the experience of dizziness account for a high proportion of PCP visits, emergency department visits, and hospitalizations among older adults (Bainbridge et al, 2008). Risk factors typically mentioned for falls include visual problems, polypharmacy, cognitive deficits, hypotension, and balance problems. Rarely is hearing loss mentioned, although it is well documented that persons with diminished hearing levels have an increased risk for falls. As dizziness affects more than 50% of older adults and is the most common reason adults over age 70 go to the physician, Tusa (2009) underscores the importance of taking a complete history when older adults complain of dizziness. Key items on which physicians should focus when taking a history include the symptoms of dizziness and the circumstances in which dizziness occurs; physicians must have an appreciation for the many causes and symptoms of dizziness including vestibular dysfunction (**Tables 10.5 and 10.6**). Finally, it is also important to discuss with physicians some facts about the fear

Table 10.6 Symptoms and Circumstances Associated with Dizziness that the History Should Uncover

Symptoms
  Imbalance, unsteadiness while walking
  Lightheadedness
  Sense of rocking or swaying as if on a ship
  Sense of spinning inside of head, rocking
  Illusion of visual motion
Accompanying symptoms
  Nausea and vomiting (vestibular origin)
  Motion sickness
  Vertigo
Circumstances leading to dizziness
  Provoked by certain movement such as standing up after lying down
  Lying down
  Turning over in bed
  Moving one's eyes with head stationary (anxiety)
  Without provocation (vestibular origin)
  Exacerbated by head movement (vestibular origin)

Source: Data from Tusa, R. (2009). Dizziness. *Medical Clinics of North America*, 263–271.

of falling that is so common among older adults who have already fallen. Fear of falling is more common in women than men, increases in people with gait abnormalities and walking disorders, and can lead to dependency, depression, and a reduced quality of life.

> **Pearl**
>
> Dysequilibrium, imbalance, or unsteadiness when walking are all considered symptoms of dizziness, and it is incumbent upon PCPs to ask the patient to describe any sensation of dizziness, as this will help in achieving a definitive diagnosis.

Behavioral Implications of Anatomical and Physiological Changes

There are several factors relating to hearing impairment beyond the audiometric data that should be discussed, especially the individual variability in terms of hearing loss. The fact that not every older adult experiences hearing difficulties is a critical point, as is the fact that those older adults who do experience a challenge in terms of speech understanding may have a physiological basis for their difficulties. Physicians should also recognize that the difficulty in understanding that older adults often experience cannot be predicted from the audiogram alone, underscoring the need for a thorough evaluation that includes tests of cognitive function and tests that uncover audibility and speech-understanding problems deriving from age-related changes in the peripheral and central auditory systems. It is also important to highlight the following points:

1. Pure-tone hearing sensitivity tends to be greatest in the frequencies above 1000 Hz (e.g., sounds such as /s/, /sh/, /th/) (Russo & Pichora-Fuller, 2008).
2. The hearing loss tends to be bilateral, symmetrical, and sensorineural (due to damage to sensory cells and nerve).
3. The odds of hearing loss are higher in men than in women, and the prevalence of hearing loss is lower in blacks than in whites (Lee, Matthews, Dubno, & Mills, 2005).
4. It is often difficult to tease out the hearing loss associated exclusively with aging from that associated with noise exposure or ototoxicity.
5. Hearing loss seems to be setting in at younger ages, and the prevalence of hearing loss is increasing among individuals younger than 65 years of age (Lee et al, 2005)
6. Among residents of nursing facilities, the sensorineural hearing loss tends to be more significant, and more prevalent, affecting 70 to 80% of residents. Hearing loss is prevalent among the homebound and those receiving palliative care, as these individuals tend to be older and have a multitude of medical problems contributing to declines in hearing and understanding.
7. Speech-understanding difficulties are exacerbated in challenging acoustic environments, such as reverberant and noisy rooms.
8. Distance between the speaker and the listener can erode speech understanding.
9. Characteristics of the speaker's voice, the complexity of the message, the listener's knowledge of the language, the use of gestures, and the availability of contextual information affect speech understanding (Gates et al, 2008)
10. Speech understanding is compromised when speech is presented without the benefit of contextual information, when multiple speakers are talking, when the speaker is not nearby, and when the speaker is looking down, such as at the computer, so that facial cues will be absent.
11. Older adults benefit from hearing aids, with persons with pure-tone averages poorer than 35 dB HL deriving greater benefit from hearing aids in terms of handicap reduction than do those with pure-tone averages better than 25 dB HL, and older adults with central auditory processing dysfunction (CAPD) exhibit less benefit from hearing aids than do those without CAPD and may require hearing assistance technologies.
12. The younger the person is when purchasing hearing aids, the easier it is to adapt, and the less the effects of auditory deprivation.
13. Hearing-aid use reduces the probability that auditory deprivation effects will set in (Silverman, Silman, Emmer, Schoepflin, & Lutolf, 2006).
14. Dual sensory impairment (visual and auditory deficits) pose great risks to personal safety.

> **Pearl**
>
> The classic complaint of older adults with presbycusis, namely, "I can hear people talking but cannot understand what they saying, especially in noisy situations," very aptly describes the problems that derive from the reduction in transmission, reception, and perception of the speech signal attributable to sensorineural hearing loss.

The consequences of the degenerative changes throughout the peripheral and central auditory systems discussed above are delineated in **Table 10.7,** which can serve as a checklist of the challenges posed by hearing impairment.

Here are some examples of scenarios of patient behaviors that physicians may note that suggest that the patient has a hearing impairment with attendant consequences:

1. As you approach the patient in the waiting room, you notice the patient is speaking at a very loud level to the accompanying family member. This may be indicative of a moderate to severe sensorineural hearing loss, resulting in difficulty hearing oneself speak.
2. You are taking the case history or doing a diagnostic test for depression, and the patient provides an incorrect or unrelated answer to your question or takes a long time to answer your question.
3. You are examining the patient and listening to the heart and lungs, and you ask the patient to inhale and exhale. The patient either does not respond consistently or asks you to repeat what you have said.
4. When you are discussing your findings with the patient, he turns his ear toward you to better hear what you are saying.

Table 10.7 Implications of Physiological Changes for Hearing and Understanding

Part of the Ear	Physiological Change	Implication for Function[*]
Inner ear (cochlea)	Degenerative changes beginning in the basilar portion	• Difficulty hearing subtle sounds associated with the entry or exit of another person into the room when attention is focused elsewhere • Inability to hear weak, high-pitched sounds • Difficulty hearing subtle sounds associated with the entry or exit of another person into the room when attention is focused elsewhere • When a talker turns partly or wholly away, there is a loss of essential consonant information, which is often distressing • Diminished enjoyment of music • Understanding a young child's speech over the telephone is often difficult
Cochlea, eighth nerve, auditory brainstem pathways, temporal lobe	Degenerative changes from the periphery in the cochlea extending centrally to the auditory brainstem pathways and the auditory processing region of the brain	• Difficulty understanding some speakers more than others, especially those who drop voice level at the end of sentences and those with a high-pitched and weak voice
Structural and functional integrity of brainstem pathways and the cortex is disordered		• Difficulty hearing and understanding in the presence of auditory stressors such as noise and other difficult listening situations (Gates, Anderson, Feeney, McCurry, & Larson, 2008); louder does not translate to fully audible or intelligible; listeners require more favorable signal-to-noise ratio than do younger individuals for aided speech understanding • Speed of information processing is slow; additional time necessary to respond to questions
Deficiency in the way in which auditory impulses are transmitted to higher brain centers		• Declines in central auditory processing are predictive of clinical dementia • Right-ear advantage or difficulty understanding speech in presence of competing message, especially in the left ear • Difficulty understanding speech in adverse listening situations especially when individuals have a mild memory loss but with none of the criteria associated with a diagnosis of Alzheimer-type dementia (Gates et al, 2008); once speech is audible, the brain may not be able to make full use of information immediately due to such cognitive factors as divided attention challenges and decrements in speed of processing • Listening to young talkers even with a hearing aid can be an insuperable challenge; diminished cognitive function hampers understanding in challenging listening environments; require a more favorable signal-to-noise ratio than do young adults to understand the speech of others. • Difficulty adjusting to or admitting communication failure; feign comprehension
Deficit in analysis of auditory information due to dysfunction within the auditory brainstem pathways and auditory cortex Central auditory processing		• Difficulty in challenging listening conditions: multiple talkers, with strangers, people with accents, when a new topic is introduced, complex tasks, many concurrent activities, rapid speech; remember less in situations with unfavorable signal-to-noise ratios • Communicating in adverse listening situations requires a great deal of effort, and this effort may reduce recall of information; older adults using hearing aids have better emotional and social well- being and greater longevity

Sources: Data from Walton, J., & Burkhard, R. (2001). Neurophysiological manifestations of aging in the peripheral and central auditory nervous system. Anatomical and neurochemical bases of presbycusis. In P. Hoff & C. Mobbs (Eds.), *Functional neurobiology of aging* (pp. 581–596). San Diego: Academic Press 581–596; and Willott, J. F., Hnath Chisolm, T., & Lister, J. J. (2001, Sep-Oct). Modulation of presbycusis: Current status and future directions. *Audiology and Neuro-Otology, 6,* 231–249.

Psychosocial Consequences of Decrements in Hearing and Speech Understanding

The behavioral implications of the hearing and speech-understanding difficulties characterizing older adults are considerable. Most relevant to physicians is how the functional changes have an impact on many facets of life, including engagement, safety, responsivity, affect, and well-being; an untreated hearing loss may affect one's quality of care (Landefeld, Winker, & Chernof, 2009). **Table 10.8** lists the signs of a moderate to profound hearing impairment. The ways in which the patient's untreated hearing loss affects the patient's interactions with the physician and the patient's compliance with treatment must be underscored. The impact of the patient's hearing loss on the physician's attempt to arrive at a valid diagnosis must be addressed, including how it interferes with a valid assessment of cognitive status and affective disorders such as depression, which is so prevalent in older adults. The way in which hearing loss and vestibular dysfunction compromise safety at home and the ability to meet personal demands and perform activities of daily living (ADLs) and instrumental ADLs (IADLs) should be addressed with specific examples and solutions (Chisolm et al, 2007a; Dalton et al, 2003; Kochkin, 2005; Wu, Chin, & Tong, 2004).

Evidence-based clinical examples are paramount, including the findings of Dalton and colleagues (2003), who reported that older adults with moderate to severe hearing loss were more likely than individuals without hearing loss to have impaired ADLs and IADLs. Their finding that severe hearing loss had a significant association with decreased function in the mental and physical component scores of the Short-Form Health Survey (SF-36) is important to address as well. Also, it should be underscored that the myth that hearing loss is harmless has been debunked; if a hearing loss is left untreated, it can be costly to the patient and the family members in terms of the patient's cognitive status, affect, and safety. Here again, evidence that untreated hearing loss is costly from an economic vantage point and is associated with lost wages and lower income in retirement should be presented (Wu et al, 2004). Kochkin's (2005) findings of a link between household income and hearing loss severity, with individuals reporting mild hearing loss reporting a household income of $36,400 and persons with severe loss reporting an income of $33,600, is rather illuminating.

Because population aging is worldwide phenomenon, the adverse effects of untreated hearing impairment found in studies from abroad are also pertinent. For example, a recent study conducted in a geriatric medicine clinic in Singapore found that of subjects with self-reported hearing difficulty and a failure score on the pure-tone screen test, 70% indicated that they would be happier if their hearing were normal, 40% indicated that their hearing difficulty made them feel frustrated, and 43% admitted to feeling sad because of their hearing handicap (Smith, Mitchell, Wang, & Leeder, 2005). Further, in light of the profound effects of untreated hearing impairment, physicians may find it noteworthy that the Australian government is designing a comprehensive approach to managing age-related hearing loss because hearing impairment is the second highest cause of disability in Australian men.

Pearl

Hearing loss interferes with medical diagnosis, treatment, management, and interventions in emergency rooms; compromises compliance with pharmacological regimens; and interferes with therapeutic interventions, compromising quality of care.

◆ Interventions for the Hearing Impaired

Hearing Aids

Informing PCPs about hearing technologies and interventions is perhaps the most important task of their partnering audiologists, and the use of case scenarios might be very helpful. Case scenarios can highlight situations in which physicians might utilize recommendations regarding communication strategies and hearing interventions. A general overview of the categories of technology available and of the communication strategies should precede the interactive activities and should be embedded in the case-based presentations. Further evidence of the value of our interventions can include a discussion of neural plasticity associated with auditory input from hearing aids and resulting improvements in sound perception. Evidence from data on sensory deprivation should serve as a strong inducement for physicians to refer older adults for a consult with an audiologist. Always keep in mind the importance of evidence-based discussions, especially as they pertain to nonmedical treatments such as hearing aids and cochlear implants.

Hearing aids remain a mystery to many physicians, and their value is underappreciated. Therefore, it is important to discuss some basic points about hearing aids, emphasizing the evidence on their value. Physicians should come away with an understanding of why it is important that they encourage patients with recognized hearing impairments to see an audiolo-

---

Table 10.8 Signs that Physicians Should Note Regarding Possible Hearing Loss Exhibited by Hearing-Impaired Patients

- Cannot hear or understand you when you ask them to enter your office for the appointment
- Not very talkative
- Does not reply when spoken to
- Does not respond appropriately to questions you are asking
- Does not understand you when you speak with them on the telephone
- Looks closely at your face or lips when you speak
- May appear confused when giving an inappropriate response
- May have a hearing aid but does not use it
- May strain to understand or place hand behind ear in an attempt to amplify your voice
- Needs occasional repetition or a louder speaking voice to understand
- Needs frequent prompting, multiple repetitions, or restatements of what was said
- Not able to understand what is being said; asks you to write the message down to facilitate understanding
- Appears to have difficulty understanding fast speech and accented speech

gist and why it is important also to refer patients who have hearing aids but do not use them. That so many patients are lost to follow-up is a matter that physicians can be instrumental in helping us to address. It may be worthwhile for them to know that the new generation of digital hearing aids used by most new hearing-aid users have several features that address the concerns raised in the past. Not only do they improve audibility, but also they are less visible and more comfortable in the ear, and they can be manipulated to provide appropriate gain at selective frequencies, to differentially compress high-intensity sounds, and to filter out background noise. Many aids have directional microphone technology that picks up speech coming in front of the speaker and eliminates unwanted noise from behind the speaker. There is a mechanism that tells patients when to change the battery, and a mechanism for controlling feedback (Johnson, 2008; Kirkwood, 2007). Also, there is emerging evidence that hearing-aid use can forestall the onset of cognitive aging, and, in combination with auditory and cognitive-based interventions, may promote cognitive plasticity in the areas of the brain responsible for executive functions.

It is of utmost importance that PCPs appreciate that hearing aids are designed to meet the needs of individuals with varying auditory and nonauditory needs, and that people with sensorineural hearing loss due to aging are prime candidates. The high-tech features in both low- and high-end hearing aids enable audiologists to custom tailor the response of the hearing instrument to the consumer's lifestyle, listening needs, and financial situation, which is an important point to emphasize. I suggest showing images of older adults with the various styles of hearing aid in the ear, as this will make the concepts being discussed more tangible. Emphasize that if patients express dissatisfaction with their units, they should be encouraged to return to the audiologist, as there is a good deal of flexibility built into present-day hearing aids. The important role of physicians in encouraging patients to consider hearing aids should be underscored, and audiological and nonaudiological factors predictive of success should be discussed, as physicians should engage patients in a conversation about the appropriateness of hearing aids for their patient and about their value and utility.

The advantages of fitting both ears with hearing aids rather than just one, especially in noisy situations, should be explained, as should the fact that hearing aids reduce the effort necessary to communicate in noise, and hence they influence cognitive capacity as patients have less divided attention and tend to remember more of what they have been told. Further, it might be helpful to explain that because older adults often require a more favorable signal-to-noise ratio than do younger adults, hearing aids now include noise reduction and directional microphones to improve the signal-to-noise ratios. Using patient testimonies as to the value of hearing aids and some form of audiological rehabilitation can be very powerful curriculum materials, especially if it is a typical older adult with comorbidities such as diabetes, arthritis, or heart disease, to which the physician can relate. Vignettes of patients or audiologists emphasizing the positive impact of hearing aids on quality of life, the benefits derived from wearing two hearing aids in the case of bilateral hearing loss, the importance of wearing hearing aids on a regular basis, and the value added when hearing aids are delivered in the context of a holistic re-

habilitation program are powerful. Evidence supporting these points can also go a long way toward influencing physicians to modify their perceptions and put their new learning into practice. For example, the data on brain plasticity, wherein functional representation of the brain is altered when the hearing impaired are taught to effectively relearn and use the new speech input provided by hearing aids through some form of listening training designed to enhance auditory and sensory deprivation, are powerful (Sweetow, 2007). Specifically, a link between lack of amplification and decrements in speech understanding over time in unaided ears of adults with sensorineural hearing loss is very persuasive and requires discussion (Chisolm, Abrams, & McArdle, 2004). Further, new findings about the contribution of hearing aids to cognitive plasticity and function are very important. It is essential that physicians understand the down side of not wearing or using hearing aids, namely decrements in auditory processing in the unaided ear and in cognitive function in general.

Finally, as evidence-based discussions carry a good deal of weight, sharing data from the cost-utility analyses that confirm that the most favorable outcomes are achieved when hearing aids are dispensed in the context of a comprehensive rehabilitation program is of utmost importance (Chisolm et al, 2004). Further, of the various approaches to audiological rehabilitation (AR), group programs that focus on counseling emphasize that communication strategies training and computer-assisted techniques to enhance perceptual learning are of proven cost utility and effectiveness, and patients should be encouraged to ask about these options when they see the audiologist (Boothroyd, 2006, 2007; Sweetow, 2007). The findings from the systematic review recently completed by Hawkins (2005), which concluded that there is reasonably good evidence that hearing-related quality of life is improved when adults participate in counseling-based group AR programs, are powerful (Boothroyd, 2006). Further, the emergence of Web-based and computer-based approaches to auditory training such as LACE (listening and communication enhancement) should be mentioned so that patients are prepped to inquire about this when they see an audiologist. **Table 10.9** summarizes the value of hearing aids in conjunction with counseling-oriented AR.

Pearl

Emerging evidence suggests that hearing aids preserve function and slow cognitive decline.

Implantable Devices

The fact that cochlear implants (CIs) and bone-anchored hearing aids (BAHAs) are a realistic option for healthy, older adults with severe to profound hearing loss for whom hearing aids are not conferring enhanced quality of life in important social environments should be addressed using case vignettes to help make important points. Physicians must understand the basic principles behind CI and BAHA along with candidacy considerations (Chisolm, Noe, McArdle, & Abrams, 2007b). Several manufacturer sites include You Tube video of how implantable

Table 10.9 The Value of Integrated Audiological Rehabilitation Programs in the Fitting of Hearing Aids

- Provide an understanding of hearing aids, their care, and maintenance
- Promote realistic expectations regarding the value and capabilities of hearing aids
- Maximize sensory input by providing the best possible visual and auditory signal
- Help the patient understand the psychological and social problems resulting from hearing impairment and the contribution of hearing aids to these domains of function
- Help maximize sensory integration by making the best use of the amplified auditory signal and the visible signal
- Promote use of cognitive processes necessary to derive meaning from incomplete sensory messages
- Promote an understanding of how to create a positive communication environment with communication partners.
- Develop within the individual assertive and interactive ways of communicating and repairing breakdowns
- Empower the hearing impaired and help them to become proactive
- Engage members of the individual's support system, especially the communication partner

devices work, which can be very helpful as they explain how CIs and BAHA devices work in general and from a surgical perspective. Physicians should be reminded to consider personal factors such as lifestyle (e.g., the patient remains employed and active), and health status (good physical health), and should be encouraged to make a referral for an older adult who is experiencing more and more difficulty communicating with the use of hearing aids (Chisolm et al, 2007b). Physicians should understand that older adults, especially late-deafened adults, are excellent candidates from an audiological perspective, as they learn to associate the signal provided by an implant with sounds they remember from their years of experience when they were part of the hearing world (Leung et al, 2005). Here again, the evidence that suggests that CIs provide improved access to verbal communication, environmental sounds, enhanced telephone communication, and enjoyment of music must be underscored (Chisolm et al, 2007b). Testimonials from patients who have been successfully implanted can help to convince physicians to make an appropriate referral to an experienced CI team. In my view the testimonials should be from patients with whom you have worked rather than those prepared by the manufacturers. In terms of candidacy, medical, audiological, cognitive considerations should be presented.

Regarding BAHAs, physicians should understand that some of their patients who present with chronic infections of the middle ear resulting in mixed or conductive hearing loss or with single-sided deafness (SSD), perhaps as a result of surgery on a vestibular schwannoma, and are not pleased with their experience with hearing aids might be candidates for a BAHA. Here too they should come to understand the mechanism behind the BAHA, namely that it is a Food and Drug Administration (FDA)-approved surgically implantable device for unilateral deafness that works on a principle similar to that of bone-conduction hearing aids. Simply put, the BAHA delivers sound into the skull by means of sound vibration. Specific cases wherein the BAHA has been successful should be dis-

cussed, as in the case of an older adult with long-standing conductive hearing loss with chronically discharging ears, or persons with complete or near-complete SSD or deafness in one ear who are in good health and lead active lives. Further, older adults with SSD who have not experienced much success with hearing aids should consider speaking with an otolaryngologist to determine their candidacy. The fact that prior to proceeding with the surgical procedure, individuals can try the BAHA to gain a feel for the experience hearing via bone conduction is an excellent reason for physicians to refer the appropriate candidate to a physician who performs the surgical procedure. Recent reports suggest that BAHAs have successfully reduced the emotional and social handicap experienced by persons with SSD from a variety of etiologies.

Hearing-Assistance Technologies

Physicians should understand that the benefits derived from hearing aids or implantable devices can be augmented with the use of hearing-assistance technologies (HATs), which are auditory and nonauditory devices that help individuals in a variety of listening situations, including interfacing with the physician. The value of signal-alerting technologies in terms of home safety should be emphasized as well (Olsen, 2008). As physicians may be providing counseling to their patients following in-office hearing screenings, telecommunication systems and media devices should be described in brief. That older adults require a more favorable signal-to-noise ratio to understand speech, especially in a room with poor acoustics and when the speech source is far from the listener, is the most important principle to be communicated. It is important that physicians understand that the further away from the sound source the listener is, the softer the sound level, the less clear the speech signal, and the more difficult it is to understand (Olsen, 2008). Physicians should understand the advantages of HATs over hearing aids, and that because most older adults with hearing impairment do not use hearing aids, these devices can be helpful during the medical encounter. Collectively, HATs rely on auditory, visual, or tactile information to augment speech understanding and to help monitor environmental sounds. HATs are recommended based on an individual's communication needs, such as in small-group face-to-face communication, electronic media, telephone use, environmental alerting needs, large-group communication, noisy environments, or for home use when personal safety is compromised due to a severe hearing impairment with or without cognitive problems. HATs that are appropriate for interpersonal communication are destined to be used as a complement to or in lieu of hearing aids or cochlear implants, and signal alerting technology is critical for patients who cannot hear the telephone ring or the smoke alarm when it sounds.

Physicians should be informed that personal amplifiers are ideal when communicating with older adults with untreated hearing impairment in various settings, such as the emergency room, during routine medical intakes, during inpatient hospital visits, or when examining the homebound patients. Physicians must come to understand that although hearing aids are beneficial, hearing aids alone may be insufficient for patients to access auditory events. Also, the majority of older adults do not use them, and the listening environments in which physicians encounter their patients are too demanding for hearing-impaired patients. Demonstrating how HATs can help to overcome some of the environmental barriers to successful communication, such as noise and distance, is a very powerful experience for physicians. Using hearing aid "Apps" paired with insert earphones with their patients can be very convincing and the use of this should be underscored.

The discussion about HATs should be brief but targeted, focusing on the four distinct categories of devices, the different modes of sound transmission, and the different types of signal delivery modalities. The value of hearing loops should be included in this conversation. The discussion should include examples of the devices, and in the case of the frequency-modulated (FM) system (with receiver, neck loop, and Bluetooth, a short-range wireless networking technology that facilitates communication between devices), physicians should experience the value in terms of enhancing speech understanding in a large room or in a separate room. The four categories of devices are (1) sound-enhancement technology, (2) television/media devices (television reception), (3) telecommunications technology (telephone reception), and (4) signal-alerting technology (reception of environmental warning sounds).

Sound-enhancement technology should be emphasized because it enables a person with hearing impairment to understand speech clearly when the speaker is at a considerable distance from the listener; thus, it can be indispensable during encounters with the physician. Sound-enhancement technologies differ in the way in which the signal is transmitted to the ear of the listener; the microphone is placed close to the sound source, within 6 inches, which picks up the signal, and via one of several modes of transmission, sends the signal to the listener's ears, overcoming the barriers posed by distance and environmental noise. The intensity of the signal relative to the noise (signal-to-noise ratio) becomes more favorable. Signals can be transmitted to the listener via a hard-wired connection between the microphone/amplifier/receiver and the headphones or via wireless radio transmission of signals (e.g., FM signal, Bluetooth, or infrared light).

The virtues and limitations of hardwired and wireless systems should be discussed and each should be demonstrated. It should be emphasized that personal amplifiers are ideal for use during an intake, when communicating at bedside with persons with hearing impairment, during diagnostic or screening tests, and when providing important recommendations to patients for whom treatment compliance is essential. If the patient is exhibiting difficulty understanding what the physician is saying, the physician should simply use a personal amplifier. Instructions for placement of the headset/earphone should be given and demonstrated or an "app" with a good microphone and earphones, as these technologies are unfamiliar to most physicians. I also recommend discussing the variety of amplified stethoscopes available for physicians. **Fig. 10.1** displays the Audiologist's Choice Amplified Bluetooth Stethoscope, which is very flexible.

Points to discuss regarding portable personal wireless systems are that the systems include a personal FM receiver and a neck loop with a telecoil-equipped hearing aid. The systems can be used with or without a hearing aid (requires telecoil, and neck loop, or Bluetooth accessory and compatibility); they are more costly than hardwired systems, although prices are

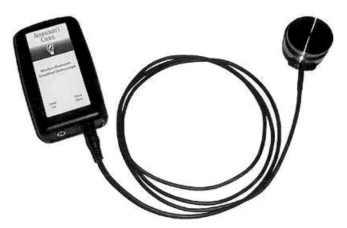

Fig. 10.1 Audiologist's Choice Amplified Bluetooth Stethoscope. (From Oaktree Products. Reprinted by permission.)

dropping, as more users purchase these devices for routine use; they facilitate listening in noisy environments, in large rooms with poor acoustics, or when the speaker is at a distance and the listener cannot understand what the speaker is saying; and they can be used with hearing aids. These systems are ideal when communicating with an older hearing-impaired adults with moderately severe to severe sensorineural hearing loss or auditory processing problems. Patients with hearing aids often experience excellent speech understanding with these devices. **Table 10.10** lists the instructions for using personal amplifiers with patients.

Telecommunication options should be specified because many physicians have patients who are hearing impaired and

Table 10.10 Instructions for Audiologists Demonstrating the Use of Personal Amplifiers (Hard Wired or Wireless) to Patients

- Explain your rationale for using the system with the patient
- Check that batteries are inserted and are active
- With the patient's permission, slowly place the headphones over the patient's ears
- Turn up the volume gradually to a comfortable loudness for the patient
  - Slowly increase the loudness using the volume control
  - Each time you increase the loudness, ask the patient if your voice is comfortably loud
- Place the *Pocket Talker*
  - in the patient's pocket, or
  - on a table next to the patient with the microphone as close as possible to sound source;

Or

- Attach the receiver to the patient's clothing
- Use an extension connector for the headphones, if the cord needs to be lengthened
- When the receiver and amplifier are on, the light should be on
- When the receiver and amplifier are turned off, the light should go off
- To turn off, turn the volume control until you hear a click and the light goes off
- If the system whistles, then move the microphone away from the headphones
- Replace the batteries as needed

Sources: From http://www.williamssound.com/productdetail.aspx?product _id=92; and http://www.williamssound.com/productdetail.aspx?product_id =372.

have difficulty understanding information that is often conveyed over the telephone. The availability of amplified telephones; the value of email, especially for those who have poor receptive skills; and telecommunication relay service options (e.g., text to voice, Internet protocol [IP] relay services, video relay services [VRS], or text telephone known as a telecommunication systems for the deaf [TDD]) should all be described briefly (Hidalgo et al, 2008). The value of and access to caption telephones (e.g., Cap-Tel) should be discussed. It is important to emphasize that while physicians are reluctant to communicate via email, it is an excellent form of telecommunication technology for persons with hearing impairment who are unable to communicate comfortably or productively over the telephone. Bluetooth technology, open canal hearing aids, and hearing-aid–compatible cellular phones allow hearing-aid users to comfortably speak on the phones while wearing hearing aids, and should be mentioned to physicians who may wish to explore these options with their patients. Of course hearing loop technology should be emphasized.

The purpose of signal-alerting technology (e.g., warns, signals, or alerts a person with a hearing loss) and the principles of operation should be discussed as well. It uses loud sounds, visual signals, or tactile signals to alert those with severe hearing impairment. It may be worthwhile describing the vibrator placed under the pillow to awaken the person with hearing loss in the morning, the strobe light attached to a smoke alarm to alert the hearing-impaired person to a fire, and the vibrating wristwatches used to alert the hearing impaired (Hidalgo et al, 2008). Emphasize that signal-alerting devices can be purchased at several Websites and are invaluable for hearing-impaired persons who are homebound, for persons with cognitive impairments, and for residents of nursing facilities who have hearing loss. Physicians should be informed that audiologists are an excellent resource, as they are well equipped to guide persons and institutions to the system that will best meet their needs and to arrange for the purchase of the necessary assistive listening devices.

Screening Protocols

Screening for hearing loss and referral for follow-up are essential components of a comprehensive physical for older adults joining Medicare for the first time. Thus, this section is integral to educational outreach curricula for physicians (American Academy of Family Physicians, 2005; Cohen, Labadie & Haynes, 2005; Yueh, Shapiro, MacLean, & Shekelle, 2003). The high prevalence and functional consequences of hearing impairment, coupled with mounting evidence suggesting that at least 25% of persons between 65 and 75 years of age have undiagnosed hearing loss that may be detectable via a routine physical examination, render the low rate of screening in primary care (12.9%) rather disheartening (Cohen et al, 2005; Danhauer et al, 2008; Johnson et al, 2008; Kochkin, 2005; Newman & Sandridge, 2004). Only 20% of Americans who could benefit from a hearing aid actually have or use one. Older adults are more likely to seek evaluation and treatment for hearing loss when physicians recommend that they do so (Cox, Alexander, & Gray, 2005; Kochkin, 2005). Tinnitus and injuries from falls often accompany adult-onset hearing loss. These prevalent conditions have dramatic functional conse-

quences in older adults, especially in those with such chronic conditions as cardiovascular disease and diabetes. These conditions should be included as part of any discussion of screening (Nondahl et al, 2002; Wallhagen, Pettengill, & Whiteside, 2006).

Most physicians do not screen older adults for hearing impairment because of reimbursement obstacles and because of a limited understanding of approaches to cost-effectively screening for these conditions in this population (Yueh et al, 2003). Routine screening for hearing loss, tinnitus, and vestibular dysfunction should be part of the training of PCPs, as they are the entry point into the health care system for the elderly, and especially given the availability of technologies and interventions to overcome the functional and emotional consequences.

Pearl

Health-related quality of life of older adults is improved when PCPs screen for hearing and balance problems (Solodar & Chappell, 2005).

The survey of 95 PCPs conducted by Johnson et al (2008) should inform the discussion of screening for otological functional impairments. The goal of this 35–item survey was to quantify physician's knowledge about hearing and balance function, attitudes toward hearing/balance screening and referral, and knowledge of hearing/balance interventions. The authors included copies of the Dizziness Handicap Inventory (DHI) and the screening version of the Hearing Handicap Inventory for the Elderly (HHIE-S), as the patient's self-reported hearing functioning and risk for falls was an integral part of the history to be taken as part of the now defunct Medicare benefit for new enrollees. The majority of respondents were internists in private practice for at least 15 years who saw older adults as a routine part of their practice; 72% of respondents said they screen for hearing and balance problems when they suspect a problem or when patients complain of a problem. We know from the literature that older adults underreport symptoms if not asked, and rarely complain about hearing or balance problems. Thus, these problems are likely to be missed if a patient complaint is the sole trigger for eliciting them. The majority of respondents were not familiar with the DHI or the HHIE-S.

It was noteworthy that the PCPs who responded indicated that when they suspect a problem, they refer the patient to an otologist, an audiologist, or a physical therapist. It was a relief to learn that 78% said they refer to an audiologist and 5% indicated that they refer to an otologist. Their data underscored the importance of making physicians aware of the evidence supporting the efficacy of self-report tools for identifying otological functional impairments such as hearing loss, tinnitus, and balance related problems (Johnson, 2008). Further, the majority of PCPs were unaware of nonmedical treatments available for hearing impairment, yet the majority did acknowledge that vestibular rehabilitation is effective for treating some balance problems. Finally, barriers toward hearing and balance screening emerged that need to be addressed, and these were primarily in the realm of process and financing. Respondents

Table 10.11 The Hearing Handicap Inventory for Individuals 65+: Screening Form (HHIE-S)

Instructions: The purpose of this questionnaire is to identify the problems your hearing loss may be causing you. Please select YES, SOMETIMES, or NO for each question. Do not skip a question if you avoid a situation because of your hearing problem. If you use a hearing aid, please answer the way you hear with a hearing aid.

Does a hearing problem cause you to feel embarrassed when you meet new people?	○ Yes	○ Sometimes	○ No
Does a hearing problem cause you to feel frustrated when talking to members of your family?	○ Yes	○ Sometimes	○ No
Do you have difficulty when someone speaks in a whisper?	○ Yes	○ Sometimes	○ No
Do you feel handicapped by a hearing problem?	○ Yes	○ Sometimes	○ No
Does a hearing problem cause you difficulty when visiting friends, relatives, or neighbors?	○ Yes	○ Sometimes	○ No
Does a hearing problem cause you to attend religious services less often than you would like?	○ Yes	○ Sometimes	○ No
Does a hearing problem cause you to have arguments with family members?	○ Yes	○ Sometimes	○ No
Does a hearing problem cause you difficulty when listening to TV or radio?	○ Yes	○ Sometimes	○ No
Do you feel that any difficulty with your hearing limits or hampers your personal or social life?	○ Yes	○ Sometimes	○ No
Does a hearing problem cause you difficulty when in a restaurant with relatives or friends?	○ Yes	○ Sometimes	○ No

Note: Score in excess of 8 triggers a referral to an audiologist.

expressed concerns with the time-consuming nature of the screening process and the fact that reimbursement for preventive services such as routine screening for hearing and risk of falls is minimal.

In lieu of the HHIE-S (**Table 10.11**) (Ventry & Weinstein, 1982, 1983; Yueh et al, 2003) and the DHI, I developed a questionnaire with Craig Newman and Sharon Sandridge that we call the Screening for Otologic Functional Impairments in the Elderly (SOFIE; **Table 10.12**). It consists of questions on hearing loss, dizziness, and tinnitus taken from parent inventories including the dizziness, tinnitus, and hearing handicap inventories. Test-retest reliability of the SOFIE is based on a sample of 14 respondents with a mean age of 69 years and mean three-frequency pure-tone averages of 31 dB HL in the better ear and 34 dB HL in the poorer ear. Respondents are asked to answer yes, no, or sometimes to three questions about each otological condition, and they rate the severity of each condition they report experiencing. The advantage of the SOFIE is that it combines the most sensitive questions on the parent questionnaires, making it briefer and less time-consuming to administer without sacrificing accuracy and it too is high in reliability.

Preliminary data suggest that mean SOFIE scores correlate with recommendations for hearing-aid use, with individuals recommended for hearing aids having higher SOFIE scores (mean of 10) and mean four-frequency pure-tone averages of 41 dB HL for the poorer ear and 36 dB HL for the better ear. In contrast, the mean SOFIE score on those not recommended was 4, with mean four-frequency pure-tone averages of 20 dB HL for the poorer ear and 18 dB HL for the better ear. The data thus far suggest that responses to the three questions within each condition have a very direct correlation to the total score on the screening and full versions of the Tinnitus Handicap Inventory (THI), the Dizziness Handicap Inventory (DHI), and the Hearing Handicap Inventory (HHI). The questionnaire is helpful, especially in a medical setting, if the goal is to identify individuals with other chronic conditions who may also have an otological condition that requires attention.

I recommend pairing the self-report with an objective screen, namely the Audioscope, which delivers pure tones at 40 dB HL at four frequencies: 500, 1000, 2000, and 4000 Hz. During the in-service training, be sure to bring the Audioscope and discuss frequencies (e.g., 1000, 2000 Hz) to be screened,

the hearing level at which screening should take place (e.g., 40 dB HL), and the pass-fail criterion. Instructions are important as well, emphasizing that the patient should be instructed to raise his or her finger or hand when the tone is heard, assuming they have dexterity and mobility in the arm and fingers. The patient's response should be time-locked to the presentation of the stimulus signaled by a red indicator light on the Audioscope. Make sure to underscore that calibration is important and that Welch-Allyn, the manufacturer, will arrange to calibrate. Also, conditioning is important. Make sure to include some practice (i.e., conditioning trials) with the physicians so that they understand the subtleties necessary to obtain valid responses from older adults to the presence or absence of tonal stimuli. Also, discuss the value of the otoscope and the importance of checking for cerumen, as this is a prevalent condition and can interfere with hearing and with the function of hearing aids. A good portion of the in-service training with physicians should be on overviewing screening efforts directed at identifying older adults at risk for otological functional impairments that may entail consequences for which effective treatments including risk reduction strategies are available.

As part of the discussion of screening, it is important to distinguish between the role of the audiologist, a hearing health care specialist who provides assistance to persons with hearing problems, and the role of the otolaryngologist, a medical doctor who diagnoses and treats medical diseases of the ear that may be causing a hearing problem. Make sure to emphasize that if medical treatment is not indicated, persons with hearing loss should be referred to an audiologist, but persons with balance problems or tinnitus should be referred to an otolaryngologist for a workup regarding the etiology and possible treatment. Emphasize that referral by a physician to an audiologist increases the likelihood that an older adult will purchase audiological services in the form of hearing tests, hearing aids, and audiological rehabilitation (Solodar & Chappell, 2005). Make sure to discuss targeted interventions for those referred following the hearing screening. Possible interventions, depending on the outcome of a screening, are referral for an audiological evaluation, referral to the audiologist and consideration of assistive devices for telephone and television, hearing-aid provision, hearing-aid orientation and counseling, audiological rehabilitation including speech reading, and

Table 10.12 Screening for Otologic Functional Impairments in the Elderly (SOFIE)

Instructions: The purpose of this questionnaire is to identify any problems you are having that may relate to your ears, including hearing difficulties, dizziness, or tinnitus (ringing/buzzing/noises in your ears/head). Please circle *Yes, Sometimes,* or *No* for each question. If you use hearing aids, please answer the way you hear while using the hearing aids. If you are not experiencing any difficulties, please indicate by marking *No.*

D-1	Because of feelings of dizziness, is it difficult for you to walk around the house in the dark?	Yes	Sometimes	No
D-2	Does dizziness interfere with your job or household responsibilities?	Yes	Sometimes	No
D-3	Does bending over increase your feeling of dizziness?	Yes	Sometimes	No

Dizziness score

H-1	Does a hearing problem cause you difficulty when listening to the television or radio?	Yes	Sometimes	No
H-2	Does your hearing problem cause you to feel frustrated when talking to members of your family?	Yes	Sometimes	No
H-3	Does a hearing problem cause you difficulty when visiting with friends, relatives, or neighbors?	Yes	Sometimes	No

Hearing score

T-1	Do you feel that you can no longer cope with your tinnitus?	Yes	Sometimes	No
T-2	Because of tinnitus, do you have trouble falling asleep or staying asleep at night?	Yes	Sometimes	No
T-3	Do you feel that you cannot escape your tinnitus?	Yes	Sometimes	No

Tinnitus score

G-1	Do you feel that any difficulty with your hearing, dizziness, or tinnitus significantly restricts your participation in social activities such as going to restaurants, dancing, movies, or other events?	Yes	Sometimes	No

Global Score

Total Score

On a scale of 1 to 10, please circle the number that would correspond with the severity of the given problem.

	Not at all Severe									Extremely Severe
Dizziness:	0	1	2	3	4	5	6	7	8	9	10
Hearing:	0	1	2	3	4	5	6	7	8	9	10
Tinnitus:	0	1	2	3	4	5	6	7	8	9	10

cochlear implant or BAHA. The many articles in JAMA on screening written by physicians should be distributed.

Communicating with the Hearing Impaired

Another important part of the curriculum to be developed for physicians is how to communicate effectively with patients given the environmental context and audiological findings. Before reviewing factors responsible for effective communication and strategies to be adapted, it is important to define communication and its role in diagnosis and outcomes. Communication is such an important component of patient care that physician-patient communication is considered a measureable clinical skill that graduates from medical school must master (Teutsch, 2003). Recognizing the need to teach and measure this clinical skill, a component of the accreditation process for residency programs is documentation of adequate interpersonal and communications skills resulting in effective information exchange between physicians and patients and their families. In fact, it is critical to emphasize that quality communication between patient and provider is integral to the effective delivery of medical care from the perspectives of diagnostic accuracy and health outcomes (shared decision making). Emphasize that counseling about unhealthy or risky behaviors, dosage of prescription medicines, palliative care,

and health proxies are a few examples where communication skills are called upon during the physician-patient encounter. The five A's of patient counseling—assess, advise, agree, assist, and arrange—are discussed in Chapter 7. All five require effective communication skills if health outcomes are to be maximized, if clinicians are to be credible and reliable professionals, and if patients are to be satisfied with the quality of their care. I have created some tables that may be helpful to distribute during a lecture to physicians. Prior to distributing and discussing the factors which contribute to effective communication and strategies for maximizing communication, emphasize the importance of eye contact and active listening during encounters with the patient. **Table 10.13** lists factors that

Table 10.13 Factors Influencing Communication

Speaker Variables	Personal Variables	Environmental Variables
Rate of speech	Visual acuity	Noise
Loudness of speaker	Mental status	Lighting
Accent	Listening skills	Visual distractions
Visibility of lips/face	Attention span	Glare
Mouth movements	Severity of hearing loss; aids for hearing	

Table 10.14 Environmental Tips for Promoting Communication Before Speaking with the Patient

- Reduce noise:
  - Select a quiet room away from street noises
  - Turn off the TV, radio, iPod, cell phone, and anything else that can be noisy
  - Shut the windows, if necessary
  - Shut the door, if necessary
- Arrange seating as follows:
  - You should be facing the patient
  - You should be sitting within 3 to 6 feet of the patient
  - The patient should sit with his/her back to the wall so sound is not coming from all sides
- A small table should be between you and the patient or next to the patient so that:
  - A pad of paper and a pen can be placed on the table for communication in writing, if necessary
  - A Pocket Talker or hearing aid can be placed on the table to make the communication easier, whenever necessary
- Arrange lighting as follows:
  - The room is well lit
  - The light is on your face
  - The light does not create glare in the patient's eyes

influence the adequacy of communication. **Table 10.14** is a checklist of the environmental barriers that can be manipulated to help to promote communication. **Table 10.15** lists tips for communicating.

◆ Conclusion

Hearing and balance problems are increasingly common, with the costs and consequences becoming a huge burden when these problems are untreated (Agrawal et al, 2009) (**Table 10.16**). 30 to 50% of older adults suffer from a handicapping hearing impairment that interferes with the quality of their lives. Also, fall-related injuries are increasing. Adults over 55 years of age make up 81% of all hearing-aid users, yet the majority of older adults with hearing loss do not use hearing aids. The stigma associated with hearing-aid use coupled with persistent complaints from experienced users about difficulty hearing in public places, especially noisy environments, have kept penetration rates stable but low over time. Technologically sophisticated hearing aids, in combination with some form of audiological rehabilitation, are more effective than ever and are a boon to older adults who are living longer and retiring early yet continue to be confronted by difficulty understanding the speech of others, especially in noise. Evidence is available demonstrating the improved audibility and enhanced speech understanding in noisy and reverberant environments afforded by today's digital hearing instruments, which reduce feedback and extraneous noise, and include directional microphone technology that automatically picks up speech while suppressing unwanted noise emanating from behind the speaker. This improved communication translates into beneficial effects on health-related quality of life. The availability of hearing assistance technologies that compensate for the shortcomings remaining with hearing aids is another avenue for persons with hearing impairment to pursue. The physician has reliable, valid, and inexpensive tools at his or her disposal to

Table 10.15 Tips for Communicating

Beginning by asking if the patient can understand what you are saying, and then consider the following:
1. Face the patient directly.
2. Be sure to look directly at the patient, preferably at eye level, before starting to speak.
3. If the patient wears a hearing aid, ensure that it is securely in the correct ear and turned on.
4. Check for visual impairment; ask "Can you read a newspaper?" If the patient wears eyeglasses, ensure that the glasses are on and clean.
5. Make sure the patient can see you and that the television is turned off.
6. Establish eye contact and face patient.
7. Make sure you do not turn your face away in the middle of a sentence.
8. Use patient's preferred communication method (this may be verbal, written, lip reading, or American Sign Language).
9. When speaking with the patient, make sure your face is at the same level as the patient's.
10. Be sure the patient is aware of you before you start talking.
11. If the patient is turned away from you or turns away from you, alert the patient with a gentle touch.
12. Ensure only one person at a time is talking to the patient.
13. Allow adequate time for the patient to listen and respond.
14. Say the patient's first name and then continue the sentence.
15. Avoid information overload.
16. Use multiple modalities.
17. Repeat, clarify, and confirm.
18. Use a personal amplifier or smart phone amplifier "app" if patient appears to have a hearing loss (e.g., soundAMP R).
19. Make sure the patient can see your lips and face.
20. If the patient wears glasses, ask the patient to wear them during the conversation.
21. If the patient doesn't understand you, then repeat (not quickly) or say things in another way (rephrase).
22. Don't move around while speaking with the patient.
23. Be patient when repeating instructions; don't look frustrated if you have to repeat yourself.
24. Check to make sure you are being understood.
25. A patient's nodding "yes" while you speak does not mean that the patient understands.

identify persons with hearing problems who require and can benefit from the expertise of audiologists. Working together, physicians and audiologists can reduce the burden of hearing loss and can promote the quality of life and care of the increasing population of older adults suffering from handicapping hearing impairment and mutlimorbidities. A wonderful primer for physicians as a supplement to any educational programming can be found in Newman and Sandridge (2004).

The ability to communicate effectively has taken on great importance as we move through the twenty-first century. Patient satisfaction and good outcomes are increasingly valued and tied to effective communication as part of the medical encounter. If we are to succeed at increasing the hearing health care knowledge base of physicians, the educational program must be interactive, and must include clear objectives, skill-building activities, and content that is appropriate to the objective, namely promoting the quality of patient care (Ockene & Zapka, 2000). Web-based interactive case scenarios that provide immediate feedback should be developed, as this approach provides an effective way to engage physicians and to

Table 10.16 Demographics of Hearing Loss, Tinnitus, and Falls in Older Adults

1. Hearing loss is the third most prevalent chronic condition in older Americans, with prevalence estimates ranging from 40 to 80% depending on age; the majority of hearing-aid users are satisfied with their hearing aids, but noise remains a problem that can be addressed with communication strategies training and use of hearing-assistance technologies (HATs).
2. Prevalence estimates of tinnitus, a possible symptom of problems including hearing loss, allergies, and exposure to ototoxic medication, range from 10 to 15% in older adults.
3. Abnormal central auditory processing test results are observed in older adults with memory loss but free of a diagnosis of Alzheimer-type dementia.
4. Hearing loss, tinnitus, and falls contribute to the high prevalence of comorbidity in older adults.
5. Risk for hearing impairment is associated with gender (males), educational status (low), industrial or military occupation, smoking, diabetes mellitus, heart disease, and advanced age.
6. The likelihood of falling is 7-fold higher in persons 80 years of age or older as compared with persons in their 40s; hearing impairment is a risk factor for falls.
7. Older adults with hearing loss are at risk for falls, which are the leading cause of deaths related to injury among people 65 years of age or older, and gait and balance problems are a common cause.
8. Hearing loss is correlated with social isolation.

Table 10.17 Environmental Adaptations in the Medical Office and With Staff

1. Speak in a room away from street noise.
2. Close windows, if necessary, when counseling the patient.
2. Arrange seating so that physician is always facing the patient and remove all barriers or obstacles that may degrade the spoken message.
3. Make sure the office is well lighted.
4. Make sure to avoid focusing light on the patient's eyes when speaking.
5. Maintain a distance of 3 to 6 feet from the patient during any conversation.
6. If patient is homebound or in a hospital room, place a small table either between or next to the patient and the physician to support the personal amplifier if used and to provide a writing surface should you use multiple modalities when counseling and instructing patient regarding recommended follow-up steps.
7. If patient is homebound or in a hospital room, speak in an area devoid of family members who might distract the patient's attention.
8. If patient is homebound or in a hospital room, make sure to turn off the radio, TV, and other sound sources when speaking.
9. Make sure the receptionists and billing staff in the offices look at the patients and not at the computer when they are checking them in or processing papers and make sure they speak slowly on the telephone.
10. Use e-mail to confirm appointments especially for the hearing impaired.
11. Use a Pocket Talker or a Smartphone App such as soundAMP R with a good set of in-ear earphones and a good external microphone such as Blue Microphone Mikey (if compatible).

help build the skills needed for patient education, counseling, and compliance with treatments. We must pay heed to the fact that physicians have limited time to devote to continuing education, and a hybrid approach that combines interactivity with face-to-face sessions may hold promise, as indicated in evidence-based studies of methodology used to promote implementation of clinical practice guidelines (Zapka, Goins, Pbert, & Ockene, 2004). An effective way to impress upon physicians the value of continuing education regarding hearing health care is by emphasizing demographics, consequences of hearing impairment, and the value of audiological interventions such as practicing communication behaviors that will facilitate compliance with medical interventions. **Table 10.17**

summarizes points to be emphasized to help physicians realize the clinical utility of expanding their knowledge base regarding hearing health care. Finally, I highly recommend the recent article by Pacala and Yueh (2012) for all PCPs, along with material on hearing loops such as a recent article in *Sound and Communication* (http://www.hearingloss.org/sites/default/files/docs/Sound_Communications_Article_growing_population.pdf).

References

Agrawal, Y., Carey, J. P., Della Santina, C. C., Schubert, M. C., & Minor, L. B. (2009, May). Disorders of balance and vestibular function in US adults: data from the National Health and Nutrition Examination Survey, 2001–2004. *Archives of Internal Medicine, 169*(10), 938–944.

Agrawal, Y., Platz, E. A., & Niparko, J. K. (2008, Jul). Prevalence of hearing loss and differences by demographic characteristics among US adults: data from the National Health and Nutrition Examination Survey, 1999-2004. *Archives of Internal Medicine, 168*(14), 1522–1530.

Ahmad, N., & Seidman, M. (2004). Tinnitus in the older adult: epidemiology, pathophysiology and treatment options. *Drugs & Aging, 21*(5), 297–305.

American Academy of Family Physicians(2005). Scientific assembly. http://www.medscape.com/viewcollection/4576

Bainbridge, K. E., Hoffman, H. J., & Cowie, C. C. (2008, Jul). Diabetes and hearing impairment in the United States: audiometric evidence from the National Health and Nutrition Examination Survey, 1999 to 2004. *Annals of Internal Medicine, 149*(1), 1–10.

Bishop, T., & Morrison, S. (2007). Geriatric palliative care—Part II: Communication and goals of care. *Clinical Geriatrics, 15,* 27–32.

Boothroyd, A. (2006). *Adult aural rehabilitation: What is it and does it work?* Paper presented at the State of the Science Conference on optimizing the benefit of hearing aids and cochlear implants for adults: The role of aural rehabilitation and evidence for its success, September 18–20, Gallaudet University, Washington, DC

Boothroyd, A. (2007, Jun). Adult aural rehabilitation: what is it and does it work? *Trends in Amplification, 11*(2), 63–71.

Brooks, D. (2010). The geezers' crusade. *New York Times,* February 2, p. A27

Chisolm, T. H., Abrams, H. B., & McArdle, R. (2004, Oct). Short- and long-term outcomes of adult audiological rehabilitation. *Ear and Hearing, 25*(5), 464–477.

Chisolm, T. H., Johnson, C. E., Danhauer, J. L., Portz, L. J., Abrams, H. B., Lesner, S., et al. (2007a, Feb). A systematic review of health-related quality of life and hearing aids: final report of the American Academy of Audiology Task Force On the Health-Related Quality of Life Benefits of Amplification in Adults. *Journal of the American Academy of Audiology, 18*(2), 151–183.

Chisolm, T. H., Noe, C. M., McArdle, R., & Abrams, H. (2007b, Jun). Evidence for the use of hearing assistive technology by adults: the role of the FM system. *Trends in Amplification, 11*(2), 73–89.

Cohen, S. M., Labadie, R. F., & Haynes, D. S. (2005, Jan). Primary care approach to hearing loss: the hidden disability. *Ear, Nose, & Throat Journal, 84*(1), 26, 29–31, 44.

Cox, R. M., Alexander, G. C., & Gray, G. A. (2005, Dec). Hearing aid patients in private practice and public health (Veterans Affairs) clinics: are they different? *Ear and Hearing, 26*(6), 513–528.

Crews, J. E., & Campbell, V. A. (2004, May). Vision impairment and hearing loss among community-dwelling older Americans: implications for health and functioning. *American Journal of Public Health, 94*(5), 823–829.

Dalton, D. S., Cruickshanks, K. J., Klein, B. E., Klein, R., Wiley, T. L., & Nondahl, D. M. (2003, Oct). The impact of hearing loss on quality of life in older adults. *The Gerontologist, 43*(5), 661–668.

Danhauer, J. L., Celani, K. E., & Johnson, C. E. (2008, Jun). Use of a hearing and balance screening survey with local primary care physicians. *American Journal of Audiology, 17*(1), 3–13.

Department of Health and Human Services (DHHS). (2008). The Secretary's Advisory Committee on National Health Promotion and Disease Prevention Objectives for 2020. Phase I report

Disogra, R. (2008). Adverse drug reactions and audiology practice. *Audiol Today, 20*, 60–70.

Eleazer, G. P., & Brummel-Smith, K. (2009, May). Commentary: Aging America: meeting the needs of older Americans and the crisis in geriatrics. *Academic Medicine, 84*(5), 542–544.

Gates, G. A., Anderson, M. L., Feeney, M. P., McCurry, S. M., & Larson, E. B. (2008, Jul). Central auditory dysfunction in older persons with memory impairment or Alzheimer dementia. *Arch of Otolaryngol—Head & Neck Surg, 134*(7), 771–777.

Grimshaw, J. M., & Russell, I. T. (1994, Mar). Achieving health gain through clinical guidelines II: Ensuring guidelines change medical practice. *Quality in Health Care, 3*(1), 45–52.

Hawkins, D. B. (2005, Jul-Aug). Effectiveness of counseling-based adult group aural rehabilitation programs: a systematic review of the evidence. *Journal of the American Academy of Audiology, 16*(7), 485–493.

Heine, C., & Browning, C. J. (2002, Oct). Communication and psychosocial consequences of sensory loss in older adults: overview and rehabilitation directions. *Disability and Rehabilitation, 24*(15), 763–773.

Hidalgo, J. L., Gras, C. B., Lapeira, J. M., Martínez, I. P., Verdejo, M. A., Rabadán, F. E., et al. (2008, Sep-Oct). The Hearing-Dependent Daily Activities Scale to evaluate impact of hearing loss in older people. *Annals of Family Medicine, 6*(5), 441–447.

Johnson, C. E., Danhauer, J. L., Koch, L. L., Celani, K. E., Lopez, I. P., & Williams, V. A. (2008, Feb). Hearing and balance screening and referrals for Medicare patients: a national survey of primary care physicians. *Journal of the American Academy of Audiology, 19*(2), 171–190.

Johnson, E. (2008). Despite having more advanced features, hearing aids hold line on retail price. *Hearing Journal, 61*, 42–48.

Kaźmierczak, H., & Doroszewska, G. (2001). Metabolic disorders in vertigo, tinnitus, and hearing loss. *The International Tinnitus Journal, 7*(1), 54–58.

Khan, K. S., & Coomarasamy, A. (2006). A hierarchy of effective teaching and learning to acquire competence in evidenced-based medicine. *BMC Medical Education, 6*, 59.

Kirkwood, D. (2007). Bucking bad economic news, hearing aid sales rise by 5.4% on way to record year. *Hearing Journal, 60*, 11–16.

Kochkin, S. (2005). Hearing loss and its impact on household income. *Hearing Review, 12*, 16–24.

Kochkin, S., & Marketrak, V. I. I. (2007). Obstacles to adult non-user adoption of hearing aids. *Hearing Journal. 60*, 27–43.

Lam, B. L., Lee, D. J., Gómez-Marín, O., Zheng, D. D., & Caban, A. J. (2006, Jan). Concurrent visual and hearing impairment and risk of mortality: the National Health Interview Survey. *Archives of Ophthalmology, 124*(1), 95–101.

Landefeld, C. S., Winker, M. A., & Chernof, B. (2009, Dec). Clinical care in the aging century—announcing "Care of the aging patient: from evidence to action". *JAMA, 302*(24), 2703–2704.

Lee, F. S., Matthews, L. J., Dubno, J. R., & Mills, J. H. (2005, Feb). Longitudinal study of pure-tone thresholds in older persons. *Ear and Hearing, 26*(1), 1–11.

Leung, J., Wang, N. Y., Yeagle, J. D., Chinnici, J., Bowditch, S., Francis, H. W., et al. (2005, Dec). Predictive models for cochlear implantation in elderly candidates. *Arch of Otolaryngol—Head & Neck Surg, 131*(12), 1049–1054.

Lieb, C. (2009). Principles of adult learning. http://honolulu.hawaii.edu/intranet/committees/FacDevCom/guidebk/teachtip/adults-2.htm

Mathers, C., Smith, A., & Concha, M.(2003). Global burden of hearing loss in the year 2000. [Internet]. Geneva: World Health Organization. http://who.int/healthinfo/statistics/bod_hearingloss.pdf

Meikle, M. B., Stewart, B. J., Griest, S. E., & Henry, J. A. (2008, Sep). Tinnitus outcomes assessment. *Trends in Amplification, 12*(3), 223–235.

Newman, C. W., & Sandridge, S. A. (2004, Mar). Hearing loss is often undiscovered, but screening is easy. *Cleveland Clinic Journal of Medicine, 71*(3), 225–232.

Nondahl, D. M., Cruickshanks, K. J., Wiley, T. L., Klein, R., Klein, B. E., & Tweed, T. S. (2002, Jun). Prevalence and 5-year incidence of tinnitus among older adults: the epidemiology of hearing loss study. *Journal of the American Academy of Audiology, 13*(6), 323–331.

Ockene, J. K., & Zapka, J. G. (2000, Aug). Provider education to promote implementation of clinical practice guidelines. *Chest, 118*(2, Suppl), 33S–39S.

Olsen, W. (2008). *Mayo Clinic on better hearing and balance.* Rochester, MN: Mayo Clinic

Pacala, J. T., & Yueh, B. (2012, Mar). Hearing deficits in the older patient: "I didn't notice anything". *JAMA, 307*(11), 1185–1194.

Rawool, V., & Harrington, B. (2007). Middle ear admittance and hearing abnormalities in individuals with osteoarthritis. *Audiology and Neuro-Otology, 12*, 127–136.

Roland, P. S., Smith, T. L., Schwartz, S. R., Rosenfeld, R. M., Ballachanda, B., Earll, J. M., et al. (2008, Sep). Clinical practice guideline: cerumen impaction. *Otolaryngology—Head and Neck Surgery, 139*(3, Suppl 2), S1–S21.

Rubenstein, L. Z. (2006, Sep). Falls in older people: epidemiology, risk factors and strategies for prevention. *Age and Ageing, 35*(Suppl 2), ii37–ii41 10.1093/ageing/afl084.

Russo, F. A., & Pichora-Fuller, M. K. (2008, Oct). Tune in or tune out: age-related differences in listening to speech in music. *Ear and Hearing, 29*(5), 746–760.

Silverman, C. A., Silman, S., Emmer, M. B., Schoepflin, J. R., & Lutolf, J. J. (2006, Nov-Dec). Auditory deprivation in adults with asymmetric, sensorineural hearing impairment. *Journal of the American Academy of Audiology, 17*(10), 747–762.

Smith, J. L., Mitchell, P., Wang, J. J., & Leeder, S. R. (2005). A health policy for hearing impairment in older Australians: what should it include? *Australia and New Zealand Health Policy, 2*, 31.

Solodar, H., & Chappell, J. (2005). "Welcome to Medicare" preventative exam includes hearing and balance screening. *Audiology Today, 17*, 49.

Stewart, R., & Wingfield, A. (2009, Feb). Hearing loss and cognitive effort in older adults' report accuracy for verbal materials. *Journal of the American Academy of Audiology, 20*(2), 147–154.

Sweetow, R. (2007). Instead of hearing aid evaluation, let's assess functional communication ability. *Hearing Journal, 60*, 26–31.

Teutsch, C. (2003, Sep). Patient-doctor communication. *The Medical Clinics of North America, 87*(5), 1115–1145.

Tinetti, M. E., Baker, D. I., King, M., Gottschalk, M., Murphy, T. E., Acampora, D., et al. (2008, Jul). Effect of dissemination of evidence in reducing injuries from falls. *The New England Journal of Medicine, 359*(3), 252–261.

Tusa, R. (2009). Dizziness. *Medical Clinics of North America,* 263–271

U.S. Preventive Services Task Force (2012a). Screening for Hearing Loss in Older Adults. http://www.uspreventiveservicestaskforce.org/uspstf/uspshear.htm. Retrieved August 29, 2012.

U.S. Preventive Services Task Force (2012b). Prevention of Falls in Community-Dwelling Older Adults. http://www.uspreventiveservicestaskforce.org/uspstf11/fallsprevention/fallsprevsum.htm. Retrieved August 29, 2012.

Ventry, I. M., & Weinstein, B. E. (1982, May-Jun). The hearing handicap inventory for the elderly: a new tool. *Ear and Hearing, 3*(3), 128–134.

Ventry, I. M., & Weinstein, B. E. (1983, Jul). Identification of elderly people with hearing problems. *ASHA, 25*(7), 37–42.

Wallhagen, M. I., Pettengill, E., & Whiteside, M. (2006, Oct). Sensory impairment in older adults: Part 1: Hearing loss. *The American Journal of Nursing, 106*(10), 40–48, quiz 48–49.

Walton, J., & Burkhard, R. (2001). Neurophysiological manifestations of aging in the peripheral and central auditory nervous system. Anatomical and neurochemical bases of presbycusis. In P. Hoff & C. Mobbs (Eds.), *Functional neurobiology of aging* (pp. 581–596). San Diego: Academic Press 581–596

Willott, J. F., Hnath Chisolm, T., & Lister, J. J. (2001, Sep-Oct). Modulation of presbycusis: current status and future directions. *Audiology & Neuro-Otology, 6*(5), 231–249.

Wu, H. Y., Chin, J. J., & Tong, H. M. (2004, Feb). Screening for hearing impairment in a cohort of elderly patients attending a hospital geriatric medicine service. *Singapore Medical Journal, 45*(2), 79–84.

Yueh, B., Shapiro, N., MacLean, C. H., & Shekelle, P. G. (2003, Apr). Screening and management of adult hearing loss in primary care: scientific review. *JAMA, 289*(15), 1976–1985.

Zapka, J., Goins, K. V., Pbert, L., & Ockene, J. K. (2004, Jul). Translating efficacy research to effectiveness studies in practice: lessons from research to promote smoking cessation in community health centers. *Health Promotion Practice, 5*(3), 245–255.

◆ Appendix 10.1: Case Scenario

There are occasions when individuals who were previously functioning well with their hearing aids can experience a decline in performance. Mr. Osborne, an 80-year-old accountant who continues to work part time, recently has been a little forgetful, and his family has noticed that he is taking considerably more time to process information than in the past. Regarding his physical health status, he smokes approximately one pack of cigarettes per day, and recently was prescribed Prozac because of a recent onset of mild depression with the passing of his wife of 45 years. He had worn analogue, behind-the-ear hearing aids for 10 years and until recently was quite satisfied with them. They were helping to alleviate his difficulties understanding speech, attributable to his bilateral, moderately to moderately severe, high-frequency sensorineural hearing loss, which he first noted on his 65th birthday. Pure-tone test results at his most recent examination revealed that his hearing loss had remained stable over the years. His speech understanding ability in quiet was good under earphones, but speech in the presence of noise was fair in the right ear, poor in the left ear, and very poor in the sound field when tested with the hearing aids and with visual cues to facilitate understanding. The audiologist administered the Mini-Mental Status Examination because Mr. Osborne appeared to respond inconsistently and inaccurately to selected questions, and his score suggests possible nascent cognitive issues.

Noteworthy is the pattern of findings on the Hearing Handicap Inventory for the Elderly (HHIE), which confirmed Mr. Osborne's subjective complaints in that he no longer was benefiting from the hearing aids. The baseline score on the HHIE was 50%, which he obtained prior to hearing aids, the score improved to 24% after the initial hearing-aid fitting. The audiologist regularly administered the HHIE when Mr. Osborne returned for follow-up evaluations, and the score remained at 20 to 24%, suggesting considerable reduction (improvement) in psychosocial handicap attributable to hearing-aid use from the baseline, but also some residual disability. At Mr. Osborne's most recent visit, the HHIE score returned to 52%, confirming limited hearing-aid benefit and considerable residual disability. The audiologist suggested the patient return to his physician because of concerns regarding cognitive status, and recommended high-end digital behind-the-ear (BTE) aids with a remote wireless FM receiver as an accessory to facilitate speech understanding in noise. The advantages of remote wireless technology include elimination of the negative effects of talker distance, room noise, and room reverberation, and the improved signal-to-noise ratio achieved by bringing the microphone closer to the source of sound. Essentially, FM systems bridge the acoustical space between the sound source and the listener by eliminating the detrimental effects on speech understanding, distance, noise, and reverberation.

Mr. Osborne, at the urging of his son, agreed to give the BTE aid with a remote wireless receiver a try, and was immediately impressed with the clarity of the signal, especially with excessive noise present in the background. Mr. Osborne was counseled on how to use the hearing aids, and upon a follow-up visit was happy to report that speech understanding in the most difficult situations had improved dramatically. The HHIE-S score of 28% verified that Mr. Osborne was deriving substantial benefit from the wireless technology. The audiologist consulted with the physician, who evaluated the dosing of the medication, which was adjusted, and cognitive status and affect seemed to improve accordingly.

Chapter 11

Long-Term-Care Services

If only I could hear, it would not be so bad to be 104 years of age; after all I survived WW I, WW II, the Vietnam War, and the attack on the World Trade Center in 2001.

—R.K., assisted-living resident

If only the staff knew that most of us cannot hear when they speak to us, it would make a world of difference.

—F.P., 91-year-old nursing home resident

◆ Learning Objectives

After reading this chapter, you should be able to

- understand the long-term-care continuum;
- explain how long-term care is organized;
- state characteristics of individuals eligible for long-term care;
- deliver audiological services in nursing facilities; and
- understand the role of audiologists in home-care settings.

◆ Overview

Long-term care is a broad term that encompasses a wide range of populations, services, and funding sources. Long-term care can be delivered in institutions or in the home. In contrast to institutional long-term care, the demand for community-based long-term care (CBLTC) is on the rise, as functionally impaired older adults increasingly choose to remain in the community, requiring services that can help them remain at home (Hayashi & Leff, 2009). Institutional long-term care refers to the array of health and social services provided in institutions over an extended period of time to individuals who have chronic, long-term, and complex conditions; are functionally impaired; and, for the most part, are elderly (Evashwick, 1993; Morgan & Kunkel, 2011). The broad range of services may be continuous or intermittent, but are generally delivered for a sustained period of time to people who are limited in their ability to function independently. The functional disabilities are variable, may be permanent or temporary, and may be physical or mental. The need for long-term care may also be to assist those with terminal illness (Samos, Aguilar, &

Ouslander, 2010). Functional dependency is typically defined in terms of the ability to perform essential activities of daily living (ADL) (e.g., eating, dressing, or getting out of bed) or activities necessary to remain independent, known as instrumental activities of daily living (IADL), which include shopping, cooking, housekeeping, and managing household finances (Morgan & Kunkel, 2011). **Table 11.1** lists functions that fall under the rubric of ADL and IADL. There are two basic types of long-term care in institutions in the United States, namely nursing homes (NHs) or assisted-living facilities (ALFs) (Samos et al, 2010). National spending on nursing home care amounts to approximately $83 billion annually.

In contrast to institutionally based long-term care, CBLTC is more decentralized, with little federal regulation. Referring to nursing, personal care, and social services, the term *CBLTC* is often used interchangeably with home care, personal care services, home and community-based services, and home visits (Hayashi & Leff, 2009). The primary goal of CBLTC is to help meet the needs of older adults who choose to remain in the community. Typically, home-care services involve some form of postacute hospital care or rehabilitation. Home health care services are either skilled or unskilled, with the need first arising following hospital discharge coupled with the need for highly advanced technological care required in the home. Services tend to be provided by community-based agencies. Unskilled care is typically delivered by family members who are unpaid, with 26 million informal caregivers in the U.S. providing the bulk of the services. Skilled home health care refers to services delivered by a variety of health care professionals including nurses and physical, occupational, and speech therapists. National spending on home care delivered by more formal, skilled caregivers amounts to $32 billion. Home health care agencies are reimbursed for the skilled services they provide to homebound individuals. Assessments regarding the need for nursing home placement are frequently done in the hospital, whereas level of care assessments for CBLTC are often performed in the patient's home or in continuing care retirement communities when a decision regarding the need to change from independent living to assisted living or to skilled care is indicated (Grant, Fey, Fedus, & Campbell, 2011).

In assessing level of care, a key concept is safety within the context of the community, and the assessment typically includes collecting data about preexisting conditions, patient

Table 11.1 Activities of Daily Living and Instrumental Activities of Daily Living

Basic activities of daily living: self-care tasks (National Research Council, 2010)

1. Feeding
2. Dressing
3. Ambulation
4. Toileting
5. Bathing
6. Transferring (moving from one surface to another)
7. Continence
8. Grooming
9. Communication

Instrumental activities of daily living (IADL): activities necessary to live independently in the community

1. Writing
2. Reading
3. Meal preparation
4. Housework (e.g., cleaning)
5. Shopping
6. Laundry
7. Climbing steps
8. Using the telephone
9. Managing medication
10. Managing finances
11. Ability to travel (use public transportation)
12. Household management

Sources: From Kane, R., Ouslander, J., & Abrass, I. (1994). *Essentials of clinical geriatrics* (3rd ed.). New York: McGraw-Hill; and National Research Council (NRC). (2010). The role of human factors in home health care: Workshop summary. In S. Olson (Ed.), *Committee on the Role of Human Factors in Home Health Care. Committee on Human-Systems Integration, Division of Behavioral and Social Sciences and Education.* Washington, DC: National Academies Press.

safety, ADL and IADL function, and cognitive function. In my view, hearing status can interfere with administration of the level of care assessment and thus may undermine the validity of the assessment, so audiologists must make sure that those doing the assessments understand how to communicate with the hearing impaired and can recognize when a hearing loss exists so as to control for it during the assessment (e.g., use a personal amplifier or screen for hearing loss).

Pearl

The essential element in defining the need for long-term care is functional capacity. Long-term care implies dependence of an individual on the services of another person (Kane, Ouslander, & Abrass, 1994). In 2007, nearly 7 million older Americans required some form of long-term care due to functional impairments from a chronic medical condition or illness (Hayashi & Leff, 2009).

◆ Institutional Long-Term Care

Given increases in life expectancy and technological advances, it is projected that 35% of Americans 65 years of age or over will require some form of nursing home care in their lifetime; 18% will likely live in a nursing home for at least 1 year, and 5%

for at least 5 years. In the United Kingdom, it is projected that between 2003 and 2051 the number of care home places will rise by 150% because of the rise in prevalence of dementia (Bowman, 2010). Today 2% of Americans aged 65 to 84 years and 14% of those 85 years of age or older reside in nursing homes, totaling 1.8 million residents (Samos et al, 2010). It is noteworthy that since the first edition of this book, the proportion of older adults living in nursing homes has decreased dramatically among individuals 75 years of age and older due to a trend toward aging in place.

Almost half of all residents of nursing homes are 85 years of age or older, with the majority being women (Samos et al, 2010). The racial disparity among residents in terms of age is noteworthy, in that black residents are twice as likely as white residents to be under age 65 (21.9% versus 10%), and black residents are less likely to be aged 85 years or older (30.2% versus 47.7%) (Jones, Dwyer, Bercovitz, & Strahan, 2009). Of the nursing home population reported to be of Hispanic or Latino origin, 22.8% are under age 65 years, and 24.6% are aged 85 years or older, totaling 47.4%, which is comparable to the total of 46.1% of residents in these two age groups who are not of Hispanic or Latino descent. The interaction between gender and race among nursing home residents is also of interest. Of all nursing home residents, 71.2% are women, and 59.5% of Hispanic or Latino nursing home residents are women, as compared with 71.6% of their non–Hispanic or Latino counterparts. Similarly, among black residents, 63.5% are women, as compared with 72.6% of their white counterparts. These trends are likely due to the lack of availability of informal support systems, economic factors, health disparities, and differences in health literacy.

The majority of residents of nursing homes have some form of dementia, more than half are wheelchair bound, and 80% need help with four or five ADLs (Samos et al, 2010). The primary characteristic of those being admitted to nursing facilities is functional decline associated with a decrease in strength and balance, cognitive changes, and impairment in IADL (Rapp & Rapp, 2009). Stroke, Parkinson's disease, Alzheimer's disease, and diabetes mellitus are risk factors for the aforementioned functional declines. Additionally, lack of availability of an informal support system increases the potential need for institutional care. Interestingly, more than half of all residents who were interviewed as part of the National Nursing Home Survey were either totally dependent or required extensive assistance in bathing, dressing, toileting, and transferring (Jones et al, 2009). According to results of the 2004 National Nursing Home Survey, mental disorders were the second leading primary diagnosis among residents at admission (16.4%) and at the time of interview (21.9%), with 14% of residents having had a primary admission diagnosis for diseases of the nervous system and sense organs. Of interest and of relevance to audiologists is that 33.9% of all residents had at least one reported fall in the 180 days prior to the interview, and 8.9% of residents had fallen in the 30 days prior to the interview. Interestingly, nursing home residents aged 65 years or older were more likely than those under age 65 to have fallen in the 180 days prior to the interview. Because dizziness often contributes to falls, and older individuals with hearing impairment are prone to dizziness, it is important to assess hearing status in these individuals.

Falls occur in nursing homes at an average rate of 1.5 falls per resident annually. The odds of a resident falling increases dramatically within 2 days of a new prescription or increase in dosage for a non–selective serotonin reuptake inhibitor (SSRI) antidepressant, especially in residents taking several medications (Berry et al, 2011).

According to the 2004 National Nursing Home Survey, there are 16,100 nursing homes in the U.S. with 1.7 million beds (Jones et al, 2009). The majority of nursing homes are proprietary (62%), with 31% operating as voluntary and not-for-profit. Nursing care at nursing facilities is provided by registered nurses, licensed practical nurses, certified nursing assistants, nurses' aides, and orderlies, and of these workers, the majority tend to be employees of the nursing home rather than contract workers. The majority of the nursing services are provided by certified nursing assistants. Despite the high prevalence of hearing impairment among nursing home residents, the curriculum for most nursing professionals working in nursing facilities includes little information about hearing impairment; hence, audiologists must consider options for educating professionals so as to promote good quality of care delivered to residents.

Nursing homes operate under both federal and state law. In general, federal law mandates the framework for what states must do, with states often imposing additional regulations. Additionally, state agencies may issue further regulations to supplement state laws. The basis for state nursing home regulations is the federal 1987 Omnibus Budget Reconciliation Act [OBRA 87; OBRA (1987)]. OBRA 87 applies to long-term facilities receiving Medicare or Medicaid funding. Interestingly, federal law describes nursing homes as skilled nursing facilities (SNFs) under the Medicare program, and nursing facilities (NFs) under the Medicaid program (Code of Federal Regulations [CFR] 483.5). Nursing homes are licensed under the Medicare or Medicaid program, or both. It is mandated that nursing homes care for their residents in a manner and in an environment that promotes maintenance or enhancement of each resident's quality of life, with emphasis placed on dignity, choice, and self-determination for residents (CFR 483.15). Nursing homes must provide the care and services necessary to attain or maintain the highest practicable physical, mental, and psychosocial well-being in accordance with the comprehensive assessment and plan of care (CFR 483.25) (Electronic Code of Federal Regulations [e-CFR], 2011). Federal law also stipulates the participation of the resident, the resident's family, or the resident's legal representative in preparation of the resident care plan. Under section 483.25, the law stipulates that nursing home residents must receive proper treatment and assistive devices to maintain vision and hearing abilities. The facility must, if necessary, assist the resident in making appointments and arrange for transportation to and from the office of the professional who specializes in the treatment of hearing impairment or the provision of hearing-assistance technologies.

Ability to perform ADL and IADL is the primary index of magnitude of functional disability. The prevalence of functional disability, defined according to ability to perform the ADL, increases dramatically with age. Functional disabilities and chronic illness (e.g., hearing impairment) are interrelated, and both increase in prevalence with age (Evashwick, 1993). Chronic diseases such as arthritis, hypertension, and hearing loss tend to be accompanied by functional disabilities.

Consumers of institutional long-term care (i.e., in nursing homes) can be divided into two types: those needing short-term care and those requiring longer or permanent long-term care (Evashwick, 1993). Persons requiring short-term care tend to be those with subacute illness, those who are medically ill, those who are terminal, or those who are undergoing rehabilitation. In contrast, individuals who require extended time periods for convalescence fall into the second group, typically referred to as long stayers (Samos et al, 2010). Long stayers tend to have physical or cognitive impairment and many have impairments of both cognitive and physical function. Short stayers are typically in a nursing home for between 1 and 6 months, whereas long-stayers tend to remain for 6 months to 2 years. The traditional long-term-care population includes individuals with ongoing and multiple health, mental health, or social problems who are unable to care for themselves. Individuals requiring short-term care or the long stayers benefit from the services of audiologists, given the rights of nursing home residents as enumerated in the Nursing Home Residents' Bill of Rights. According to the Bill of Rights, residents must be engaged in decisions regarding their care plan and must be fully informed in advance of any changes in care, treatment, or their status in the facility, and they must be treated with dignity. Clearly, the ability to communicate with older residents who are likely to be hearing impaired is an important consideration if resident rights are to be met.

Assessment Protocols in Nursing Homes

Nursing homes are heavily governed by federal and state regulations to ensure adequate care, yet despite this at least 20% are cited annually for serious deficiencies that place the resident at risk (Stefanacci, 2010). Under OBRA 87, which became a federal law in 1990, nursing homes participating in Medicare and Medicaid must monitor residents using the Resident Assessment Instrument (RAI). The comprehensive assessment tool mandated by the Nursing Home Reform Act guides individualized care planning (Lubinski & Frattali, 1993). The RAI consists of (1) a multidimensional assessment known as the Minimum Data Set (MDS), and (2) the Resident Assessment Protocols (RAPs). A federally mandated needs assessment, the MDS is performed upon admission and quarterly thereafter (Berry et al, 2011). MDS assessment items cover dimensions ranging from hearing and cognitive status, history of recent falls, and physical function, to depression and well-being, with checklists for common geriatric diagnoses, symptoms, and syndromes.

Table 11.2 Conditions Assessed by the Resident Assessment Plan

Delirium
Cognitive loss/dementia
Visual function
Communication
ADL/functional rehabilitation
Urinary incontinence
Psychosocial well-being
Mood state
Behavior symptoms
Activities
Falls
Nutrition
Feeding tubes
Dehydration/fluid maintenance
Dental care
Pressure ulcers
Psychotropic drug use
Physical restraint

Source: From Samos, L., Aguilar, E., & Ouslander, J. (2010). Institutional Long-Term Care in the United States. In H. Fillit, K. Rockwood, & K. Woodhouse (Eds.), *Brockelhurst's textbook of geriatric medicine and gerontology* (7th ed.). Philadelphia: Saunders Elsevier.

Table 11.3 Tool Kit Used for Nursing Home Staff When Making Resident Visits

Stethoscope
Pocket oto-ophthalmoscope
Cerumen spoon
Reflex hammer
Monofilament
Personal digital assistant (PDA) with drug reference and medical calculations
Prescription pad
Bandage scissor
Mirror
Pen

Source: From Rapp, M., & Rapp, K. (2009). Nursing facility care. In J. Halter, J. Ouslander, M. Tinetti, S. Studenski, K. High, & S. Asthana (Eds.), *Hazzard's geriatric medicine and gerontology* (6th ed.). New York: McGraw-Hill.

The RAI drives clinical care in nursing homes. A registered nurse coordinates the intake, and a multidisciplinary team, including nursing, social services, dietary, rehab/restorative activities, pharmacy, and medical staff, partners with the resident and family member to ensure the accuracy of the assessment and care planning process. The MDS prescribes resident assessment in the following areas: ADL, cognition, continence, mood, vision, communication, activities, and psychosocial well-being (Stefanacci, 2010). As noted above, the MDS requires assessment of communication/hearing patterns and psychosocial well-being, among other areas of function. Depending on responses to items on the MDS, residents are "triggered" into a RAP as potentially having a related problem, risk factor, or potential for improved function. The RAPs are designed to guide nursing facility staff in identifying and developing care plans for patient problems (Phillips, Hawes, Mor, Fries, & Morris, 1998). OBRA 87 requires a registered nurse to coordinate the assessment with the MDS, with appropriate input from health professionals. Through the MDS, risks for decline are identified, triggering further assessment on one or more of the RAIs RAP. The RAP addresses the conditions listed in **Table 11.2**, and is used to identify treatable causes of problems prevalent in nursing home residents (Stefanacci, 2010). The resident plan of care is considered a dynamic interdisciplinary document; the initial plan must be implemented within 24 hours of admission to the facility. Ideally, a more formal plan of care is to be completed no later than the 21st day of the resident's stay. Interestingly, a study of over 200 nursing homes revealed that the rate of decline in ADL, social engagement, and cognitive function was reduced following the introduction of the coordinated resident assessment. If nursing homes had an audiologist on staff, I am confident that the rate of decline in social engagement and cognitive function would be further reduced from auditory/communication-based interventions.

The initial plan of care must include physicians' orders and additional assessments/interventions as outlined by the ad-

mitting nurse/charge nurse to ensure resident safety (Shipman, 2011). According to Samos et al (2010), input from team members is variable, and care planning is often not coordinated. Audiologists have a responsibility to educate nurses about how to recognize persons with hearing impairment, how to communicate with them, and when to refer them to audiology, as the ability to understand staff during the intake and throughout one's stay is key to accurate diagnosis and quality care. Rapp and Rapp (2009) list the supplies and equipment used by physicians and nursing staff to monitor patients and to ensure the day runs efficiently. The contents of the pocket tool kit they recommend is included as **Table 11.3**. Note that Rapp and Rapp recommend that ear exams be conducted, as a cerumen spoon is included in the list but not an otoscope or Audioscope. I would like to see a Pocket Talker added to the tool kit, as one can assume that most residents will have hearing loss, and communicating with the resident will be much easier for those who do not have a hearing aid or are not wearing hearing aids.

The Centers for Medicare and Medicaid Services (CMS) is the component of the U.S. Department of Health and Human Services that oversees the Medicare and Medicaid programs. A large portion of Medicare and Medicaid dollars is used each year to cover nursing home care and services for the elderly. Further, CMS is responsible for establishing quality-of-care standards and conditions of participation for Medicare and Medicaid programs. CMS contracts with quality improvement organizations to assist nursing homes in making improvements in priority areas (CMS, 2007). States are responsible for licensing nursing homes, and states contract with CMS to monitor nursing homes that wish to become eligible to provide care to Medicare and Medicaid beneficiaries (Medicare, 2008). CMS is interested in promoting quality in nursing home care, and there are now Web-based report cards on nursing home care. Additionally, the certification process has been expanded and overhauled. More specifically, CMS has launched several initiatives designed to improve the effectiveness of the survey process and of complaint investigations, including, for example, a pilot of a background check system and improved fire safety regulations (Stefanacci, 2010).

In a continuing effort to improve quality of care, Quality Improvement Organizations (QIOs) in each state are contracted

Table 11.4 Selected Components of Nursing Home Culture Change and Implications for Hearing Health Care

1. Opportunities to gather for socialization and activities
2. Natural light
3. New technologies (e.g., loop system, TV ears)
4. Natural sounds that are audible
5. Contact with other generations (group FM systems)
6. Group bonding with communication
7. Nurture the human spirit (hearing is important)

Source: From Samos, L., Aguilar, E., & Ouslander, J. (2010). Institutional Long-Term Care in the United States. In H. Fillit, K. Rockwood, & K. Woodhouse (Eds.), *Brockelhurst's textbook of geriatric medicine and gerontology* (7th ed.). Philadelphia: Saunders Elsevier.

Table 11.5 Services Offered by Nursing Facilities

1. Nursing, personal care and related services, and specialized rehabilitative services to attain or maintain the highest practicable physical, mental, and psychosocial well-being of each resident
2. Medically related social services to attain or maintain the highest practicable physical, mental, and psychosocial well-being of each resident
3. Pharmaceutical services
4. Dietary, food, and nutrition services
5. Ongoing programs, directed by a qualified professional, of activities designed to meet the interests and the physical, mental, and psychosocial well-being of each resident
6. Routine dental services
7. Treatment and services required by mentally ill and mentally retarded individuals
8. Recreational and social services
9. Religious services
10. Financial management services

to assist nursing homes in their quality improvement efforts (Samos et al, 2010). Some of the focuses of the QIO initiative are to reduce depression in residents, to improve staff satisfaction, to reduce staff turnover, and to promote person-centered care. The use of hearing assistance technologies, including personal amplifiers and loop systems installed in selected areas, would likely help promote staff satisfaction, as it would facilitate communication with residents. Further, available evidence suggests that hearing interventions can reduce depression in older adults with hearing impairment. Similarly, in the nursing home industry, the buzz term is *culture change*, which means empowering staff to deliver patient-centered care, to improve quality of life for residents, and to modify the environment of the nursing home. I am convinced that audiologists have an important role to play in this regard as well. **Table 11.4** includes key components of the culture change initiative and the potential place of audiological services.

Nursing Home Personnel and Services

It is helpful for audiologists to understand the role of key personnel staffing nursing homes, as these are the individuals with whom the hearing-impaired residents will interact. Medicare and Medicaid regulations require that all nursing facilities hire and appoint a physician who is an independent contractor who typically devotes 2 to 4 hours a week to administrative matters. The primary role of the medical director is to ensure that medical care is coordinated and resident care policies implemented (Rapp & Rapp, 2009). The medical director also participates in the development of policies and procedures relevant to medical care delivery, and coordinates medical quality improvement programs. Attending physicians are expected to visit and approve orders for each resident every 30 days for the first 90 days and then every 60 days thereafter. During their resident visits, the physician or primary care provider is expected to address concerns raised by residents, family members, nursing, or rehabilitation staff, and here the role of the audiologist in educating staff and family about hearing loss can be key. Further, the primary care provider is responsible for determining the potential for functional improvement from therapy and to document therapeutic goals and objectives. The medical director interfaces with key personnel, including the facility administrator, who is responsible for fiscal matters, and the director of nursing, who coordinates and manages resident nursing care.

Nursing personnel have very distinct responsibilities, ranging from the MDS nurse, who is responsible for coordinating completion of the MDS, to the charge nurse, who supervises nursing assistance, carries out physician orders, and contacts physicians when there is a change in patient status (Rapp & Rapp, 2009). As part of the Older Americans Act, all nursing homes have an ombudsman available to residents who is basically an advocate for residents and their families. Certified nursing assistants provide most of the direct care for ADL to residents, and the restorative nurses' aides report to either nursing or physical therapy and are responsible for continuing restorative care when physical and occupational therapy services are completed. Each of the above professionals should have a basic understanding of the symptoms of hearing loss, when to refer residents for a hearing exam, how to communicate with the hearing impaired, and how to operate basic hearing instruments. The in-service coordinator who is typically a nurse is responsible for helping employees acquire and maintain skills essential to the efficient and efficacious administration of nursing homes.

Nursing facilities must provide or arrange for the provision of services, many of which are listed in **Table 11.5**. According to the rules and regulations governing the long-term-care facilities that are listed in the Federal Register, nursing facilities are obliged to provide or obtain from an outside resource the rehabilitative service (e.g., audiology) if required as part of the resident's comprehensive plan of care. Audiological services certainly fall under the purview of specialized rehabilitative services to attain or maintain the highest practicable physical, mental, and psychosocial well-being. Audiologists working in nursing facilities must think of themselves as rehabilitation specialists as well as diagnosticians. In a later section of this chapter the MDS and associated care plan for hearing is discussed at length.

Hearing Status of Nursing Home Residents

It is estimated that 70 to 90% of elderly residents in long-term-care facilities have some degree of hearing impairment. Yet despite this high prevalence, there is significant underuse of hearing aids or other assistive devices, especially among those with dementia (Cohen-Mansfield & Taylor, 2004a; Garahan, Waller, Houghton, Tisdale, & Runge, 1992; Schow & Nerbonne, 1980). The high prevalence of disabling hearing loss is primarily due to the fact that the majority of residents are over 85 years of age, and, as discussed in previous chapters, there is a direct correlation between age and hearing loss severity. Further, the majority of residents suffer from medical conditions, including diabetes and cardiovascular disease, and cognitive impairments, all of which have a comorbidity with hearing loss. The prevalence of senile dementia among residents is high, with the proportion expected to increase given the trend toward nursing home placement for persons with dementia who are unable to care for themselves. The effects of dementia leave residents unable to fulfill many of their personal needs because of perceptual problems, communication difficulties, and an inability to manipulate their environment. The goals of treatment should then be to uncover and address the person's unmet needs.

Lin (2011) reported on the relation between hearing loss and cognitive function in a sample of 60- to 69-year-olds who were part of the National Health and Nutritional Examination Survey (NHANES). All participants included in the nationally representative data set underwent audiometry and tests of cognitive function, which included a nonverbal test of executive function and psychomotor speed. Apparently, performance on the Digit Symbol Substitution Test (DSST) is one of the first to decline prior to the onset of dementia. The DSST is a component of the Wechsler Adult Intelligence Scale (WAIS). Given the age of the sample, the majority of subjects had normal hearing, whereas 30% had a mild to moderate hearing loss. Only 6.7% of participants were hearing-aid users, which is not surprising as the majority of persons with hearing loss had mild impairment. Interestingly, poorer hearing was associated with lower DSST scores, and this correlation remained after controlling for age, sex, and hearing-aid use. Even among those with mild hearing loss, a 10-dB increase in hearing loss was associated with a DSST score difference of –1.5. Most interesting was that hearing-aid use was associated with better cognitive scores on the DSST. These findings, coupled with the mean age of nursing home residents, the high prevalence of cognitive problems among nursing home residents, and the mean hearing levels of persons in their 80s, suggest that many residents of nursing homes will have a co-occurrence of cognitive and hearing loss. Treating hearing loss may be effective in forestalling cognitive decline.

Hearing loss in nursing home residents is typically moderate to moderately severe, whereas in the noninstitutionalized population hearing loss tends to be mild to moderate. Many of the residents have auditory processing problems that tend to be more severe than the hearing impairment would suggest. Garahan et al (1992) reported that 52% of the residents they evaluated had moderate to severe hearing loss (average of 1000 to 2000 Hz). The majority of residents with moderate to severe hearing impairment perceived themselves to be handicapped. Interestingly, nurses tended to underestimate the extent of handicap relative to the residents' judgments. This is not surprising given the limited interpersonal contact nurses tend to have with residents, which suggests that the validity of nurses' judgments of hearing status is questionable, underlining the importance of audiologists or speech-language pathologists in the identification process. Nearly half of the residents with moderate to severe hearing impairment did not have a record of documented hearing impairment. Despite the high prevalence of hearing loss, barriers to hearing-aid use in nursing homes are multifactorial, involving a lack of system commitment to utilization of hearing aids and hearing-aid design, issues of fit and cost, and lack of knowledge regarding value and use (Cohen-Mansfield & Taylor, 2004b).

In 1987 Congress legislated sweeping changes in certified nursing homes, which included passage of OBRA, requiring nursing homes certified for Medicare coverage to screen all newly admitted residents for hearing loss, among other sensory and communication functions. Although OBRA does not specify the professional needed to assess hearing status of newly admitted residents, it is not atypical for facilities to contract with audiologists in private practice or hearing-instrument specialists to deliver services (Bloom, 1994; Center for Excellence in Assisted Living [CEAL], 2010). OBRA mandated a minimum set of standards of care and resident rights, with an emphasis on quality of life and quality of care (CEAL, 2010). Specifically, it mandated a uniform assessment strategy for all nursing home residents and is structured to trigger consideration of selected functional health problems that will ultimately lead to care planning for the resident. The use of a uniform geriatric assessment tool has been found to increase the rate at which residents' care problems are addressed. Incorporated into OBRA was the Nursing Home Reform Act, which is a series of amendments to the federal budget that changed the focus of long-term care from process evaluations to an emphasis on patient care outcomes, the caring process, and resident feelings (Evashwick, 1993). As will be discussed in a later section, OBRA (1987) is relevant to audiologists in that it requires a structured resident assessment and care plan including consideration of hearing status and communicative function

---

Pearl

Managing behavioral symptoms and helping residents to establish meaningful social engagement are important treatment goals for residents if quality of care and quality of life are to become a mandated reality. Communication function is at the heart of transforming nursing homes into facilities with physical environments and service delivery that are conducive to delivery of quality care.

Assisted-Living Facilities (ALFs)

As institutional long-term care also takes place in ALFs, the characteristics of these facilities are of relevance to audiologists. Introduced in the late 1980s, ALFs are designed to allow older adults to age in place with dignity and to enjoy their independence as long as possible. The concept of assisted living came about because of a desire on the part of the consumer for an alternative to a nursing home. The term *assisted living* describes a wide range of housing and service models with a focus on resident choice, independence, privacy, and dignity. Consumer demand for combining housing with services has contributed to a 5% decline in the proportion of nursing facility residents 65 years of age and older between 1994 to 2004, with a corresponding increase in the number of ALFs throughout the country. A key reason for the popularity of ALFs is the desire for little federal regulation, which allows for consumers to drive the movement and to satisfy the desire to age in place (NRC, 2010).

In general, residents of ALFs do not require the intensive medical and nursing care required of those in nursing homes, as they can typically perform ADL independently or with a little assistance (Samos, Aguilar, & Ouslander, 2010). According to a survey conducted by the National Center for Assisted Living, there are more than 36,000 ALFs in the U.S., with the average age of residents being 83 years (Samos, Aguilar, & Ouslander, 2010). The majority of persons residing in ALFs are women. Key services provided in ALFs include meals, social services, housekeeping, recreational and spiritual activities, assistance with medication management, and social services. To meet the scheduled and unscheduled needs of residents, ALFs provide awake staff 24 hours per day (National Research Council [NRC], 2010). ALFs are philosophically distinct from NHs, as the cost is paid privately by residents and family members, thus for the most part ALFs are out of the reach of low-income individuals (Morgan & Kunkel, 2011). As residents of ALFs increasingly require some assistance with ADL and IADL, some are beginning to resemble nursing homes without the level of regulatory oversight.

As promoting resident dignity, autonomy, independence, and quality of life is central to the mission of ALFs, the ability to communicate with other residents and personnel is vital to the well-being of residents of ALFs. Thus, audiologists have an important role to play in the lives of ALF residents. Person-centered care (PCC) is a core principle driving the evolution of ALFs, and the latter concept is important to audiologists as personal choice through relationships and a sense of community is the vehicle for achieving PCC (CEAL, 2010). According to CEAL (2010), PCC has a three-pronged focus: (1) changes in the physical environment (i.e., need to create a feeling of residing in one's home); (2) service delivery (resident directed); and (3) core values (dignity, respect, choice, and independence). PCC recognizes that residents' well-being will be optimized through meaningful activity and opportunities that ensure that residents achieve a sense of self-worth in their everyday living experience and physical environment. To ensure that these goals are achieved, residents of ALFs are personally involved in directing their living arrangements and ensuring that services are delivered in a manner that best meets their needs (Bowers, 2009). **Table 11.6** lists the elements and essence of PCC and the role of hearing/communication in achieving the outcomes at the heart of PCC.

Pearl

A nurturing environment in which to live and a positive environment in which to work are at the heart of the definition of PCC.

Table 11.6 Elements Fundamental to Person-Centered Care and Relationship to Hearing

Element	Interpretation	Relevance of Hearing Status
A comprehensive and ongoing process	Is the operation and function of ALFs continually being monitored, assessed, and transformed. Is staff accountable? Are stakeholders involved?	Residents are stakeholders and must be involved in discussions regarding changes to the facility; ability to communicate is key.
Adoption of nurturing and empowering practices as part of service delivery	Is the resident empowered to drive the everyday operation of the facility?	Resident and staff must be able to communicate to achieve this element.
Enable residents to experience a purpose and meaning in their daily lives	Activities must be engaging, interpersonal interactions must be ongoing, relationships must evolve, and each resident must be valued; activities must support psychological well-being.	The ability to communicate with other residents, staff, and family members is central to a sense of purpose in life; ALFs must enhance relationships and reciprocity, mutual enjoyment, and adequate communication skills are at the heart of relationships.
Relationship-based culture and environment	The residence operates with a culture of mutual respect for residents' unique interests, preferences, and talents.	The ability to hear and communicate is the driver of a person- or resident-oriented ALF.
A home environment that feels safe and comfortable	The staff is essential in creating the environment necessary to thrive in an ALF.	The work culture must be one that fosters a sense of community, consistency, familiarity, and one that is conducive to staff socializing with residents; hearing status is key.
Quality of care	Good quality of care assumes that residents are well cared for in terms of health care, hygiene, housekeeping, and nutritional status.	The resident must communicate effectively with the staff, and communication must be bidirectional.
Quality of life	Are routines of residents respected and meaningful, and is life experience respected?	Residents needs and preferences drive the operation of the facility.

Abbreviation: ALF, assisted-living facility.
Source: From Center for Excellence in Assisted Living (CEAL). (2010). *Person-centered care in assisted living: An informational guide.* http://www.theceal.org/assets/pdf/person-centered%20care%20in%20assisted%20living.pdf.

◆ Community-Based Long-Term Care (Home Care)

Home care, a cost-effective alternative to hospital or institutional care, entails a broad spectrum of health care and social services provided in the home or other residential settings (Richardson, 1998). Bringing health care to people in their homes has significant benefits including reduced cost, convenience, and improved well-being (NRC, 2010). The rise in the proportion of people considered to be home health care recipients helps to make health and medical care delivered in the home more effective and efficient, allowing for aging in place with dignity. Recent studies have shown that older adults strongly prefer to continue living in their own homes (National Association of Home Builders Research Center, 2010). More than two thirds of home health care recipients are over the age of 65 (National Association for Home Care & Hospice [NAHCH], 2008). According to the National Association for Home Care, home-care organizations, which include home health care agencies, home-care aide organization, and hospices, have been providing services for over 100 years. There were 14,500 home health and hospice agencies in the U.S. in 2007, with expenditures exceeding $57.6 billion; 75% of these were home-care agencies, 15% provided hospice care only, and 10% were considered mixed agencies. The most common model of home health care involves a home health agency (HHA) that is certified to provide care under the rules established by Medicare (Hayashi & Leff, 2009). Currently, 56% of HHAs are free standing, whereas 18% are hospital based (NAHCH, 2008). Medicare added hospice benefits in 1983, and currently there are 3257 Medicare-certified hospices. There are a large number of HHAs, home-care aide organizations, and hospices that do not participate in Medicare.

Home health agencies differ by ownership type, ranging from proprietary to voluntary nonprofit to government and other ownership. Operated under private commercial ownership, proprietary HHAs are for profit, whereas voluntary nonprofit agencies are operated under voluntary or nonprofit auspices such as by religious organizations, and government agencies are operated under federal, state, or local government agencies (Park-Lee & Decker, 2010). Approximately 75% of all HHAs are proprietary, with 81% Medicare certified.

Pearl

Total employment in home health care has grown from 695,000 in 1996 to 913,300 in 2007 (U.S. Bureau of Labor Statistics, 2008).

Home health care involves at least two basic types of care delivered in a person's home: medically related services, often referred to as "home health care"; and services related to personal care or social needs (e.g., homemaking and chore services) (Kane et al, 1994; Richardson, 1998). Home health-care services consist of visits by health care professionals and include (1) nursing care; (2) physical, occupational, or speech therapy; (3) medical social services; and (4) home health aide services. Physician services are also offered by most agencies. For medically related services, a plan of care must be prescribed by a physician, and the care provided in the home must be supervised by a professional (e.g., a nurse). In contrast, personal care services, usually referred to as "home care," are semiskilled or nonskilled services that are designed to assist with the tasks of bathing, grooming, light housekeeping, meal preparation, laundry, and grocery shopping.

The triad of individuals engaged in health care in the home include the residents (i.e., the recipients of care), informal providers of care (informal caregivers), and formal caregivers. Informal caregivers are typically not paid, whereas formal caregivers are paid and are likely to have health care training, although it is not always specific to the provision of care in the home. Individuals with disabilities represent a significant population of people who engage in or are recipients of care at home. Formal caregivers include physicians, nurses, physician assistants, nurse practitioners, practitioners, social workers, physical and occupational therapists, speech-language pathologists, pharmacists, and home health aides (NRC, 2010). Of all health professionals involved in health delivery in the home, home health aides and registered nurses are the most numerous and visible. Interestingly, registered nurses and licensed practical nurses are certified and credentialed to work in the home, whereas credentialing for the dominant workers, namely home health aides/personal assistants, is limited. In 2007, agencies that provided home health care only were less likely than mixed agencies (e.g., provide hospice and home care) to provide speech therapy or audiology (67.0% compared with 89.5%), occupational therapy (74.1% compared with 89.8%), homemaker or companion services (37.8% compared with 56.6%), and durable medical equipment and supplies (13.6% compared with 56.0%) (Park-Lee & Decker, 2010). However, provision of physical therapy, personal care, and skilled nursing services did not differ by agency type. Home-care agencies specify that speech therapy or audiology services such as evaluation, treatment, and monitoring of specific communication disorders must be delivered by a certified or licensed speech-language pathologist or audiologist.

Home health aides employed by Medicare- and Medicaid-certified agencies must complete 75 hours of classroom and practical training and pass a competency test covering 12 subject areas including communication skills and basic nutrition (Institute of Medicine, 2008). Supervised by nurses or by speech, occupational, or physical therapists, home health aides can work for up to 4 months before completing their training (NRC, 2010). Audiologists have an important role to play in developing curricula on communication to ensure that home health aides are well versed in working with older adults with hearing impairment. **Table 11.7** shows the total number of skilled home health care workers by occupational status, confirming that home health aides make up the bulk of the home-care work force. **Table 11.8** shows that speech therapists and audiologists are included as services offered by selected home health agencies.

Health care tasks carried on in the home and delivered by caregivers can be divided into four distinct categories: (1) health maintenance—promoting general health and well-being, preventing disease or disability; (2) episodic care—optimizing outcomes of health events that pertain to pregnancy, childbirth, and mild or acute illness or injury; (3) chronic care—managing ongoing treatment of chronic disease or impairment;

Table 11.7 Number of Home Health Care Workers in Medicare-Certified Agencies by Occupational Status in 2006

Employment Status	Number of Employees
Registered nurses	126,453
Licensed practical nurses	56,610
Physical therapists	21,196
Home-care aides	458,685
Occupational therapists	6,272
Social workers	12,564
Other	183,320
Total	865,100

Source: From U.S. Bureau of Labor Statistics. (2008) National Industry Occupational Employment Matrix, data for 2006. In *Basic statistics about home care: Updated 2008.* http://www.nahc.org/facts/08hc_stats.pdf.

Table 11.8 Selected Services Offered by Agencies Providing Home Care and Hospice Care (Mixed) (1996 Through 2007)

Service
Skilled nursing
Physical therapy
Speech therapy or audiology
Occupational therapy
Physician services
Medical social services
Dietary and nutrition services
Pastoral services
Homemaker services
Referral services
Durable medical services

Source: From Park-Lee, E., & Decker, F. (2010). *Comparison of home and hospice care agencies by organizational characteristics and services provided: United States, 2007.* National Health Statistics Report No. 30. Hyattsville, MD: National Center for Health Statistics.

and (4) end-of-life care—addressing physical and psychological dimensions of dying (NRC, 2010). Given the level of the care delivered in the home and the important role played by formal and informal caregivers, there must be a productive partnership for the benefit of the care recipient. It remains a challenge to develop curricula designed to educate formal caregivers about strategies for including family members in health care provision in the home.

Informal caregivers carry a good deal of responsibility for their family members who choose to age in place. Approximately 2.7 to 36 million informal caregivers provide care to disabled older adults (Giovannetti & Wolff, 2010). Physical characteristics of informal caregivers, such as cognitive status and hearing, vision, and physical capabilities, are important and must be sufficient to provide effective service delivery. Sensory capabilities can influence the responsiveness and efficacy of care, especially the medically oriented care that involves dispensing medication, administering injections, and providing wound care. Informal caregivers typically accompany the home bound to medical appointments and are actively involved in communicating with health care professionals, underscoring their need to hear and understand (Wolff & Roter, 2008). In light of the weight of the responsibility on informal caregivers, skills training is playing an increasingly important role. The ability of caregivers to cope with the challenges of caregiving and to provide the appropriate assistance is a consideration for audiologists when working with older adults who are homebound. Their hearing status is important, and their knowledge of how to communicate with the hearing impaired and how to assist with the technology being used in the home is integral to care. Schulz and Tompkins (2010) have demonstrated that interventions that simultaneously target the caregiver and care recipient are quite effective in enhancing caregiver function. Although there is no reimbursement for caregiver education, it is well accepted that hearing-aid orientation and counseling sessions and rehabilitation should include an informal caregiver.

Health-related services provided by home health agencies differ dramatically from those offered by nursing facilities, primarily due to the case mix. Skilled home-health services include skilled nursing care; skilled therapies such as speech, occupational, and physical therapy; medical social work; and nutritional counseling. Skilled nursing care accounts for the

bulk of the reimbursable visits (Hughes, 1996). Often, several services are offered to one patient, requiring use of a multidisciplinary team. Team members visit the patient at different times and coordinate the paperwork required on each patient (Evashwick, 1993). In contrast, home health care services, specifically homemaker care, tend to consist of personal care, bathing and grooming, meal preparation, shopping, transportation, and household chores. Medicare-certified agencies are bound to the Outcome and Assessment Information Set (OASIS), and the HHA must certify each care recipient's medical, functional, and socioeconomic status, which determines the amount of reimbursement the agency will receive (Hayashi & Leff, 2009).

Pearl

As the number of residents in nursing homes is decreasing (Hetzel & Smith, 2001) and the number of persons receiving care in their homes is increasing, home-care agencies are adopting delivery systems to accommodate this change and are becoming more reliant on remote care technologies. The use of some form of telehealth is seen as both cost-effective and accessible, especially for the increasing number of homebound older adults (Engle, 2009; Wohlstadter, 2010).

Private HHAs are not bound by Medicare rules, although they do offer the same professional services plus numerous others (Evashwick, 1996). Noncertified agencies provide 24-hour care and daily care, as well as specialty services. These agencies also offer homemaker care services, including meal preparation, home repair, shopping, and housekeeping. Physician prescription is not required for these services. Private home-care agencies are staffed by a pool of health care professionals, home health aides, or homemakers who, for the most part, work on an as-needed basis. These agencies charge hourly rates, and typically a minimum number of hours is required. For the most part, audiologists do not work for Medicare-certified HHAs, yet many recipients of home health care have handicapping hearing impairments. It is incumbent

Table 11.9 Hearing Impairment Checklist for Recipients of Home Health Care Services

Name: _____   Age: _____

Hearing aids/implant: **Right ear:** Yes or No   **Left ear:** Yes or No

Assistive device: Specify type: _____

Item	YES	NO
1. Does the patient have the television volume raised to a very loud level?		
2. Does the patient ask people to repeat themselves when they speak?		
3. Does the patient answer when the doorbell rings, the telephone rings, or when someone knocks at the door?		
4. Does the patient misunderstand when spoken to by formal or informal caregivers?		
5. Do family members report that the patient frequently does not hear or misunderstands what they say?		
6. Does the patient complain of difficulty hearing/understanding?		
7. Does the patient own hearing aids that he or she does not wear?		
8. Does the patient have impacted cerumen in one or both ears?		

Recommendation and disposition: _____

on audiologists to educate the registered nurses, speech-language pathologists, and home health aides (i.e., the professionals who account for the majority of all staff in Medicare-certified agencies) about symptoms of hearing loss and referral criteria so that their clients are referred for the hearing health care services from which they can benefit. I did some consulting work for an HHA and in this capacity was responsible for identifying individuals requiring audiological services. My recommendations were to be based on my impressions from the patients' medical records. But this was an impossible task, as there was little evidence regarding hearing status in the charts. So I developed a brief checklist for home health personnel to help them identify individuals with potentially handicapping hearing loss (**Table 11.9**). If the answer to any of the questions is yes, the resident should be referred for audiological services.

Whenever feasible financially and geographically, one home visit is necessary for individuals identified as having a hearing impairment, as certain environmental modifications may be necessary to make sure that the home is safe. Hearing Assistance Technologies (HATs) that might be installed include an amplified telephone, alerting devices such as a visible smoke alarm or carbon monoxide detector, a vibrating or flashing alarm clock, and a visual display device that attaches to the door and emits a flashing light when someone knocks. If a home visit is not possible, a comprehensive assessment of the client's lifestyle, living arrangements, and listening difficulties should be completed to assist in decisions regarding installation of auxiliary assistive devices in the home. Telehealth technology could be instrumental in viewing a home to decide upon environmental modifications integral to safety.

Pearl

Homebound patients with hearing impairments and hearing aids must be reminded to wear their hearing aids at home to enable them to hear environmental and warning sounds. Audiologists must educate the other professionals working with the homebound about threats to safety in the home posed by significant hearing loss.

◆ Telehealth

The terms *telemedicine, telecare,* and *telehealth* fall within the sphere of gerontechnology, which entails information exchange between older persons/patients and health and care staff when they are in different settings or sites. Thanks to technical advances and societal demographic pressures, it is often used to bridge the transfer of care from hospital discharge to the home setting (Craig & Miskelly, 2010). Focusing on clinical data exchange, telemedicine refers to the use of electronic information and communications technologies to provide and support health care when distance separates the health care provider and recipient, and computer technology is the interface between the provider and the recipient (Dang, Golden, Cheung, & Roos, 2010). It is typically used to access off-site databases or to transmit diagnostic images that are then examined or interpreted at a remote site (Craig & Miskelly, 2010). Defined as the use of telecommunication technologies to provide access to health information and services across a geographical distance, the term *telehealth* increasingly refers to provision of preventive, rehabilitative, and educational health care services through telecommunication devices when patient and provider are in different locations (Flynn, 2010; Glueckauf, Nickelson, Whitton, &Loomis, 2004). According to the Agency for Healthcare Research and Quality (2001), telehealth which may or may not be delivered by physicians, involves the use of telecommunication technology for the delivery of medical diagnostics, to facilitate medical research across distances, for patient monitoring (e.g., vital signs monitoring), and for therapeutic purposes when distance separates the user from the health care provider (Dixon, Hook, & McGowan, 2008). Telehealth implies the use of telecommunication technologies to provide health care services and access to medical information for training and education. It provides for a wider stream of information not only to health care professionals but to consumers as well, with the goal being to increase awareness and to educate consumers about health-related issues (Barlow, Singh, Bayer, & Curry, 2007; Craig & Miskelly, 2010).

The terms *telemedicine, telehealth,* and *telecare* are often used interchangeably, but there are subtle distinctions. For example, when the focus is on social support in the patients' homes, home telecare is the primary focus, entailing provision of care in a home-based setting with the objective of providing primary support for the patient (Flynn, 2010). The rationale is that home telecare helps to promote independence, increased compliance, and improved quality of life and care to its users while reducing overall health care costs to society (Barlow et al, 2007).

Telehealth delivery can take many forms, including interactive communication devices such as videoconferencing, cameras connected inside and outside of the home for transmission of still images, and remote monitoring of vital signs. Typically, it is used for specialist referral services, patient consultations, remote patient monitoring of vital signs or of the home for safety and security purposes, medical education, and provision of consumer medical information and support through the telephone or Internet (Barlow et al, 2007). I have found telehealth to be useful as it has enabled me to provide corrective feedback and guidance to individuals in their homes who have difficulty inserting or removing hearing aids. I envision it being helpful to provide reminders about hearing-aid insertion, changing batteries, wearing hearing aids in the home (Rogers & Fisk, 2004).

Telehealth is delivered either asynchronously or synchronously; the latter is most applicable with older adults. Synchronous applications, referred to as "real-time data transfer," entails a two-way exchange between the care recipient and the provider in real time, thereby allowing the health care professional to assess the patient from a distance (Dang et al, 2010). It usually involves teleconferencing or two-way interactive television technology (Wohlstadter, 2010). Tele-rehabilitation, tele–mental health, and telecardiology tend to be delivered synchronously. I know of HHAs that use videoconferencing for delivery of therapeutic speech-language pathology services to the homebound, which is exceedingly well received.

"Store and forward" or "asynchronous" telehealth involves using technology to obtain clinical data from one location, storing it, and then sending it to a second location where the data can be evaluated for use in diagnosis and consultations (Wohlstadter, 2010). Store and forward data, which typically include digital images, email correspondence, and video and sound files, are used by specialists in dermatology, radiology, and ophthalmology because the technology allows for evaluation of cases without regard to schedule, appointment time, or clinic location (Brown, 2005; Wohlstadter, 2010).

An emerging area, e-health, involves delivery and dissemination of information and support services via the Internet. Delivery of health care information and health care resources over the Internet to older adults can only flourish if Web site design and navigation take into account the vision, dexterity, and cognitive changes that challenge the ability of older adults to use the Internet effectively. Further, for telecare or e-health to be effective, patients must be willing to forgo face-to-face communication with their health care provider and embrace the use of communication technology and medical devices either in their own home or at a remote location (Demiris, Speedie, & Hicks, 2004; Wohlstadter, 2010). A key to acceptance of e-health and telehealth is user-friendly technology that is reliable and not too costly. **Table 11.10** lists some of the potential advantages of e-health in hearing health care.

Table 11.10 Potential Role and Advantages of Telehealth in Hearing Health Care

1. Resource for information about hearing loss, hearing aids, hearing assistance technologies
2. Resource for preventive hearing health care including screening for self-reported hearing problems
3. Improve patient adherence via automated text message reminders pertaining to use and function of personal amplifiers, hearing aids, etc.
4. Online support groups
5. Monitor use of rehabilitative software such as the Listening and Communication Enhancement (LACE) software
6. Sense of security knowing that one has direct access to health care provider
7. Cost and time savings
8. Improved accessibility and convenience

Sources: From Dang, S., Golden, A., Cheung, H., & Roos, B. (2010). Telemedicine applications in geriatrics. In H. Fillit, K. Rockwood, & K. Woodhouse (Eds.), *Brockelhurst's textbook of geriatric medicine and gerontology* (7th ed.). Philadelphia: Saunders Elsevier; and Wohlstadter, J. (2010). *The state of telehealth in the delivery of hearing healthcare services to the elderly: A systematic literature review.* Capstone paper submitted in partial fulfillment of Doctor of Audiology Program at the Graduate Center, City University of New York.

Pearl

Telehealth encompasses delivery of health-promotion and disease-prevention services.

Rehabilitation conducted through telehealth and home education programs has been shown to provide patients with a greater sense of accomplishment and more positive feelings about their potential capabilities (Flynn, 2010). More specifically, from the perspective of the patient, potential advantages of telehealth include improved patient adherence, empowered patient participation in care, decreased need for the care recipient to travel, and treatment changes through patient feedback without office visits (Dang et al, 2010). From the perspective of the provider, telehealth offers more efficient use of clinician time, enhanced ability for follow-up, and enhanced access to care. Use of videoconferencing or text messaging can facilitate compliance and adherence to treatment regimens. The latter is an area requiring greater exploration by audiologists. The opportunity for ongoing interactions that are individualized and provide a lens into the person's home environment can be so important for older hearing-impaired adults who typically have difficulties in the home to which the audiologist is rarely privy. Interestingly, a 2008 Philips National Study on the Future of Technology and Telehealth in Home Care revealed that 64% of home health agencies reported that care managers were receptive to implementing telehealth, and over 71% of home-care agencies that use patient satisfaction monitoring services found that telehealth improved patient satisfaction with care (Engle, 2009).

Catherine Flynn (2010) one of my Au.D. students and a recent graduate, conducted a systematic review of the literature on the perceptions of telecare by adults with chronic illnesses and chronic conditions in the hope that the studies would inform the design of telehealth programs to be used in the delivery of hearing health care. She analyzed 19 studies exploring satisfaction with telecare and found that perceptions regarding telecare were overwhelmingly positive in the samples studied. The most widely used telecare delivery modes in her review were synchronous, and included vital sign monitoring devices, and communicating remotely using videoconferencing equipment, televisions, or telephones. Some of the studies were of questionable validity, because of subjects' hearing status and because telephones were the primary modality. In contrast, studies using videoconferencing were less problematic, as this allows for visualization of the provider's face to facilitate speech reading. The most commonly reported advantages of telecare delivery models included greater sense of security, less waiting time in the reception area, more frequent and direct access to the health care provider, and cost and time savings, and above all telecare enabled patients to remain healthy and manage their illness. There were also several disadvantages, including anxiety over having to be monitored regularly and the inconvenience of having to report vital signs at the same time daily. Reimbursement also remains a significant barrier to overcome prior to implementing telehealth. A system needs to be created to adequately compensate providers for their direct contact with the patients, as the lack of Medicare reimbursement is a huge disincentive to embrace telehealth. Further, ethical issues, including compliance with the Health Insurance Portability and Accountability Act (HIPAA), need to be addressed, and legal issues limit the ability to implement telehealth practices due to interstate licensure issues, for example (Dang et al, 2010). Finally, there remains a need for studies comparing the effectiveness, acceptability, and quality of telehealth services as compared with more traditional delivery.

◆ Tool Kit for the Delivery of Audiology Services in Long-Term-Care Settings

Home Care

Audiological services for homebound individuals are only covered to the extent that Medicare covers diagnostic services.

Hence, audiologists typically do not usually do home visits but do have a role to play in home care. Although audiologist are only peripherally involved in the delivery of services to homebound individuals, their role in ongoing education of physicians, nurses, home health aides, and home-care professionals (especially speech-language pathologists and physical therapists) regarding case finding, strategies for communicating with the hearing impaired, and tips on hearing-aid use and assistive technologies is critical. Speech-language pathologists (SLPs) hired by HHAs are considered experts on hearing, and so audiologists must educate formal caregivers such as SLPs, physical therapists, home health aides, and nurses about hearing health care, as the majority of homebound older adults are likely to have a hearing impairment that will interfere with the delivery of services. Formal caregivers are likely to encounter (1) homebound clients who may have been evaluated and received an amplification device prior to hospitalization and discharge and now require assistance; (2) homebound clients who are functionally impaired for a short time and may be identified through a brief screening as requiring the services of the audiologist once they can safely leave the home; or (3) persons who are functionally impaired on a permanent basis and could benefit from hearing assistance technology in the home to ensure that the environment is safe and that health professionals can be understood by the patients. Education of caregivers must focus on the likely scenarios to be encountered when working with these individuals.

I worked with colleagues in audiology (Carol Silverman) and colleagues in psychology (Bert Flugman and Seymour Spiegel), as part of a series of worker development grants, to develop a series of curricula addressing the knowledge and skills required of formal caregivers involved in home care. **Table 11.11** summarizes the basic knowledge and skills required by the professionals who are most likely to be working with the hearing impaired. As is evident, the skill set varies dramatically by occupation. Nurses primarily are responsible for the intake and for overseeing patient care, and therefore they need to be able to recognize a patient with hearing impairment to make the appropriate referral. Hence, basic tools for a hearing screening

Table 11.11 Knowledge and Skills Required of Selected Health Care Professionals Working with the Hearing Impaired Who Are Recipients of Home-Care Services

Knowledge and Skills	Nurses	Physical Therapists	Speech-Language Pathologists	Nurses' Aides
Universal precautions*	Yes	No	No	Yes
Basic anatomy of the ear and disease of the ear	Yes	Yes	Yes	No
Type and degree of hearing loss and associated symptoms	Yes	Yes	Yes	No
Basic hearing-aid styles	Yes	Yes	Yes	Yes
Operation of hearing aids	Yes	Yes	Yes	Yes
Maintenance and troubleshooting of hearing aids	No	No	Yes	No
Use of communication aids such as the Pocket Talker or television ears	Yes	Yes	Yes	Yes
Basic operation of cochlear implants or bone-anchored hearing aids	Yes	Yes	Yes	Yes
Maintenance of cochlear implants or bone-anchored hearing aids	No	No	Yes	Yes
Recognizing a patient with hearing impairment	Yes	Yes	Yes	Yes
Communicating with a patient with hearing impairment	Yes	Yes	Yes	Yes

*Handle hearing aids/earmolds with disinfectant wipes, use a disinfectant towelette (e.g., Audiowipes) to wipe the hearing aid with disinfectant before handling another hearing aid; when using an otoscope or the Audioscope, make sure to disinfect the speculum before each use or use disposable specula for otoscopic examinations.

Source: Adapted from Weinstein, B., Silverman, C., Flugman, B., & Spiegel, S. (2009). In-service training module for selected home care employees working with the homebound hearing impaired elderly. Unpublished report.

are important if case finding is to become a reality. Knowledge of anatomy of the ear and basic disorders is important, with an emphasis on tinnitus and dizziness as a contributing factor to falls, and cerumen impaction. Nurses also need to know about hearing technologies for communicating with the elderly; these devices will prove indispensable when doing home visits. Nurses also need to know how to communicate with the hearing impaired, as this will be critical when conducting the initial assessment and intake. Finally, universal precautions must be practiced by all health care workers.

In contrast to nurses, nurses' aides have little formal education, yet they are the primary formal caregiver who spends the most time with the homebound. Hence, they must have considerable familiarity with communication strategies and with the basic operation of hearing aids, including battery and hearing-aid insertion and removal, and manipulation of the volume control. If they are responsible for bathing the homebound patient, they also must know about taking precautions with hearing aids, cochlear implants, and bone-anchored hearing aids (e.g., avoidance of moisture).

Speech-language pathologists are often considered the expert on communication, and professionals may assume that they are conversant with all things related to hearing, so it is important that they are well versed in the basics of audiology, hearing screening, hearing technologies, and communication strategies.

Physical therapists work at length with the homebound, especially those prone to falls. They must know how to communicate with the hearing impaired, and should be versed in the anatomy of the inner ear, especially the vestibular system as it pertains to dizziness. They must be conversant with the communication strategies they will need during their regular sessions.

I cannot underscore enough the importance of imparting information about hearing to these professionals, as this information will contribute to improving the quality of care and lives of the homebound. Knowledge of communication strategies also is critical when nurses and home health aides are working in hospices, but that is beyond the scope of this chapter.

Case finding, or the identification of individuals who need an audiological referral, is made possible by hospital discharge planners, intake nurses, physicians, and other home-care providers. Audiologists should educate the nurses and referring physicians about appropriate strategies for identifying individuals who may require audiological services. The Welch Allyn Audioscope, which emits a 40 dB HL tone at 500, 1000, 2000, and 4000 Hz, is ideal for bedside screening for hearing impairment, and can be used to identify persons with impacted cerumen who may require a referral for cerumen management. In my view, even before the OASIS is completed, nurses or physicians should conduct a hearing screen and perform visual inspection of the ear. If the patient fails the screen, the nurse or physician should refer the patient and in the interim make sure to use a personal amplifier when performing the intake, as it will help with the flow of the assessment and will ensure that responses are reliable and valid. If a homebound older adult has recently received a hearing aid, the nurse should be instructed to place a note in the chart maintained by the HHA with specifics about troubleshooting hearing aids, a

Table 11.12 Tips for Communicating with Hearing-Impaired Patient (Included in a Medical Record)

- Get the resident's attention by gently touching his or her shoulder or raising a finger.
- Face the resident. Do not walk away while talking, and do not talk from outside the resident's room.
- Eliminate distractions: no food, cigars, or cigarettes when speaking.
- Rephrase what you have said if repetitions do not clarify.
- Speak using a slightly slower rate and pause between lengthy sentences.
- Supplement communication with gestures, reading, and writing modalities.
- Use a hardwired amplification system when speaking to residents who do not use hearing aids.
- Enunciate difficult words.
- Pay attention to the resident for puzzled looks that may suggest that there was a communication breakdown.
- Speak slightly louder than normal.
- Make sure the hearing aid is turned on and that batteries are working.
- Slow down but do not exaggerate when you speak.
- *Speak* to the hearing impaired, do not *shout*—this distorts the sound and look of speech.
- *Do not* underestimate the resident's intelligence.
- Keep your hands away from your face when talking.
- Recognize that hard-of-hearing people understand less when they are tired or ill, so be patient.
- Make sure televisions and radios are turned off when communicating and that people are not speaking on a cellular phone in the background.

checklist about hearing-aid care and operation, and a list of strategies to be used by the staff when communicating with the hearing impaired (**Table 11.12**). I also urge audiologists to target marketing and educational efforts at HHAs, as they can be an important referral source. Older adults who ultimately recover and no longer need formal caregiver and homemaker services are good candidates for hearing health care services.

An important aspect of home care is documentation. Record keeping must meet all agency, regulatory, and reimbursement requirements (American Speech-Language-Hearing Association [ASHA], 1994). All entries should be legible (no corrections), accurate, and comprehensive. All telephone contacts with the patient, family, and other members of the multidisciplinary team should be documented. Retain copies of all correspondence with or about the patient being treated. It is important to document each visit as well as canceled or rescheduled appointments. For new hearing-aid users, it is helpful to keep records of the hearing aid dispensed (e.g., serial numbers of each hearing aid), and to document limitations of the treatment process. The patient should be given all warranties pertaining to the hearing aids as well as options for insuring the units.

Home health care is a nontraditional setting for audiologists, given the fact that Medicare does not reimburse for routine diagnostic or treatment services delivered to homebound individuals, unless indicated for medical reasons. However, hospitalized patients referred for home-care services have a high probability of having a hearing impairment that may interfere with the delivery of services in general and with recovery of functional health in particular. Audiologists should strive to contract with HHAs to, at the very least, educate staff members about how best to interact with the hearing impaired, how to identify a hearing-impaired older adult, and how to maintain hearing aids/hearing assistance technologies used by recipients of home-care benefits. The ability to communicate should be considered an important outcome for home-care beneficiaries.

Nursing Facilities

Although nursing homes are not a primary work setting for audiologists, those who do find themselves in these settings have a scope of practice that includes diagnostic and therapeutic services delivered to a heterogeneous population in a nontraditional environment. The procedures comprising the audiological assessment and intervention must be moderated by the overall goals of nursing home care, the residents' length of stay (short stay or long stay), and the requirements of OBRA. The focus of care at all times must be on maintaining the resident's functional independence, autonomy, quality of life, comfort, and dignity (Kane et al, 1994). Quality of care is an integral part of the federal regulation governing nursing home care, and it is dependent on the ability of staff to communicate with residents. To be eligible for Medicare and Medicaid funding, nursing homes must provide care that will help residents attain the highest practicable physical, mental, and psychosocial well-being and quality of life. The approach to the delivery of audiological services should be outcome oriented, with the role of the audiologist at every stage being to gain an understanding of the resident's function, perceived needs, abilities, and limitations. The challenge to the audiologist is to apply standard procedures to a typically frail older adult in nonstandard settings to attain a complete picture of hearing status and audiological rehabilitation needs. Also, audiologists must attempt to work as part of a team that includes health care professionals who have little formal training in audiology and therefore must come to respect and work collaboratively with audiologists to benefit residents.

Upon admission, nursing home residents must undergo a comprehensive assessment using the RAI. At the bare minimum, the assessment must include evaluation of communication, well-being, and cognitive patterns—all functions of which hearing status is integrally related but rarely assessed as part of the RAI. In my view, the first step in the delivery of hearing health care services to residents of nursing facilities is a hear-

ing screening to identify residents with impaired hearing or a hearing disorder in need of audiological or medical services to ensure their health, safety, and maximal level of functioning (Ammentorp, Gossett, & Euchner, 1991). Screening results and any referrals should be documented in the patient's medical record. The initial assessment in nursing facilities is typically through the MDS administered routinely to all residents to obtain a comprehensive approach to assessment, problem identification, and individualized care planning. Initial admission assessment must occur within 14 days of admission. The team leader/primary nurse coordinates the resident assessment. The MDS assessment tool has several sections with over 450 assessment items in categories ranging from communication/ hearing patterns to mood and behavior patterns and cognitive patterns. RAPs are triggered by specific resident responses from one or a combination of MDS elements. Outcomes in such areas as index of social engagement, level of depression, and level of cognition emerge from the MDS data.

Included in Section B of the MDS is an assessment of hearing, speech, and vision. The manual provides excellent steps to be followed when the nurse assesses the resident's hearing status. It specifically states that should the resident use a "hearing appliance," it should be operational and used during the assessment, and the examiner must document whether a hearing aid or hearing appliance was worn during the assessment. Further, the examiner is encouraged to ask the resident how he/she hears in different situations (e.g., hearing staff members, talking to visitors, using telephone, watching TV, attending activities). Similarly, the examiner is asked to consult the resident's family, direct care staff, activities personnel, and speech or hearing specialists to gain a better understanding of a potential hearing problem. Further, the examiner is expected to observe the resident during verbal interactions and when he or she interacts with other residents, family, or staff members throughout the day at the nursing facility. Finally, the instructions list communication strategies to be used when speaking with the resident, including the need to speak clearly, to make sure the resident can see the examiner's face when speaking, to use a loud tone, to speak slowly or to use gestures, and to speak in a quiet area. The manual suggests that if any of these modifications are necessary, the resident may have a hearing problem. The instructions and the examination of hearing status is much more sophisticated than when the MDS was first created when I served on an ASHA team involved in developing the items in the section on communication.

Included in the hearing section of the manual is a statement that hearing ability is assessed to document the resident's ability to hear (with assistive hearing devices, if they are used), understand, and communicate with others, and to determine whether the resident experiences vision limitations or difficulties related to diseases common in aged persons. The resident's ability to hear with a hearing aid (if one is used) is judged on a four-point scale ranging from being adequate to being highly impaired. If residents are unable to respond to a standard hearing assessment due to cognitive impairment, the manual suggests that the examiner observe them in their normal environment to see if they respond by turning their head when a noise is made at a normal level or at a loud level, or whether the resident does not appear to respond at all.

Table 11.13 Care Plan for Residents Identified as Having a Hearing Problem on the Minimum Data Set (MDS)

1. Address reversible causes of hearing difficulty (such as cerumen impaction).
2. Evaluate potential benefit from hearing-assistive devices.
3. Offer assistance to residents with hearing difficulties to avoid social isolation.
4. Consider other communication strategies for persons with hearing loss that is not reversible or is not completely corrected with hearing devices.
5. Adjust environment by reducing background noise, such as by lowering the sound volume on televisions or radios, because a noisy environment can inhibit opportunities for effective communication.

Source: From Centers for Medicare and Medicaid Services (CMS). (2011). *Section B: Hearing, speech, and vision.* CMS's RAI MDS 3.0 manual. http://www.aodsoftware.com/docs/mds3raimanual/MDS_3.0_Chapter_3_-_Section_B_V1.05_May_2011.pdf.

Contained within the CMS RAI MDS manual is a rationale for including a question on hearing and on hearing-aid ownership. The authors acknowledge that problems with hearing can impact quality of life (e.g., contribute to sensory deprivation, social isolation, mood and behavior disorders), and unaddressed hearing impairment can be mistaken for cognitive impairment or confusion. Regarding documentation about hearing-aid ownership and function, the narrative in the section on hearing points out that many residents without hearing aids or other hearing appliances could benefit from them, and that many persons who benefit from and own hearing aids do not have them on arrival at the nursing home, or the hearing aid they have is not functional (CMS, 2011). **Table 11.13** lists five options for addressing hearing loss should one exist, and **Table 11.14** lists care plans for hearing-aid users included in the MDS manual.

Phillips et al (1998) sampled 254 nursing facilities in a variety of metropolitan areas across the country, and found changes in the prevalence of key care processes over the first 3 years that OBRA was in effect. Specifically, in 1990, prior to use of the RAI, 80% of residents reportedly had a hearing loss but did not have or use hearing aids, whereas in 1993 the percentage dropped to 70%. Similarly, residents were less likely to deteriorate functionally and cognitively during the initial period that the RAI was in use. The authors concluded that comprehensive functional assessment data alerted staff to the need for selected interventions and led to improvements in selected areas of function. Audiologists must maintain their visibility in nursing facilities and do ongoing in-service training sessions to remind the staff of the importance of assessing hearing status, especially in residents with comorbidities including diabetes, Alzheimer's disease, cognitive decline, cardiovascular disease, and vision problems, as well as in residents with a history of falling. Due to the high turnover, staff members need constant reminders regarding how to recognize individuals with hearing problems, and how to assist and encourage residents in the use of their hearing aids or personal amplifiers.

Pearl

Although many residents may be difficult to test because of their medical or cognitive status, they can certainly benefit from the use of devices to improve communications with medical staff, other residents, and family members, and these devices should be field tested on site.

Audiological Assessment in Nursing Homes

Residents referred for assessment of hearing status should undergo an assessment that addresses the information in the care plan. This section links the care plan to the audiological assessment. If the care plan states that reversible causes of hearing difficulty such as cerumen impaction should be addressed, then this is a trigger for a complete audiological evaluation that should begin with a review of the medical record to see if there are possible medical factors contributing to the hearing loss such as ototoxic medication or a new diagnosis of diabetes. I typically administer the Mini-Mental State Examination (MMSE), using a personal amplifier, to gain a feel for the client's cognitive status, given the link between cognition and hearing status. Although it does not directly address functional issues, the MMSE is a baseline screening test for cognitive status that entails brief questions and tasks that sample orientation, immediate and delayed word recall, attention and calculation, naming, repetition, responses to verbal and written commands, writing, and visuoconstructional abilities (Folstein, Folstein, & McHugh, 1975). Alternatively, information from the resident's chart regarding mental status also figures into a decision regarding intervention options. The following exams and tests should also be done:

Table 11.14 Care Plan for Residents with Hearing Aids

1. For residents with hearing aids, use and maintenance should be included in care planning and medical record.
2. Residents who do not have adequate hearing without a hearing aid should be asked about their history of hearing-aid use.
3. Residents who do not have adequate hearing despite wearing a hearing aid should be reevaluated with the device or should undergo a hearing assessment.
4. If the resident is unable to respond when wearing the hearing aid, the examiner is asked to check with family and care staff about the hearing aid or hearing appliance.

Source: From Centers for Medicare and Medicaid Services (CMS). (2011). *Section B: Hearing, speech, and vision.* CMS's RAI MDS 3.0 manual. http://www.aodsoftware.com/docs/mds3raimanual/MDS_3.0_Chapter_3_-_Section_B_V1.05_May_2011.pdf.

1. An otoscopic examination of the external ear canal and tympanic membrane. The audiologist should make sure to study the features of the outer ear, given the susceptibility of residents to collapsed canals, impacted cerumen, and tumorous growth. In my view, cerumen management should not be attempted by audiologists in nursing homes, given the frail status and complexity of medical conditions characterizing most residents, and the availability of attending physicians, nurses, nurse practitioners to address this problem.

2. Air-conduction (AC) testing at 250, 500, 1000, 2000, 3000, 4000, and 6000 Hz using insert earphones. The purpose of AC testing is to determine hearing loss type and severity, to identify residents with senile dementia who have underlying hearing loss that may exacerbate the cognitive problems, and to identify candidates for intervention. The diagnosis of senile dementia may be confounded by the presence of hearing loss, and so ruling hearing loss in or out is critical for these individuals. Lin et al (2011) found that hearing loss is associated with incident all-cause dementia.

3. Bone-conduction (BC) testing in a soundproof room at 250 to 4000 Hz. In the event that an unexplained high-frequency air–bone gap is present, the audiologist should check carefully for collapsed canals or possible acoustic radiation from the oscillator. Immittance testing should be substituted for bone conduction testing if the acoustic environment is not sound treated. Immittance testing will help to uncover possible medically reversible causes of hearing loss (i.e., middle ear problems) as stated in the care plan.

4. Speech reception or detection thresholds testing, to determine a recognition level for speech information and to determine reliability/validity of air conduction test results. This is especially important as test reliability and validity may be jeopardized in residents with cognitive problems. Often a speech detection threshold is the only measure of speech recognition that can be obtained because of compromised cognitive status, but this information can guide the audiologist in terms of management decisions.

5. Speech-recognition testing using sentences or simple questions presented at normal conversational level. The goal is to determine the resident's functionality. I would assess speech understanding with and without visual cues, as this addresses a concern raised in the care plan about whether the use of communication strategies such as facing the speaker when communicating can facilitate speech understanding. Testing with and without visual cues should be done in quiet and with some background noise, as the benefits of using visual cues can more easily be underscored during counseling. I highly recommend using functionally relevant test material to assess the adequacy of the resident's functional-communication capacity, as the primary purpose of word-recognition testing for residents of nursing facilities is to ensure that hearing/understanding is adequate for communication with other residents, caregivers, and staff members, and to determine if speech understanding problems are so severe that they may contribute to social isolation. A secondary goal is to identify those persons in need of some form of hearing assistance, including hearing aids, personal amplifiers, telephone devices, media devices, or warning devices. If enough residents have hearing aids with a t-coil, a loop system in a common room might be a cost-effective investment in terms of quality of life and care.

If behavioral testing could not be completed or results are of questionable validity, otoacoustic emissions screening or auditory brainstem response testing could be fruitful; however, it is unlikely that nursing homes have such costly instrumentation on the premises.

At the conclusion of the testing, a reliable and valid scale that assesses functional communication status should be administered, as responses may help uncover the impact of hearing problems on hearing-related quality of life. Insights into communicative function should also be gleaned from a formal and an informal caregiver, as this could assist with care planning.

Prior to concluding testing, I try to administer the MMSE with and without amplification (e.g., personal amplifier or hearing aid) to residents with a significant hearing loss, as this allows me to quickly gain insight into whether amplification impacts on the resident's orientation and mental status. I have worked with several residents with undiagnosed severe hearing loss for whom the quality of their responses to the items on the MMSE differed dramatically once my voice was made audible. Many of these residents may not be candidates for hearing aids, but certainly should be using a hardwired assistive-listening device when communicating with staff, family members, or other residents.

When testing is completed, it is imperative that audiometric findings are documented in the medical record, and all residents with a hearing loss should have an indicator on the outside of the medical record and a visible indicator outside the room if the severity of their hearing loss precludes hearing emergency sounds such as a smoke or fire alarm. Hearing status should be monitored annually to determine whether any significant change has taken place, or more frequently when symptoms arise.

Referral and Intervention Options: Hearing Aids

Following the audiological assessment, and consistent with case planning in the MDS, the audiologist should make one of two referrals: (1) a medical referral, if otoscopic examination or audiometric tests are indicative of a possible medical condition requiring treatment, such as impacted cerumen or possible external otitis, or the need for medical clearance for a hearing-aid fitting; or (2) referral for a trial with audiological rehabilitation if audiometric findings, and cognitive, physical, and psychosocial conditions, suggest that the resident can use and benefit from a hearing aid/replacement hearing aid or assistive device, the latter being preferable for those who are not experiences hearing-aid users. The decision regarding candidacy for a hearing aid should take into account the audiological data, input from the nursing and rehabilitative staff, input from the resident, and input from family members. Financing of the hearing aid is often critical, and the ability to use the hearing aid independently must be an important consideration, as staff members are often too busy to assist residents with the care, use, and maintenance of hearing aids.

Audiological rehabilitation with hearing aids should be restorative and maintenance oriented, using a holistic approach that takes into account physical, sociological, psychological, cognitive, and communicative capabilities. Restoration as applied in long-term-care settings entails assisting residents in doing as much as they can, as well as they can, for as long as they can (Hegner & Caldwell, 1994). Maintenance is aimed at preventing further functional loss and limitation, assisting the resident in achieving as high a level of adequate communication as possible, which will ultimately foster improved quality of care. Properly fit basic or "low-tech" hearing aids or hearing assistance technologies can achieve these goals; high-end hearing aids are not necessary for the listening needs of most residents of nursing homes. If hearing aids are recommended, care should be taken to recommend a hearing aid with an earmold/dome that can be easily maintained, inserted, and removed by the resident or staff members, and is not prone to blockage by specks of cerumen. A lengthy field trial should be conducted and feedback from family members, the resident, and staff should be obtained to determine the utility and value of hearing aids for the resident. Extended warranties or supplemental insurance for loss and damage should be considered. Similarly, an informal caregiver should be included in the rehabilitation process and should be encouraged to attend the hearing-aid fitting and orientation sessions to ensure that he/she understands how to operate and maintain the hearing aid. It is especially important to emphasize the limitations of hearing-aid use and the importance of selected communication strategies, and to instill realistic expectations. Suggestions for how best to communicate with the hearing-impaired resident should be emphasized, including tips listed in **Table 11.12**.

At the time of the hearing-aid fitting, it is important for the audiologist to verify the hearing-aid response using real-ear technology, if available. Informal conversations between the resident and a staff member or between residents are a powerful way to verify the adequacy of the hearing-aid fit. New hearing-aid users should be scheduled for a post-fitting session within 1 week of the fitting to determine if the resident is deriving communicative, psychosocial, and functional benefit from the hearing aid. When the perceived benefit is at odds with real-ear data, the audiologist must make a decision as to the adequacy of the response, paying attention to the input from the resident and caregiver as well as the real-ear data. The resident should be seen on a weekly basis for approximately 1 month before a determination is made as to the value of the hearing aid for the resident. At each session, the fit should be verified, and the resident should be counseled about the operation and use of the hearing aid, and how best to communicate with others. The resident or caregiver should demonstrate how to operate and troubleshoot the hearing aid. These ongoing hearing-aid orientation sessions are important to optimize the benefits of hearing-aid use and to make adjustments based on feedback and the audiologist's observations. It is critical that the orientation sessions be patient-centered, with particular attention being paid to the resident's communication needs within the given facility or listening environment. Hearing-aid users should be given a set of large-print instructions describing hearing-aid care, maintenance, use, insertion, removal, and operation. Residents and caregivers should be given a list of helpful hints for adjusting to and maintaining hearing aids such as the checklists shown in **Tables 11.15 and 11.16**. The checklists should be reviewed with the resident and caregiver at each session. Safety and infection-control procedures should be in effect before, during, and after the hearing-aid fitting. Finally, the audiologist should maintain a list of residents obtaining hearing aids. The list should include the resident's name, hearing-aid model and serial number, battery type, the ear(s) fitted, and the date of fitting. The hearing aid should be imprinted with the resident's name in the event it is misplaced.

Table 11.15 Helpful Hints for Patients Adjusting to Hearing Aids

- Be patient and allow time to adjust to hearing aids. Hearing aids require time for adaptation and to attain maximum performance potential.
- Take advantage of services offered by the audiologist.
- Do not get discouraged if the hearing aid does not restore hearing to normal. Return to the audiologist for reassurance and counseling regarding realistic expectations. Understand that hearing aids *will not* restore hearing capabilities to normal.
- Gradually adjust to loud, incoming signals by first using the hearing aid in quiet and in small groups, later moving to larger, less favorable listening situations.
- Understand the audiogram in terms of the particular speech sounds and words that may be problematic and in terms of the effect of noise on speech understanding. This will help make sense of some of the misunderstandings.
- Understand that hearing aids will not filter out all background noise, and certain listening environments will continue to present a significant listening challenge.
- Tell people you have a hearing loss and ask for repetition if the speech of others is unclear.

Special Consideration

Hearing-aid malfunction due to cerumen is a major problem in nursing homes. Wax guards are especially important for this population; however, residents are limited in their ability to routinely remove and replace them, and staff members are often too busy to attend to these matters.

Pearl

A successful hearing-aid fitting depends in large part on the resident's level of dependency and the availability of a caregiver to assist the resident in inserting and adjusting to the hearing aid.

Referral and Intervention Options: Alternatives to Hearing Aids

The majority of residents of nursing facilities do not use or are not candidates for hearing aids. Interestingly, only 5 to 10% of residents at any one time use hearing aids. Several nonaudiological factors including lifestyle variables, financial considerations, manual dexterity, listening needs, and cognitive status account for their lack of acceptance. Cognitive impairment in particular may render residents unable to consistently wear hearing aids. Older residents who are withdrawn, isolated, and rarely interact with others may be adverse to hearing-aid use. Also, the structure and staffing of nursing facilities may limit the utilization of hearing aids because residents are reliant on nurses and aides for insertion, removal, and maintenance of hearing aids. If these staff members are not available or willing to assist residents, hearing aids cannot be utilized.

Because hearing aids are not a sustainable option in this setting, there is an important place for hearing assistance technologies or "rehabilitation technology" in nursing facilities. Sound-enhancement devices available as hardwire, wireless, FM, or audio-induction loop systems are ideal for one-on-one

Table 11.16 Hearing-Aid Maintenance Tips

- Hearing aids should be kept dry and free of debris and cerumen.
- Hearing aid should not be worn in the shower, when applying hair spray, or when sleeping.
- Battery should be removed when hearing aid is taken out of the ear and checked before reinserting.
- Hearing aid should be stored in a safe place and in the same place each night, preferably in a drawer.
- Prior to inserting hearing aid, check opening for wax buildup. If present, clean opening with a wax pick and arrange to have the ear checked for impacted cerumen.
- Confirm that this is the correct hearing aid and that it is placed in the correct ear.

communication (e.g., when talking to nursing staff), large- or small-group situations (e.g., recreational therapy), and television or radio listening. In particular, hardwire systems can facilitate resident-to-resident, resident-to-staff, or informal caregiver-to-resident interactions. These inexpensive systems are durable and easy to use, and make communication exchanges easier and more meaningful. An additional advantage of hardwire systems is that they represent a visible symbol of hearing loss, signaling to other residents and staff that it is necessary to modify communication techniques to ensure understanding. This will minimize misunderstandings and the tendency for people who have significant hearing loss to be ignored. Wireless devices are ideal for residents who enjoy television viewing. If the lounge area within the nursing facility is equipped with a television, the facility should make sure to include a transmitter along with several receivers to enable residents to enjoy television viewing, and possibly a loop system for residents with a T-coil on their hearing aids. Infrared systems have been installed successfully in large listening rooms such as auditoriums, activity rooms, and places of worship, enabling large numbers of residents to follow the speaker free of noise and free of the disadvantage posed by distance.

A variety of telecommunication technologies that enhance speech understanding over the telephone are ideal for use in nursing facilities, including in-line amplifiers installed in each resident's telephone. Assistance with sending and receiving text messages is a 21st century option for the projected increase in residents with cellular phones. Finally, alerting devices should be used throughout the nursing facility, especially in large areas where residents congregate. Telephone alerting devices and smoke detectors with strobe lights or vibrotactile stimulation should be in rooms with persons with hearing impairment. Individuals with hearing loss, nursing facility staff, family members, and administrators should be informed of the availability and advantages of rehabilitation technology. The fact that these devices can be used to bring facilities into compliance with the Americans with Disabilities Act, helping to create a barrier-free environment for the hearing impaired, should be emphasized.

Pearl

Personal amplifiers are less costly than hearing aids and may provide sufficient auditory benefit for individuals with limited financial resources or who do not warrant full-time hearing-aid usage.

Special Consideration

Audiologists should consult with the nursing facility administration to ensure that the facility is in compliance with the Americans with Disabilities Act. It is our professional responsibility to ensure this law is implemented so that residents who are hard of hearing or deaf have equal access to services in nursing facilities.

Hearing-Aid Maintenance Program

The hearing-aid maintenance program is a system in place for ensuring that hearing aids given to residents are used on a regular basis, are maintained, and are secured when not in use. This is especially important because of the high rate of hearing-aid loss and damage in nursing facilities. The hearing-aid maintenance program for each nursing home resident with hearing loss should be included in the comprehensive care plan (CCP). A list that includes (1) the resident's name and room number, (2) the hearing-aid model and serial number, (3) the battery type, (4) the ear(s) fitted, and (5) the need for notification in the event of emergency should be posted at the nursing station to provide a quick and easy reference. When residents receive hearing aids, they should automatically be placed on a maintenance program. This program includes periodic checks conducted by the audiologist, a nurse's aide, or a volunteer to ensure that the aid remains clean and in good working order, is worn on a regular basis, has a working battery, and is turned on when worn by the patient. Typically, residents will either not wear their hearing aids or will have them in the ears but not have them turned on or the battery will be dead.

Documentation is especially important in nursing facilities. All contacts with the resident, information about the dispensed product, canceled appointments, and rescheduled appointments should be noted in the chart. Instructions for the staff should be specified as well. An effort should be made to incorporate an index of the quality of service provided to the resident. For example, the audiologist should document if the resident uses an assistive-listening device on a regular basis when communicating with family members. Similarly, the audiologist should include as a chart entry whether the resident is able to use the hearing aid independently and is more coherent and communicative.

Pearl

Documenting the value of audiological services is important, as it demonstrates to the facility the importance of contracting with an audiologist for hearing health care services.

Caregiver Education

The audiologist should provide regular and periodic in-service training for the entire nursing home staff, including caregivers involved in direct care, to provide carryover about hearing-aid use into the daily lives of the residents. In-service programs should be scheduled periodically and regularly to ensure that all staff members (e.g., aides, recreational therapists, and social workers) have the opportunity to attend. Most of the hands-on care in nursing homes is provided by nurses' aides who are typically poorly educated, poorly paid, and may speak limited English. Nursing homes employ very few registered and licensed nurses (Ouslander, 1998). Hence, aides are the primary targets of our in-service efforts. Recall that shifts for aides and nurses can be 12 hours or 8 hours, requiring the need for in-service programs to be scheduled during the day and in the evening. Further, turnover in nursing facilities is quite high, underlining the importance of regularly scheduled sessions. Audiologists are encouraged to take advantage of technology such as videotape playback units and computers to demonstrate and reinforce important points. Talking about particular residents often helps the hospital staff to remember important points about hearing-aid use and operation and a particular resident's experience with amplification. Hands-on experience with hearing aids and assistive technology and interactivity is important as well. All sessions should be practical and relevant to the attendees. Finally, I find that applying the Health Belief Model when outlining the content of the in-service session is important. Thus, it is important to emphasize the following:

1. Residents of nursing facilities are particularly susceptible to hearing loss because of their age (e.g., briefly discuss etiologies of hearing loss experienced by older adults).
2. Hearing impairment experienced by older adults has been documented to be handicapping in terms of the ability to communicate with family, caregivers, and other residents.
3. Unremediated hearing impairment can have significant psychosocial consequences, including depression, confusion, isolation, and dementia.
4. Amplification devices including hearing aids and hearing assistance technologies can reverse the negative psychosocial consequences of hearing impairment.
5. Amplification devices can make it easier for staff members when communicating with the hearing impaired.
6. Amplification plays an important role in the diagnosis of cognitive status, in the management of the cognitively impaired, and during a routine intake. Social workers, physicians, nurses, and aides should be encouraged to use hardwired systems or wireless systems when communicating with residents. This will certainly promote easier communication.

In addition to the above, audiologists should review the basics of hearing aids, assistive technologies and implantable devices including the following:

1. Styles, parts, and functions of hearing aids, cochlear implants, and assistive technologies
2. Batteries (storage, dangers of battery ingestion, types, and insertion)
3. Hearing-aid maintenance and troubleshooting procedures of hearing aids and implantable devices
4. Feedback: causes and prevention
5. Realistic expectations about hearing aids
6. Methods to facilitate communication
7. Procedures to report lost hearing aids

At the beginning or end of each in-service session, it is important to emphasize that staff members are key to realizing the functional communication potential of hearing-impaired residents and that hearing aids and assistive devices are designed to enable residents to (1) maintain hearing abilities, (2) effectively communicate their needs and requests, and (3) participate in social communication. If these goals are accomplished, the quality of life for nursing-home residents will be enhanced, indirectly impacting positively on the morale and functioning of nursing facilities.

Pearl

Periodic in-service sessions are key to the success of a hearing health care program in a nursing facility. Cooperative and informed staff members make the difference for hearing-impaired residents.

Garahan et al (1992) recommend designating one nurse at each nursing facility as the hearing health care specialist. Responsibilities would include ensuring that residents needing hearing assessment are scheduled and evaluated, otoscopics/cerumen management, hearing-aid management and maintenance, staff training, and distribution of assistive-listening devices. Training a single nurse would most likely result in an increase in hearing-aid/assistive-listening device utilization and promote communication among residents and staff.

Hearing health care is critical to the quality of life and care of residents of nursing facilities. To accomplish this, the audiologist should be involved in the assessment of the resident's continuing care and contribute to a written care plan for meeting communicative needs. Audiologists should work closely with the speech-language pathologists who are responsible for following up on residents in the absence of the audiologist. Aides, nurses, and therapists should be considered important partners as well, as they help to ensure carryover of information and inclusion of recommendations into the daily lives and routines of the residents.

Special Consideration

Audiologists should strive to become part of the multidisciplinary team assigned to prescribe care for patients.

◆ Conclusion

The goal of long-term care is to enable older adults to do the most they can for themselves, given their physical and mental limitations (Evashwick, 1993). Increasingly, individuals who need long-term care are cared for in their homes by informal or formal networks. The majority of recipients of long-term-care services are of advanced age; hence, they have a high probability of having an unremediated hearing impairment. Audiologists have an important role to play in the long-term-care continuum. Most important is educating providers and payers of long-term care, including the individual, about the integral role that the ability to hear, understand, and communicate can play in the lives of individuals with chronic multi-faceted problems. For this population, the goal should be the provision of amplification systems that will enable one-to-one communication, television listening, telecommunication accessibility, and safety in their living space. As baby boomers become senior citizens, they will be better educated, more sophisticated technologically, more vocal, and more demanding as consumers. They must come to learn that audiologists offer products and services that will enhance the quality of their prolonged lives.

References

Agency for Healthcare Research and Quality. (2001). *Telemedicine for the Medicare population: Update.* http://www.ahrq.gov/downloads/pub/evidence/pdf/telemedup/telemedup.pdf

American Speech-Language Hearing Association (ASHA). (1994). Professional liability and risk management for the audiology and speech-language pathology professions. *American Speech-Language-Hearing Association, 36* (Suppl 12), 25–38

Ammentorp, W., Gossett, K., & Euchner, P. (1991). *Quality assurance for long-term care providers.* Newbury Park, CA: Sage

Barlow, J., Singh, D., Bayer, S., & Curry, R. (2007). A systematic review of the benefits of home telecare for frail elderly people and those with long-term conditions. *Journal of Telemedicine and Telecare, 13,* 172–179

Berry, S. D., Zhang, Y., Lipsitz, L. A., Mittleman, M. A., Solomon, D. H., & Kiel, D. P. (2011, Oct). Antidepressant prescriptions: an acute window for falls in the nursing home. *Journals of Gerontology, Series A, Biological Sciences and Medical Sciences, 66,* 1124–1130

Bloom, S. (1994). Hearing care in nursing homes offers daunting challenges, special rewards. *Hearing Journal, 47,* 13–20

Bowers, B. (2009). *Implementing change in long term care: A practical guide to transformation.* New York: Commonwealth Fund

Bowman, C. (2010). Long-term care in the United Kingdom. In H. Fillit, K. Rockwood, & K. Woodhouse (Eds.), *Brockelhurst's textbook of geriatric medicine and gerontology* (7th ed.). Philadelphia: Saunders Elsevier

Brown, N. A. (2005). Information on telemedicine. *Journal of Telemedicine and Telecare, 11,* 117–126

Center for Excellence in Assisted Living (CEAL). (2010). *Person-centered care in assisted living: An informational guide.* http://www.theceal.org/assets/pdf/person-centered%20care%20in%20assisted%20living.pdf

Centers for Medicare and Medicaid Services (CMS). (2007). *2007 action plan for (further improvement) in nursing home quality.* https://www.cms.gov/SurveyCertificationGenInfo/downloads/2007ActionPlan.pdf

Centers for Medicare and Medicaid Services (CMS). (2011). *Section B: Hearing, speech, and vision. CMS's RAI MDS 3.0 manual.* http://www.aodsoftware.com/docs/mds3raimanual/MDS_3.0_Chapter_3_-_Section_B_V1.05_May_2011.pdf

Cohen-Mansfield, J., & Taylor, J. W. (2004a, Sep-Oct). Hearing aid use in nursing homes. Part 1: Prevalence rates of hearing impairment and hearing aid use. Journal of the American Medical Directors Association, 5, 283–288

Cohen-Mansfield, J., & Taylor, J. W. (2004b). Hearing aid use in nursing homes. Part 2: Barriers to effective utilization of hearing aids. Journal of the American Medical Directors Association, 5, 289–296

Craig, D., & Miskelly, R. (2010). *Telecare/telehealth (BGS Best Practice Guide).* http://www.epractice.eu/files/Telecare_Telehealth%20-%20British%20Geriatrics%20Society%20(BGS)%20Best%20Practice%20Guide.pdf

Dang, S., Golden, A., Cheung, H., & Roos, B. (2010). Telemedicine applications in geriatrics. In H. Fillit, K. Rockwood & K. Woodhouse (Eds.), *Brockelhurst's textbook of geriatric medicine and gerontology* (7th ed.). Philadelphia: Saunders Elsevier

Demiris, G., Speedie, S. M., & Hicks, L. L. (2004, Dec). Assessment of patients' acceptance of and satisfaction with teledermatology. *Journal of Medical Systems, 28,* 575–579

Dixon B. E., Hook J. M., & McGowan J. J. (2008). *Using telehealth to improve quality and safety: Findings from the AHRQ portfolio.* Contract No. 290-04-0016. AHRQ National Resource Center for Health IT

Electronic Code of Federal Regulations (2011). *Part 483: Requirements for states and long-term-care facilities.* http://ecfr.gpoaccess.gov/cgi/t/text/text-idx?c=ecfr&sid=e3979b25f8d8b29c78b1b3f6c66dbdaa&rgn=div5&view=text&node=42:5.0.1.1.2&idno=42#42:5.0.1.1.2.2.7.8

Engle, W. (2009). The approaching telehealth revolution in home care. *Telehealth Information Exchange.* http://tie.telemed.org/articles/article.asp?path=articles&article=telehealthRevolution_wengle_tie09.xml

Evashwick, C. (1993). The continuum of long-term care services. In S. Williams & P. Torrens (Eds.), *Introduction to health services* (4th ed.). Albany: Delmar

Evashwick, C. (1996). *The Continuum of long-term care: An integrated systems approach.* Albany: Delmar

Flynn, C. (2010). *A systematic review of perception of telecare by patients with chronic conditions: Implications for audiology.* Capstone paper submitted in partial fulfillment of Doctor of Audiology Program at the Graduate Center, City University of New York

Folstein, M. F., Folstein, S. E., & McHugh, P. R. (1975, Nov). "Mini-mental state". A practical method for grading the cognitive state of patients for the clinician. *Journal of Psychiatric Research, 12,* 189–198

Garahan, M. B., Waller, J. A., Houghton, M., Tisdale, W. A., & Runge, C. F. (1992, Feb). Hearing loss prevalence and management in nursing home residents. *American Geriatrics Society, 40,* 130–134

Giovannetti, E. R., & Wolff, J. L. (2010, Sep). Cross-survey differences in national estimates of numbers of caregivers of disabled older adults. *Milbank Quarterly, 88,* 310–349

Glueckauf, R. L., Nickelson, D. W., Whitton, J., & Loomis, J. S. (2004). Telehealth and healthcare psychology: Current developments in telecommunications regulatory practices, and research. In R. G. Frank, A. Baum, & J. Wallander (Eds.), *Handbook of clinical health psychology* (vol. 3). Washington, DC: American Psychological Association

Grant, R., Fey, J., Fedus, D., & Campbell, J. (2011). Contextual factors influencing level of care decisions for geriatric patients. *Clinical Geriatrics, 19,* 32–35

Hayashi, J., & Leff, B. (2009). Community-based long term care and home care. In J. Halter, J. Ouslander, M. Tinetti, S. Studenski, K. High, & S. Asthana (Eds.), *Hazzard's geriatric medicine and gerontology* (6th ed.). New York: McGraw-Hill

Hegner, B., & Caldwell, E. (1994). *Assisting in long-term care* (2nd ed.). Albany: Delmar

Hetzel, L., & Smith, A. (2001). *The 65 years and over population: 2000.* Suitland, MD: U.S. Census Bureau

Hughes, S. (1996). Home health. In C. Evashwick (Ed.), *The continuum of long-term care: An integrated systems approach.* Albany: Delmar

Institute of Medicine. (2008). *Retooling for an aging America: Building the health care workforce. Committee on the Future Health Care Workforce for Older Americans. Board on Health Care Services.* Washington, DC: National Academies Press

Jones, A. L., Dwyer, L. L., Bercovitz, A. R., & Strahan, G. W. (2009). The National Nursing Home Survey: 2004 overview. National Center for Health Statistics. *Vital and Health Statistics, Series 13, Data from the National Health Survey, 13,* 167

Kane, R., Ouslander, J., & Abrass, I. (1994). *Essentials of clinical geriatrics* (3rd ed.). New York: McGraw-Hill

Lin, F. (2011). Hearing loss and cognition among older adults in the United States. *Journal of Gerontology, Series A, Biological Sciences and Medical Sciences, 66A,* 1131–1136

Lin, F. R., Metter, E. J., O'Brien, R. J., Resnick, S. M., Zonderman, A. B., & Ferrucci, L. (2011, Feb). Hearing loss and incident dementia. *Archives of Neurology, 68,* 214–220

Lubinski, R., & Frattali, C. (1993, Jan). Nursing home reform. The resident assessment instrument. *American Speech-Language-Hearing Association, 35,* 59–62

Medicare. (2008). *Nursing homes.* http://www.medicare.gov/nursing/about inspections.asp

Morgan, L., & Kunkel, S. (2011). *Aging, society and the life course.* New York: Springer

National Association of Home Builders Research Center. (2010). *The national older adult housing survey. A secondary analysis of findings.* http://www.toolbase.org/pdf/casestudies/noahsecondaryanalysis.pdf

National Association for Home Care and Hospice (NAHCH). (2008). *Basic statistics about home care.* http://www.nahc.org/facts/08HC_stats.pdf

National Research Council (NRC). (2010). The role of human factors in home health care: Workshop summary. In S. Olson (Ed.), *Committee on the Role of Human Factors in Home Health Care. Committee on Human-Systems Integration, Division of Behavioral and Social Sciences and Education.* Washington, DC: National Academies Press

Omnibus Budget Reconciliation Act (OBRA). (1987). U.S. Public Law 100-203.101 Stat. 1330. Codified at 42 U.S.C.A. Sec. 1396 (Supplement 1989)

Ouslander, J. (1998). The American nursing home. In: R. Tanis, H. Fillit, & J. Brocklehurst (Eds.), *Brocklehurst's Textbook of Geriatric Medicine and Gerontology.* London: Churchill Livingstone

Park-Lee, E., & Decker, F. (2010). *Comparison of home and hospice care agencies by organizational characteristics and services provided: United States, 2007.*

National Health Statistics Report No. 30. Hyattsville, MD: National Center for Health Statistics

Phillips, C., Hawes, C., Mor, V., Fries, B., & Morris, J. (1998). Geriatric assessment in nursing homes in the United States: Impact of a national program. *Generations (San Francisco, California), 21,* 15–21

Rapp, M., & Rapp, K. (2009). Nursing facility care. In J. Halter, J. Ouslander, M. Tinetti, S. Studenski, K. High, & S. Asthana (Eds.), *Hazzard's geriatric medicine and gerontology* (6th ed.). New York: McGraw-Hill

Richardson, H. (1998). Long-term care. In: A. Kovner (Ed.), *Jonas's health care delivery in the United States* (5th ed.). New York: Springer

Rogers, W. A., & Fisk, A. D. (2004). Psychological science and intelligent home technology: Supporting functional independence of older adults. *Psychological Science Agenda, 18.* http://www.apa.org/science/about/psa/2004/02/rogers.aspx

Samos, L., Aguilar, E., & Ouslander, J. (2010). Institutional Long-Term Care in the United States. In H. Fillit, K. Rockwood, & K. Woodhouse (Eds.), *Brockelhurst's textbook of geriatric medicine and gerontology* (7th ed.). Philadelphia: Saunders Elsevier

Schow, R. L., & Nerbonne, M. A. (1980, Feb). Hearing levels among elderly nursing home residents. *Journal of Speech and Hearing Research, 45,* 124–132

Schulz, R., & Tompkins, C. (2010). Informal caregivers in the United States: Prevalence, characteristics, and ability to provide care. In S. Olson, National Research Council (Eds.), *The role of human factors in home health care: Workshop summary* (pp. 118–144). Committee on the Role of Human Factors in Home Health Care. Committee on Human-Systems Integration, Division of Behavioral and Social Sciences and Education. Washington, DC: The National Academies Press

Shipman, P. (2011). *Resident Assessment Instrument (RAI)/Minimum Data Set (MDS) policy.* http://www.nursinghomehelp.org/QI01RAIpolicyfinal6.06.pdf

Stefanacci, R. (2010). Managed care for older Americans. In H. Fillit, K. Rockwood, & K. Woodhouse (Eds.), *Brockelhurst's textbook of geriatric medicine and gerontology* (7th ed.). Philadelphia: Saunders Elsevier

U.S. Bureau of Labor Statistics. (2008) National Industry Occupational Employment Matrix, data for 2006. In *Basic statistics about home care: Updated 2008.* http://www.nahc.org/facts/08hc_stats.pdf

Weinstein, B., Silverman, C., Flugman, B., & Spiegel, S. (2009). *In-service training module for selected home care employees working with the homebound hearing impaired elderly.* Unpublished report

Wohlstadter, J. (2010). *The state of telehealth in the delivery of hearing healthcare services to the elderly: A systematic literature review.* Capstone paper submitted in partial fulfillment of Doctor of Audiology Program at the Graduate Center, City University of New York

Wolff, J. L., & Roter, D. L. (2008, Jul). Hidden in plain sight: medical visit companions as a resource for vulnerable older adults. *Archives of Internal Medicine, 168,* 1409–1415

Chapter 12

Financing Health Care

The Social HMO program represents an alternative option for addressing gaps in the Medicare benefit package and for integrating care into a more seamless system. Social HMOs are required to cover all Medicare Part A and B services as well as an expanded package of benefits including case management, prescription drugs, eyeglasses, hearing aids, and dental care. Each of these services is critical to help the elderly maintain independence in the community, prevent further progression of chronic conditions, and, in many cases, avoid costly institutionalization.

—*Walter Leutz (1998)*

◆ Learning Objectives

After reading this chapter, you should be able to

- integrate your knowledge of Medicare and Medicaid into your practice;
- apply the long-term-care benefits under Medicare and Medicaid;
- understand managed care and Medicare managed care; and
- explain funding of audiological services under Medicare and managed care.

◆ Overview

This chapter provides audiologists with a brief perspective on the complicated and ever-changing financing of health care. Audiologists must have an appreciation for the amount of money spent on health care, for what the money buys, and how money is paid out. More important, the government's role in health care is of critical concern, as navigating the system is the key to the survival of audiologists in this ever-changing health care environment. Having a broad perspective will also assist audiologists who are actively engaged in increasing funding for hearing health care services.

Health care is a large and rapidly growing segment of the United States economy. In 2009 the U.S. spent $2.5 trillion on health care, and at the current rate of growth expenditures is expected to exceed $4.4 trillion by 2018 (Truffer et al, 2010). From 1970 to 2010, health care expenditures jumped from 7% to 17.6% of the U.S. gross domestic product (GDP), an increase

far out of line with other wealthy democracies, where costs have risen but still average only 9% of the GDP (Starr, 2011). Interestingly, health care's share of the GDP is expected to be 0.3% higher in 2019. Several factors, including advances in technology, increase in the aging population, administrative costs, and fee-for-service reimbursement account for the economic trends characterizing the health care system in the U.S. (Morgan & Kunkel, 2011). One final explanation for the expenditures is a shift in the focus of treatment for elders from curing to slowing down the progression of diseases and chronic conditions and to reducing the functional limitations resulting from multiple chronic conditions that plague this population. The increase in health costs has driven insurance rates up faster than median incomes, and therefore the proportion of the population without coverage has risen from between 10% and 12% in the early 1970s to 16.3% in 2010, or to 50 million people.

Pearl

Older adults with multiple chronic conditions have more physician visits such that, among Medicare beneficiaries, those with three or more chronic conditions have on average 11 physician visits per year. Medicare beneficiaries with zero, one, two, and three and more chronic conditions accumulated expenditures of $3079, $7879, $16,402, and $35,701, respectively (Schneider, O'Donnell, & Dean, 2009).

The health care system for older adults relies heavily on third-party, private, and government insurance programs (Morgan & Kunkel, 2011). More specifically, private health insurance coverage for older adults is provided by managed care organizations (MCOs), private indemnity insurers, and Medicare Advantage Plans (Part C), whereas public health insurance programs include Medicare, Medicaid, the Veterans Administration, and Tricare for military retirees (Boult, 2009). Administered by the Centers for Medicare and Medicaid Services (CMS), the Medicare program reimburses health care organizations and professionals for providing health care services to adults over age 65, the disabled, and those suffering from end-stage renal disease. Medicaid is a joint federal–state health insurance program for young and old Americans on limited incomes who meet the assets test. The Veterans Health Admin-

Table 12.1 Features of Selected Public and Private Health Insurance Plans

Insurance Coverage	Type	Features	Financial Arrangements
Medicare Fee for Service	Public	Comprises two fee-for-service programs (Plans A and B), each of which pays a predetermined amount for health-related goods and services	Older Americans who have had Medicare taxes deducted from their pay checks for more than 10 years are entitled to Part A without paying a premium; eligible beneficiaries must enroll in and pay a monthly premium for Part B
Medicaid	Public	Pays supplemental health insurance to low-income Medicare beneficiaries	Most state Medicaid programs pay the Part B premiums
Medicare Managed Care (Part C) 22–26% of Medicare beneficiaries enrolled	Private	Medicare managed care plans have lower deductibles, premiums, and copayments than Medicare fee-for-service (FFS) and offer benefits not included in the FFS plans, including hearing aids, eyeglasses, health education, and health-promotion programs	Each November, Medicare beneficiaries can join any Medicare Advantage plan, and each January Medicare Advantage plan holders can change their provider network, premiums, or benefits; under Medicare Advantage plans, Medicare buys coverage for its beneficiaries from private plans and monthly payments are made
Veterans Health Administration (VHA)	Public	VHA stratifies veterans into eight priority groups based on several variables including income and history of illness or injury during military service, and each priority group has a different benefits package; veterans who simultaneously enroll in Medicare and Medicaid have access to non-VA physicians and medications not listed on the VA formulary	According to the stratification system, veterans with at least a 50% service-connected disability that causes them to be unemployed do not have to make copayments
Medigap insurance*	Covers co-insurance, deductibles, and some benefits not covered by Medicare	Covers preventive care not covered by Medicare (up to $120) but does not cover hearing aids, eyeglasses, or long-term care in a nursing home	Out-of-pocket expenses can range from $40 to $400

*It is important to determine if a Medicare Advantage plan will cover more of what the beneficiary needs at less cost.
Source: Adapted from Boult, C. (2009). The health care system. In J. Halter, J. Ouslander, M. Tinetti, S. Studenski, K. High, & S. Asthana (Eds.), *Hazzard's geriatric medicine and gerontology* (6th ed.). New York: McGraw-Hill.

istration (VHA) insures and provides comprehensive health care for honorably discharged military veterans. Finally, older Americans who choose private health insurance have their coverage provided by MCOs, private indemnity insurers such as "Medigap" or long-term-care insurance, and Medicare Part C providers. Typically MCOs include health maintenance organizations (HMOs) that offer either Medicare Advantage plans, preferred provider organizations (PPOs), or point-of-service plans. The term *managed care* refers to a system in which payment is made to the provider or health plan that is then responsible for providing a particular group of services (Stefanacci, 2010). Due in part to the Medicare Modernization Act (MMA), which was passed in 2003, participation in Medicare managed care has increased steadily over the years. In contrast, whereas long-term-care insurance could help defray the high cost of long-term care, only 5% of Americans have long-term-care insurance policies, most likely due to the high cost of the premiums. **Table 12.1** summarizes some of the features of the various options to which older adults are entitled.

Pearl

More than half of Medicare beneficiaries have multiple chronic conditions and account for 96% of annual Medicare spending.

◆ Medicare

A federal health insurance program for people over 65 years of age, the disabled, and those individuals suffering from end-stage renal disease, the Medicare program was enacted in 1965, representing the first entry of the federal government into the provision of State Health Insurance (Koch, 1993). Established under Title XVIII, Health Insurance for the Aged and Disabled, of the Social Security Act, Medicare provides a range of medical care benefits to persons over 65 years of age (Knickman & Thorpe, 1998). Medicare is virtually universal for adults over 65 years. Today, nearly 40 million Americans rely on Medicare for their health care. Under the leadership of President Johnson, the 1965 legislation had three elements. As originally enacted it comprised two fee-for-service plans: Part A, the hospital–insurance program, financed by a dedicated payroll tax currently split between employer and employee; and Part B, a voluntary insurance program subsidized out of general revenues that covers physician bills for older adults. Parts A and B pay predetermined amounts for specified health-related goods and services including hospital, hospice, post-acute care in skilled nursing facilities, and medically necessary home care. The legislation also included a mixed federal–state program that provides funds to the states to pay a share of medical costs for the poor who qualified for welfare (Starr, 2011). It is notable that Medicare's share of the federal budget rose from 8.5% in 1990 to 15.1% in 2010, and it is projected to reach 17.4% of the federal budget in 2020 (this figure is likely to increase). Since the late 1990s, Medicare's costs per beneficiary have grown more slowly than that of private insurers. Notably, there are geographic variations in Medicare spending due to differences in physician–practice patterns, including differences in decisions about hospitalization, surgery, and drug prescribing. Medicare spending per beneficiary runs nearly 50% higher in some regions than in others (Starr, 2011). It is projected that Medicare expenditures will climb from $207 billion in 2007 to between $2.2 and $3 trillion by the year 2030. Accordingly, this spending will become a much larger part of the federal budget, potentially affecting the funding of other important programs such as justice, health and safety, and environmental protection.

Medicare Part A, which contracts with regional insurance companies referred to as "intermediaries," is considered insurance for inpatient hospital services, hospice, skilled nursing care in a Medicare-approved facility, and, to a limited extent, home care. Those not eligible for Medicare because payroll taxes were not deducted from their paychecks can purchase Part A coverage but at a steep monthly premium. Part A is typically referred to as hospital insurance, as it covers room, board, and all nursing services when the beneficiary is hospitalized (Morgan & Kunkel, 2011).

Pearl

Today, Medicare beneficiaries pay a large percentage of their health care costs from their own pockets.

Part B is a voluntary supplemental medical insurance program paid for in part by the individual subscriber through premiums and deductibles. It helps cover physician services, some preventive services, hospital outpatient care, diagnostic laboratory tests, and outpatient physical, speech, and occupational therapy. It also covers some home health care and helps pay for covered services and supplies when they are medically necessary, including ambulance services and vaccinations. It does not cover dental care, cosmetic surgery, orthopedic services, and hearing and vision services. Under Part B, those services, including diagnostic testing, not provided directly by physicians (e.g., audiology) require a referral by a physician,

physician assistant, or nurse practitioner (if allowed by state law). For Medicare Part B, premiums in 2012 rise from $99.00 a month for some individual seniors with incomes of $85,000 or below to as high as $319.70 a month for those making more than $214,000. The monthly premium is automatically deducted from monthly Social Security checks for beneficiaries currently receiving Social Security. Typically, Medicare pays 80% of the fee medical fee and the beneficiary pays 20%. The 20% collected from the patient is considered a co-insurance payment. Physicians have the option to participate in the Medicare fee-for-service (FFS) program, and if they do they must submit a claim to the Part B carrier indicating that they accept the preestablished fee for the indicated service (Boult, 2009). Physicians who choose not to participate bill the patient directly for a specified amount, which is set relative to the amount allowed by Medicare.

Also known as Medicare Advantage, Medicare Part C, is another plan a beneficiary may choose as part of their Medicare options. Medicare Advantage plans tend to offer extra benefits not covered by Medicare and they are permitted to charge extra premiums for these services. Similar to an HMO or a PPO, Part C is offered by private insurance companies that are approved by Medicare. When beneficiaries join a Medicare Advantage plan, the plan will provide their Medicare Part A and Part B. Beginning in 2006, Medicare Advantage plans are required to offer at least one plan option that covers the Part D drug benefit. In 2010, 79% of Medicare Advantage plans offered prescription drug coverage. It is important to note the beneficiaries who join a Medicare Advantage plan cannot use a Medigap policy. Several companies provide Medicare Advantage plans. United Health Care, a large provider of Medicare Advantage plans with over 2 million members, recently updated its benefit plan and accordingly received a good deal of negative press for their online diagnostic, treatment, and distribution model for hearing health care. Interestingly, some plans do cover hearing, vision, dental, and wellness services.

The Medicare Advantage plans grew out of the Balanced Budget Act (BBA) of 1997 and the passage of the Medicare Prescription Drug Improvement and Modernization Act of 2003. **Table 12.2** describes four types of Medicare Advantage plans. In 2010, Medicare payment to private plans accounted for 22% of total Medicare spending; a majority of the 47 million Medicare enrollees are in an FFS plan, with only 22% in a Medicare Advantage plan. However, the number of beneficiaries enrolled in private plans has more than doubled from 5.3 million in 2005 to 11.1 million in 2010 (Kaiser Family Foundation, 2010). Notably, enrollment is growing most rapidly in the private FFS plans, yet 80% of beneficiaries enrolled in a Medicare Advantage plan are in HMOs or PPOs, which have comprehensive networks of providers but differ in terms of out-of-network benefits. A key feature of HMO and PPO plans is care management services intended to promote better coordination and more effective use of health care (Congressional Budget Office [CBO], 2007). Private FFS plans do not maintain a network of providers. They pay providers fee-for-service rates. PFFS enrollment and plans are focused in urban settings. According to the Congressional Budget Office, spending for Medicare Advantage is projected to total nearly $1.5 trillion from 2007 through 2017, more than a quarter of all spending for benefits

Table 12.2 Types of Medicare Advantage Plans

Type of Plan	Features of Plan
Local coordinate care plans that are either health maintenance organizations (HMOs) or preferred provider organizations (PPOs)	HMO beneficiaries can only go to doctors, hospitals, and specialists that are part of the plan's network, whereas PPOs permit out-of-network care but charge higher copayments when beneficiaries do so. In an HMO there is no coverage if the beneficiary goes out of network unless care is due to an emergency.
Regional preferred provider organization (PPO)	There are a fixed number of regional PPOs and they all must offer Part D prescription coverage.
Private fee-for-service (PFFS) plan	These plans cover all Medicare-covered care, but the plan (not Medicare) decides how much providers will be paid and how much the enrollee will pay. If the enrollee goes to a provider that accepts the private FFS plan's payment terms, the care is covered. Beneficiaries may have to pay up to 15% more than the traditional Medicare-approved amount to a plan provider.
Special needs Medicare Advantage plan (SNP)	A coordinated care plan restricted to beneficiaries who meet selected criteria: (1) they are dually entitled to Medicare and Medicaid; (2) they live in an institutional setting (or would otherwise require an institutional level of care); or (3) they have certain chronic or disabling conditions.

under Parts A and B (CBO, 2007). Finally, with regard to audiology, MCOs contract directly with audiologists or they employ audiologists. Hearing and balance diagnostic test benefits must conform to the level of Part B Medicare services.

In 2003 Medicare Part D, as part of the Medicare Prescription Drug Improvement and Modernization Act, was signed into law. Coverage became available in 2006 (Morgan & Kunkel, 2011). Every Medicare beneficiary is entitled to this coverage but participation is voluntary. Interestingly, in 2009, 90% of beneficiaries had some form of prescription drug coverage, with 60% having coverage through Medicare Part D or a Medicare Advantage drug plan (Neuman & Cubanski, 2009). **Table 12.3** summarizes Medicare Parts A, B, C, and D. It is worth noting that Medicare covers preventive services including colon cancer screening, glaucoma screening, diabetes screening, and smoking cessation counseling. Sadly, the one-time hearing screening and education benefit as part of the Welcome to Medicare Exam is no longer included as a benefit.

Pearl

Medicare Advantage is the program through which private plans participate in Medicare. The Medicare beneficiary must participate in some cost sharing. Under Medicare, audiology services are limited by law to a diagnostic-only service. Medicare is a major payer of health care for older adults, with the majority of dollars spent on hospitals and doctors. Audiology is considered a diagnostic test benefit under Medicare and is limited to the Current Procedural Terminology (CPT) codes.

Medicare has a national fee schedule that sets fees for physician services delivered in a variety of settings, including physician offices, hospitals, skilled nursing facilities, hospices, beneficiaries' homes, or in clinical laboratories. Payment rates for a given service are based on a complex formula that includes three components: Relative Value Units (RVUs), which

Table 12.3 The ABCDs of Medicare

Part A	Part B	Part C	Part D
Hospital insurance that helps cover inpatient care in hospitals, skilled nursing facilities, hospices, and home health care	Medical insurance (outpatient care) helps cover medically necessary services like physicians' services, outpatient care, home health services, and other services, including physical, occupational, and speech therapy; also covers some preventive services	Provider network, includes both Parts A and B; options offered by private companies approved by Medicare; Medicare Advantage plans provide all of Part A and Part B coverage, and may offer extra coverage, such as vision, hearing, dental, and health and wellness programs; many plans include Medicare prescription drug coverage (Part D)	Prescription drug coverage; if beneficiary wants prescription drug coverage and it is offered by the plan, beneficiaries can get it through the plan; if plan does not offer drug coverage, individuals can choose and join a prescription drug plan; beneficiaries are entitled to Medicare prescription drug coverage either by joining a Medicare prescription drug plan or by joining a Medicare Advantage plan that offers drug coverage; both types of Medicare drug coverage are called "Medicare drug plans"
Financed by payroll taxes, primarily	Monthly premium based on income	Monthly premium varies by plan	Monthly premium varies by plan and income

Table 12.4 Relative Value Units (RVUs) for Three Types of Resources That Define the Fee for the Physician Service

Type of Resource	Description of Factors Considered in the Calculation
Physician work	Time, technical skill, effort, stress to provide a service, mental effort, and judgment
Practice expense	Expenses for the building, space, equipment, office supplies, and nonphysician clinical and nonclinical labor
Professional liability	Cost of malpractice insurance premiums

Source: From Dummit, L. (2009). The basics—relative value units (RVUs). WWW.nhpf.org.

assigns relative values to services based on several variables; a conversion factor (CF); and a geographic practice cost index (GPCI), which helps to account for geographic variations in the cost of practicing medicine in different settings. In short, the formula used to calculate payment rates and the relative value assigned for a given service are adjusted according to geography and multiplied by a national conversion factor to arrive at the dollar amount (Knickman & Thorpe, 1998). The Medicare Physician Fee Schedule (MPFS), which is the responsibility of CMS, is updated on a regular basis. Congress requires that CMS review the RVUs no less frequently than every 5 years, and it must develop RVUs for new services made available to beneficiaries (Dummit, 2009). With regard to RVUs, the resources used to deliver services, which include the physician's work (e.g., time, technical skill), the expenses of the physician's practice (e.g., overhead, practice expenses), and professional liability insurance costs, tend to define the fee (Dummit, 2009; Knickman & Thorpe, 1998). The specific type of resources that will determine the RVUs are listed in **Table 12.4**. In contrast to relative values for physicians, most audiology codes have not been assigned a professional work value. However, over the past few years, professional work values have been systematically assigned for the audiologist's time and effort, and transferred out of the practice expense component. The latter remains a work in progress (American Speech-Language-Hearing Association [ASHA], 2011a).

Pearl

Medicare recognizes audiological testing as a covered diagnostic service and will reimburse when a physician orders the testing to obtain information for a diagnostic medical evaluation or to determine the appropriate medical or surgical treatment for a hearing loss or related medical condition.

The CPT codes and the Healthcare Common Procedure Coding System (HCPCS) define the physician services, which, as noted above, can range from services that require considerable amounts of time to those requiring little time and minimal resources (Dummit, 2009). With regard to audiology, most CPT codes represent "typical" visit lengths or typical times necessary to conduct a typical test. Audiology services under Part B have reimbursement rates established by the MPFS regardless of provider setting, except for outpatient audiology services provided in hospitals. Finally, Medicare and the Ameri-

can Medical Association (AMA) establish rules for using specific CPT codes. The Medicare rule always supersedes the AMA rule when billing Medicare. Regarding billing for diagnostic versus therapeutic services, CMS is quite stringent and explicit.

Pearl

Audiologists who engage in cerumen management should have patients sign the Advance Beneficiary Notice (ABN), as this enables patients to make an informed decision about the item or service for which they may have to pay out-of-pocket. This signed form should be placed in the patient's medical record.

The Social Security Act, section 1861(II)(3), defines the term *audiology services* as hearing and balance assessment services furnished by a qualified audiologist. It is noteworthy that in Chapter 15, Section 80.3 of the Medicare Benefit Policy Manual, hearing and balance assessment services are termed "audiology services," regardless of whether they are furnished by an audiologist, physician, or nonphysician practitioner (NPP). Audiology services must be furnished by an audiologist, yet physicians may also furnish audiology services, and technicians or other qualified staff may furnish those parts of a service that do not require professional skills under the direct supervision of physicians. Hearing and balance assessment services that are furnished to hospital outpatients are covered as "diagnostic services" under section 1861(s)(2)(C). They are payable under the Hospital Outpatient Prospective Payment System (HOPPS) or other payment methodology applicable to the provider furnishing the services (ASHA, 2011a).

Regarding outpatient services, Medicare payments are determined by the HOPPS, and payment for hearing and balance diagnostic assessments (e.g., pure-tone tests, tinnitus assessment, central auditory function tests, caloric testing) is determined by assignment of the CPT code to an Ambulatory Payment Classification (APC) (ASHA, 2011a). APCs are categorical listings of procedures for which reimbursement is a flat fee for each CPT procedure in the APC. Private third-party payers can often be billed by CPT code without conversion to the APC listing, depending on the specific contract with the respective payers. As audiologists are keenly aware, there is no provision for Medicare to pay audiologists for therapeutic audiological services.

Another condition for Medicare reimbursement is that orders are required for audiology services delivered in any and all settings. Coverage and payment for hearing and balance diagnostic tests are determined by the reason the tests were performed, rather than by the diagnosis associated with the patient's condition. Further, payment is determined by the fee associated with a specific procedure (the CPT code) in the particular settings. (The CPT coding is organized by descriptor and includes vestibular function studies, audiometric tests, electrophysiological/audiometric tests, audiology-related aural rehabilitation, and implant services.) In contrast, hospital outpatient audiology services are paid under the Outpatient Prospective Payment System. The fee schedule is updated annually. In the 2010 fee schedule, CMS stressed that time spent on counseling, establishment of interventional goals, and evaluation of rehabilitative potential for remediation is not billable. Also noteworthy is that all Part B services require the beneficiary to pay a 20% copayment, and the fee schedule does not deduct the copayment amount. Hence, the actual payment by Medicare is less than that which is shown in fee schedule (ASHA, 2011a).

The scope of coverage of audiological services has remained the same for decades. Independently practicing audiologists have their services covered under Medicare only through the diagnostic test benefit, and such a diagnostic test continues to be covered only if it is ordered by a physician. A physician referral must be included in the patient's clinical record and is always required for audiometric or vestibular testing if the billing is in the name of the audiologist, even if the audiologist shares office space with the physician under a lease or other arrangement. For the audiologist to be reimbursed, the physician must order testing to obtain additional information necessary for evaluation of the need for, or determination of the appropriate type of, medical or surgical treatment for a hearing deficit or a related medical problem. In certain venues, hearing tests can be covered for diagnosis of such conditions as cochlear deafness, sensorineural deafness, tinnitus, ear trauma, and vertigo. There is no provision for coverage of therapeutic services performed by privately practicing audiologists or audiologists on the staff of a non–physician-directed clinic.

It is important to note that audiologists who work in a variety of settings including private practice, hospitals, physician offices, university clinics, rehabilitation centers, and skilled nursing facilities are eligible to participate in Medicare, with documentation requirements differing somewhat by setting. For example, for an outpatient evaluation in either a private practice or in a hospital outpatient department, extensive documentation is required. It should include a history noting the patient's chief complaints, why the patient came to the audiologists, and information justifying what was done for the patient. In addition, the provider must document the results of the testing, and in the interpretation it is important to note the implications of the results. Ending with the conclusions and recommendations is important. The outpatient evaluation must have an original or electronic signature. In contrast, outpatient services rendered in a physician's office should include the audiogram and notes that can be included on the same page. The documentation must be detailed enough to discuss what was done, the results, and the recommendations. The ASHA Web site has coding and reimbursement modules that I highly recommend (http://www.asha.org/practice/reimbursement/modules/) for more detail on Medicare documentation and policy.

A voluntary program designed to improve quality of care to Medicare beneficiaries, the Medicare Physician Quality Reporting System program is a payment system that incentivizes audiologists to report data on "quality" measures for professional services furnished to beneficiaries. As of this writing, the CMS is considering including 264 individual quality measures and retiring 14 measures of which 2 are audiology related. Interestingly, audiologists are listed as practitioners along with other professionals including physician assistants, clinical social workers, clinical psychologists, and nutrition professionals, who are eligible to participate in Physician Quality Reporting System. Listed along with therapists eligible to participate are physical therapists, speech-language therapists, and occupational therapists (CMS, 2011). To participate in the 2011 Physician Quality Reporting System, eligible professionals may choose to report information on individual Physician Quality Reporting System quality measures or report to one of the following: (1) to CMS on a Medicare Part B claim, (2) to a qualified Physician Quality Reporting System registry, or (3) to CMS via a qualified electronic health record (EHR) product. Professionals who meet the criteria for satisfactory submission of Physician Quality Reporting System quality measures data will qualify to earn a Physician Quality Reporting System incentive payment equal to 1.0% of their total estimated Medicare Part B Physician Fee Schedule (PFS) allowed charges for covered professional services furnished during that reporting period. According to CMS (2011), reporting is voluntary from 2010 through 2015, and the incentive payment for satisfactorily reporting on measures is 0.5% of all allowable Medicare charges for the reporting period between 2012 and 2014 as set forth in the Affordable Care Act (ACA). Starting in 2015, eligible professionals who do not satisfactorily report on quality measures will be subject to a payment reduction of –1.5%.

The CMS has announced a transition from ICD-9 code sets to ICD-10 diagnosis codes, which was to go into effect for all health care services provided in the U.S. on or after October 1, 2013, however as of this writing the date has been delayed. Specifically, on August 24, 2012, the Department of Health and Human Services (HHS) confirmed a one-year delay in the implementation compliance date for the International Classification of Diseases, 10th Edition (ICD-10) codes. The new implementation date is October 1, 2014. Hence, on the latter date we will be required to use the new ICD-10 system, which replaces the ICD-9-CM.

In general, coding under the ICD-10 will be more specific because of problems inherent with the ICD-9 code sets, which

Table 12.5   International Classification of Diseases ICD-10 Versus ICD-9 Code Sets (ASHA, 2011a; ASHA, 2011b)

Type of Coding	ICD-9	ICD-10 (Proposed)
Diagnosis coding	Uses three to five characters and first character is a letter (E or V) or a number (e.g., 496 or V55.3)	Codes can be 3 to 7 characters (ICD-10-CM) in length the first character is alpha, the second is numeric and the third through seventh can be either alpha or numeric (e.g., H91.11 = presbucusis, right ear
Inpatient procedure coding	Uses three to four numeric digits and lacks detail Consists of approximately 13,000 codes	Uses 7 alphanumeric digits (ICD-10-PCS) Codes are more specific Laterality or side of the body affected has been added to relevant codes Codes reflect modern medicine and updated medical terminology Consists of approximately 68,000 available codes

provided very limited data about beneficiaries, medical conditions, and hospital inpatient procedures. As shown in **Table 12.5**, the number of codes will increase dramatically necessitating new superbill/encounter forms. Two basic differences in formatting between ICD-9 and ICD-10 in terms of the coding are listed in **Table 12.5**. The advantages of the ICD-10-CM (clinical modification) code set according to CMS (2011) include an improved ability to monitor resource allocation, to set health policy, to track public health and risks, and to measure the quality, safety, and efficacy of care.

Medicare is very specific regarding billing for services delivered by an Au.D. student. Specifically, according to the Center for Medicare Management, Medicare requires that the supervising audiologist remain in the room guiding the student in service delivery when the student is participating in the provision of audiological services. A supervising audiologist cannot be engaged in treating another patient or doing other tasks at the same time. The supervising audiologist bears responsibility for the services rendered and, as such, must sign all documentation. The language used by Medicare is that the student who is participating in field experience must be under "line-of-sight" level of supervision by the audiologist and engaged only in that patient's assessment at all times (ASHA, 2011b). The question often arises regarding whether the physician must see the patient before recommending a hearing test. Because the system is set up on the basis of "medical necessity," a physician should examine the patient first to determine if additional information is needed for diagnosis. If so, the referral for diagnostic audiology is made, and the physician will then use the results to determine a diagnosis. The referral "order" or communication from the treating physician/practitioner can be done in written or by telephone or e-mail. If the order is via telephone, the treating physician and the audiologist must document the telephone call in the patient's medical record.

The Welcome to Medicare preventive health visit is an excellent program, but unfortunately it no longer includes a hearing screening in its menu of preventive services. Our professional organizations should inquire why hearing services were eliminated and make every effort to advocate for the return of this benefit. Medicare covers all the costs of the one-time, comprehensive Welcome to Medicare preventive visit during the first 12 months that beneficiaries have Part B. As part of this preventive visit, which is free to Medicare beneficiaries whose physician accepts assignment, patients undergo a complete physical that includes vision screening and extensive preventive screening as part of their Part B benefit. Covered

preventive services include but are not limited to diabetes screening (one or two tests per year for those at high risk), cardiovascular screening (every 5 years), glaucoma testing, bone mass measurement, nutrition therapy, and smoking cessation therapy. Beneficiaries who have had Part B for longer than 12 months are entitled to a yearly "wellness" visit to develop or update their personalized plan to prevent disease based on their current health status and on risk factors.

Pearl

Audiology procedures are classified under the Social Security Act as "other diagnostic tests." The term *diagnostic test* includes diagnostic x-ray tests and laboratory tests. The term *Medigap,* or gap filler insurance, refers to private insurance policies purchased by individuals or made available by employers to cover charges not covered by Medicare.

◆ Medicaid

Medicaid, a welfare program for which individuals qualify depending on need and poverty level, was enacted into law in 1965 as Title XIX of the Social Security Act. Eligibility depends on income, assets, and resources. Medicaid is part of the existing federal–state welfare structure to assist indigent individuals who fit into an eligibility group recognized by federal and state law (Koch, 1993). Recipients must prove their eligibility, and thus it has no entitlement feature. It is a state-administered program, with each state setting its own guidelines regarding eligibility and scope and duration of service benefits, subject to broad guidelines established by the federal government. Audiology is recognized as a covered service under the Medicaid program. However, according to Title XIX, every state Medicaid program must provide specific basic health services including but not limited to home health services for persons eligible for skilled nursing facility (SNF) services. Optional services include eyeglasses, hearing aids, dental care, prescribed drugs, and clinic services. Each state determines the payment rate for services provided to Medicaid recipients. It is important to underscore that federal Medicaid regulations require that a patient receive a referral from a physician or other licensed practitioner of the healing arts (ASHA, 2011a). Over 15% of older adults, nearly 6.3 million, rely on Medicaid-funded services. According to national data for 2005, Medicaid payments for services for 4.9 million older adults averaged $13,675 per person.

◆ Financing Long-Term Care

The federal government is the largest purchaser of long-term-care services (Morgan & Kunkel, 2011). Specifically, Medicare and Medicaid are the principal payers for long-term-care services at nursing homes and in home- and community-based settings. In 2004, Medicaid paid for over 41% of the total cost of care for persons using nursing facility or home health services, and Medicare covered 25% of long-term-care expenditures. National data for 2005 showed that Medicaid payments for nursing facility services totaled $44.7 billion for more than 1.7 million beneficiaries of these services. This translates into an average expenditure of $26,234 per nursing home beneficiary. Similarly, Medicaid payments for home health services totaled $5.4 billion for 1.2 million beneficiaries, an average expenditure of $4510 per home health care beneficiary. Medicare beneficiaries with low incomes and limited resources may be eligible for Medicaid, in which case the Medicare health care coverage is supplemented by services that are available under a state's Medicaid program. These services may include nursing facility care beyond the 100-day limit covered by Medicare, prescription drugs, eyeglasses, and even hearing aids. According to the CMS estimates in 2007, Medicaid provided some level of supplemental health coverage for 8.1 million Medicare beneficiaries (Social Security Administration [SSA], 2008).

State Medicaid programs, private long-term-care insurers, and other programs that provide long-term-care benefits typically use ability to perform activities of daily living (ADL) and instrumental activities of daily living (IADL) as the litmus test for long-term-care benefits. Further, insurers commonly pay benefits when an individual's cognitive impairment is so severe that supervision is required to protect the person's health and safety. According to the CBO, funds for long-term-care come from two broad sources of financing: personal resources (consisting of out-of-pocket spending and private long-term-care insurance), and government programs (primarily Medicare and Medicaid). Another significant source of financing is donated, or informal, care, because most impaired seniors rely on help from family and friends and not on purchased services.

If only services in which dollars change hands are taken into account, Medicaid and Medicare together are responsible for the majority of long-term-care expenditures. Medicare primarily funds short stays in nursing facilities, skilled home care, hospices, and short-term mental health services. Medicare beneficiaries must meet stringent criteria for the Medicare SNF benefit. Medicare is the major public payer for home care. The Medicare home health benefit will pay for services as long as a physician certifies that the individual is homebound and has a skilled nursing need (i.e., has a condition that restricts the ability to leave home, except with the assistance of another person or the aid of a supportive device) (Kane, Ouslander, & Abrass, 1994). More specifically, a skilled nursing need requires that care is part-time and provided by a specialist such as a nurse, physical therapist, or speech pathologist. Hence, Medicare pays for the following types of home health benefits: skilled nursing care on a part-time or intermittent basis, home health aide services, physical therapy, occupational therapy, and speech-language therapy to help regain and strengthen speech skills. With regard to reimbursement, the traditional model for home care is that a home health care agency that is certified to provide care under Medicare employs nurses, therapists, and aides, contracts with them for their services, and assigns them to a variety of cases. However, home health agencies can also be paid privately by the recipient of the services. Medicare beneficiaries must be recertified for multiple 60-day periods as long as skilled nursing care is necessary and for the home health agency to be reimbursed.

Medicare expenditures for home health care far exceed those of Medicaid, even though Medicaid does finance some forms of home health and hospice care. Because Medicaid is a state program, each state has different rules for who can qualify for home care. In most states, Medicaid will pay for some forms of in-home care and hospice care. Depending on state policy, Medicaid spending on home health services can be extensive, potentially including services by nurses, home health aides, social workers, housekeepers, and various therapists. The bulk of Medicaid home care expenditures are for personal care services (Burwell, Crown, O'Shaugnessy, & Price, 1996). **Table 12.6** summarizes long-term-care financing.

Pearl

Based on the aging of the U.S. population, in 2050, total public and private expenditures fort long-term care are expected to account for an additional 1% to 1.5% of GDP.

◆ Financing for Hearing Aids

As hearing aids are costly and are not covered by Medicare, many older adults cannot afford them. The Better Hearing Institute has an extensive list of agencies and organizations that help to fund hearing aids (http://www.betterhearing.org/hearing_loss_resources/financial_assistance/index.cfm). Listed on this Web site are speech and hearing clinics, agencies (e.g., Easter Seals, Kiwanis Club), and organizations (e.g., Hear Now, H.E.A.R. Project) that provide some form of financial assistance for hearing aids. For example, the H.E.A.R. Project provides financial assistance for hearing aids and FM systems for Colorado residents who do not qualify for Medicaid. Kiwanis Clubs provide members with discounts on hearing aids, and through the Starkey Sound Choice program participating hearing aid providers can obtain financing for hearing aids for their patients. The Veterans Administration ensures access to audiology services including but not limited to hearing aids for veterans with a service-connected disability, for veterans who have hearing impairment severe enough that it interferes with their ability to participate actively in their own medical treatment and to reduce the impact of dual sensory impairment, and for veterans who have significant functional or cognitive impairments affecting their ability to perform ADL.

Another option for consumers is the hearing aid program deriving from the partnership between the AARP and HearUSA, typically referred to as the AARP Hearing Care Program. The plan offers uniform pricing for AARP members. The features and benefits of the program include (1) 20% savings on a wide range of digital hearing aids; (2) a 90-day money-back guarantee; (3) a 3-year manufacturer's warranty; (4) a free

Table 12.6   Federal Programs Supporting Long-Term Care Services

Federal Program	Services Covered	Eligibility
Medicare eligible	100 days of skilled nursing facility care; home health, hospice	All persons 65+ years and others with chronic medical conditions
Medicaid	Skilled nursing facility, home health care; optional services vary from state to state and may include dental care, private-duty nurses, eyeglasses, hearing aids, medical transportation	Aged, blind, disabled persons
Title XX of Social Security Act* (Block Grants to states for Social Services and Elder Justice)	Various social services as defined by the state, including home-maker, home health aide, personal care, home-delivered meals	No federal requirements; states may have a means test—goal is to increase state flexibility in using Social Service grants

*Federal funds that enable each state to furnish financial assistance to needy older adults.
Sources: From Evashwick, C. (1993). The continuum of long-term care services. In S. Williams & P. Torrens (Eds.), *Introduction to health services* (4th ed.). Albany: Delmar; and Kane, R., Ouslander, J., & Abrass, I. (1994). *Essentials of clinical geriatrics* (3rd ed.). New York: McGraw-Hill.

3-year supply of hearing-aid batteries; (5) free directional microphones; and (6) a 1-year extended follow-up care program at no charge to AARP members, which includes otoscopy, reprogramming, hearing aid cleaning and check, and counseling. As of this writing, the Hearing Care Program through HearUSA is available in nearly every state except for California, Minnesota, Oklahoma, and Rhode Island. By way of disclosure, the AARP Web site, which describes the arrangement Hear USA has worked out with AARP, states the following: "AARP does not recommend health related products, services, insurance or programs. You are strongly encouraged to evaluate your needs." HearUSA includes a series of questions (most taken from the Hearing Handicap Inventory for the Elderly) on its Web site (http://aarp.hearusa.com/HearUSAMainMenu/Hearing Evaluation.aspx) that it recommends to viewers to help them begin to consider whether they have a hearing problem warranting professional attention. Audiology Online (http://www.audiologyonline.com/ceus/recordedcoursedetails.asp?class_id=18110) provides a free 40- minute introduction by Cindy Beyer of HearUSA to the hearing care program for those interested in learning more about the plan.

◆ Conclusion

This chapter is not an exhaustive discussion of health care financing, but rather addresses issues pertaining to reimbursement for audiology. Health-care financing patterns are continually changing, and audiologists in private practice or in university, hospital, or rehabilitation settings must keep abreast of information in this arena. The Internet is an ideal source for

information on health care financing, as information is constantly being updated, reflecting the rapid pace at which governmental regulations change. **Table 12.7** provides tips for audiologists regarding advocacy and financing for audiological services.

Table 12.7   Tips for Audiologists Regarding Financing of Hearing Health Care for Older Adults

- Form alliances with primary care providers, geriatric care providers, nurse practitioners, physical therapists, occupational therapists, and speech-language pathologists.
- Pressure professional associations to advocate to reinstitute the Welcome to Medicare first-time hearing health care benefit.
- Become an informed and up-to-date provider.
- Learn contract negotiation skills.
- Develop an outcome-oriented quality improvement system.
- Equip your office with professional testing and hearing-aid fitting equipment, and market your practice by showing the proportion of patients who benefit from your services.
- Join a network that provides centralized contract administration, utilization data, satisfaction information, patient complaint procedures, billing, and collection of fees.
- Educate consumers about the expertise of audiologists and the importance of audiological testing to determine hearing status and need for intervention.
- Market services to agencies offering Medicare Advantage plans that they market to older adults.
- Collecting and disseminating outcome data can help to justify the cost of digital hearing aids with their many features.

Sources: Adapted from Michaud, L. (1997). Gaining access to the managed care market. Hearing Journal, 50, 62–64; and Griffin, K., & Fazen, M. (1993). A managed care strategy for practitioners. In *Quality improvement digest* (pp. 1–7). Rockville, MD: American Speech-Language-Hearing Association.

References

American Speech-Language-Hearing Association (ASHA). (2011a). *2011 Medicare fee schedule.* http://www.asha.org/practice/reimbursement/medicare/feeschedule/

American Speech-Language-Hearing Association (ASHA). (2011b). *Medicare coverage of students & clinical fellows: audiology.* http://www.asha.org/practice/reimbursement/medicare/student_participation.htm

Barker, W. (1998). Geriatrics in North America. In R. Tanis, H. Fillit, & J. Brockelhurst (Eds.), *Brockelhurst's textbook of geriatric medicine and gerontology* (5th ed.). London: Churchill-Livingstone

Boult, C. (2009). The health care system. In J. Halter, J. Ouslander, M. Tinetti, S. Studenski, K. High, & S. Asthana (Eds.), *Hazzard's geriatric medicine and gerontology* (6th ed.). New York: McGraw-Hill

Burwell, B., Crown, W., O'Shaugnessy, C., & Price, R. (1996). Financing long-term care. In C. Evashwick (Ed.), *The continuum of long-term care: An integrated systems approach.* Albany: Delmar

Centers for Medicare and Medicaid Services (CMS). (2011). *Physician Quality Reporting System, formerly known as the Physician Quality Reporting Initiative.* https://www.cms.gov/pqrs/

Congressional Budget Office (CBO). (2007). *Medicare Advantage: Private health plans in Medicare.* http://www.cbo.gov/ftpdocs/82xx/doc8268/06-28-medicare_advantage.pdf

Dummit, L. (2009). *The basics—relative value units (RVUs).* WWW.nhpf.org

Evashwick, C. (1993). The continuum of long-term care services. In S. Williams & P. Torrens (Eds.), *Introduction to health services* (4th ed.). Albany: Delmar

Griffin, K., & Fazen, M. (1993). A managed care strategy for practitioners. In *Quality improvement digest* (pp. 1–7). Rockville, MD: American Speech-Language-Hearing Association

Kaiser Family Foundation. (2010). *Medicare.* http://www.kff.org/medicare/upload/2052-14.pdf

Kane, R., Ouslander, J., & Abrass, I. (1994). *Essentials of clinical geriatrics* (3rd ed.). New York: McGraw-Hill

Knickman, J., & Thorpe, K. (1998). Financing for health care. In A. Kovner (Ed.), *Jonas's health care delivery in the United States.* New York: Springer

Koch, A. (1993). Financing health services. In: S. Williams & P. Torrens (Eds.), *Introduction to health services.* Albany: Delmar

Leutz, W. (1998). *National Bipartisan Commission on the Future of Medicare.* http://thomas.loc.gov/medicare/leutztest.html

Michaud, L. (1997). Gaining access to the managed care market. *Hearing Journal, 50,* 62–64

Morgan, L., & Kunkel, S. (2011). *Aging, society, and the life course.* New York: Springer

Neuman, P., & Cubanski, J. (2009, Jul). Medicare Part D update—Lessons learned and unfinished business. *New England Journal of Medicine, 361,* 406–414

Schneider, K. M., O'Donnell, B. E., & Dean, D. (2009). Prevalence of multiple chronic conditions in the United States' Medicare population. *Health and Quality of Life Outcomes, 7,* 82

Social Security Administration (SSA). (2008). *Annual Statistical Supplement (Washington, D.C.), 2008.* http://www.ssa.gov/policy/docs/statcomps/supplement/2008/medicaid.html

Starr, P. (2011). *The Medicare bind.* http://prospect.org/article/medicare-bind-0-

Stefanacci, R. (2010). Managed care for older Americans. In H. Fillit, K. Rockwood, & K. Woodhouse (Eds.), *Brockelhurst's textbook of geriatric medicine and gerontology* (7th ed.). Philadelphia: Saunders Elsevier

Truffer, C. J., Keehan, S., Smith, S., Cylus, J., Sisko, A., Poisal, J. A., et al. (2010, Mar-Apr). Health spending projections through 2019: The recession's impact continues. *Health Affairs (Project Hope), 29,* 522–529

Index

Note: Page numbers followed by a *t* or an *f* indicate tables or figures, respectively.